Cardiovascular Magnetic Resonance Imaging: Contemporary Cardiology

Cardiovascular Magnetic Resonance Imaging: Contemporary Cardiology

Edited by Zachary Garcia

hayle medical

New York

Hayle Medical,
750 Third Avenue, 9th Floor,
New York, NY 10017, USA

Visit us on the World Wide Web at:
www.haylemedical.com

ISBN: 978-1-63241-556-1

Cataloging-in-Publication Data

Cardiovascular magnetic resonance imaging : contemporary cardiology / edited by Zachary Garcia.
    p. cm.
Includes bibliographical references and index.
ISBN 978-1-63241-556-1
1. Cardiovascular system--Magnetic resonance imaging. 2. Medical radiology.
3. Cardiology. I. Garcia, Zachary.
RC670.5.M33 C37 2019
616.107 548--dc23

Table of Contents

Preface

Over the recent decade, advancements and applications have progressed exponentially. This has led to the increased interest in this field and projects are being conducted to enhance knowledge. The main objective of this book is to present some of the critical challenges and provide insights into possible solutions. This book will answer the varied questions that arise in the field and also provide an increased scope for furthering studies.

Cardiovascular magnetic resonance imaging or cardiac MRI is a non-invasive imaging technology used for the assessment of the cardiovascular system. It has a significant role in evidence-based therapeutic and diagnostic pathways in cardiovascular disease, especially the surgical planning in complex heart diseases. It has applications in the assessment of cardiovascular disorders, such as myocarditis, cardiomyopathies, myocardial ischemia and viability, congenital heart disease, besides others. The development of CMR is an active area of research and is witnessing innovation in terms of better and improved techniques. This book explores all the important aspects of cardiovascular magnetic resonance imaging in the present day scenario. The various studies that are constantly contributing towards advancing technologies and the evolution of this field are examined in detail. Students, researchers, experts and all associated with cardiology and medical imaging will benefit alike from this book.

I hope that this book, with its visionary approach, will be a valuable addition and will promote interest among readers. Each of the authors has provided their extraordinary competence in their specific fields by providing different perspectives as they come from diverse nations and regions. I thank them for their contributions.

Editor

Test-retest variability of left ventricular 4D flow cardiovascular magnetic resonance measurements in healthy subjects

Victoria M. Stoll[1]*![ORCID], Margaret Loudon[1], Jonatan Eriksson[2], Malenka M. Bissell[1], Petter Dyverfeldt[2], Tino Ebbers[2], Saul G. Myerson[1], Stefan Neubauer[1], Carl-Johan Carlhäll[2] and Aaron T. Hess[1]

Abstract

Background: Quantification and visualisation of left ventricular (LV) blood flow is afforded by three-dimensional, time resolved phase contrast cardiovascular magnetic resonance (CMR 4D flow). However, few data exist upon the repeatability and variability of these parameters in a healthy population. We aimed to assess the repeatability and variability over time of LV 4D CMR flow measurements.

Methods: Forty five controls underwent CMR 4D flow data acquisition. Of these, 10 underwent a second scan within the same visit (scan-rescan), 25 returned for a second visit (interval scan; median interval 52 days, IQR 28–57 days). The LV-end diastolic volume (EDV) was divided into four flow components: 1) Direct flow: inflow that passes directly to ejection; 2) Retained inflow: inflow that enters and resides within the LV; 3) Delayed ejection flow: starts within the LV and is ejected and 4) Residual volume: blood that resides within the LV for > 2 cardiac cycles. Each flow components' volume was related to the EDV (volume-ratio). The kinetic energy at end-diastole (ED) was measured and divided by the components' volume.

Results: The dominant flow component in all 45 controls was the direct flow (volume ratio 38 ± 4%) followed by the residual volume (30 ± 4%), then delayed ejection flow (16 ± 3%) and retained inflow (16 ± 4%). The kinetic energy at ED for each component was direct flow (7.8 ± 3.0 microJ/ml), retained inflow (4.1 ± 2.0 microJ/ml), delayed ejection flow (6.3 ± 2.3 microJ/ml) and the residual volume (1.2 ± 0.5 microJ/ml). The coefficients of variation for the scan-rescan ranged from 2.5%–9.2% for the flow components' volume ratio and between 13.5%–17.7% for the kinetic energy. The interval scan results showed higher coefficients of variation with values from 6.2–16.1% for the flow components' volume ratio and 16.9–29.0% for the kinetic energy of the flow components.

Conclusion: LV flow components' volume and their associated kinetic energy values are repeatable and stable within a population over time. However, the variability of these measurements in individuals over time is greater than can be attributed to sources of error in the data acquisition and analysis, suggesting that additional physiological factors may influence LV flow measurements.

Keywords: Left ventricular, 4D flow, Repeatability, Variability, Kinetic energy

---

* Correspondence: Victoria.stoll@cardiov.ox.ac.uk
[1]University of Oxford Centre for Clinical Magnetic Resonance Research (OCMR), Division of Cardiovascular Medicine, Radcliffe Department of Medicine, Oxford, UK
Full list of author information is available at the end of the article

Background

The main purpose of the cardiovascular system is to drive, control and maintain blood flow through the heart and vessels [1]. Insights into intra-cardiac blood flow are now afforded by the use of retrospectively electrocardiogram (ECG) gated, three-dimensional (3D), time resolved flow encoded cardiovascular magnetic resonance (CMR) (3D + time = 4D flow) [2–6]. The 4D flow within the left ventricle (LV) can be separated into four functional flow components and the kinetic energy (KE) of the blood throughout the cardiac cycle can be quantified [3, 7, 8]. In healthy hearts these functional flow components have specific routes and energetics that may represent important aspects of normal ventricular function [9]. Typically a third of the inflow to the LV passes directly through to the aorta in healthy hearts allowing a preservation of LV inflow KE, which may assist with an efficient systolic ejection phase. Alterations in LV blood flow components have been found in patients with early compensated dilated cardiomyopathy, where a substantial proportion of the inflow is retained within the LV and there is an associated decrease in preservation of the LV inflow KE [8]. These findings suggest that the volume and KE of the 4D flow components may be sensitive biomarkers for the early detection of cardiac pathology. 4D flow also provides a potential future tool for the evaluation of therapeutic interventions [10]. However the use of 4D flow components for early diagnosis and monitoring of changes in individual patients requires an understanding of the intra-subject repeatability of the measures and the variability of these parameters over time.

To date, studies reporting healthy control data have enrolled small numbers, typically 6–17 participants with data acquired at a single time point [3–5, 8] and none have assessed the stability of LV 4D flow components over time. Thus, this study aims to understand the stability of the volume and KE profiles of LV flow components in healthy participants. In order to achieve this we first assessed the repeatability of the 4D flow data acquisition, post-processing and analysis in order to understand the error associated with the technique. Subsequently we determined how these components change over time by repeating a data acquisition after a period of a few weeks.

Methods

Study population

Forty five healthy subjects were prospectively recruited specifically for the aims of this study. All participants had no contraindication to CMR scanning, no history of cardiac disease, nor symptoms of cardiac disease. This study was approved by the local research ethics committee and written informed consent was obtained from each participant.

Ten of the participants underwent two 4D flow data acquisitions within the same study visit to assess 'scan-rescan' repeatability. Between each data acquisition the participant was removed completely from the scanner so each data set was acquired with the same potential real-life sources of variance, including subtle changes in subject positioning in the CMR system. Twenty five of the participants returned for a second 'interval' 4D flow data acquisition at least 10 days later ($52 \pm$ IQR 28–57 days). The participants in the scan-rescan and interval groups were different as this study was conducted in two phases. Additional file 1: Table S1 shows that the two groups were similar for cardiac function measurements.

Anthropometric measurements

Height and weight were recorded and body mass index (BMI) calculated. Blood pressure was recorded as an average of 3 supine measurements taken over 10 min (DINA-MAP-1846-SX, Critikon Corporation; General Electric Healthcare, Waukesha, Wisconsin, USA). Heart rate was recorded at the time of the short axis stack acquisition.

Cardiovascular magnetic resonance protocol

Each participant underwent CMR imaging on a 3 Tesla system (Trio, Siemens Healthineers Erlangen, Germany) using a 32 channel cardiac coil. All images were ECG-gated. Images for LV volumes were acquired using retrospectively gated balanced steady-state free precession (bSSFP) cine sequences scan parameters were echo time 1.5 ms, repetition time 3 ms and flip angle 50°. Slice thickness was 8 mm with contiguous slice position for the short axis stack. Each cine slice was acquired during a single breath hold, as a free breathing method was not available, this protocol allowed shorter breath holds (which will be helpful when this technique is utilised in patients), and easier repetition if any mis-triggering or breathing artefact occurred during data acquisition. Cine images were analysed using cmr42 (Circle Cardiovascular Imaging Inc., Calgary, Canada) as previously described [11].

4D flow data acquisitions were acquired during free breathing, using a retrospectively ECG triggered, respiratory navigator gated three dimensional (3D), three directional, time resolved phase contrast CMR sequence with data measured over many cardiac cycles. The echo time was 2.75 ms with a repetition time of 4.3 ms and temporal resolution of 52 ms. The flip angle was 7°, read field of view 390 mm and voxel size 3x3x3 mm³. The velocity encoding was 100 cm/s. The field-of-view (FOV) was sagittal and adjusted for each subject to fully encompass the whole heart. The data acquisition times were between 15 and 20 min. While the data are presented as a single cardiac cycle they capture the complete cardiac cycle which means they can be used to form a closed loop where the first and last frame are also consecutive frames. For illustration: if the 4D flow loop is concatenated after itself (doubling the number of time frames) the data will appear continuous and to have captured two cardiac cycles.

Post processing and data analysis

Background phase offsets were corrected with a third-order polynomial fit. Data quality control steps were applied as previously described [3] using automated customised Matlab software (The Mathworks Inc., Natick, Massachusetts, USA). Velocity data was converted into a file format compatible with commercially available visualisation software (EnSight, CEI Inc., Research Triangle Park, North Carolina, USA).

All data sets were analysed using a method previously described by Eriksson et al. [3, 5]. The LV endocardium was manually segmented from short-axis images at end diastole (ED) and end systole (ES), using freely available software (Segment, version 1.9 R2842) [12]. The ED and ES timeframes were determined by visual inspection of the open or closed positions of the aortic and mitral valves and the LV size in the long and short axis images. The segmentation at ED is resampled to give a volume with isotropic voxels equal to the size of the flow data voxels. A pathline is emitted from the centre of each voxel included in the LV segmentation. Pathlines are created forwards and backwards in time until the preceding or subsequent ES, respectively. A pathline is a probabilistic path a finite volume of blood takes through space as a function of time. Combined these forward and backward pathlines represent the entire LV end diastolic volume (EDV) tracked over one complete cardiac cycle. The positions of all pathlines at the time of ES relative to the LV cavity, as defined by the segmentation at ES, are then used to divide them into four functional flow components: direct flow, retained inflow, delayed ejection flow and residual volume as described previously [3, 5, 8]. Direct flow is defined as blood that enters and exits the LV in the analysed cardiac cycle, retained inflow enters the LV but does not exit during the same cardiac cycle, whilst delayed ejection flow starts within the LV but exits during the analysed cardiac cycle and residual volume is the component that resides within the LV for at least 2 cardiac cycles, these are illustrated in Fig. 1a. Accuracy of this quantification was evaluated by comparing the LV inflow components (direct flow and retained inflow) to the LV outflow components (direct flow and delayed ejection flow), any data sets with > 10% difference would have been excluded from further analysis for quality control, however no datasets met this criteria so all acquired datasets were included in the further analysis.

The KE of these flow components can be calculated throughout the cardiac cycle by utilising $KE = \frac{1}{2} \cdot \rho_{blood} \cdot V_{pathline} \cdot v_{pathline}^2$, where ρ_{blood} is blood density, $V_{pathline}$ the volume of blood that a pathline is emitted from, equal to one voxel, and $v_{pathline}$ the velocity of the pathline at a given time point. The KE for each component is the sum of all pathlines in the group. The KE values were calculated over the cardiac cycle and reported at ED, as the KE values at this time-point reflect the preservation of the inflowing KE prior to the rapid ejection of blood during systole. The KE at ED for each component was then divided by the components volume to give a KE per millilitre value, therefore removing any variation due to LV cavity size.

Intra- and inter-observer variability

Intra-observer variability was determined by an operator experienced in CMR who conducted two blinded assessments of 10 randomly selected data sets, with each assessment separated by more than one month. Inter-observer variability was conducted independently by a second observer experienced in CMR with the same 10 datasets.

Statistical analysis

Statistical analysis was performed with SPSS (version 22, International Business Machines, Armonk, New York, USA). Data were tested for normality using the D'Agostino and Pearson omnibus normality test and values are presented as mean ± standard deviations, unless otherwise specified. For 2 group comparisons the Student's t test was used for normally distributed data or Mann Whitney U test was used for non-normally distributed data. Repeated measures ANOVA with post hoc Tukeys's multiple comparisons test or Friedman test with post hoc Dunn's multiple comparison tests were performed for normally and non-normally distributed multiple groups respectively. P values < 0.05 were considered significant. Correlation was assessed using the Pearson or Spearman method as appropriate. Repeatability was assessed by consideration of the absolute difference between the results obtained from scan 1 and 2 for each subject. The coefficient of variance (CoV) was calculated for each subject, using the root mean square method [13]. The average CoV for a group for scan-rescan and interval scan repeatability was calculated by summing the squares of the variance for each subject, then taking the mean of the CoVs for all subjects and then square rooting this value. Mann Whitney tests were conducted to compare the CoV for the scan-rescan results to the CoV for the interval scan results. Bland-Altman plots [14] were used to display the differences between the paired datasets.

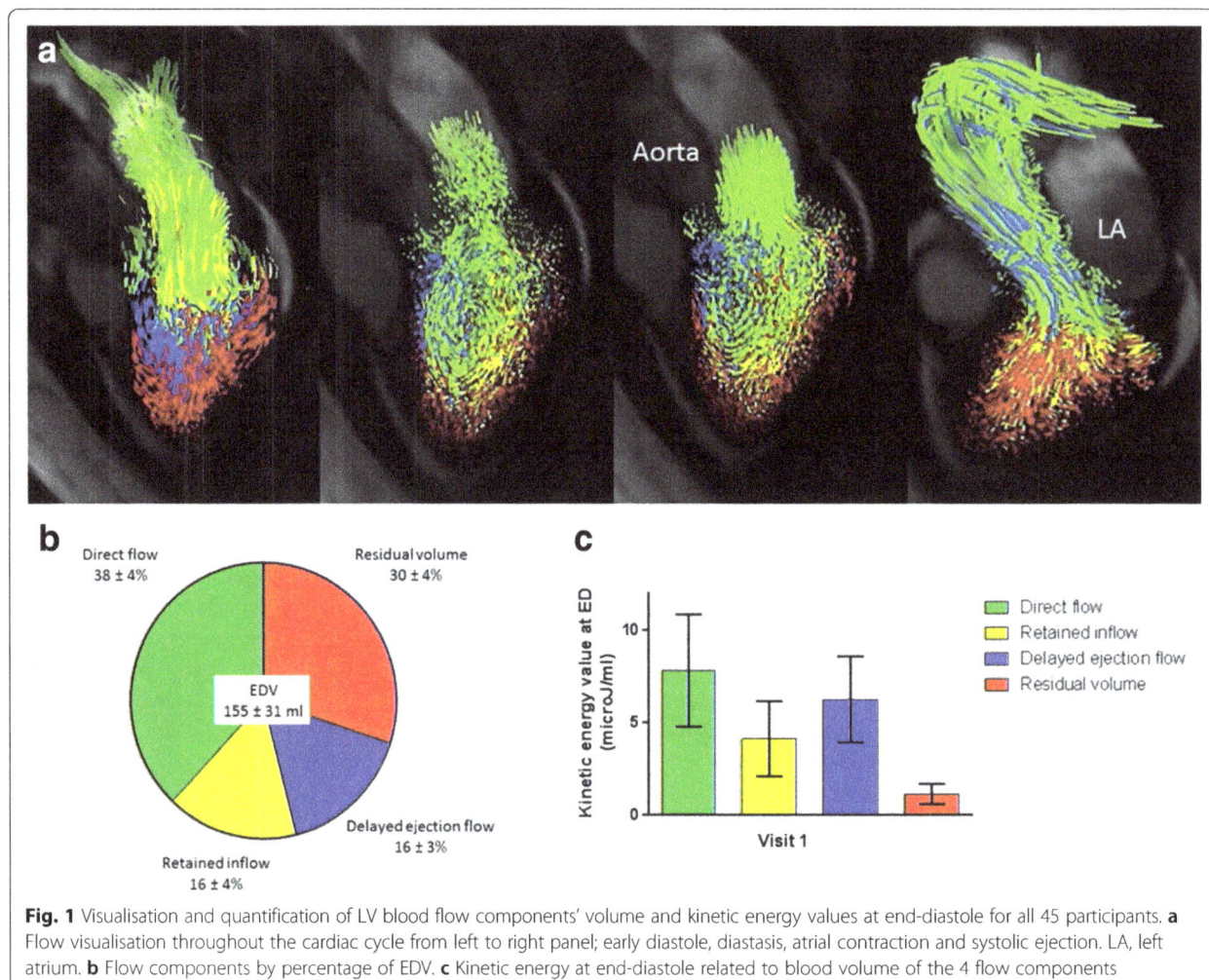

Fig. 1 Visualisation and quantification of LV blood flow components' volume and kinetic energy values at end-diastole for all 45 participants. **a** Flow visualisation throughout the cardiac cycle from left to right panel; early diastole, diastasis, atrial contraction and systolic ejection. LA, left atrium. **b** Flow components by percentage of EDV. **c** Kinetic energy at end-diastole related to blood volume of the 4 flow components

Results

Participant characteristics

Forty-five participants were recruited; mean age 54 ± 14 years (range 24–75 years) and 27 (59%) male. Demographic, anthropometric and routine CMR measurements are shown in Table 1. All LV volumes were within the normal range [15] and the mean ejection fraction was $66 \pm 4\%$.

4D flow components' volume and kinetic energy

All 80 data acquisitions passed data quality checks, with no significant difference in inflow versus ejected volume (inflow 82 ± 21 ml, outflow 81 ± 22 ml, $P = 0.57$).

Figure 1a demonstrates the visualised flow components, whilst Fig. 1b shows the average proportion of the 4 flow components as a percentage of the EDV for all 45 participants. The average contribution of each flow component, from largest to smallest, was: direct flow ($38 \pm 4\%$), residual volume ($30 \pm 4\%$), retained inflow ($16 \pm 4\%$) and delayed ejection flow ($16 \pm 3\%$). The results in Table 2 of repeated measures ANOVA comparisons with Tukey post-hoc testing demonstrate that the 4 flow components volumes were all significantly different to each other except for the retained inflow and delayed ejection flow.

The kinetic energy at ED in proportion to blood volume for each flow component is shown in Fig. 1c. The ED kinetic energy of each flow component, ordered from largest to smallest was: direct flow (7.8 ± 3.0 microJ/ml), delayed ejection flow (6.3 ± 2.3 microJ/ml), retained inflow (4.1 ± 2.0 microJ/ml) and residual volume (1.2 ± 0.5 microJ/ml). The mean KE at ED was statistically significantly different between all flow components, as found by comparison with Friedman test with post hoc Dunn's testing demonstrated in Table 2.

Intra and inter-observer variability

The results from the intra and inter-observer variability for the flow components as a percentage of the EDV are shown in Table 3. The coefficients of variation for the different flow components were low and similar for both intra and inter-observer results (range intra-observer 3.6–6.1%, vs

Table 1 Demographic, anthropometric and routine CMR measurements

	Controls N = 45
Age, years	54 ± 14 (range 24–75)
Male, %	59
Systolic blood pressure, mmHg	133 ± 20
Diastolic blood pressure, mmHg	78 ± 10
BMI, kg/m^2	24.7 ± 3.8
Heart rate, beats per minute	65 ± 13
CMR data	
LV ejection fraction, %	66 ± 4
LV end diastolic volume, ml	155 ± 31
LV EDV indexed BSA, ml/m^2	82 ± 14
LV end systolic volume, ml	52 ± 13
LV stroke volume, ml	103 ± 21
Cardiac output, L/min	6.5 ± 1.4

Values are mean ± standard deviations
BMI indicates Body mass index, CMR Cardiovascular magnetic resonance, LV Left ventricle, EDV End diastolic volume, BSA Body surface area

inter-observer 2.6–5.7%), suggesting good intra and inter-observer variability.

Scan-rescan repeatability

Ten subjects underwent 2 data acquisitions within the same study visit; Bland-Altman plots are shown in Fig. 2a for the relative volume and kinetic energy value at ED for each flow component. The observed mean difference values and coefficient of variation (CoV) for these results are summarised in Table 4. The flow component with the lowest CoV was the direct flow (2.5%), whilst the most variable flow component as a percentage of the EDV was the delayed ejection flow (CoV 9.2%). The kinetic energy

Table 2 Multiple comparisons following repeated measures ANOVA for flow components as a percentage of EDV and Friedman test for KE at ED

	Mean ± SD	Retained inflow (P value)	Delayed ejection flow (P value)	Residual volume (P value)
Multiple comparisons for volume, % EDV				
Direct flow, % EDV	38 ± 4	< 0.001	< 0.001	< 0.001
Retained inflow, % EDV	16 ± 4	–	0.7534	< 0.001
Delayed ejection flow, % EDV	16 ± 3	0.7534	–	< 0.001
Residual volume, % EDV	30 ± 4	< 0.001	< 0.001	–
Multiple comparisons for KE at ED, µJ/ml				
Direct flow, µJ/ml	7.8 ± 3.0	< 0.001	0.0256	< 0.001
Retained inflow, µJ/ml	4.1 ± 2.0	–	0.0049	< 0.001
Delayed ejection flow, µJ/ml	6.3 ± 2.3	0.0049	–	< 0.001
Residual volume, µJ/ml	1.2 ± 0.5	< 0.001	< 0.001	–

SD indicates Standard deviation, EDV End-diastolic volume, KE Kinetic energy

Table 3 Intra and Inter-observer variability

	Intra-observer (Investigator 1)			Inter-observer (Investigator 2)	
	Analysis 1.1	Analysis 1.2	CoV	Analysis 2	CoV
Direct flow, % EDV	38 ± 4	37 ± 5	3.9	36 ± 5	5.7
Retained inflow, % EDV	14 ± 3	15 ± 3	3.6	15 ± 3	2.6
Delayed ejection flow, % EDV	17 ± 3	17 ± 3	6.1	18 ± 3	4.8
Residual volume, % EDV	31 ± 3	30 ± 3	3.5	31 ± 4	5.0
Ejection fraction, %	70 ± 3	69 ± 3	4.0	67 ± 4	4.1
EDV, ml	162 ± 46	166 ± 44	4.3	154 ± 40	5.8
ESV, ml	50 ± 16	51 ± 17	5.7	51 ± 16	5.6

CoV Coefficient of variation, EDV End diastolic volume, ESV End systolic volume

values had higher coefficients of variation than those for the percentage of each flow component; with a range of 13.5% for direct flow to 17.7% for delayed ejection flow.

Interval scans: Evaluation of variability and physiological variability

A total of 25 participants returned for a second scan after a median interval period of 52 days (IQR 28–57 days). The average proportion of each flow component as a percentage of the EDV did not differ significantly between visits, nor did the mean kinetic energy per millilitre at ED, as shown in Fig. 3. Figure 2b shows the Bland-Altman plots for the flow components' volume and kinetic energy values; observed mean difference values and coefficients of variation are provided in Table 3. The 95% confidence intervals and CoV for each parameter measured are increased compared to those for the 10 scan-rescan datasets. As before the most stable flow parameter by percentage of EDV was the direct flow (CoV 6.2%) and the most variable component was the retained inflow (CoV 16.1%). The coefficients of variation for the KE values were again higher than those for the flow components as a percentage of EDV. The least variable parameter was the direct flow kinetic energy (CoV 16.9%), whilst the residual volume was the most variable with a CoV of 29.0%.

In order to understand whether the variability seen in each flow component volume and associated KE value, between the interval scans, was related to physiological parameters the changes in these results were correlated against each other. The mean difference between scan 1 and 2 was calculated for heart rate (2 ± 7 beats/min), LV EDV (3 ± 11 ml), stroke volume (1 ± 9 ml), LV ejection fraction (EF) (1 ± 3%) and cardiac output (10 ± 90 ml). There were no correlations seen between any of the flow component percentages or KE changes with the change in stroke volume, LV EDV or cardiac output. The change in the KE of the delayed ejection flow correlated weakly to the change in EF ($r = 0.435$, $P = 0.03$). Correlations were seen between the change in heart rate and the breakdown of flow components as a percentage of the EDV (direct flow r

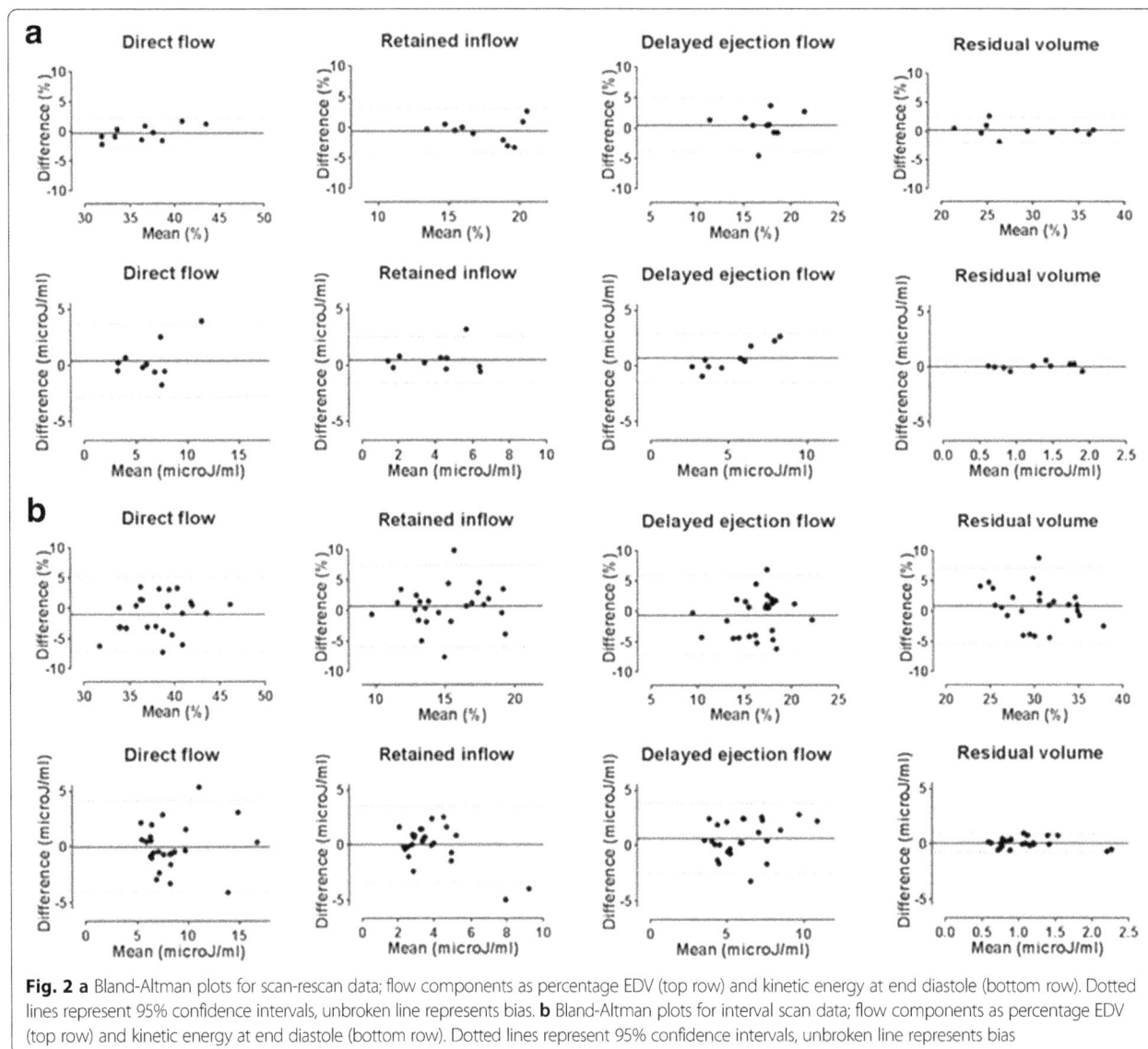

Fig. 2 a Bland-Altman plots for scan-rescan data; flow components as percentage EDV (top row) and kinetic energy at end diastole (bottom row). Dotted lines represent 95% confidence intervals, unbroken line represents bias. **b** Bland-Altman plots for interval scan data; flow components as percentage EDV (top row) and kinetic energy at end diastole (bottom row). Dotted lines represent 95% confidence intervals, unbroken line represents bias

$= 0.509$, $P = 0.009$, retained inflow $r = 0.424$, $P = 0.035$, delayed ejection flow $r = 0.500$, $P = 0.009$ and residual volume $r = 0.414$, $P = 0.04$).

Discussion

This study presents results from the largest cohort to date of healthy subjects for the quantification of LV flow components' volume and KE values. The baseline data are in agreement with those from previous studies [3, 5, 7] with direct flow being the largest flow component, as a percentage of the EDV. The direct flow is also the component that possesses the highest kinetic energy value at ED. We found the retained inflow and delayed ejection flow components to be very similar as a proportion of the EDV, which provides a reassuring data quality control as they are inter-related components. These components are inter-related as much of the incoming retained inflow is ejected during the

subsequent cardiac cycle as the delayed ejection flow, furthermore the volumes must be the same to preserve the cardiac volume. We successfully conducted scan-rescan data acquisitions to assess for repeatability and post-processing variability as well as interval scans to assess for the additional effect of physiological variability.

Repeatability of data acquisition and post-processing

To our knowledge this is the first study to report 4D flow data from scan-rescan data acquisitions, where the aim was to attempt to quantify the magnitude of variation that is due to inherent sources of error in the data acquisition, post-processing and analysis. The scan-rescan repeatability was good for the flow components as a proportion of the EDV and slightly more variable for the KE values. The coefficients of variation we found for our flow component

Table 4 Repeatability of measurements comparing scan-rescan and interval scans

	Scan-rescan		Interval scans		
	Observed mean difference (95% confidence interval)	CoV	Observed mean difference (95% confidence interval)	CoV	P value between CoV for scan-rescan and interval scans
End diastolic volume, ml	6.6 (−11.9 to 25.1)	4.6	1.1 (−19.2 to 21.4)	4.6	0.65
End systolic volume, ml	1.4 (−7.3 to 10.2)	6.8	−1.0 (−13.3 to 11.3)	9.5	0.11
Left ventricular ejection fraction, %	0.4 (−5.5 to 6.5)	3.0	1.1 (−5.2 to 7.3)	3.3	0.12
Heart rate, bpm	4.3 (−6.9 to 15.5)	7.6	1.7 (−11.7 to 15.1)	6.8	0.18
Volume ratios					
Direct flow, % EDV	−0.2 (−2.8 to 2.3)	2.5	−1.0 (−7.1 to 5.1)	6.2	0.10
Retained inflow, % EDV	−0.5 (−4.1 to 3.0)	6.6	0.7 (−6.0 to 7.5)	16.1	0.04
Delayed ejection flow, % EDV	0.6 (−3.9 to 5.0)	9.2	−0.6 (−7.2 to 6.0)	15.0	0.07
Residual volume, % EDV	0.2 (−2.0 to 2.4)	3.0	0.9 (−5.4 to 7.2)	8.0	0.007
Kinetic energy					
Direct flow KE at ED, μJ/ml	0.4 (−2.8 to 3.7)	13.5	−0.01 (−4.2 to 4.2)	16.9	0.40
Retained inflow KE at ED, μJ/ml	0.5 (−1.6 to 2.6)	13.8	0.03 (−3.5 to 3.5)	20.4	0.13
Delayed ejection flow KE at ED, μJ/ml	0.7 (−1.5 to 3.0)	17.7	0.6 (−2.5 to 3.8)	27.5	0.16
Residual volume KE at ED, μJ/ml	0.06 (−0.5 to 0.6)	15.4	0.1 (−0.8 to 0.9)	29.0	0.23

CoV Coefficient of variation, *EDV* End diastolic volume, *bpm* Beats per minute

volumes were of a similar magnitude to those found in LV volumes calculated by cine CMR for conventional LV parameters including LV EDV, LV ESV and LV EF that found coefficients of variation between 4.1–10.3% [16].

Analysis of the influence of the post-processing steps including LV segmentation and selection of the appropriate time frame for ED and ES was assessed via the intra and inter-observer variability. The coefficients of variation for the flow component proportions were very similar between the intra and inter-observer variability results. These results are in agreement with previous studies assessing intra and inter-observer variability for cine CMR LV volumes [16, 17] and a study assessing flow component proportions that showed no difference in the group means and standard deviation [3]. These findings are expected; the main influence the operator has upon the post processing of the data is the contouring of the short axis ventricular images at ED and ES, which is then used to create the mask for analysis of the flow data. Both investigators undertaking analysis in this study are experienced at placing LV contours and were trained in the same CMR unit so will have similar

contouring styles. The intra-observer coefficient of variation for the flow components as a proportion of the EDV was similar to that obtained for the scan-rescan data analysis suggesting that much of the variability in the results will be from the data analysis steps and not the data acquisition itself.

Influence of physiological variability upon interval scans

The flow components as a percentage of the EDV and the KE of each component at ED were not significantly different between visit 1 and 2 across the group, however on a per participant basis there was greater variability between visit 1 and 2.. As expected the coefficients of variation were higher for all measured parameters for the 2 scans performed at an interval compared to the 2 scans performed in the same study visit. The results from the scan-rescan data acquisitions provide an estimation of the variability in 4D flow data acquisition, post-processing and analysis. The additional variability seen with the interval scans over scan-rescan suggests that as well as the differences in data acquisition, post processing and analysis there are additional influencing factors. We hypothesised that the increased variability was most likely due to a degree of normal physiological variability. We found that the change in heart rate recorded between the 2 interval scans correlated modestly to the changes seen in the flow components as a proportion of the EDV. This is an interesting finding and may be explained by the longstanding physiological observation that changes in heart rate predominantly affect the diastolic phase of the cardiac cycle, as the systolic phase is of a relatively fixed duration [18]. Hence, it may be that as the heart rate changes the proportions of the flow components alter to adapt to the new length of the diastolic period, whilst still maintaining an efficient systolic ejection phase. This may be an important physiological adaptation for exercise, which would be interesting to assess in future studies, including in disease states. However, the correlations with heart rate alone were only modest, suggesting further additional physiological factors such as fluid status, vascular tone and hormonal influences may be implicated in the variability seen for interval data acquisitions.

Individual flow components

Direct flow was consistently the largest component with the highest possession of energy at ED; it was also the least variable of the four flow components in both composition and KE values. The direct flow represents the blood that transits directly from the left atrium via the LV cavity to be ejected into the aorta within the same cardiac cycle. Previous studies have demonstrated that the direct flow follows an efficient pathway to the LV outflow tract with the shortest distance, more favourable angle and

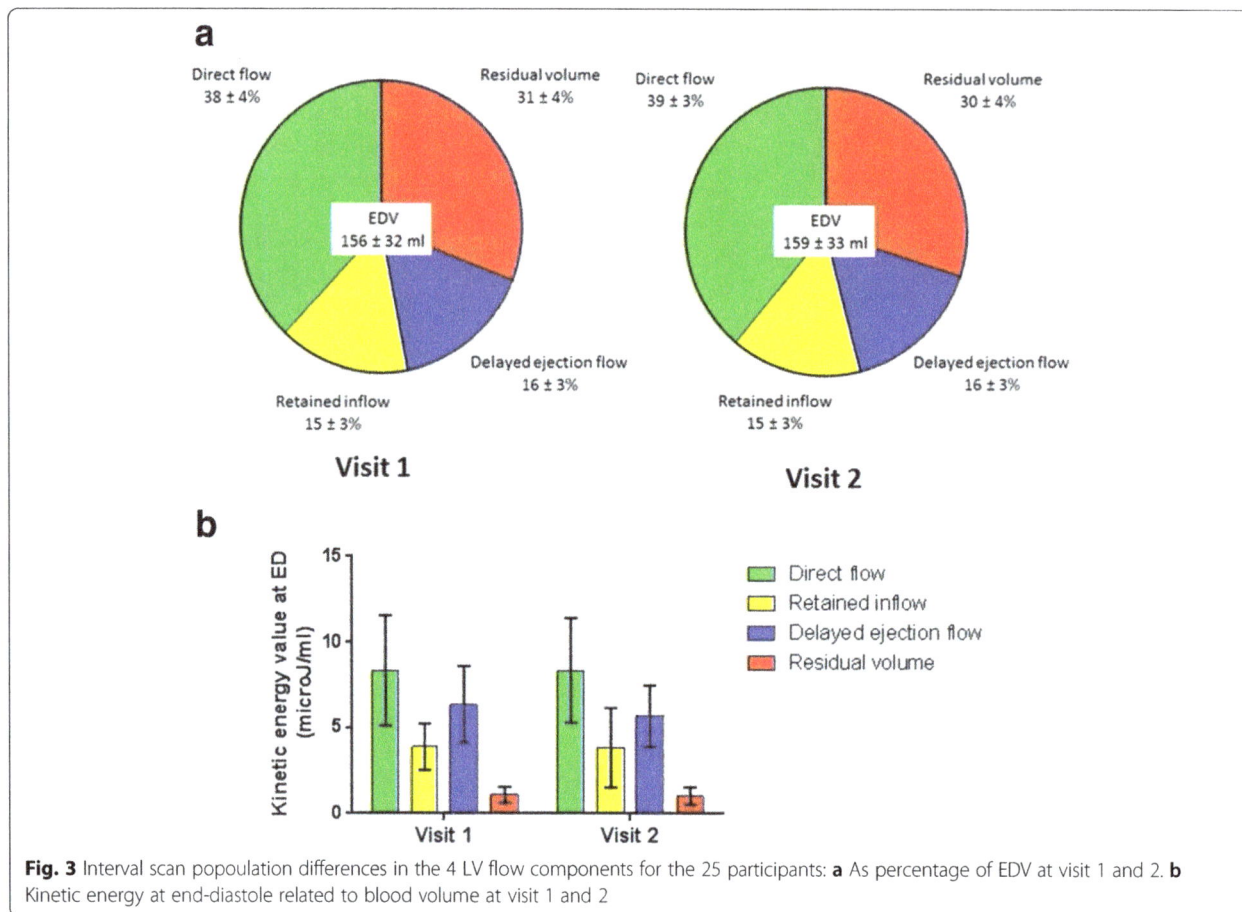

Fig. 3 Interval scan popoulation differences in the 4 LV flow components for the 25 participants: **a** As percentage of EDV at visit 1 and 2. **b** Kinetic energy at end-diastole related to blood volume at visit 1 and 2

increased linear momentum in comparison to the other flow components [7]. This suggests that in a healthy heart the percentage of blood pumped via the efficient shorter pathway taken by the direct flow component is relatively consistent; this may allow conservation of the KE of this component, which may be important in reducing the additional energy that is required for its ejection during systole. The residual volume was the second most stable component over time in terms of composition, but possessed the most variable amount of KE. The residual volume is located at the periphery of the LV cavity, outlining the functional border of the chamber, providing a fluid-fluid interface that interacts with the exchanging blood flow [9]. The location and stability in terms of the percentage of the residual volume could imply it is a static component of the LV blood flow volume. However the variability of the KE it possesses suggests it remains part of the dynamic interactions that occur with the incoming and outgoing cardiac blood flow within the LV cavity during each cardiac cycle. This may be an important factor in preventing blood stasis and thrombus formation within the healthy heart.

The KE for the retained inflow component at ED was significantly lower than that of the delayed ejection flow. This finding is in keeping with the notion proposed by *Bolger* et al. [5] that the retained inflow blood has to decelerate at the end of diastole and then acquire additional kinetic energy prior to ejection during a subsequent systole (as part of the delayed ejection flow). Previous studies have demonstrated a late diastolic boost in the KE of the delayed ejection flow, which was presumed to result from transfer of energy from the inflow components, so it may be that the KE is interchanged predominantly from the retained inflow to the delayed ejection flow. The amount of energy present within the delayed ejection flow at ED was not significantly different to the energy possessed by the direct flow; suggesting that a threshold level of kinetic energy favours ejection of blood from the LV during systole.

Clinical applications

The applicability of 4D flow to assess the severity of cardiac disease has been previously demonstrated in patients with clinically compensated mild heart failure secondary to dilated cardiomyopathy [8] and ischaemic cardiomyopathy [19]. The use of this technique in longitudinal clinical studies is now required to assess how these parameters change over time in patients with heart disease and whether 4D flow parameters provide additional information to current imaging techniques in monitoring these patients.

Limitations

The 4D flow data acquisitions undertaken in this study were conducted at rest. Given the relationship between the change in heart rate and the flow components as a percentage of the EDV it would be interesting to assess whether these proportions vary to a greater degree in an exercising heart. Blood flow within the heart is a dynamic process and 4D flow data is acquired over many heart beats with the end data representing the blood flow over an averaged cardiac cycle. In order to understand further if haemodynamic changes during the data acquisition influenced the final results continuous monitoring of heart rate and central blood pressure would be needed. For these measurements to be reliable they would need to be invasive which we felt would be too high a burden for our participants. The findings presented here are from a single study site and although they are in keeping with previous studies, future studies comparing the same study participants at different sites would provide additional validation of the 4D flow LV flow components' volume and KE profiles. The two study groups (scan-rescan versus interval scan) consisted of different participants. We cannot exclude an influence of this upon the results seen, but as both groups had normal cardiac function and similar flow parameters we would expect any variability to be the same between these two groups. Finally the participants enrolled in this study were all healthy subjects and the reproducibility of this technique in patients with cardiac disease remains to be investigated. However it is unlikely that this technique will have less variability over time in patients with heart disease than controls, so this data may still act as an aid in assessing the significance of any changes in 4D flow parameters seen with longitudinal studies.

Conclusions

This study provides an increased understanding of the variability of blood flow within the healthy heart. LV flow components' relative volume and kinetic energy values are repeatable and are stable within a population over time. However, the variability of these measures in individuals over time is greater than can be attributed to inherent sources of error in the data acquisition, post processing and analysis, suggesting that additional physiological factors may influence the volume and KE profiles of the flow components. The assessment of intra-cardiac blood flow may become helpful in examining disease states and quantification of the variability of the results from this technique prior to this use is important.

Abbreviations

4D flow: Four dimensional flow; BMI: Body mass index; bSSFP: balanced steady-state free precession; CMR: Cardiovascular magnetic resonance; CoV: Coefficient of variation; ECG: electrocardiogram; ED: End diastole; EDV: End diastolic volumes; ES: End systole; FoV: Field of view; KE: Kinetic energy; LV: Left ventricular

Acknowledgements

The authors gratefully acknowledge Hayley Harvey for her help and support with participant recruitment and Jane Francis for her assistance with image acquisition.

Funding

VS (Ref FS/12/14/29354) and MMB are supported by British Heart Foundation Clinical Research Training Fellowships. ATH is supported by the Medical Research Council. ML, SGM and SN are funded by the National Institute for Health Research (NIHR) Oxford Biomedical Research Centre Programme. SN and ATH acknowledge support of the Oxford British Heart Foundation Centre of Research Excellence. PD acknowledges support from the Swedish Research Council. TE acknowledges support of the European Research Council (Heart4flow, 310612). CJC is funded by the Swedish Heart and Lung Foundation.

Authors' contributions

VS designed the study, recruited and scanned all participants, undertook analysis and preparation of the manuscript. ML undertook inter-observer variability analysis with VS. JE, PE, TE and CJC designed and provided support with use of the analysis tool for this study. MMB was involved in data acquisition and interpretation. ATH wrote the CMR 4D flow sequence and provided assistance with data acquisition and interpretation. SGM and SN participated in study design and data interpretation. All authors participated in manuscript revision including reading and approving the final manuscript.

Competing interests

The authors declare that they have no competing interests.

Author details

[1]University of Oxford Centre for Clinical Magnetic Resonance Research (OCMR), Division of Cardiovascular Medicine, Radcliffe Department of Medicine, Oxford, UK. [2]Division of Cardiovascular Medicine, Linköping University, Linköping, Sweden.

References

1. Richter Y, Edelman ER. Cardiology is flow. Circulation. 2006;113(23):2679–82.
2. Calkoen EE, de Koning PJ, Blom NA, Kroft LJ, de Roos A, Wolterbeek R, Roest AA, Westenberg JJ. Disturbed Intracardiac flow organization after Atrioventricular Septal defect correction as assessed with 4D flow magnetic resonance imaging and quantitative particle tracing. Investig Radiol. 2015; 50(12):850–7.
3. Eriksson J, Carlhall CJ, Dyverfeldt P, Engvall J, Bolger AF, Ebbers T. Semi-automatic quantification of 4D left ventricular blood flow. J Cardiovasc Magn R. 2010;12.
4. Wigstrom L, Ebbers T, Fyrenius A, Karlsson M, Engvall J, Wranne B, Bolger AF. Particle trace visualization of intracardiac flow using time-resolved 3D phase contrast MRI. Magnet Reson Med. 1999;41(4):793–9.
5. Bolger AF, Heiberg E, Karlsson M, Wigstrom L, Engvall J, Sigfridsson A,

   Ebbers T, Kvitting JPE, Carlhall CJ, Wranne B. Transit of blood flow through
   the human left ventricle mapped by cardiovascular magnetic resonance. J
   Cardiovasc Magn R. 2007;9(5):741–7.

6. Nilsson A, Bloch KM, Carlsson M, Heiberg E, Stahlberg F. Variable
   velocity encoding in a three-dimensional, three-directional phase
   contrast sequence: evaluation in phantom and volunteers. J Magn
   Reson Imaging. 2012;36(6):1450–9.

7. Eriksson J, Dyverfeldt P, Engvall J, Bolger AF, Ebbers T, Carlhall CJ.
   Quantification of presystolic blood flow organization and energetics in the
   human left ventricle. Am J Physiol-Heart C. 2011;300(6):H2135–41.

8. Eriksson J, Bolger AF, Ebbers T, Carlhall CJ. Four-dimensional blood flow-
   specific markers of LV dysfunction in dilated cardiomyopathy. Eur Heart J-
   Card Img. 2013;14(5):417–24.

9. Carlhall CJ, Bolger A. Passing strange flow in the failing ventricle. Circ-Heart
   Fail. 2010;3(2):326–31.

10. Markl M, Bonk C, Klausmann D, Stalder AF, Frydrychowicz A, Hennig J,
    Beyersdorf F. Three-dimensional magnetic resonance flow analysis in a
    ventricular assist device. J Thorac Cardiov Sur. 2007;134(6):1471–6.

11. Rider OJ, Lewandowski A, Nethononda R, Petersen SE, Francis JM, Pitcher A,
    Holloway CJ, Dass S, Banerjee R, Byrne JP, et al. Gender-specific differences
    in left ventricular remodelling in obesity: insights from cardiovascular
    magnetic resonance imaging. Eur Heart J. 2013;34(4):292–9.

12. Heiberg E, Sjogren J, Ugander M, Carlsson M, Engblom H, Arheden H.
    Design and validation of segment–freely available software for
    cardiovascular image analysis. BMC Med Imaging. 2010;10:1.

13. Hyslop NP, White WH. Estimating precision using duplicate measurements. J
    Air Waste Manag Assoc. 2009;59(9):1032–9.

14. Bland JM, Altman DG. Statistical methods for assessing agreement between
    two methods of clinical measurement. Lancet. 1986;1(8476):307–10.

15. Petersen SE, Aung N, Sanghvi MM, Zemrak F, Fung K, Paiva JM, Francis JM,
    Khanji MY, Lukaschuk E, Lee AM, et al. Reference ranges for cardiac structure
    and function using cardiovascular magnetic resonance (CMR) in Caucasians
    from the UK biobank population cohort. J Cardiovasc Magn R. 2017;19.

16. Bogaert JG, Bosmans HT, Rademakers FE, Bellon EP, Herregods MC,
    Verschakelen JA, Van de Werf F, Marchal GJ. Left ventricular quantification
    with breath-hold MR imaging: comparison with echocardiography. MAGMA.
    1995;3(1):5–12.

17. Hudsmith LE, Petersen SE, Francis JM, Robson MD, Neubauer S. Normal
    human left and right ventricular and left atrial dimensions using steady
    state free precession magnetic resonance imaging. J Cardiovasc Magn R.
    2005;7(5):775–82.

18. Boudoulas H, Rittgers SE, Lewis RP, Leier CV, Weissler AM: Changes in
    diastolic time with various pharmacologic agents - implications for
    myocardial perfusion. Circulation 1978, 58(4):247-247.

19. Svalbring E, Fredriksson A, Eriksson J, Dyverfeldt P, Ebbers T, Bolger AF,
    Engvall J, Carlhall CJ. Altered diastolic flow patterns and kinetic energy in
    subtle left ventricular remodeling and dysfunction detected by 4D flow MRI.
    PLoS One. 2016;11(8):e0161391.

2

Impact of surgical pulmonary valve replacement on ventricular strain and synchrony in patients with repaired tetralogy of Fallot: a cardiovascular magnetic resonance feature tracking study

Sowmya Balasubramanian[1,2]* [ID], David M. Harrild[1,2], Basavaraj Kerur[1], Edward Marcus[1,2], Pedro del Nido[3,4], Tal Geva[1,2] and Andrew J. Powell[1,2]

Abstract

Background: In patients with repaired tetralogy of Fallot (TOF), a better understanding of the impact of surgical pulmonary valve replacement (PVR) on ventricular mechanics may lead to improved indications and outcomes. Therefore, we used cardiovascular magnetic resonance (CMR) feature tracking analysis to quantify ventricular strain and synchrony in repaired TOF patients before and after PVR.

Methods: Thirty-six repaired TOF patients (median age 22.4 years) prospectively underwent CMR a mean of 4.5 ± 3.8 months before PVR surgery and 7.3 ± 2.1 months after PVR surgery. Feature tracking analysis on cine steady-state free precession images was used to measure right ventricular (RV) and left ventricular (LV) circumferential strain from short-axis views at basal, mid-ventricular, and apical levels; and longitudinal strain from 4-chamber views. Intraventricular synchrony was quantified using the maximum difference in time-to-peak strain, the standard deviation of the time-to-peak, and cross correlation delay (CCD) metrics; interventricular synchrony was assessed using the CCD metric.

Results: Following PVR, RV end-diastolic volume, end-systolic volume, and ejection fraction declined, and LV end-diastolic volume and end-systolic volume both increased with no significant change in the LV ejection fraction. LV global basal and apical circumferential strains, and basal synchrony improved. RV global circumferential and longitudinal strains were unchanged, and there was a varied impact on synchrony across the locations. Interventricular synchrony worsened at the midventricular level but was unchanged at the base and apex, and on 4-chamber views.

Conclusions: Surgical PVR in repaired TOF patients led to improved LV global strain and no change in RV global strain. LV and RV synchrony parameters improved or were unchanged, and interventricular synchrony worsened at the midventricular level.

Keywords: Tetralogy of fallot, Pulmonary valve replacement, Feature tracking, Myocardial strain, Ventricular synchrony

* Correspondence: sowmyab@med.umich.edu
Dr. Mark Fogel served as a Guest Editor for this manuscript.
[1]Department of Cardiology, Boston Children's Hospital, Boston, USA
[2]Department of Pediatrics, Harvard Medical School, Boston, USA
Full list of author information is available at the end of the article

Background

Young children undergoing surgical repair of tetralogy of Fallot (TOF) have excellent short-term survival [1]; however, they experience significant morbidity and mortality related to biventricular dysfunction and arrhythmia in their adult years [2–4]. These sequelae are believed to be in part related to chronic pulmonary regurgitation (PR) caused by efforts to relieve pulmonary valve stenosis with the initial repair. Thus, surgical pulmonary valve replacement (PVR) is often performed subsequently to improve the long-term outcome [5, 6]. Although a reduction in PR, right ventricular (RV) end-diastolic volume (EDV), and RV end-systolic volume (ESV) is observed, the beneficial impact of PVR on ventricular systolic function, exercise capacity, arrhythmia, and survival is uncertain [6–9].

A better understanding of the effects of surgical PVR on ventricular function may lead to improved indications and outcomes for the procedure. In particular, areas that merit further investigation are regional ventricular mechanics and synchrony. In repaired TOF patients, right bundle branch block is nearly universal and several studies have documented dyssynchronous ventricular contraction [10–12]. Moreover, left ventricular (LV) dysfunction is seen in conjunction with RV dysfunction suggesting adverse ventricular-ventricular interactions [3, 13, 14]. Nevertheless, our knowledge of regional ventricular mechanics in this patient group remains rudimentary, in part because robust techniques for its assessment have not been applied.

Feature tracking is an image processing technology that quantifies myocardial tissue deformation, and has been increasingly employed to aid cardiac resynchronization therapy [15, 16]. This technique has primarily been applied to ultrasound images; however, recent work has adapted and validated its use with cardiovascular magnetic resonance (CMR) images in both the right and left ventricles [12, 17–21]. CMR offers the advantage over echocardiography of consistent high-quality imaging of both ventricles in patients with repaired TOF.

Our group previously published a prospective, randomized study comparing 2 techniques for surgical PVR: PVR alone versus PVR plus RV remodeling with the resection of scar tissue [22]. No significant difference was observed in the primary outcome–change in RV ejection fraction (EF) measured by CMR–or in any of the secondary outcomes at 6-month postoperative follow-up. In this study, we performed feature tracking image analysis on data from the trial cohort to determine the impact of surgical PVR on strain and ventricular synchrony in patients with repaired TOF.

Methods

Subjects

Subjects in this study were all participants in a previously reported prospective, randomized, single-center trial comparing 2 techniques for surgical PVR [22]. These patients were > 10 years of age with repaired TOF or similar physiology presenting for PVR between February 2004 and October 2008. Other inclusion criteria in the prior study included chronic PR (regurgitation fraction by CMR ≥25%) and at least 2 of the following conditions: RV EDV index ≥160 ml/m^2, RV ESV index ≥70 ml/m^2, RV EF ≤45%, LV EDV index ≤65 ml/m^2, RV outflow aneurysm, or a clinical criterion such as exercise intolerance, symptoms and signs of heart failure, or cardiac medications. Exclusion criteria included any of the following: severe RV outflow obstruction, severe RV hypertension with RV pressure ≥ systemic pressure, and contraindications to preoperative CMR. Patients were randomized to PVR alone or a combination of PVR with RV remodeling surgery. The study protocol included a pre-operative and a 6-month post-operative CMR study.

For the current study, we analyzed the database of the prospective trial, selected only those patients with TOF, and performed feature tracking analysis of the CMR images. The Boston Children's Hospital Committee on Clinical Investigation granted permission for this study and waived the requirement for informed consent.

CMR

The CMR protocol used for patients with repaired TOF has been previously published [23]. Briefly, studies were performed with a 1.5-T whole body scanner (Achieva, Phillips Healthcare Systems, Best, the Netherlands or TwinSpeed, GE Healthcare, Milwaukee, Wisconsin, USA) using surface coils selected based on patient size. The scanner manufacturer was different for the pre- and post-PVR CMR study in 4 patients. Imaging included breath-hold, electrocardiographically-gated, balanced steady-state free precession cine CMR acquisitions in 4-chamber and short-axis planes. A total of 12–14 slices were obtained in the short-axis plane to completely cover both ventricles. In all views, 30 images per cardiac cycle were acquired which yielded a temporal resolution of 20–40 ms, depending on heart rate. Ventricular volumes and blood flow were measured using commercially available software (QMASS and QFLOW, Medis, Leiden, the Netherlands) [23].

Strain analysis

Feature tracking analysis for determination of strain was performed using commercially available software (Diogenes v. 1.1.02, TomTec Imaging Systems, Unterschleissheim, Germany), as previously described [12]. Circumferential strains for the LV and RV were measured from short-axis views at 3 levels: basal, mid-ventricular, and apical. The mid-ventricular level was first identified, and the basal and apical slices were specified to be equidistant from the mid-ventricular slice. The LV outflow tract was not included in the basal slice. Pre- and post-PVR images on each subject were compared to ensure similar slice locations. For short-axis views, the myocardium of each ventricle was divided equally into 6 segments at the mid and basal locations, and 4 segments at the apical location (Fig. 1a). Longitudinal strains for the LV and RV were measured from the 4-chamber view with division into 6 segments (Fig. 1b). Global peak strain for each view was calculated as the average of the peak strains for each segmental curve [17, 24]. Strain measurements were performed by the same investigator in all patients in order to promote consistency. In addition, they were repeated by that investigator and performed by a second investigator in a random sample of patients to assess intraobserver and interobserver agreement. Note that strain is calculated as follows: (final length – initial length) / initial length. Thus, shortening in the longitudinal and circumferential directions yields a negative strain number, and that the more negative the number, the better the shortening.

Synchrony analysis

Various ventricular synchrony parameters based on feature tracking measurements have been reported; however, there is no consensus on the optimal approach. Hence, we used 3 techniques that have been reported in the literature as measures of ventricular synchrony [17, 25, 26]. Three ventricular synchrony parameters were calculated for each ventricle on each of the 3 short-axis views and the 4-chamber view based on the

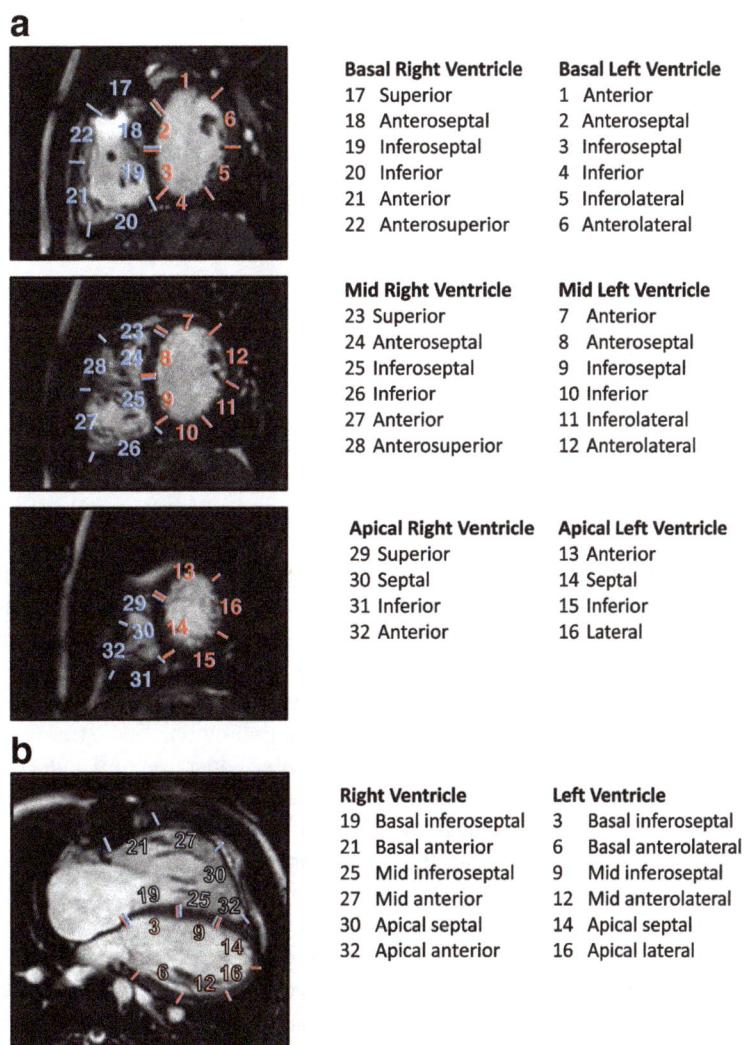

Fig. 1 Schematic diagram illustrating the division of the right ventricle (RV) and left ventricle (LV) myocardium into segments on short-axis (**a**) and 4-chamber views (**b**)

strain versus time data: 1) the maximum difference in time-to-peak strain among any 2 of the segments (latest versus earliest segment), 2) the standard deviation of the time-to-peak strain values for all segments, and 3) the cross-correlation delay (CCD). The time to peak strain was measured from the QRS trigger to the peak strain time. Using a custom built virtual instrument (LabVIEW 8.2, National Instruments, Austin, Texas, USA), the CCD was measured by iteratively shifting 1 curve in time relative to a second curve in a stepwise fashion, and calculating the normalized correlation co-efficient between the curves for each time shift [25, 27]. The time shift that resulted in the maximum correl-ation coefficient was defined as the CCD between the 2 curves. Rather than relying on just the peak points, CCD takes into account the entire strain versus time curve to determine the temporal offset. For each ven-tricle on each of the 4 views, the CCDs were measured between opposing segments, and the largest value of the opposing segment CCDs was reported. In addition, the interventricular CCD on each of the 4 views was calculated by comparing the global strain versus time curves for the LV and RV.

Statistical analysis

All collected data were tested for normalcy using the Shapiro-Wilk test. Continuous data are presented as median (range) and mean ± standard deviation. A two-tailed paired t-test was used to compare pre- and post-PVR strain and synchrony parameters. A p-value ≤0.05 was considered statistically significant. The intra-class correlation coefficient (ICC) and mean difference were used to assess intraobserver and interobserver agreement.

Results

Patients

Of the 64 patients in the initial prospective trial, 36 had a diagnosis of TOF as well as pre- and post-operative CMR studies with suitable image quality for strain ana-lysis. These patients constitute the study group, and their demographic and clinical data are summarized in Table 1. Thirteen patients were randomized to the PVR alone group and 23 to the PVR with RV remodeling sur-gery group. CMR examinations occurred at a mean of 4.5 ± 3.8 (range 0.03–12.7) months before PVR surgery and 7.3 ± 2.1 (range 5.2–10.8) months after surgery.

Diagnostic testing results

Key diagnostic testing results pre- and post-PVR are shown in Table 2. As expected, PVR led to virtual elim-ination of PR, and a significant decline in RV EDV and ESV. These changes yielded a slight decline in RV EF. The LV EDV and ESV both increased slightly with no

Table 1 Patient characteristics (n = 36)

Male	23 (64%)
Prior aortopulmonary shunt	10 (28%)
Age at initial complete repair (years)	1.5 (0.0–19.4)
Age at PVR (years)	22.4 (12.3–57.7)
Cardiac symptoms prior to PVR	21 (58%)
NYHA Class I or II prior to PVR	33 (92%)
NYHA Class III or IV prior to PVR	3 (8%)
Prescribed cardiac medications prior to PVR	16 (44%)
Additional procedures with PVR	
Closure of patent foramen ovale or atrial septal defect	8 (22%)
Pulmonary artery plasty	10 (28%)
Tricuspid annuloplasty	6 (17%)
Cryoablation	2 (6%)
Maze procedure	4 (11%)
Closure of ventricular septal defect	3 (8%)
Other	4 (11%)

Data presented as n (%) or median (range)
PVR pulmonary valve replacement

significant change in the LV EF. There was no significant change in QRS duration or the heart rate at the time of CMR.

Strain analysis

Global strain values pre- and post-PVR are shown in Fig. 2. In the LV, global circumferential strain at the base and apex improved following PVR; strain at the mid ventricle also tended to improve but this did not reach statistical significance. Global longitudinal strain was unchanged. In the RV, global circumferential strain at all 3 levels and global longitudinal strain were unchanged.

The impact of PVR on segmental strain in the LV and RV is shown in Fig. 3. Overall, changes in regional stain were minimal. Significant differences in circumferential LV strain were seen in 2 of 16 segments, and these were both improvements. Longitudinal strain changed in 1 of 6 segments and this was a decline. Significant differences in circumferential RV strain were seen in 2 of 16 segments, 1 increase and 1 decrease. Longitudinal strain changed in 1 of 6 segments and this was a decline.

Synchrony analysis

Synchrony parameters derived from the segmental strain versus time curves pre- and post-PVR are shown in Table 3. For LV circumferential strain, all 3 parameters showed significantly improved synchrony post-PVR at the base. At the mid and apex levels, all parameters tended to improve and some met the significance threshold. There were no significant synchrony changes based on longitudinal strain.

Table 2 Diagnostic testing results pre- and post-PVR ($n = 36$)

Parameter	Pre-PVR	Post-PVR	P-value
Electrocardiogram			
QRS duration (ms)	153 ± 38	152 ± 39	0.99
Exercise Testing			
Peak VO$_2$ (ml/kg/min)	26 ± 9	25 ± 8	0.31
Echocardiography			
≤ Mild tricuspid regurgitation	33	35	
≥ Moderate tricuspid regurgitation	3	1	
RV systolic pressure by tricuspid regurgitation jet velocity	35 ± 15	25 ± 7	0.009
CMR			
Heart rate	75 ± 11	73 ± 13	0.38
LV EDV$_i$ (ml/m^2)	88 ± 17	93 ± 17	0.01
LV ESV$_i$ (ml/m^2)	37 ± 10	40 ± 12	0.02
LV ejection fraction (%)	58 ± 8	57 ± 7	0.35
RV EDV$_i$ (ml/m^2)	194 ± 34	119 ± 16	< 0.001
RV ESV$_i$ (ml/m^2)	100 ± 24	65 ± 16	< 0.001
RV ejection fraction (%)	49 ± 7	46 ± 7	0.02
Pulmonary regurgitation fraction (%)	48 ± 10	4 ± 5	< 0.0001

EDV end-diastolic volume, *ESV* end-systolic volume, *LV* left ventricular, *PVR* pulmonary valve replacement, *RV* right ventricular

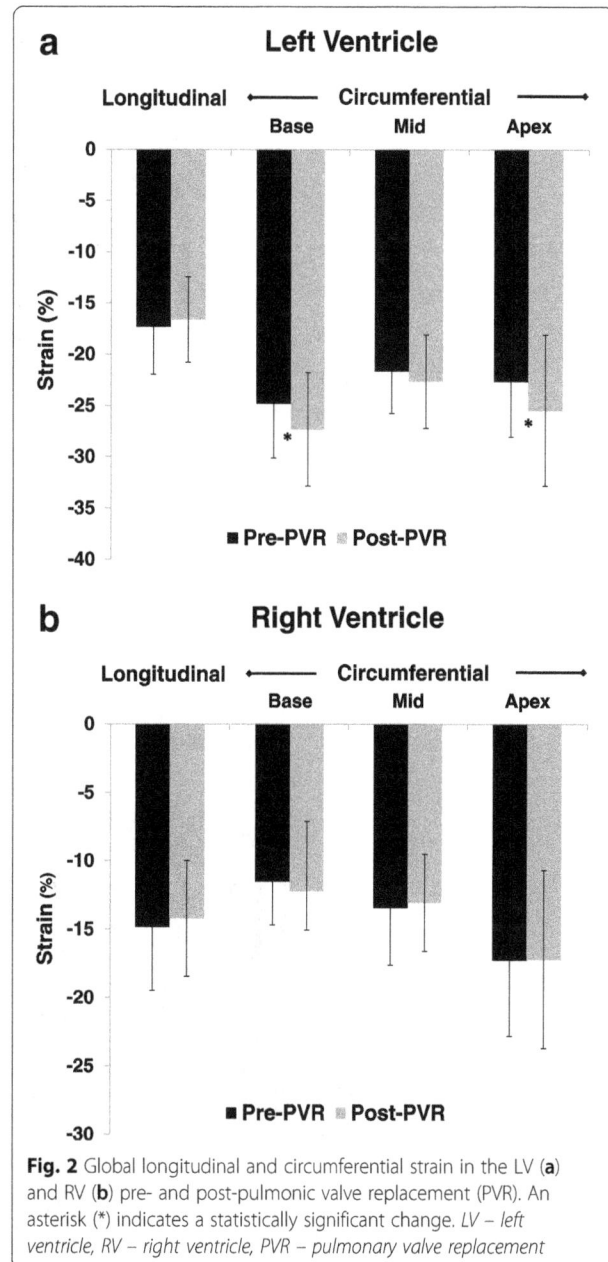

Fig. 2 Global longitudinal and circumferential strain in the LV (**a**) and RV (**b**) pre- and post-pulmonic valve replacement (PVR). An asterisk (*) indicates a statistically significant change. *LV – left ventricle, RV – right ventricle, PVR – pulmonary valve replacement*

For the RV, both of the time-to-peak parameters showed significantly improved synchrony at the base and worsened at the apex and longitudinally. At the mid location, there were no significant synchrony changes.

In addition to the synchrony parameters reported above, the raw time-to-peak strain values (rather than differences) for each segment were compared pre- and post-PVR. This analysis provides information on how PVR affects the timing of contraction relative to the cardiac cycle rather than assessing synchrony per se. All LV segments with a statistically significant change in time-to-peak strain following PVR were increases and these were 2 of the 6 longitudinal and 7 of 16 circumferential segments (Fig. 4a). Similarly, all RV segments with a statistically significant change in time-to-peak strain after PVR were increases, and these were 1 of the 6 longitudinal and 4 of the 16 circumferential segments (Fig. 4b).

Interventricular synchrony was assessed by comparing the global strain versus time curves for the LV and RV on each of the 4 views, and calculating the CCDs. The LV peak strain preceded RV peak strain in 128 of 144 segments (89%) pre-PVR and in 127 of the 144 segments (88%) post PVR. The interventricular CCD significantly increased after PVR at the mid-ventricular level (50.4 ± 26.4 ms vs. 66.7 ± 29.1 ms, $p = 0.002$), as a result of slightly earlier LV peak strain. There was no change in the interventricular CCD at the base (76.5 ±

53.8 ms vs. 90.5 ± 56.2 ms, $p = 0.62$), the apex (46.8 ± 34.4 ms vs. 49.0 ± 33.2 ms, $p = 0.73$), or the 4-chamber view (61.8 ± 109.6 ms vs. 52.3 ± 86.7 ms, $p = 0.69$).

Intraobserver and interobserver agreement

Table 4 shows the intraobserver and interobserver agreement results for global strain and synchrony parameters. Intraobserver agreement was good for LV circumferential and longitudinal strain, and for RV circumferential strain (all ICCs ≥0.93), and acceptable for RV longitudinal strain (ICC 0.85). Interobserver agreement for these parameters was lower. Compared to global strains, time-to-peak strain and CCD generally had lower ICCs;

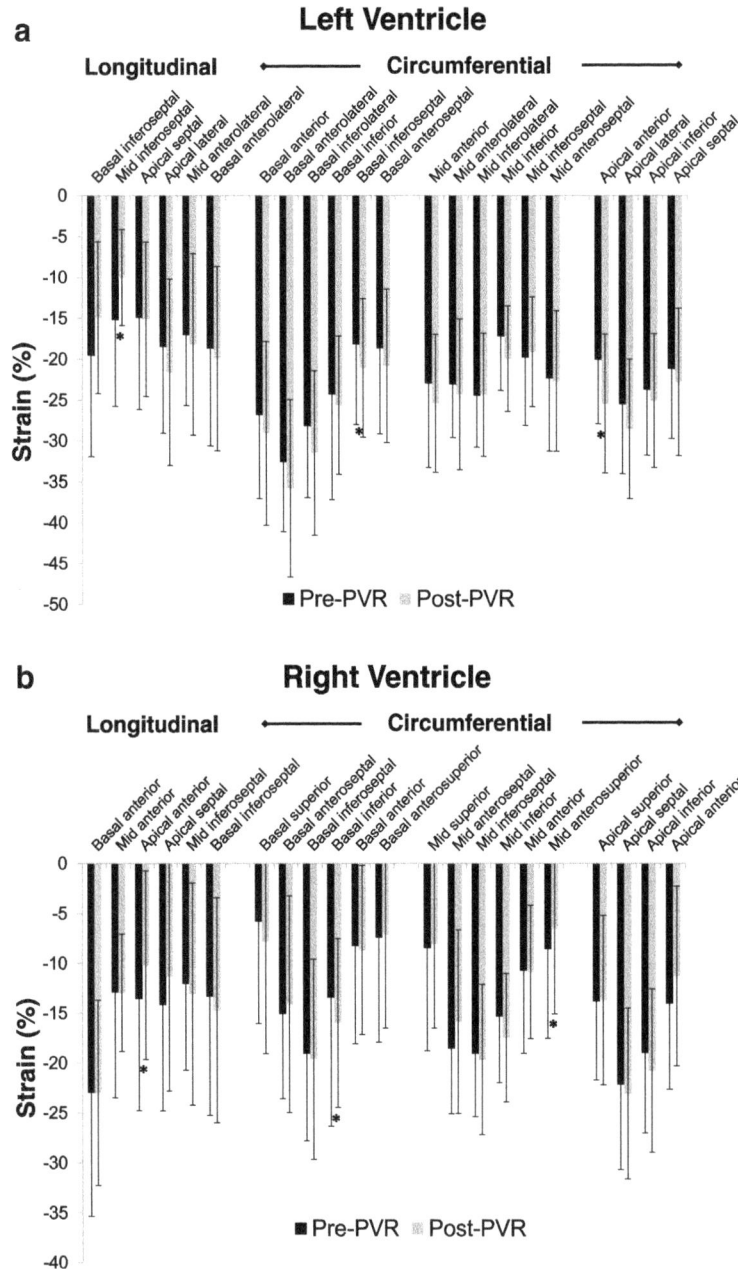

Fig. 3 Segmental longitudinal and circumferential strain in the LV (**a**) and RV (**b**) pre- and post-PVR. An asterisk (*) indicates a statistically significant change. *LV – left ventricle, RV – right ventricle, PVR – pulmonary valve replacement*

nevertheless, intraobserver ICCs for these LV synchrony parameters were all ≥0.73. Agreement for RV synchrony values derived from longitudinal strain curves was only fair.

Discussion
This is the first study to use CMR to assess the impact of surgical PVR on myocardial strain and synchrony in patients with repaired TOF. At a mean of 7 months following PVR, LV global basal and apical strain, and basal

synchrony improved. PVR had no impact on RV global circumferential and longitudinal strains, and a varied impact on synchrony across the locations. Interventricular synchrony worsened at the midventricular level but was unchanged at the base and apex, and on 4-chamber views. These results provide new insight into the effects of PVR on ventricular mechanics and may prompt modifications in management.

Based on multiple studies published over the past decade in repaired TOF patients, a clear picture has

Table 3 Synchrony parameters pre- and post-PVR (n = 36)

Parameter	Pre-PVR	Post-PVR	P-value
Left ventricle			
Longitudinal strain			
Maximum difference in time-to-peak	315 ± 185	351 ± 196	0.33
Standard deviation of time-to-peak	121 ± 73	139 ± 82	0.23
Cross-correlation delay	301 ± 218	340 ± 242	0.39
Circumferential strain: base			
Maximum difference in time-to-peak	233 ± 172	151 ± 120	0.01
Standard deviation of time-to-peak	89 ± 63	58 ± 48	0.02
Cross-correlation delay	217 ± 182	107 ± 77	0.0001
Circumferential strain: mid			
Maximum difference in time-to-peak	124 ± 75	107 ± 55	0.02
Standard deviation of time-to-peak	49 ± 27	43 ± 20	0.15
Cross-correlation delay	106 ± 113	77 ± 53	0.13
Circumferential strain: apex			
Maximum difference in time-to-peak	58 ± 46	47 ± 44	0.27
Standard deviation of time-to-peak	28 ± 22	23 ± 21	0.26
Cross-correlation delay	99 ± 146	42 ± 24	0.04
Right ventricle			
Longitudinal strain			
Maximum difference in time-to-peak	249 ± 176	337 ± 170	0.02
Standard deviation of time-to-peak	97 ± 70	128 ± 64	0.02
Cross-correlation delay	258 ± 171	254 ± 179	0.91
Circumferential strain: base			
Maximum difference in time-to-peak	361 ± 198	265 ± 155	0.01
Standard deviation of time-to-peak	136 ± 70	99 ± 59	0.004
Cross-correlation delay	342 ± 285	341 ± 286	0.56
Circumferential strain: mid			
Maximum difference in time-to-peak	214 ± 133	268 ± 179	0.11
Standard deviation of time-to-peak	96 ± 55	101 ± 66	0.73
Cross-correlation delay	268 ± 216	263 ± 224	0.93
Circumferential strain: apex			
Maximum difference in time-to-peak	95 ± 84	129 ± 97	0.047
Standard deviation of time-to-peak	43 ± 37	60 ± 43	0.03
Cross-correlation delay	119 ± 148	126 ± 145	0.82

Values expressed as mean ± standard deviation in ms

emerged regarding the short-term effects of surgical PVR on ventricular volumes and EF [5, 6, 28]. On average, RV EDV decreases by 30–40%, LV EDV increases slightly, and RV and LV EF largely remain unchanged. This response was also seen in our study cohort.

Analysis of these global parameters, however, is likely insufficient to fully characterize the effects of PVR on ventricular mechanics. Myocardial deformation indices are thought to be more sensitive markers of ventricular function than volumetric parameters [12, 13, 29]. Our

finding of improved LV circumferential strain and synchrony following PVR in the absence of appreciable changes in LV EF follows this premise. The utility of echocardiography-based strain measurement techniques in repaired TOF patients is limited by diminished acoustic windows and visualization, particularly for the RV. CMR has the advantage of providing consistently high image quality for both the RV and LV myocardial walls. There are several CMR methods for myocardial deformation imaging; however, only feature tracking can be applied to standard cine images without performing additional time-consuming imaging sequences. The use of this approach for our study is further supported by reports from our group and others that have shown acceptable correlation between feature tracking and the more established myocardial tagging technique for strain measurement [18, 30, 31]. Investigations have also found that intraobserver and interobserver agreement for radial strain by CMR feature tracking is lower than that for circumferential and longitudinal strain [20, 30]. For this reason, radial strain assessment was not included in the current study. In our study, intraobserver agreement for LV and RV strain and LV synchrony parameters was good; for RV synchrony parameters, it was only fair. Interobserver agreement for several of the strain and synchrony parameters was rather low, which suggests a limited clinical role of this technique for assessing RV synchrony in particular. However, the high intraobserver reliability for most parameters is of primary importance in this study as all of the pre- and post-PVR measurements were made by a single observer.

As the optimal technique to assess ventricular synchrony is unknown, we examined the effect of PVR on 3 metrics extracted from segmental strain versus time curves—maximum difference in time-to-peak, standard deviation of time-to-peak, and CCD. In our analysis, the most robust change with PVR was a significant improvement in intraventricular RV and LV synchrony at the basal level. Interventricular synchrony did not change in 3 of the 4 views; the one statistically significant difference was a mild worsening of synchrony in the mid-ventricular view related to earlier LV contraction. QRS duration was unchanged.

Our data demonstrated for the most part concordant changes in strain and synchrony parameters in the LV supporting a causal relationship. Specifically, following PVR, most of the circumferential strain-based synchrony parameters significantly improved at the base and apex of the LV. This enhanced coordination of contraction may have contributed to the improvements in LV global circumferential strain that were also seen in the same segments. More favorable

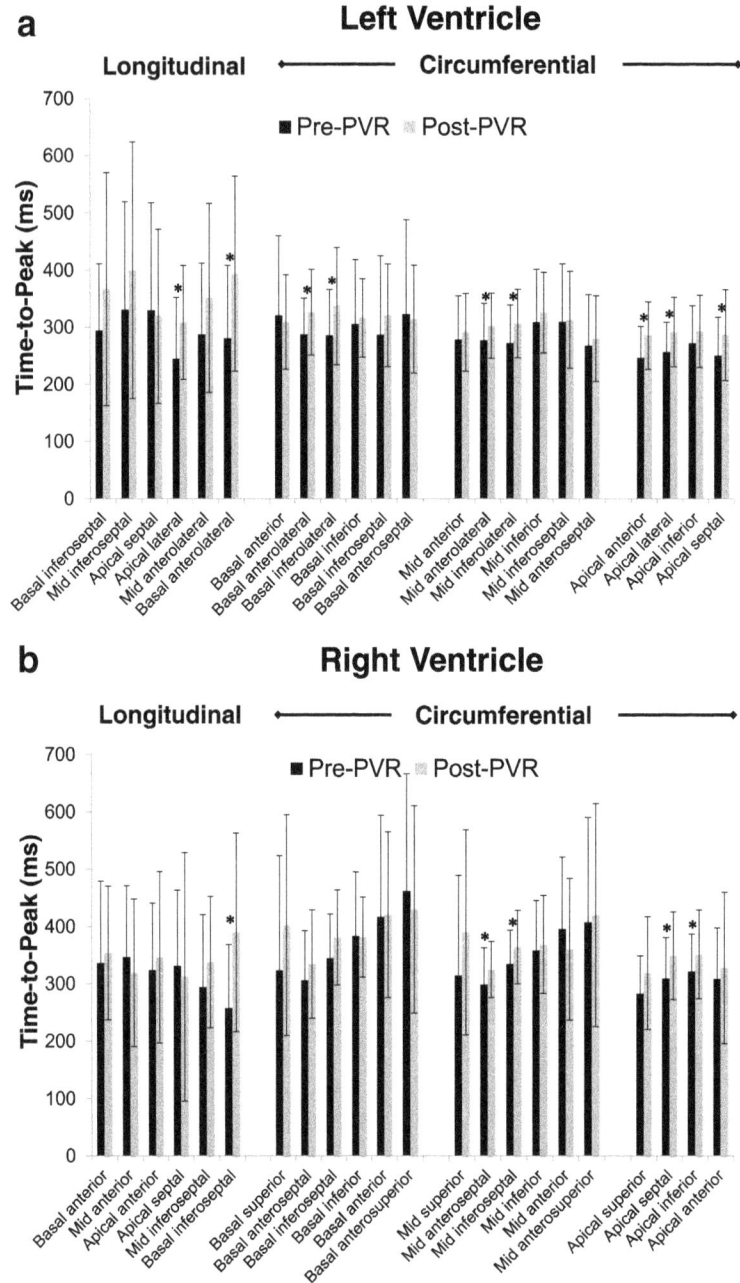

Fig. 4 Segmental time-to-peak longitudinal and circumferential strain in the LV (**a**) and RV (**b**) pre- and post-PVR. An asterisk (*) indicates a statistically significant change. *LV – left ventricle, RV – right ventricle, PVR – pulmonary valve replacement*

ventricular-ventricular interactions in diastole may also have contributed to the improved LV strain [32]. The near elimination of PR with PVR would be expected to reduce the pressure difference across the ventricular septum, and, therefore, diminish diastolic septal bowing toward the LV. The resultant improved LV filling increases preload and muscle fiber stretch leading to increased strain by the Frank–Starling mechanism. This explanation is supported by the increase in indexed LV EDV seen after PVR.

Prior studies

Only a few other reports have measured changes in strain that accompany PVR. A similar study from our group examined the impact of transcatheter pulmonary valve implantation on strain assessed by CMR feature tracking [17]. All patients (*n* = 31) had RV-to-pulmonary artery conduit dysfunction, and were divided into those with predominant pulmonary stenosis (*n* = 18) and those with predominant PR (*n* = 13). For the PR subgroup, PVR led to not only improved LV circumferential strain,

Table 4 Interobserver and intraobserver variability for global strain and synchrony parameters

Parameter	Intraobserver (*n* = 10)		Interobserver (*n* = 10)	
	Mean difference ± SD	ICC	Mean difference ± SD	ICC
Left ventricle				
Circumferential – mid				
Global strain (%)	0.25 ± 1.3	0.96	0.30 ± 1.9	0.89
Maximum difference T2P (ms)	12.5 ± 27.8	0.86	1.0 ± 38.5	0.82
Cross-correlation delay (ms)	2.8 ± 21.9	0.83	14.6 ± 31.4	0.62
Longitudinal				
Global strain (%)	0.33 ± 2.1	0.93	1.6 ± 3.7	0.75
Maximum difference T2P (ms)	102.3 ± 145	0.80	40.0 ± 154	0.67
Cross-correlation delay (ms)	25.0 ± 80.7	0.73	45.8 ± 107	0.65
Right ventricle				
Circumferential – mid				
Global strain (%)	0.40 ± 1.6	0.95	0.31 ± 2.0	0.88
Maximum difference T2P (ms)	64.0 ± 126	0.82	90.6 ± 107.9	0.61
Cross-correlation delay (ms)	104 ± 233	0.66	93.0 ± 230	0.59
Longitudinal				
Global strain (%)	1.0 ± 2.8	0.85	2.6 ± 2.2	0.76
Maximum difference T2P (ms)	146 ± 133	0.76	157 ± 158	0.66
Cross-correlation delay (ms)	22.4 ± 85.9	0.64	42.1 ± 118	0.53

ICC intraclass correlation coefficient, *T2P* time-to-peak, *SD* standard deviation

as it did in our patients with surgical PVR, but also improved longitudinal strain. This difference in longitudinal strain response may be related to the fact that even in the PR subgroup, there was some degree of pulmonary stenosis, more than in the current study population. There was no change in RV circumferential or longitudinal strain with transcatheter PVR in the PR subgroup, in agreement with our results for surgical PVR.

Prior studies assessing the impact of PVR on ventricular synchrony are also scarce. Lurz et al. examined 20 patients with RV-to-pulmonary artery conduit obstruction, most with TOF, before and after transcatheter PVR [14]. Based on tissue Doppler echocardiography from an apical 4-chamber view, the time-to-peak strain for the RV free wall decreased and for the LV free wall was unchanged, leading to significantly less interventricular mechanical delay following PVR. Again, the presence of RV outflow tract obstruction confounds the comparison to our results. However, similar to our study, the QRS duration was unchanged highlighting the importance of assessing both mechanical and electrical measures of ventricular synchrony.

Clinical implications
The clinical implications of improved LV circumferential strain and synchrony following PVR are uncertain but there are some data to suggest that this may be beneficial. Impaired LV systolic function in repaired TOF patients is

fairly common [33, 34]. Both reduced LV global function as well as deformation indices have been shown to be important independent predictors of clinical deterioration, arrhythmia, and death in adults after TOF repair [3, 4, 24, 29, 34–36]. Moreover, our group has shown that LV dyssynchrony is associated with ventricular tachycardia and death in repaired TOF patients [12]. It is thus possible that the improvements in these parameters seen with PVR may lead to a better prognosis, and further study is warranted. For the RV in TOF, global systolic dysfunction is common and associated with adverse outcomes [4, 24]. Abnormalities in RV deformational indices are also prevalent [10, 37, 38]. Our data showed no improvement in any of these parameters with PVR. This finding suggests that strategies other than PVR may need to be pursued to achieve meaningful changes in outcomes related to impaired RV function. To this end, our data supports efforts to maintain pulmonary valve function and optimize myocardial preservation at the time of initial repair as later PVR cannot be relied on to restore function. Similarly, antifibrotic pharmacologic therapy should be explored as studies have implicated fibrosis in the pathophysiology of myocardial dysfunction [39–41]. The lack of improvement in RV functional indices may be because restoration of normal loading conditions occurred after the myocardium had sustained irreversible damage. Accordingly, future studies with larger numbers should assess whether earlier PVR leads to a better RV response. Lastly, our data showed that PVR did not lead to a convincing improvement in interventricular synchrony. Thus, for repaired TOF patients in whom interventricular dyssynchrony is thought to be playing a clinically important role, cardiac resynchronization therapy [42] and not simply PVR, may be needed. Future studies which focus on patients with marked interventricular dyssynchrony who undergo PVR are needed to definitely address this proposition.

Limitations
Several limitations of this study are worth noting. Assessments were performed at a mean of 7 months following PVR. Available data suggests that RV volumes and, thus, EF remain stable between 1 and 5 years after PVR [43]. Nevertheless, we cannot exclude the possibility that changes in strain and synchrony might develop with longer follow-up even in the absence of prosthetic valve dysfunction. The distal RV outflow tract wall was not analyzed because in many patients it consisted of thin patch material from the initial TOF repair and was not amenable to feature tracking analysis. The temporal resolution of the cine CMR data was relatively low; consequently, small changes in synchrony parameters may have gone undetected. However, as the temporal resolution for each patient was similar on the pre- and post-PVR CMR studies, the synchrony changes which were identified are likely valid. The small sample size of the study may have limited the ability to detect small changes in strain and synchrony parameters. Similarly, the power of our study was not sufficient to assess the influence of age at initial repair and age at PVR on the impact of PVR. Finally, a comparison between the PVR alone versus the PVR with RV remodeling cohorts was not reported owing to the small numbers in each subgroup. We acknowledge that RV remodeling may have some impact on regional mechanics, but our study was not adequately powered to address this question.

Conclusions
In this cohort, surgical PVR in repaired TOF patients resulted in improved LV global strain and no change in RV global strain. LV synchrony parameters improved or were unchanged, RV synchrony effects varied by location, and interventricular synchrony was largely unchanged. Future studies should address longer-term changes in strain and synchrony following PVR and their relationship to clinical outcomes.

Abbreviations
CCD: cross-correlation delay; CMR: cardiovascular magnetic resonance; EDV: end-diastolic volume; EF: ejection fraction; ESV: end-systolic volume; ICC: intraclass correlation coefficient; LV: left ventricle/left ventricular; PR: pulmonary regurgitation; PVR: pulmonary valve replacement; RV: right ventricle/right ventricular; TOF: Tetralogy of Fallot

Funding
This study was supported in part by the Higgins Family Research Fund. There are no relationships with industry.

Authors' contributions
SB: Study design, data acquisition and interpretation, writing of initial and final drafts and final approval of the manuscript. DH: Development of feature tracking technique for use in the laboratory, training of personnel for data acquisition and interpretation, contribution to interobserver variability analysis, review and final approval of the manuscript. BK: Data collection and interpretation, final approval of manuscript. EM: Development of a software package using LabVIEW® for cross-correlation analysis which was used as a component of synchrony analysis in this study as well as final approval of manuscript. PN: Design of the original randomized controlled trial and review and final approval of manuscript. TG: Conception and design of the original randomized controlled trial, review and final approval of manuscript. AP: Responsible for all aspects of the study. All authors read and approved the final manuscript.

Competing interests
All authors declare that they have no competing interests.

Author details
[1]Department of Cardiology, Boston Children's Hospital, Boston, USA. [2]Department of Pediatrics, Harvard Medical School, Boston, USA. [3]Department of Cardiac Surgery, Boston Children's Hospital, Boston, USA. [4]Department of Surgery, Boston Children's Hospital, Boston, USA.

References
1. Egbe AC, Mittnacht AJ, Nguyen K, Joashi U. Risk factors for morbidity in infants undergoing tetralogy of fallot repair. Ann Pediatr Cardiol. 2014;7(1):13–8.
2. Cuypers JA, Menting ME, Konings EE, Opic P, Utens EM, Helbing WA, et al. Unnatural history of tetralogy of Fallot: prospective follow-up of 40 years after surgical correction. Circ. 2014;130(22):1944–53.
3. Geva T, Sandweiss BM, Gauvreau K, Lock JE, Powell AJ. Factors associated with impaired clinical status in long-term survivors of tetralogy of Fallot repair evaluated by magnetic resonance imaging. J Am Coll Cardiol. 2004;43(6):1068–74.
4. Valente AM, Gauvreau K, Assenza GE, Babu-Narayan SV, Schreier J, Gatzoulis MA, et al. Contemporary predictors of death and sustained ventricular tachycardia in patients with repaired tetralogy of Fallot enrolled in the INDICATOR cohort. Heart. 2014;100(3):247–53.
5. Cheung EW, Wong WH, Cheung YF. Meta-analysis of pulmonary valve replacement after operative repair of tetralogy of fallot. Am J Cardiol. 2010;106(4):552–7.
6. Ferraz Cavalcanti PE, Sa MP, Santos CA, Esmeraldo IM, de Escobar RR, de Menezes AM, et al. Pulmonary valve replacement after operative repair of tetralogy of Fallot: meta-analysis and meta-regression of 3,118 patients from 48 studies. J Am Coll Cardiol. 2013;62(23):2227–43.
7. Gengsakul A, Harris L, Bradley TJ, Webb GD, Williams WG, Siu SC, et al. The impact of pulmonary valve replacement after tetralogy of Fallot repair: a matched comparison. Eur J Cardio-thorac Surg. 2007;32(3):462–8.
8. Harrild DM, Berul CI, Cecchin F, Geva T, Gauvreau K, Pigula F, et al. Pulmonary valve replacement in tetralogy of Fallot: impact on survival and ventricular tachycardia. Circ. 2009;119(3):445–51.
9. Therrien J, Siu SC, Harris L, Dore A, Niwa K, Janousek J, et al. Impact of pulmonary valve replacement on arrhythmia propensity late after repair of tetralogy of Fallot. Circ. 2001;103(20):2489–94.
10. Dragulescu A, Friedberg MK, Grosse-Wortmann L, Redington A, Mertens L. Effect of chronic right ventricular volume overload on ventricular interaction in patients after tetralogy of Fallot repair. J Am Soc Echocardiogr. 2014;27(8):896–902.

11.　Jing L, Haggerty CM, Suever JD, Alhadad S, Prakash A, Cecchin F, et al. Patients with repaired tetralogy of Fallot suffer from intra- and inter-ventricular cardiac dyssynchrony: a cardiac magnetic resonance study. Eur Heart J Cardiovasc Imaging. 2014;15(12):1333–43.

12.　Ortega M, Triedman JK, Geva T, Harrild DM. Relation of left ventricular dyssynchrony measured by cardiac magnetic resonance tissue tracking in repaired tetralogy of fallot to ventricular tachycardia and death. Am J Cardiol. 2011;107(10):1535–40.

13.　Kempny A, Diller GP, Orwat S, Kaleschke G, Kerckhoff G, Bunck A, et al. Right ventricular-left ventricular interaction in adults with tetralogy of Fallot: a combined cardiac magnetic resonance and echocardiographic speckle tracking study. Int J Cardiol. 2012;154(3):259–64.

14.　Lurz P, Puranik R, Nordmeyer J, Muthurangu V, Hansen MS, Schievano S, et al. Improvement in left ventricular filling properties after relief of right ventricle to pulmonary artery conduit obstruction: contribution of septal motion and interventricular mechanical delay. Eur Heart J. 2009;30(18):2266–74.

15.　Tanaka H, Nesser HJ, Buck T, Oyenuga O, Janosi RA, Winter S, et al. Dyssynchrony by speckle-tracking echocardiography and response to cardiac resynchronization therapy: results of the speckle tracking and resynchronization (STAR) study. Eur Heart J. 2010;31(14):1690–700.

16.　Taylor RJ, Umar F, Panting JR, Stegemann B, Leyva F. Left ventricular lead position, mechanical activation, and myocardial scar in relation to left ventricular reverse remodeling and clinical outcomes after cardiac resynchronization therapy: a feature-tracking and contrast-enhanced cardiovascular magnetic resonance study. Heart rhythm. 2016;13(2):481–9.

17.　Harrild DM, Marcus E, Hasan B, Alexander ME, Powell AJ, Geva T, et al. Impact of transcatheter pulmonary valve replacement on biventricular strain and synchrony assessed by cardiac magnetic resonance feature tracking. Circ Cardiovasc Interv. 2013;6(6):680–7.

18.　Hor KN, Gottliebson WM, Carson C, Wash E, Cnota J, Fleck R, et al. Comparison of magnetic resonance feature tracking for strain calculation with harmonic phase imaging analysis. JACC Cardiovasc Imaging. 2010;3(2):144–51.

19.　Liu B, Dardeer AM, Moody WE, Edwards NC, Hudsmith LE, Steeds RP. Normal values for myocardial deformation within the right heart measured by feature-tracking cardiovascular magnetic resonance imaging. Int J Cardiol. 2018;252:220–3.

20.　Lu JC, Connelly JA, Zhao L, Agarwal PP, Dorfman AL. Strain measurement by cardiovascular magnetic resonance in pediatric cancer survivors: validation of feature tracking against harmonic phase imaging. Pediatr Radiol. 2014;44(9):1070–6.

21.　Vo HD, Marwick TH, Negishi K. MRI-Derived Myocardial Strain Measures in Normal Subject. JACC Cardiovasc Imaging. 2018;11(2 Pt 1):196–205.

22.　Geva T, Gauvreau K, Powell AJ, Cecchin F, Rhodes J, Geva J, et al. Randomized trial of pulmonary valve replacement with and without right ventricular remodeling surgery. Circ. 2010;122(11 Suppl):S201–8.

23.　Samyn MM, Powell AJ, Garg R, Sena L, Geva T. Range of ventricular dimensions and function by steady-state free precession cine MRI in repaired tetralogy of Fallot: right ventricular outflow tract patch vs. conduit repair. Journal of magnetic resonance imaging : JMRI. 2007;26(4):934–40.

24.　Moon TJ, Choueiter N, Geva T, Valente AM, Gauvreau K, Harrild DM. Relation of biventricular strain and dyssynchrony in repaired tetralogy of fallot measured by cardiac magnetic resonance to death and sustained ventricular tachycardia. Am J Cardiol. 2015;115(5):676–80.

25.　Fornwalt BK, Arita T, Bhasin M, Voulgaris G, Merlino JD, Leon AR, et al. Cross-correlation quantification of dyssynchrony: a new method for quantifying the synchrony of contraction and relaxation in the heart. J Am Soc Echocardiogr. 2007;20(12):1330–7.

26.　Hor KN, Wansapura JP, Al-Khalidi HR, Gottliebson WM, Taylor MD, Czosek RJ, et al. Presence of mechanical dyssynchrony in Duchenne muscular dystrophy. J Cardiovasc Magn Reson. 2011;13:12.

27.　Delfino JG, Fornwalt BK, Eisner RL, Leon AR, Oshinski JN. Cross-correlation delay to quantify myocardial dyssynchrony from phase contrast magnetic resonance (PCMR) velocity data. J Magn Reson Imaging : JMRI. 2008;28(5):1086–91.

28.　Geva T. Repaired tetralogy of Fallot: the roles of cardiovascular magnetic resonance in evaluating pathophysiology and for pulmonary valve replacement decision support. J Cardiovasc Magn Reson. 2011;13:9.

29.　Diller GP, Kempny A, Liodakis E, Alonso-Gonzalez R, Inuzuka R, Uebing A, et al. Left ventricular longitudinal function predicts life-threatening ventricular arrhythmia and death in adults with repaired tetralogy of fallot. Circ. 2012;125(20):2440–6.

30.　Harrild DM, Han Y, Geva T, Zhou J, Marcus E, Powell AJ. Comparison of cardiac MRI tissue tracking and myocardial tagging for assessment of regional ventricular strain. Int J Cardiovasc Imaging. 2012;28(8):2009–18.

31.　Moody WE, Taylor RJ, Edwards NC, Chue CD, Umar F, Taylor TJ, et al. Comparison of magnetic resonance feature tracking for systolic and diastolic strain and strain rate calculation with spatial modulation of magnetization imaging analysis. J Magnetic Reson Imaging : JMRI. 2015;41(4):1000–12.

32.　Coats L, Khambadkone S, Derrick G, Hughes M, Jones R, Mist B, et al. Physiological consequences of percutaneous pulmonary valve implantation: the different behaviour of volume- and pressure-overloaded ventricles. Eur Heart J. 2007;28(15):1886–93.

33.　Broberg CS, Aboulhosn J, Mongeon FP, Kay J, Valente AM, Khairy P, et al. Prevalence of left ventricular systolic dysfunction in adults with repaired tetralogy of fallot. Am J Cardiol. 2011;107(8):1215–20.

34.　Ghai A, Silversides C, Harris L, Webb GD, Siu SC, Therrien J. Left ventricular dysfunction is a risk factor for sudden cardiac death in adults late after repair of tetralogy of Fallot. J Am Coll Cardiol. 2002;40(9):1675–80.

35.　Knauth AL, Gauvreau K, Powell AJ, Landzberg MJ, Walsh EP, Lock JE, et al. Ventricular size and function assessed by cardiac MRI predict major adverse clinical outcomes late after tetralogy of Fallot repair. Heart. 2008;94(2):211–6.

36.　Orwat S, Diller GP, Kempny A, Radke R, Peters B, Kuhne T, et al. Myocardial deformation parameters predict outcome in patients with repaired tetralogy of Fallot. Heart. 2016;102(3):209–15.

37.　Friedberg MK, Fernandes FP, Roche SL, Slorach C, Grosse-Wortmann L, Manlhiot C, et al. Relation of right ventricular mechanics to exercise tolerance in children after tetralogy of Fallot repair. Am Heart J. 2013;165(4):551–7.

38.　Menting ME, van den Bosch AE, McGhie JS, Eindhoven JA, Cuypers JA, Witsenburg M, et al. Assessment of ventricular function in adults with repaired tetralogy of Fallot using myocardial deformation imaging. Eur Heart J Cardiovasc Imaging. 2015;16(12):1347–57.

39.　Broberg CS, Huang J, Hogberg I, McLarry J, Woods P, Burchill LJ, et al. Diffuse LV myocardial fibrosis and its clinical associations in adults with repaired tetralogy of Fallot. JACC Cardiovasc Imaging. 2016;9(1):86–7.

40.　Chen CA, Dusenbery SM, Valente AM, Powell AJ, Geva T. Myocardial ECV fraction assessed by CMR is associated with type of hemodynamic load and arrhythmia in repaired tetralogy of Fallot. JACC Cardiovasc Imaging. 2016;9(1):1–10.

41.　Pradegan N, Vida VL, Geva T, Stellin G, White MT, Sanders SP, et al. Myocardial histopathology in late-repaired and unrepaired adults with tetralogy of Fallot. Cardiovasc Pathol. 2016;25(3):225–31.

42.　Kubus P, Materna O, Tax P, Tomek V, Janousek J. Successful permanent resynchronization for failing right ventricle after repair of tetralogy of Fallot. Circ. 2014;130(22):e186–90.

43.　Hallbergson A, Gauvreau K, Powell AJ, Geva T. Right ventricular remodeling after pulmonary valve replacement: early gains, late losses. Ann Thorac Surg. 2015;99(2):660–6.

3

A comprehensive characterization of myocardial and vascular phenotype in pediatric chronic kidney disease using cardiovascular magnetic resonance imaging

Mun Hong Cheang[1,2], Nathaniel J. Barber[1,2], Abbas Khushnood[1,2], Jakob A. Hauser[1,2], Gregorz T. Kowalik[1], Jennifer A. Steeden[1], Michael A. Quail[1,2], Kjell Tullus[2], Daljit Hothi[2] and Vivek Muthurangu[1,2*]

Abstract

Background: Children with chronic kidney disease (CKD) have increased cardiovascular mortality. Identifying high-risk children who may benefit from further therapeutic intervention is difficult as cardiovascular abnormalities are subtle. Although transthoracic echocardiography may be used to detect sub-clinical abnormalities, it has well-known problems with reproducibility that limit its ability to accurately detect these changes. Cardiovascular magnetic resonance (CMR) is the reference standard method for assessing blood flow, cardiac structure and function. Furthermore, recent innovations enable the assessment of radial and longitudinal myocardial velocity, such that detection of sub-clinical changes is now possible. Thus, CMR may be ideal for cardiovascular assessment in pediatric CKD. This study aims to comprehensively assess cardiovascular function in pediatric CKD using CMR and determine its relationship with CKD severity.

Methods: A total of 120 children (40 mild, 40 moderate, 20 severe pre-dialysis CKD subjects and 20 healthy controls) underwent CMR with non-invasive blood pressure (BP) measurements. Cardiovascular parameters measured included systemic vascular resistance (SVR), total arterial compliance (TAC), left ventricular (LV) structure, ejection fraction (EF), cardiac timings, radial and longitudinal systolic and diastolic myocardial velocities. Between group comparisons and regression modelling were used to identify abnormalities in CKD and determine the effects of renal severity on myocardial function.

Results: The elevation in mean BP in CKD was accompanied by significantly increased afterload (SVR), without evidence of arterial stiffness (TAC) or increased fluid overload. Left ventricular volumes and global function were not abnormal in CKD. However, there was evidence of LV remodelling, prolongation of isovolumic relaxation time and reduced systolic and diastolic myocardial velocities.

Conclusion: Abnormal cardiovascular function is evident in pre-dialysis pediatric CKD. Novel CMR biomarkers may be useful for the detection of subtle abnormalities in this population. Further studies are needed to determine to prognostic value of these biomarkers.

Keywords: Chronic renal failure, Pediatrics, Arterial stiffness, Systemic vascular resistance, Hypertension, Myocardial impairment

* Correspondence: v.muthurangu@ucl.ac.uk
[1]Centre for Cardiovascular Imaging, UCL Institute of Cardiovascular Science, 30 Guilford Street, London WC1N 1EH, UK
[2]Great Ormond Street Hospital, London, UK

Background

Cardiovascular events are a leading cause of death in pediatric chronic kidney disease [1] (CKD). Two-dimensional transthoracic echocardiography (TTE) is conventionally used to assess the heart in children with CKD. Several TTE markers have been used as indicators of increased risk including: left ventricular (LV) hypertrophy (LVH), LV dysfunction and abnormal myocardial strain [2–4]. However, TTE can be hampered by inaccurate measurement of volumes and mass [5], as well as operator dependence.

Cardiovascular magnetic resonance (CMR) cine imaging is the reference standard method of assessing LV volumes, ejection fraction (EF) and mass [6]. Novel CMR including tissue phase mapping (TPM) to assess myocardial velocities [7] and high temporal resolution phase contrast CMR (PCMR) to measure mitral inflow velocities and cardiac timing intervals are also now available. Furthermore, CMR can be used to characterize the vasculature by combining flow measurements with simultaneously acquired blood pressure (BP) [8]. Thus, CMR offers a comprehensive method of assessing myocardial and vascular phenotype in pediatric CKD.

The objectives of this study were to i) evaluate any differences in vascular and cardiac phenotype between healthy children and those with CKD, ii) determine the relationship between vascular and cardiac phenotype and any additional effect of CKD, iii) assess the relationship between markers of renal disease and cardiovascular phenotype.

Methods

Study population

The study population consisted of 120 children: 100 with confirmed CKD (stages 1–5) and 20 healthy volunteers. The CKD patients were divided into 3 groups based on CKD stage: Mild (CKD stage 1–2), Moderate (CKD stage 3) and Severe (CKD stage 4–5). The study was powered to detect differences in mean arterial BP (MBP) between the groups (including healthy controls). For between group comparisons, a sample size of 14 children per group provided 90% power ($p < 0.05$) to detect a difference of 3 mmHg in MBP (assuming a normal MBP of 82 mmHg, and a variance of 40 mmHg [9]). The group size was increased to 20 for redundancy. In addition, we increased the population size of the mild and moderate CKD groups to 40 children in order to improve our spread of estimated glomerular filtration rate (eGFR) data points for correlation analysis.

All patients were recruited from the CKD and hypertension clinics at Great Ormond Street Hospital, London. Healthy subjects were recruited by advertising within the hospital and a detailed history was taken from the parents to ensure there was no significant medical history. Exclusion criteria were: i) age < 7 or > 18 years, ii) congenital structural heart disease or primary myocardial disease, iii) primary renovascular disease, iv) active vasculitis v) cardiac arrhythmia, vi) medical devices precluding CMR, vii) history of current or previous renal replacement therapy and viii) acutely deteriorating renal function. This study was approved by UK national research ethics service (National Research Ethics Service Committee London, London Bridge, reference: 15/LO/0213). Informed parental consent and patient assent was obtained from all participants.

All CKD participants had blood and urine tests as part of their outpatient care including: haemoglobin (Hb), urea, creatinine, electrolytes, calcium, phosphate, intact parathyroid hormone level (PTH), and urine albumin to creatinine ratio measurements. The eGFR was estimated by modified Schwartz formula. Neither blood nor urine tests were performed for healthy controls.

Imaging protocol

Imaging was performed on a 1.5 T CMR system (Avanto; Siemens Healthineers, Erlangen, Germany) with vector cardiographic gating. All CMR images were processed using in-house plug-ins developed for open-source DICOM software OsiriX [10] (Osirix Foundation, Geneva, Switzerland). All images were analyzed by the same individual, who is a CMR trained cardiologist (MC) with 5 years of CMR experience. No gadolinium- contrast was given.

Left ventricular volumes and mass

LV volumes were assessed using short axis multi-slice free-breathing real-time radial k-t SENSE balanced steady state free precision sequence sequence [11]. Scan parameters - FOV: ≈350 mm, matrix: 128 × 128, voxel size: ≈2.7 × 2.7 × 8 mm, TE/TR: ≈1.1/ ≈2.2 msec, Flip angle: 40°, acceleration factor: 8, temporal resolution: ≈36 msec. LV endocardial borders were manually traced at end-diastole and end-systole to evaluate end-diastolic volume (EDV) and end-systolic volume (ESV). Stroke volume (SV) was obtained by subtracting ESV from EDV. All ventricular volumes were indexed to body surface area (BSA). LV EF was assessed SV/LVEDV × 100.

Epicardial LV borders were manually traced in end-diastole and combined with endocardial borders to obtain LV mass (LVM). The effect of body size on LV mass was controlled by both indexing to height to the power of 2.7 ($LVMht^{2.7}$) [12] and dividing LVM by EDV to calculate mass volume ratio (MVR) [13].

The right atrial and left atrial areas were measured in diastole from 4-chamber view (using the same sequence) and indexed to BSA.

Cardiac timing and inflow velocities

LV outflow tract and mitral inflow velocities were assessed with a free-breathing high temporal resolution real-time UNFOLD-SENSE spiral PCMR sequence. This sequence has previously been validated against Doppler echocardiography [14]. Scan parameters - FOV: $\approx$450 mm, matrix: 128×128, voxel size: $\approx 3.5 \times 3.5 \times 7$ mm, TE/TR: $\approx 1.97/ \approx 7.41$ msec, flip angle: 20°, VENC: 150 m/s, acceleration factor: 10, temporal resolution: ≈ 15 ms. The imaging plane was positioned so that both the mitral inflow and LV outflow tract were imaged in the short axis.

The mitral valve orifice and LV outflow tract were manually segmented from the resultant inflow and outflow curves to obtain the isovolumic relaxation time (IRT), isovolumic contraction time (ICT) and ejection time (ET) as previously described [14]. Myocardial performance index (Tei) was calculated as the sum of ICT and IRT divided by ET. Peak early (E) and atrial (A) diastolic velocities were measured from the inflow curves.

Myocardial velocities

LV myocardial velocities was measured using a free breathing self-navigated golden-angle spiral TPM sequence planned in the mid LV short axis view [7, 15]. Scan parameters - FOV: $\approx$400 mm, matrix: 192×192, voxel size: $\approx 2.1 \times 2.1 \times 8$ mm, TE/TR: $\approx 3.51/ \approx 11.7$ msec, flip angle: 15°, respiratory navigation efficiency: 30%, scan time: $\approx$7-8 min, temporal resolution: ≈ 23 msec.

All TPM indices were measured from a mid LV short axis slice. Each acquisition produces a magnitude image and 3 phase images (in the x-, y- and z- direction). The epi- and endocardial borders were manually segmented on the magnitude image for all frames and regions of interest were transferred to the accompanying phase images. From these masked phase images, radial velocity was calculated by transforming the x and y-direction velocities to an internal polar coordinate system using the LV center of mass as a reference point [7, 15]. The longitudinal velocity was taken as the z-direction velocity. Global radial and longitudinal LV velocities were calculated by averaging velocities across the segmented LV slice for a given direction. The magnitude of the peak systolic (S′), early diastolic (E′) and late diastolic (A′) velocities were measured from the velocity-time curves. E′/A′ ratio was the ratio of longitudinal E′ over longitudinal A′ velocity. The longitudinal E/E′ ratio was obtained by dividing the mitral E wave velocity by longitudinal peak early diastolic velocity.

Aortic flow

Aortic flow assessment was performed using a breath held retrospectively-gated, spiral SENSE PCMR just above the sinotubular junction [16]. Scan parameters - FOV: $\approx$400 mm, matrix: 256×256, voxel size: $\approx 1.6 \times 5$ mm, TE/TR: $\approx 2.1/ \approx 8.0$ msec, flip angle: 25°, acceleration factor: 3, breath hold time: 4-8 s, temporal resolution: ≈ 32.0 msec.

The aorta was segmented using a semi-automatic vessel edge detection algorithm with manual operator correction. The SV was derived from the flow curve and multiplied by heart rate to calculate cardiac output (CO). The maximum (AoMax) and minimum (AoMin) cross-sectional areas of the ascending aorta over the cardiac cycle were also recorded.

Blood pressure measurement

Brachial systolic, diastolic and mean arterial BPs (SBP, DBP, MBP) were measured using a CMR compatible oscillometric sphygmomanometer (Datex Ohmeda; General Electric Healthcare, Boston, Massachusetts, USA) during CMR image acquisition. This enabled optimum combination of BP and flow data for calculation of vascular indices. All BP measurements were acquired with an appropriate sized arm cuff after the subject had been lying in the scanner for at least 10 min. Pulse pressure (PP) was the difference between SBP and DBP.

Measures of vascular characteristics

Total systemic vascular resistance (SVR) was calculated by dividing MBP by cardiac output (CO) [8]. Total arterial compliance (TAC) was calculated using a two-element windkessel model described previously [8]. Briefly, aortic flow curves were inputted into the model with measured SVR. The compliance was tuned so that pulse pressure generated by the model equaled measured pulse pressure. Ascending aortic strain (AoS) was calculated as (AoMax − AoMin)/AoMin (expressed as a percentage). Local arterial stiffness was assessed by calculating ascending aortic compliance (AoC) = AoS/pulse pressure [17].

Statistics

Statistical analyses were performed using Stata 13 (StataCorp, College Station, Texas, USA). Data were examined for normality using Shapiro-Wilk test and non-normally distributed data was transformed using a zero-skewness log transform prior to analysis. Descriptive statistics were expressed as mean ($\pm$ standard deviation) or geometric mean ($\pm$ geometric standard deviation) if data was log transformed. Between CKD group differences in vascular and cardiac phenotype were assessed using analysis of variance (ANOVA) (objective 1). Levene's test was used to assess for homogeneity of variances across the groups and Welch's correction was applied for non-homogeneous variance. Six groups of statistical tests comparing healthy controls to patients were performed in the following domains - baseline characteristics, blood pressure, vascular phenotype, global cardiac structure and function, cardiac timings and mitral velocities, and tissue phase mapping. Each group of tests was considered a single family of statistical inferences and the family-wise error rate was controlled using Bonferroni correction. The corresponding corrected critical p-values are listed in the respective tables. Post-hoc pairwise comparison was performed on parameters significantly different on ANOVA testing. The Bonferroni method was used to adjust for potential Type 1 errors in the pairwise comparisons. Spearman's correlation coefficient (rho) was used to determine the relationship between specific vascular and cardiac phenotypic markers (objective 2) that were significant on ANOVA testing. Multi-variable ANOVA models were also constructed to examine the independent effect of CKD group. Spearman's correlation coefficient was also used to determine the relationship between markers of renal disease severity - eGFR, hemoglobin (Hb) and PTH and significant abnormal cardiac and vascular indices - MVR, IRT, S ', E', MBP, SVR (objective 3). Multi-variable linear regression was used to determine the independent effect of renal severity on cardiac markers by controlling for vascular phenotype. Only patients with recent blood tests were included into models involving blood indices. A p value < 0.05 was considered statistically significant, except where Bonferroni correction was applied as indicated. Indices not statistically

different to healthy subjects have been described as 'normal'.

Results

Demographics

The CKD cohort ($n = 100$) consisted of 40 children with mild CKD (stage 1–2: eGFR 78.6 ± 8.8 ml/min/1.73 m^2), 40 children with moderate CKD (stage 3: eGFR 48.3 ± 8.4 ml/min/1.73 m^2) and 20 children with severe CKD (eGFR 19.2 ± 6.5 ml/min/1.73 m^2). Twenty-five (25%) children (mild CKD: 10, moderate CKD: 9; severe CKD: 6) had a prior diagnosis of hypertension and were on treatment (Table 1). The two most common causes of CKD were congenital abnormalities of the kidney and urinary tract ($n = 60$, 60%) and renal dysplasia ($n = 11$, 11%). All other causes represented < 10% of the population. Eight CKD children had undergone a previous nephrectomy. No children had previously received or were currently receiving renal replacement therapy as per exclusion criteria. None of the healthy subjects ($n = 20$) had any significant past medical history nor were they taking any medications. There were no differences in age, BSA or sex distribution between groups (Table 1). As expected, markers of renal function (urea, creatinine, eGFR and urine albumin/creatinine ratio) were worse in the latter CKD stages, with the most abnormal results observed in

Table 1 Demographics and Baseline Characteristics of study population

	Healthy Controls ($n = 20$)	Mild CKD ($n = 40$)	Moderate CKD ($n = 40$)	Severe CKD ($n = 20$)	P-value
Age (years)[a]	12 ± 1.3	11 ± 1.3	12 ± 1.3	13 ± 1.3	0.12
Sex (% male)	40%	38%	23%	45%	0.42
Height (cm)	162 ± 18	150 ± 17	152 ± 18	151 ± 18	0.075
Weight (kg)[a]	53 ± 1.4	43 ± 1.5	45 ± 1.5	44 ± 1.4	0.22
Body Mass Index (kg/m^2)[a]	20 ± 1.1	19 ± 1.2	20 ± 1.2	20 ± 1.1	0.77
Body Surface Area (m^2)	1.6 ± 0.32	1.4 ± 0.33	1.4 ± 0.35	1.4 ± 0.3	0.16
Hemoglobin (g/L)		132 ± 13	133 ± 16	128 ± 11	0.57
Urea (mmol/L)		5.4 ± 1.2	8.6 ± 2.5	18.0 ± 5.2	< 0.001[†]
Creatinine (umol/L)[a]		68 ± 1.2	117 ± 1.2	305 ± 1.4	< 0.001[†]
eGFR (ml/min/1.73 m^2)		79 ± 8.8	48 ± 8.4	19 ± 6.5	< 0.001
Calcium-Phosphate product (mmol^2/L^2)		3.4 ± 0.45	3.4 ± 0.39	3.5 ± 0.56	0.40
Intact parathyroid hormone (pmol/L)[a]		3.5 ± 3.2	3.7 ± 2.4	8.5 ± 2.4	0.011
Urine Albumin/ Creatinine Ratio (mg/mmol)[a]		4.7 ± 3.7	22 ± 6.2	261 ± 2.5	< 0.001
Angiotensin converting enzyme inhibitor		28%	40%	15%	0.13
Calcium Channel Blocker		5%	13%	15%	0.38
Beta-Blocker		5%	5%	20%	0.09
Aldosterone antagonist (Spironolactone)		3%	0%	0%	0.47

Bonferroni correction applied- $p < 0.003$ is considered significant
Abbreviations: CKD chronic kidney disease, eGFR estimated globular filtration rate
[a]Logarithmic transformation was applied
[†]ANOVA Welch (W) test was used. 10% of CKD patients were on 2 or more anti-hypertensive agents

the severe CKD group ($p < 0.03$). The severe CKD group also had highest parathyroid hormone (PTH) ($p = 0.01$). There was no difference in Hb between the groups ($p = 0.57$). Outline of blood and urine tests results of study population can be seen in Additional file 1: Table S1.

Vascular characteristics
The DBP, DBP centile and MBP were significantly different between the groups ($p < 0.001$, Table 2) and were elevated in all CKD groups compared to controls ($p < 0.05$) on pairwise comparison. However, there were no significant differences between the CKD groups. There were also no group differences in SBP and PP ($p \geq 0.13$), although there was a trend for SBP centile ($p = 0.08$).

The SVR was also significantly different between the groups ($p = 0.004$, Table 3). On pairwise comparison, both moderate and severe CKD groups were elevated compared to controls ($p \leq 0.014$). However, there were no significant differences in SVR between the CKD groups. Importantly, there were no group differences in TAC, local measures of ascending aorta stiffness (AoS and AoC) or cardiac output (Table 3).

Cardiac geometry and global function
There was a significant difference in MVR (a marker of LV remodeling) between the groups ($p = 0.003$, Table 4). On pairwise comparison, only the severe CKD group was significantly different from healthy subjects and all other CKD groups ($p \leq 0.034$).

The MVR correlated with all measures of BP (SBP: rho = 0.29, $p = 0.001$; MBP: rho = 0.26, $p = 0.004$; and DBP: rho = 0.19, $p = 0.036$; Fig. 1). When a model was created to study the combined effect of BP and CKD group on LV remodeling, both SBP (BP with highest univariate correlation) and CKD group were independent predictors of MVR ($p = 0.009$, $p = 0.008$ respectively).

The SVR correlated with MVR (rho = 0.3, $p < 0.001$), and remained an independent predictor of MVR ($p < 0.001$) in

a model including CKD group ($p = 0.01$). There was no correlation between MVR and TAC ($p = 0.15$). Although LVMht$^{2.7}$ did appear higher in CKD, this did not reach statistical significance ($p = 0.12$, Table 4).

There were no differences in EDV, ESV, SV, EF, RAA or LAA between the groups (Table 4).

Inflow velocities and cardiac timing intervals
The IRT (a marker of active myocardial relaxation [18]) was different across groups ($p < 0.001$, Table 5). On pairwise comparison, IRT was significantly elevated in moderate and severe CKD patients compared to controls ($p \leq 0.01$). In addition, IRT was higher in severe CKD than in mild CKD patients ($p = 0.023$).

There was a significant association between IRT and MVR (rho = 0.25, $p = 0.008$) as seen in Fig. 1. However, both MVR and CKD group were independent predictors of IRT in a multi-variable model ($p = 0.01$ and 0.007 respectively).

There were no differences in ICT, ET or Tei index between the groups. Peak transmitral E and A wave velocities and peak E/A ratio were also normal in CKD (Table 5).

Tissue phase mapping
Radial S′ velocity, a marker of systolic function, was significantly different between groups ($p = 0.003$, Table 6). Specifically, radial S′ was lower in moderate and severe CKD compared to controls ($p \leq 0.035$). There was no significant difference in longitudinal S′ between groups.

Radial S′ negatively correlated with MBP (rho = − 0.22, $p = 0.016$), DBP (rho = − 0.37, $p < 0.0001$–Fig. 2) and SVR (rho = − 0.22, $p = 0.014$), but not SBP ($p = 0.52$). Longitudinal S′ did not significantly correlate with any blood pressures. A model created to study the effects of CKD and DBP (BP with highest univariate correlation) on radial systolic velocity demonstrated that DBP was an independent predictor of radial S′ ($p = 0.001$) but CKD group was not significant ($p = 0.16$). Radial S′ also significantly correlated with LVEF (rho = 0.24, $p = 0.009$–

Table 2 Blood pressure profile of study population

	Healthy Controls (n = 20)	Mild CKD (n = 40)	Moderate CKD (n = 40)	Severe CKD (n = 20)	P-value
Systolic BP (mmhg)[a]	109 ± 1.1	113 ± 1.1	116 ± 1.1	116 ± 1.1	0.14
Systolic BP percentile[a]	33 ± 2.5	58 ± 1.7	61 ± 1.8	64 ± 1.7	0.08[†]
Diastolic BP (mmhg)[a]	53 ± 1.2	63 ± 1.2	65 ± 1.2	69 ± 1.2	< 0.001
Diastolic BP percentile[a]	17 ± 2.3	45 ± 1.9	48 ± 1.8	60 ± 1.6	< 0.001[†]
Mean BP (mmhg)	78 ± 7.8	84 ± 8.8	87 ± 9.9	89 ± 8.8	< 0.001
Pulse Pressure (mmhg)	55 ± 13	50 ± 10	51 ± 9.5	48 ± 12	0.13
Heart Rate (BPM)[a]	72 ± 1.2	75 ± 1.2	72 ± 1.2	74 ± 1.2	0.75

Bonferroni correction applied $p < 0.007$ is considered significant
Abbreviations: CKD chronic kidney disease, BP blood pressure, BPM beats per minute
[a]Logarithmic transformation was applied
[†]ANOVA Welch (W) test was used

Table 3 Vascular phenotype in CKD

	Healthy Controls (n = 20)	Mild CKD (n = 40)	Moderate CKD (n = 40)	Severe CKD (n = 20)	P-value
SVR (WU.m^2)^a	21 ± 1.3	24 ± 1.2	26 ± 1.2	26 ± 1.2	0.004
TAC (ml/mmHg. m^2.10^2)^a	52 ± 1.3	55 ± 1.2	54 ± 1.3	58 ± 1.3	0.56
AoS (%)^a	46 ± 1.5	52 ± 1.6	53 ± 1.6	51 ± 1.5	0.74
AoC (%mmHg^{-1}.10^2)^a	86 ± 1.6	108 ± 1.6	105 ± 1.7	111 ± 1.7	0.33
CO^a (l/min/m^2)	3.6 ± 1.2	3.5 ± 1.2	3.4 ± 1.2	3.4 ± 1.2	0.61

Bonferroni correction applied- $p < 0.01$ is considered significant
Abbreviations: *CKD* chronic kidney disease, *SVR* systemic vascular resistance, *TAC* total arterial compliance. *AoS* ascending aortic strain, *AoC* ascending aortic compliance, *CO* cardiac output
^{a}Logarithmic transformation was applied

Fig. 2), but there was no association between LVEF and longitudinal S′ ($p = 0.24$).

Radial E′ velocity, a marker of LV relaxation and stiffness, was significantly lower in all CKD groups compared to controls ($p ≤ 0.005$) on pairwise comparison. However, there were no significant differences between the CKD groups. There were no significant group differences in longitudinal E′ velocity in CKD (Table 6). Radial E′ was negatively correlated with DBP (rho = − 0.21, $p = 0.021$) and SVR (rho = − 0.27, $p = 0.003$). Two separate models were created to separately study the effects of CKD and DBP or SVR on radial E′. Although CKD group and SVR were independent determinants of Radial E′ ($p < 0.003$ and 0.01, respectively), DBP was not a significant predictor ($p = 0.19$).

In addition, radial and longitudinal E′ correlated negatively with IRT (rho = − 0.28, $p < 0.003$ & rho = − 0.24, $p < 0.01$ respectively). Unlike IRT, neither was associated with MVR or LVMht$^{2.7}$ ($p > 0.25$).

The E′/A′ was different between groups ($p = 0.003$, Table 6), but was only significantly reduced in moderate CKD compared to controls and mild CKD ($p ≤ 0.035$)

on pairwise comparison. There were no group differences in radial and longitudinal A′ velocities or E/E′.

Association between renal and cardiovascular biomarkers

Worsening eGFR was associated with higher MBP (rho = − 0.26, $p = 0.04$), MVR (rho = − 0.29, $p = 0.02$) and longer IRT (rho = − 0.30, $p = 0.02$). On multi-variable regression, eGFR remained a significant determinant of MVR (β = − 0.26, $p = 0.035$,) and IRT (β = − 0.28, $p = 0.043$) after adjustment for MBP ($p ≥ 0.06$). In a model with IRT as dependant variable, eGFR trended towards significant (β = − 0.25, $p = 0.052$) and MVR was significant (β = 0.27, $p = 0.039$).

Reduced Hb was also associated with a reduced radial function (Rad S′: rho = 0.35, $p < 0.005$, Rad E′: rho = 0.35, $p < 0.006$). These relationships remained significant after adjusting for the effect of afterload (MBP or SVR) in a multi-variable regression model (Rad S′ models: Hb $p = 0.001$, Rad E′ models: Hb $p = 0.001$). There were no other significant relationships between eGFR, PTH and Hb with other cardiovascular parameters.

Table 4 Cardiac structure and global function in CKD

	Healthy Controls (n = 20)	Mild CKD (n = 40)	Moderate CKD (n = 40)	Severe CKD (n = 20)	P-value
LVEDV (ml/m^2)	74 ± 11	68 ± 9.1	68 ± 10	65 ± 9.7	0.03
LVESV (ml/m^2)^a	23 ± 1.3	21 ± 1.3	20 ± 1.3	19 ± 1.3	0.13
LVSV (ml/m^2)^a	50 ± 1.1	46 ± 1.1	47 ± 1.2	46 ± 1.2	0.18
EF (%)	68 ± 4.6	68 ± 6.1	69 ± 6.7	70 ± 5.8	0.72
LVMht$^{2.7}$ (g/m$^{2.7}$)^a	21 ± 1.2	21 ± 1.3	22 ± 1.2	25 ± 1.2	0.12
MVR (g/ml)	0.7 ± 0.1	0.72 ± 0.16	0.75 ± 0.16	0.87 ± 0.17	0.003
RA Area (cm^2/m^2)	12 ± 1.8	12 ± 1.9	11 ± 2.5	11 ± 2	0.69
LA Area (cm^2/m^2)^a	12 ± 1.3	12 ± 1.2	11 ± 1.2	11 ± 1.2	0.38

Bonferroni correction applied- $p < 0.006$ is considered significant
Abbreviations: *CKD* chronic kidney disease, *LVEDV* left ventricular end-diastolic volume, *LVESV* left ventricular end-systolic volume, *LVSV* left ventricular stroke volume, *EF* ejection fraction, *LVMht(2.7)* left ventricular mass indexed to height to the power of 2.7, *MVR* left ventricular mass to volume ratio
^{a}Logarithmic transformation was applied

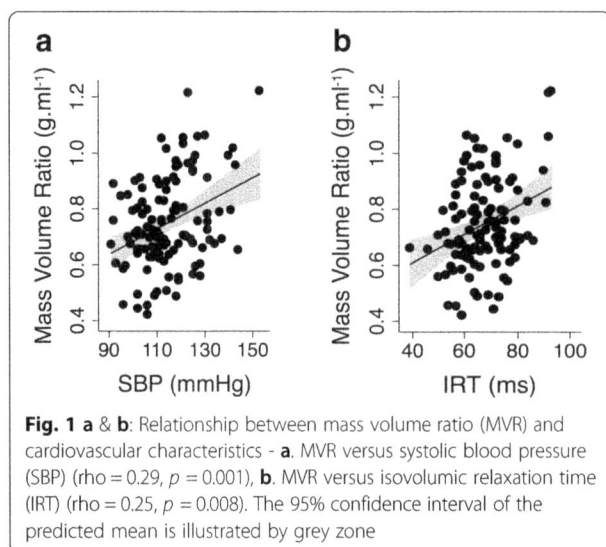

Fig. 1 a & b: Relationship between mass volume ratio (MVR) and cardiovascular characteristics - **a**. MVR versus systolic blood pressure (SBP) (rho = 0.29, p = 0.001), **b**. MVR versus isovolumic relaxation time (IRT) (rho = 0.25, p = 0.008). The 95% confidence interval of the predicted mean is illustrated by grey zone

Discussion

This is the largest study to investigate the vascular and cardiac phenotype in pre-dialysis pediatric CKD using CMR. The main findings were that children with CKD had: i) elevated BP (both MBP and DBP), ii) increased SVR, but no evidence of increased vascular stiffness, iii) higher LV MVR independent of BP, iv) abnormalities of diastolic function suggestive of reduced active relaxation and increased chamber stiffness and v) Reduced systolic velocities with preserved global systolic function. These changes appeared most marked in children with moderate and severe CKD stages.

Vascular phenotype in pediatric CKD

It is well recognized that hypertension is common in pediatric CKD [19]. However, the abnormal components of afterload have not been fully described. In this study, we found that SVR was significantly increased in all CKD groups compared to normal controls. Possible

reasons include; salt retention and abnormal renin-angiotensin stimulation [20], sympathetic overdrive [21] and endothelial dysfunction via reduced nitric oxide bio-availability [22]. Irrespective of the cause, our results suggest that vascular resistance is an important mediator of increased afterload and may be a useful target for intervention. Interestingly, we found no evidence of reduced TAC or increased aortic stiffness. This is slightly surprising as studies have shown elevated pulse wave velocity (PWV), reduced carotid distensibility and increased carotid intimal medial thickness in children with CKD [23]. However, elevated PWV is not a universal finding and even in positive studies, PWV is only mildly raised (i.e. in the 4C's study the PWV z-score was 0.33) [23]. Furthermore, changes in carotid artery characteristics do not necessarily reflect changes in the aorta [24], which is the repository for most vascular buffering. In fact, pulse pressure has been shown to be normal in other large pediatric CKD studies [25], which is in keeping with our finding of normal aortic stiffness. Of course, the vascular phenotype may be different in dialysis patients due to more extensive arterial calcification.

Other possible causes of hypertension in CKD are fluid overload or high CO. Although fluid overload is difficult to assess, we did show that RAA (a marker of fluid overload) was normal in our cohort. Furthermore, we also demonstrated that CO was not increased in CKD. Therefore, it is unlikely that these factors are important in the pathogenesis of hypertension in early CKD.

Left ventricular remodelling in CKD

In our study, we demonstrated that children in the severest CKD group had increased LV MVR compared to controls and, as eGFR fell, MVR increased. These results suggest that worsening CKD is associated with increased concentric remodelling in children. Interestingly, height indexed LV mass was not statistically different in our

Table 5 Cardiac timings and mitral inflow velocities in CKD

	Healthy Controls (n = 20)	Mild CKD (n = 40)	Moderate CKD (n = 40)	Severe CKD (n = 20)	P-value
IRT (ms)[a]	61 ± 1.2	64 ± 1.1	70 ± 1.1	72 ± 1.1	< 0.001
ICT (ms)[a]	44 ± 1.6	36 ± 1.6	33 ± 1.8	37 ± 1.8	0.24
ET (ms)	277 ± 21	275 ± 16	274 ± 19	276 ± 15	0.92
Tei[a]	0.39 ± 1.3	0.37 ± 1.2	0.38 ± 1.2	0.41 ± 1.3	0.56
E (mls)	47 ± 9.8	49 ± 11	50 ± 11	49 ± 9.7	0.87
A (mls)	19 ± 4.3	20 ± 6.7	21 ± 6.8	22 ± 5.6	0.36
E/A ratio[a]	2.6 ± 1.2	2.6 ± 1.4	2.5 ± 1.5	2.3 ± 1.3	0.63

Bonferroni correction applied- p < 0.007 is considered significant
Abbreviations: CKD chronic kidney disease, IRT isovolumic relaxation time, ICT isovolumic contraction time, ET ejection time, Tei myocardial performance index, E early transmitral mean velocity, A late transmitral mean velocity, E/A ratio E to A ratio
[a]Logarithmic transformation was applied

Table 6 Tissue Phase Mapping in CKD

	Healthy Controls (n = 20)	Mild CKD (n = 40)	Moderate CKD (n = 40)	Severe CKD (n = 20)	P-value
Rad S' (cm/s)	2.7 ± 0.31	2.6 + 0.24	2.5 ± 0.38	2.4 ± 0.31	0.003
Rad E' (cm/s)	4.2 ± 0.59	3.6 ± 0.62	3.4 ± 0.78	3.3 ± 0.53	< 0.001
Rad A' (cm/s)	1.3 ± 0.35	1.1 ± 0.34	1.2 ± 0.31	1.2 ± 0.28	0.30
Long S' (cm/s)	4.6 ± 1.6	3.9 ± 1.1	3.4 ± 1.3	3.6 ± 1.3	0.009
Long E' (cm/s)	7.9 ± 1.5	7.5 ± 2.0	6.7 ± 1.8	6.8 ± 1.4	0.046
Long A' (cm/s)	2.3 ± 0.71	2.5 ± 1.1	2.7 ± 0.85	2.5 ± 0.64	0.61
Long E'/A' ratio[a]	3.4 ± 1.3	3.2 ± 1.6	2.6 ± 1.4	2.8 ± 1.3	0.003[†]
Long E/E' ratio[a]	6 ± 1.2	6.7 ± 1.3	7.5 ± 1.4	7.3 ± 1.4	0.03

Bonferroni correction applied- p < 0.006 is considered significant
Abbreviations: *CKD* chronic kidney disease, *Rad* radial, *Long* longitudinal, *S'* systolic myocardial velocity, *E'* early diastolic myocardial velocity, *A'* late diastolic myocardial velocity, *E'/A'* E' over A' ratio, *E/E'* E over E' ratio
[a]Logarithmic transformation was applied
[†]ANOVA Welch (W) test was used

population, unlike previous TTE studies. This may be due to the well-recognized overestimation of LV mass using TTE, particularly in patients with CKD [26].

Ventricular remodelling in these children is partly explained by their hypertensive phenotype. However, both CKD group and eGFR remained significant predictors of MVR after controlling for BP. This implies that other 'uremic' processes are involved in CKD associated remodelling. Possible 'uremic' causes of hypertrophy include: anemia, hyperparathyroidism and sympathetic overactivity [24, 27, 28]. Identification of the exact stimulus may provide new targets for therapeutic intervention that may be important in remediating the increased cardiovascular risk associated with LVH [2].

Diastolic function in CKD
We found conventional transmitral inflow peak E/A to be normal in children with CKD. However, both IRT and

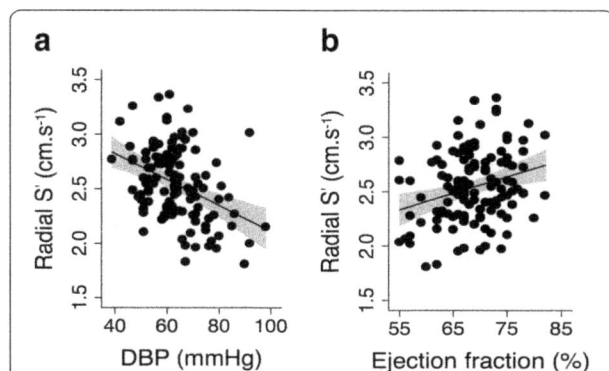

Fig. 2 a & b: Relationship between tissue phase mapping indices and conventional measures of cardiac function - **a**. Radial systolic myocardial velocity (S') versus diastolic blood pressure (DBP) (rho = − 0.37, p < 0.0001), **b**. Radial systolic myocardial velocity (S') versus ejection function (rho = 0.24, p = 0.009). The 95% confidence interval of the predicted mean is illustrated by the grey zone

radial E' were abnormal, pointing towards subtle diastolic dysfunction in moderate to severe CKD. In addition, longer IRT was associated with lower eGFR. IRT is a marker of active myocardial relaxation and correlates with invasively measured isovolumic relaxation constant [18]. Previous studies in adults have shown that active relaxation is associated with LV mass [29] and our findings are in keeping with this. However, even after controlling for MVR, CKD remains a significant predictor of IRT and eGFR trends towards significance. This suggests that CKD exerts an independent effect possibly mediated through abnormal energy or calcium handling. This could be due to myocyte/capillary mismatch resulting in a relative oxygen deficit as demonstrated in animal models [30].

Early diastolic peak velocity is a marker of both active relaxation and ventricular compliance [31]. Our demonstration of lower E', measured using TPM, is in keeping with a previous smaller study in pediatric CKD [32]. In our study, E' did not correlate with MVR or LVMht$^{2.7}$. Thus, reduced early filling cannot simply be explained by LV hypertrophy. One explanation for reduced ventricular compliance is myocardial fibrosis, which has been demonstrated in several animal models [33]. Unfortunately, it is not possible to perform post contrast T1 mapping in these patients due to the risk of nephrogenic systemic fibrosis [34]. Nevertheless, non-contrast methods are now available [34] and these could be used to quantify fibrosis in future studies. We also demonstrated that lower radial E' was associated with lower Hb. The reason for this is unclear but may be related to reduced oxygen delivery affecting the active component of relaxation.

Systolic function in CKD
Global systolic function was preserved in CKD patients with normal LVEF. However, radial S' was reduced in moderate and severe CKD, implying some

element of systolic dysfunction in the latter stages of renal disease. These findings are in keeping with previous tissue Doppler imaging and echocardiographic strain studies and illustrate the importance of assessing systolic function in a more sophisticated manner [4, 35]. The most obvious explanation for reduced S′ is that increased blood pressure limits contraction through the force velocity relationship. This is in keeping with our findings in which DBP independently predicted radial S′, unlike CKD group.

The use of CMR for cardiovascular assessment in CKD

We have demonstrated that children with CKD exhibit a specific, but subtle cardiovascular phenotype. This phenotype is characterized by: i) increased MVR, ii) increased IRT, iv) reduced radial S′ and E′ and iv) increased SVR. All of these metrics can be evaluated with TTE. In fact, due to its high temporal resolution, it is probably the most accurate method of assessing timing parameters (i.e. IRT) and tissue velocity. However, there are some limitations to TTE. In particular, TTE overestimates LVM [26] and cannot accurately estimate CO (necessary for calculation of SVR). As we have found that these two measures are abnormal in pediatric CKD, we believe there may be a role for CMR identification of abnormal cardiac and vascular phenotypes in this group of patients. Nevertheless, it is still unclear what the clinical significance of this phenotype is. The next important step is to ascertain whether it can be used to guide therapy and determine prognosis.

Limitations

An important limitation is the relatively older age of the study cohort. Although the entire cohort of CKD patients did include patients from 7 to 18 years of age, the majority of children were between the ages of 9 to 16 years. Thus, the study findings may not be as applicable to younger children. In order to ensure that the study findings can be extrapolated to all age groups, future studies should consider recruiting younger patients.

The absence of recent TTE data in the subjects is also a potential limitation in this study. Performing an TTE in tandem may have been informative for the comparison of CMR findings with an established standard clinical investigation. This would have enabled us to confirm our CMR findings of subtle systolic and diastolic impairment with TTE results. Unfortunately, this was not performed as part of the study protocol in order to minimise inconvenience to the study subjects. No recent clinical TTE data were available for comparison in this cohort either. However, despite that, our findings are in agreement with the majority of previous studies in pediatric CKD using TTE as referenced in the paper.

Another limitation is our use of mild, moderate and severe CKD grouping instead of the conventional categorization of CKD stages 1–5. This was done to ensure adequate powering for group wise differences. However, the use of conventional CKD groups would be desirable in future larger, multicenter studies.

Finally, BP measurements were carried out using an oscillometric sphygmomanometer, which may be less accurate than using manual sphygmomanometer [36]. This was because it was essential for BP measurements to be acquired simultaneously during PCMR flow acquisition for accurate assessment of vascular measures. Unfortunately, this could not be performed manually in the CMR scanner during flows acquisitions. However, BP measurement was taken with a standardized protocol for all subjects using the same machine. This meant that the measurements were comparable across the cohort.

Conclusion

It is possible to use CMR to comprehensively evaluate cardiac and vascular phenotype in children with CKD. In the future, these novel CMR indices may even be useful for identifying high-risk pediatric CKD patients. More work is needed to determine normative pediatric values. Future prospective studies will also be required to correlate these markers with prognosis in order to predict cardiovascular risk.

Abbreviations
A: Peak late diastolic (mitral inflow) velocity; A′: Peak late diastolic LV myocardial velocity; ANOVA: Analysis of variance; AoC: Ascending aortic compliance; AoMax: Maximum ascending aortic diameter; AoMin: Minimum ascending aortic diameter; AoS: Ascending aortic strain; BP: Blood pressure; BSA: Body surface area; CKD: Chronic kidney disease; CMR: Cardiovascular magnetic resonance; CO: Cardiac output; DBP: Diastolic blood pressure; E: Peak early diastolic (mitral inflow) velocity; E′: Peak early diastolic LV myocardial velocity; EDV: End-diastolic volume; EF: Ejection Fraction; eGFR: Estimated glomerular filtration rate; ESV: End-systolic volume; ET: Ejection time; FOV: Field of view; Hb: Hemoglobin; ICT: Isovolumic contraction time; IRT: Isovolumic relaxation time; LV: Left ventricle/left ventricular; LVH: Left ventricular hypertrophy; LVM: Left ventricular mass; LVMht$^{2.7}$: Left ventricular mass indexed to height to the power of 2.7; MBP: Mean blood pressure; MVR: Mass volume ratio; PCMR: Phase contrast cardiovascular magnetic resonance; PP: Pulse pressure; PTH: Parathyroid hormone; PWV: Pulse wave velocity; Rho: Spearman's coefficient; S′: Peak systolic LV myocardial velocity; SBP: Systolic blood pressure; SV: Stroke volume; SVR: Systemic vascular resistance; TAC: Total arterial compliance; TE: Echo time; TEI: Myocardial performance index; TPM: Tissue phase mapping; TR: Repetition time; TTE: Transthoracic echocardiography; VENC: Maximum measurable velocity range; β: Beta coefficient of variables in regression model

Acknowledgements
We would like to express our gratitude to our research CMR radiographers and all the doctors and nurses in the renal department in Great Ormond Street Hospital, London. This work was supported by the National Institute

for Health Research Biomedical Research Centre at Great Ormond Street Hospital for Children National Health Service Foundation Trust and University College London.

Funding
This study was funded by Kids Kidney Research, UK.

Authors' contributions
MC recruited and analysed all the patient data and was a major contributor in writing the manuscript. NB, AB, JH, GK, MQ and JS helped with data acquisition, analysis and provided valuable support towards completion of the project. KT, DH and VM provided essential input on research hypothesis, manuscript writing and project design. All authors have read and approved the final manuscript.

Competing interests
The authors declare that they have no competing interests.

References
1. Groothoff J, Gruppen M, de Groot E, Offringa M. Cardiovascular disease as a late complication of end-stage renal disease in children. Perit Dial Int. 2005; 25(Suppl 3):S123–6.
2. Paoletti E, de Nicola L, Gabbai FB, Chiodini P, Ravera M, Pieracci L, Marre S, Cassottana P, Luca S, Vettoretti S, et al. Associations of left ventricular hypertrophy and geometry with adverse outcomes in patients with CKD and hypertension. Clin J Am Soc Nephrol. 2016;11:271–9.
3. Hickson LJ, Negrotto SM, Onuigbo M, Scott CG, Rule AD, Norby SM, Albright RC, Casey ET, Dillon JJ, Pellikka PA, et al. Echocardiography criteria for structural heart disease in patients with end-stage renal disease initiating hemodialysis. J Am Coll Cardiol. 2016;67:1173–82.
4. Chinali M, Matteucci MC, Franceschini A, Doyon A, Pongiglione G, Rinelli G, Schaefer F. Advanced parameters of cardiac mechanics in children with CKD: the 4C study. Clin J Am Soc Nephrol. 2015;10:1357–63.
5. Hoffmann R, Barletta G, von Bardeleben S, Vanoverschelde JL, Kasprzak J, Greis C, Becher H. Analysis of left ventricular volumes and function: a multicenter comparison of cardiac magnetic resonance imaging, cine ventriculography, and unenhanced and contrast-enhanced two-dimensional and three-dimensional echocardiography. J Am Soc Echocardiogr. 2014;27:292–301.
6. Pennell DJ, Sechtem UP, Higgins CB, Manning WJ, Pohost GM, Rademakers FE, van Rossum AC, Shaw LJ, Yucel EK, European society of c, Soceity for cardiovascular magnetic R. Clinical indications for cardiovascular magnetic resonance (CMR): consensus panel report. J Cardiovasc Magn Reson. 2004;6:727–65.
7. Steeden JA, Knight DS, Bali S, Atkinson D, Taylor AM, Muthurangu V. Self-navigated tissue phase mapping using a golden-angle spiral acquisition-proof of concept in patients with pulmonary hypertension. Magn Reson Med. 2014;71:145–55.
8. Steeden JA, Atkinson D, Taylor AM, Muthurangu V. Assessing vascular response to exercise using a combination of real-time spiral phase contrast MR and noninvasive blood pressure measurements. J Magn Reson Imaging. 2010;31:997–1003.
9. Elmenhorst J, Hulpke-Wette M, Barta C, Dalla Pozza R, Springer S, Oberhoffer R. Percentiles for central blood pressure and pulse wave velocity in children and adolescents recorded with an oscillometric device. Atherosclerosis. 2015;238:9–16.
10. Odille F, Steeden JA, Muthurangu V, Atkinson D. Automatic segmentation propagation of the aorta in real-time phase contrast MRI using nonrigid registration. J Magn Reson Imaging. 2011;33:232–8.
11. Muthurangu V, Lurz P, Critchely JD, Deanfield JE, Taylor AM, Hansen MS. Real-time assessment of right and left ventricular volumes and function in patients with congenital heart disease by using high spatiotemporal resolution radial k-t SENSE. Radiology. 2008;248:782–91.
12. de Simone G, Devereux RB, Daniels SR, Koren MJ, Meyer RA, Laragh JH. Effect of growth on variability of left ventricular mass: assessment of allometric signals in adults and children and their capacity to predict cardiovascular risk. J Am Coll Cardiol. 1995;25:1056–62.
13. Foley RN, Parfrey PS, Harnett JD, Kent GM, Murray DC, Barre PE. The prognostic importance of left ventricular geometry in uremic cardiomyopathy. J Am Soc Nephrol. 1995;5:2024–31.
14. Kowalik GT, Knight DS, Steeden JA, Tann O, Odille F, Atkinson D, Taylor A, Muthurangu V. Assessment of cardiac time intervals using high temporal resolution real-time spiral phase contrast with UNFOLDed-SENSE. Magn Reson Med. 2015;73:749–56.
15. Knight DS, Steeden JA, Moledina S, Jones A, Coghlan JG, Muthurangu V. Left ventricular diastolic dysfunction in pulmonary hypertension predicts functional capacity and clinical worsening: a tissue phase mapping study. J Cardiovasc Magn Reson. 2015;17:116.
16. Steeden JA, Atkinson D, Hansen MS, Taylor AM, Muthurangu V. Rapid flow assessment of congenital heart disease with high-spatiotemporal-resolution gated spiral phase-contrast MR imaging. Radiology. 2011;260:79–87.
17. Laurent S, Cockcroft J, Van Bortel L, Boutouyrie P, Giannattasio C, Hayoz D, Pannier B, Vlachopoulos C, Wilkinson I, Struijker-Boudier H, European network for non-invasive investigation of large A. Expert consensus document on arterial stiffness: methodological issues and clinical applications. Eur Heart J. 2006;27:2588–605.
18. Nagueh SF, Appleton CP, Gillebert TC, Marino PN, Oh JK, Smiseth OA, Waggoner AD, Flachskampf FA, Pellikka PA, Evangelisa A. Recommendations for the evaluation of left ventricular diastolic function by echocardiography. Eur J Echocardiogr. 2009;10:165–93.
19. Wong H, Mylrea K, Feber J, Drukker A, Filler G. Prevalence of complications in children with chronic kidney disease according to KDOQI. Kidney Int. 2006;70:585–90.
20. van Biesen W, Verbeke F, Devolder I, Vanholder R. The relation between salt, volume, and hypertension: clinical evidence for forgotten but still valid basic physiology. Perit Dial Int. 2008;28:596–600.
21. Grassi G, Quarti-Trevano F, Seravalle G, Arenare F, Volpe M, Furiani S, Dell'Oro R, Mancia G. Early sympathetic activation in the initial clinical stages of chronic renal failure. Hypertension. 2011;57:846–51.
22. Vaziri ND. Effect of chronic renal failure on nitric oxide metabolism. Am J Kidney Dis. 2001;38:S74–9.
23. Schaefer F, Doyon A, Azukaitis K, Bayazit A, Canpolat N, Duzova A, Niemirska A, Sozeri B, Thurn D, Anarat A, et al. Cardiovascular phenotypes in children with CKD: the 4C study. Clin J Am Soc Nephrol. 2017;12(1):19–28. doi: https://doi.org/10.2215/CJN.01090216.
24. Mitsnefes MM, Kimball TR, Kartal J, Witt SA, Glascock BJ, Khoury PR, Daniels SR. Cardiac and vascular adaptation in pediatric patients with chronic kidney disease: role of calcium-phosphorus metabolism. J Am Soc Nephrol. 2005;16:2796–803.
25. Sinha MD, Keehn L, Milne L, Sofocleous P, Chowienczyk PJ. Decreased arterial elasticity in children with nondialysis chronic kidney disease is related to blood pressure and not to glomerular filtration rate. Hypertension. 2015;66:809–15.
26. Arnold R, Schwendinger D, Jung S, Pohl M, Jung B, Geiger J, Gimpel C. Left ventricular mass and systolic function in children with chronic kidney disease-comparing echocardiography with cardiac magnetic resonance imaging. Pediatr Nephrol. 2016;31:255–65.
27. Mitsnefes MM, Daniels SR, Schwartz SM, Meyer RA, Khoury P, Strife CF. Severe left ventricular hypertrophy in pediatric dialysis: prevalence and predictors. Pediatr Nephrol. 2000;14:898–902.
28. Floras JS. Clinical aspects of sympathetic activation and parasympathetic withdrawal in heart failure. J Am Coll Cardiol. 1993;22:72A–84A.
29. Muller-Brunotte R, Kahan T, Malmqvist K, Edner M, Swedish ibesartan left ventricular hypertrophy investigation vs a. Blood pressure and left ventricular geometric pattern determine diastolic function in hypertensive myocardial hypertrophy. J Hum Hypertens. 2003;17:841–9.
30. Amann K, Breitbach M, Ritz E, Mall G. Myocyte/capillary mismatch in the heart of uremic patients. J Am Soc Nephrol. 1998;9:1018–22.
31. Opdahl A, Remme EW, Helle-Valle T, Lyseggen E, Vartdal T, Pettersen E, Edvardsen T, Smiseth OA. Determinants of left ventricular early-diastolic lengthening velocity: independent contributions from left ventricular relaxation, restoring forces, and lengthening load. Circulation. 2009;119:2578–86.

32. Gimpel C, Jung BA, Jung S, Brado J, Schwendinger D, Burkhardt B, Pohl M, Odening KE, Geiger J, Arnold R. Magnetic resonance tissue phase mapping demonstrates altered left ventricular diastolic function in children with chronic kidney disease. Pediatr Radiol. 2017;47:169–77.

33. Khan R, Sheppard R. Fibrosis in heart disease: understanding the role of transforming growth factor-beta in cardiomyopathy, valvular disease and arrhythmia. Immunology. 2006;118:10–24.

34. Jellis CL, Kwon DH. Myocardial T1 mapping: modalities and clinical applications. Cardiovasc Diagn Ther. 2014;4:126–37.

35. Mencarelli F, Fabi M, Corazzi V, Doyon A, Masetti R, Bonetti S, Castiglioni L, Pession A, Montini G. Left ventricular mass and cardiac function in a population of children with chronic kidney disease. Pediatr Nephrol. 2014; 29:893–900.

36. Flynn JT, Pierce CB, Miller ER 3rd, Charleston J, Samuels JA, Kupferman J, Furth SL, Warady BA, Chronic Kidney Disease in Children Study G. Reliability of resting blood pressure measurement and classification using an oscillometric device in children with chronic kidney disease. J Pediatr. 2012; 160:434–40. e431

4

Quantitative cardiovascular magnetic resonance: extracellular volume, native T1 and 18F-FDG PET/CMR imaging in patients after revascularized myocardial infarction and association with markers of myocardial damage and systemic inflammation

Karl P. Kunze[1*], Ralf J. Dirschinger[2], Hans Kossmann[2], Franziska Hanus[2], Tareq Ibrahim[2,3], Karl-Ludwig Laugwitz[2,3], Markus Schwaiger[1,3], Christoph Rischpler[1,3†] and Stephan G. Nekolla[1,3†]

Abstract

Background: Characterization of tissue integrity and inflammatory processes after acute myocardial infarction (AMI) using non-invasive imaging is predictive of patient outcome. Quantitative cardiovascular magnetic resonance (CMR) techniques such as native T_1 and extracellular volume (ECV) mapping as well as ^{18}F-FDG positron emission tomography (PET) imaging targeting inflammatory cell populations are gaining acceptance, but are often applied without assessing their quantitative potential. Using simultaneously acquired PET/CMR data from patients early after AMI, this study quantitatively compares these three imaging markers and investigates links to blood markers of myocardial injury and systemic inflammatory activity.

Methods: A total of 25 patients without microvascular obstruction were retrospectively recruited. All imaging was simultaneously performed 5 ± 1 days after revascularization following AMI on an integrated 3T PET/MRI scanner. Native and post-contrast T_1 data were acquired using a modified Look-Locker inversion recovery (MOLLI) sequence, ECV maps were calculated using individually sampled hematocrit. ^{18}F-FDG PET was executed after 1 day of dietary preparation, 12 h of fasting, and administration of heparin. ECV, ^{18}F-FDG and native T_1 data were compared mutually as well as to peak counts of peripheral blood markers (creatine kinase, creatine kinase-MB, troponin, leukocytes, monocytes) and infarct size.

(Continued on next page)

* Correspondence: karl-p.kunze@tum.de
†Equal contributors
[1]Nuklearmedizinische Klinik und Poliklinik, Klinikum rechts der Isar,
Technische Universität München, Ismaninger Straße 22, 81675 Munich,
Germany
Full list of author information is available at the end of the article

(Continued from previous page)

Results: High intra-patient correlations of relative ECV, ^{18}F-FDG PET and native T_1 signal increases were observed in combination with no inter-patient correlation of maximum absolute values at the infarct center, suggesting well-colocalized but physiologically diverse processes begetting the respective image signals. Comparison of maximum image signals to markers of myocardial damage and systemic inflammation yielded highly significant correlations of ECV to peak creatine kinase-MB and overall infarct size as well as between native T_1 and peak monocyte counts.

Conclusions: Absolute native T_1 values at the infarct core early after AMI can be linked to the systemic inflammatory response independent of infarct size. Absolute ECV at the infarct core is related to both infarct size and blood markers of myocardial damage.

Keywords: Myocardial infarction, T_1 mapping, Inflammation, Extracellular volume, PET/MRI

Background

The development of quantitative cardiovascular magnetic resonance (CMR) imaging techniques as a means for myocardial tissue characterization has seen a number of advances in recent years. Due to their relative robustness [1], especially extracellular volume (ECV) mapping and contrast media free native T_1 mapping are being translated into clinical applications [2, 3] and both have shown promising results with respect to infiltrative and fibrotic cardiac diseases [4–6]. For acute myocardial infarction (AMI), equivalence or superiority of quantitative mapping approaches over qualitative techniques with respect to the delineation of the Area At Risk (AAR) [7, 8] and the prediction of functional outcome have been shown for native T_1 [9, 10] and ECV [11] mapping. While there is ongoing discussion about the limits of detection for absolute changes of ECV in more subtle disease processes [12, 13], studies involving ECV and native T_1 mapping often make only limited use of absolute values. Both mapping techniques have usually been evaluated as more sensitive or accurate versions of late gadolinium enhancement (LGE) or T_2-weighted imaging for the determination of infarct size or AAR in the context of AMI [7, 8, 10, 11, 14]. This however neglects part of the quantitative potential of ECV and T_1 mapping, which for the first time allow non-invasive CMR of the local severity of myocardial injury and edematous processes as opposed to only measuring their extent.

The assessment of post-AMI inflammatory processes have recently also come into the focus of positron emission tomography (PET) imaging, where ^{18}F-fluorodeoxyglucose (^{18}F-FDG) is used in combination with metabolic preparation to target cardiac infiltration by inflammatory cells [15, 16]. However, there is still uncertainty with respect to the contribution of infiltrative inflammatory cells and altered metabolism by post-ischemic but viable cardiomyocytes to the ^{18}F-FDG imaging signal when applied in a clinical setting [15]. In this context, simultaneous PET/CMR imaging offers the potential for a deeper understanding of quantitative

methods from both modalities and their relation to physiology [17, 18].

The study at hand employs PET/CMR to quantitatively investigate the relationship of the three imaging markers ^{18}F-FDG uptake, native T_1 and ECV in the context of a complex tissue state consisting of diverse processes including inflammation, edema and cellular tissue damage after revascularized AMI. In addition, blood markers of myocardial damage and blood counts of inflammatory cells have been obtained following the acute event. Consequently, quantitative regional results from the three imaging methods under investigation are compared among themselves as well as with peripheral blood parameters. It is investigated to what degree the three imaging methods indicate independent features of the post-ischemic healing process, and to what degree these features are co-localized.

Proceeding in this fashion, it is the goal of this manuscript to highlight the potential in making full use of available quantitative information from cardiac multimodality imaging for a better understanding of image signals and their relation to pathophysiology.

Methods

Patient cohort

Patients that were retrospectively enrolled for this investigation ($n = 25$) represent a large subgroup of a cohort from a previously published study [15], which has focused on global measures of ^{18}F-FDG uptake and LGE and their relationship to functional outcome. All patients underwent examination on a clinical 3T PET/MRI scanner (Biograph mMR, Siemens Healthineers, Erlangen, Germany) 5 ± 1 days after myocardial infarction and subsequent, successful revascularization (Thrombolysis in Myocardial Infarction (TIMI) grade ≥ 2, average: 2.9). The study was approved by the local ethics committee, performed in agreement with the Declaration of Helsinki, and all participants gave written and informed consent. Criteria for retrospective enrollment were membership in the final study cohort reported in [15] and availability of native and post contrast T_1 data. Additionally, patients showing signs of microvascular obstruction (MVO) in LGE images were excluded from quantitative analysis, as the necessary contrast agent equilibration for ECV mapping is not attainable. Also, segmentation of MVO border zones was deemed not practicable in these cases due to the differences in spatial resolution between PET and CMR images, and quantitative values would not have been comparable to results from transmural segmentation. A detailed description of the criteria for retrospective enrollment similar to the corresponding statements in [15] is given in Table 1.

PET imaging
^{18}F-FDG PET was performed with patients receiving a low-carbohydrate diet the day before imaging, followed by a 12-h fasting period in order to suppress physiological myocardial FDG uptake. 30 min before ^{18}F-FDG injection, patients received unfractionated heparin (50 UI/kg body weight intravenously) to further suppress physiological myocardial FDG uptake [15]. A list-mode PET scan in 3D mode was started 144 ± 39 min after intravenous injection of 311 ± 72 MBq of ^{18}F-FDG. Correction of emission data was performed for randoms, scatter, dead time and attenuation. Attenuation correction was accomplished using 2-point Dixon sequence as previously described [19]. Parts of the body truncated in the attenuation map due to the limited field-of-view were recovered from PET emission data using the maximum likelihood reconstruction of attenuation and activity (MLAA) technique [20]. For reconstruction, a 3D attenuation-weighted ordered-subsets expectation maximization iterative reconstruction algorithm (AW-OSEM 3D) was used with three iterations and 21 subsets, Gaussian smoothing at 4 mm full width at half maximum, matrix size 344×344, zoom 1 and a resulting spatial resolution of 5 mm. For quantitative analysis, ^{18}F-FDG image signals were expressed as standardized uptake values based on lean body mass

Table 1 Criteria for Retrospective Enrollment

	n
Original cohort in [15]	49
Received ^{18}F-FDG imaging and T_1 mapping	45
Exclusion due to	n out of 45
Unsuccessful suppression of physiological ^{18}F-FDG uptake	3
Previous infarctions revealed during imaging	2
Para-venous ^{18}F-FDG injection	1
Acute pneumonia	1
Non-diagnostic T_1 data	2
MVO at infarct core	11
Retrospectively enrolled	25

(SUV LBM) or - for comparison to blood markers - also as tissue-to-background ratio (TBR) normalized to blood signal taken from an LV-centric region of interest.

CMR imaging
As part of a comprehensive resting-state CMR exam, native and post-contrast T_1 maps were acquired using a MOLLI prototype sequence in three short axis slices per patient. Acquisition (3(3)3(3)6) scheme [21]), retrospective motion correction and registration of native and post-contrast MOLLI data was performed as previously described [22]. If necessary, additional manual motion correction was applied to the T_1 image series as it was acquired in shallow breathing. After registration, ECV maps were calculated from the resulting T_1 maps using individually measured hematocrit. LGE images covering the complete left-ventricular (LV) myocardium were acquired directly following post contrast T_1 maps after a cumulative dose of 0.2 mmol/kg Gd-DTPA (Magnevist, Bayer Healthcare, Berlin, Germany).

PET/CMR image analysis
For PET/CMR image registration, the MunichHeart software [23] was used to fuse ^{18}F-FDG PET images with ECV and native T_1 maps. Manual alignment was performed between ungated PET data and individually motion-corrected CMR data if necessary. Manual segmentation on the basis of ECV maps was performed for the most infarct-centric of the three acquired slices, which was determined on the basis of LGE images covering the whole left ventricle. Basal and mid-ventricular slices were segmented into 32 sectors (16 for apical slices), equally spaced along a centerline between endo and-epicardial borders without additional morphological reference. This segmentation was applied to the registered ECV, native T_1 and ^{18}F-FDG PET images of that slice. For each patient, segmentation of the chosen slice therefore resulted in 32 transmural sector values (16 for apical slices) for each of the three image signals under investigation as shown in Fig. 1. An average of the two highest sector values was taken as representing maximum insult severity for each patient and each image signal in the sense of an "imaging biopsy". These maximum values were determined independently for each imaging method, and therefore do not necessarily refer to the exact same intra-slice location (see Fig. 1). For the quantitative analysis of remote regions, three sectors as distal as possible to the sector with the highest value were chosen manually. Therefore, for each patient, the remote value of ECV, native T1 and ^{18}F-FDG uptake respectively refers to the average from the so-defined remote sectors, and the maximum value refers to the average of the two highest sector values. Additional measures of infarct size in % of LV volume were

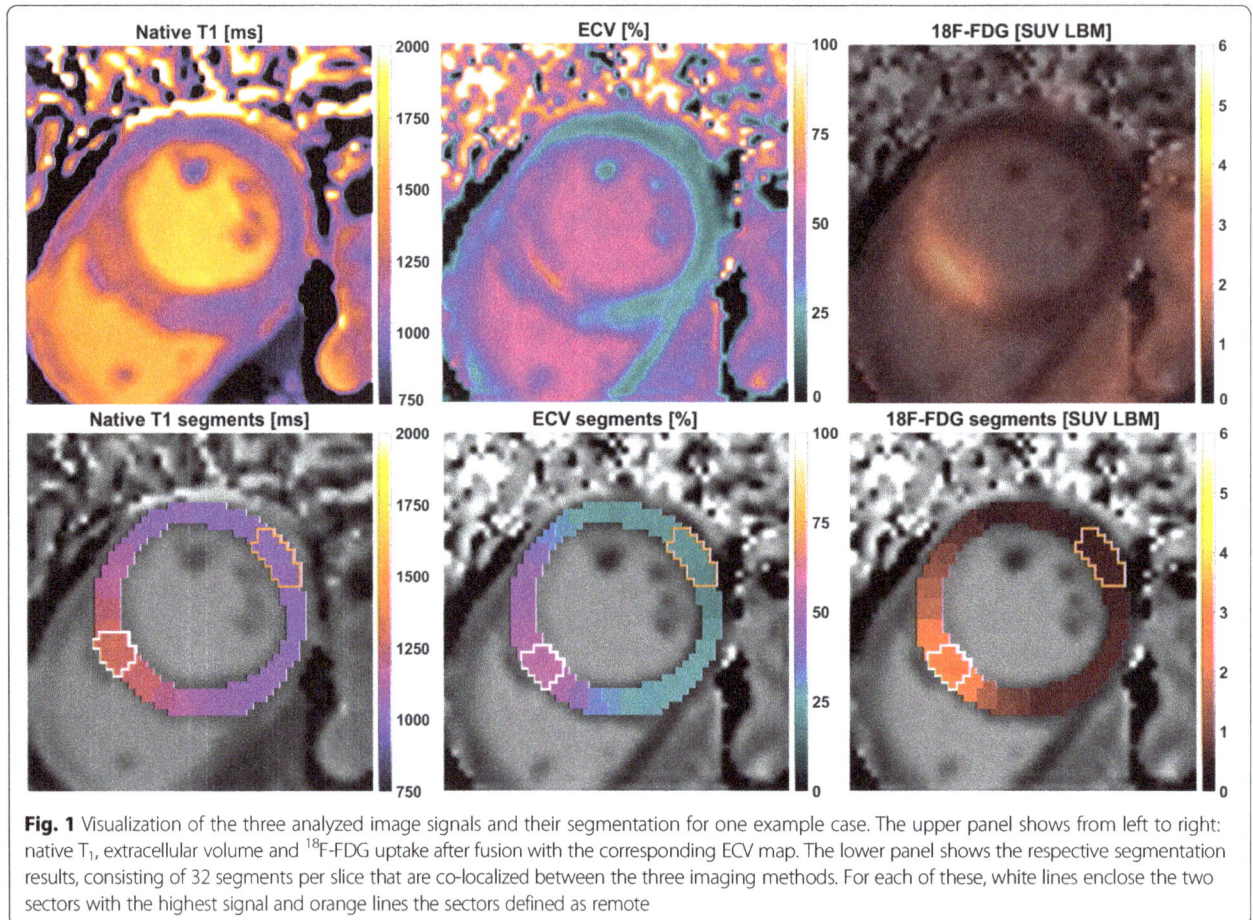

Fig. 1 Visualization of the three analyzed image signals and their segmentation for one example case. The upper panel shows from left to right: native T_1, extracellular volume and ^{18}F-FDG uptake after fusion with the corresponding ECV map. The lower panel shows the respective segmentation results, consisting of 32 segments per slice that are co-localized between the three imaging methods. For each of these, white lines enclose the two sectors with the highest signal and orange lines the sectors defined as remote

obtained by manual delineation of enhancement regions in the LGE images as described previously [15].

Blood analysis

Daily blood sampling was performed for up to 6 days after revascularization. Peak levels of blood parameters creatine kinase (CK), creatine kinase-MB (CK-MB), troponin T as well as peak leukocyte and monocyte counts were taken from this sampling period as previously reported [15].

Data analysis and statistics

Data processing and statistical analysis were executed in Matlab R2017a (Mathworks, Natick, Massachusetts, USA). Between-subject correlations represent a correlation of per-subject means, within-subject correlations were calculated using multiple regression (analysis of covariance). R- and p-values are given as Pearson correlation coefficients with a 5% significance level.

Results

Patient cohort

The physiological characteristics of the final patient cohort ($n = 25$) are shown in Table 2. A total of 42

individual segments from four patients were excluded before quantitative analysis due to small susceptibility artifacts in the T_1 maps ($n = 3$) or breathing artifacts in the PET attenuation map ($n = 1$).

Table 2 Patient Characteristics

Characteristics	
Final [n] (%)	25 (100)
Male [n] (%)	22 (88)
Age [y]	66 ± 10
Pain to PCI [h]	7.2 ± 7.1
PCI to scan [d]	4.9 ± 1.4
HR at scan [bpm]	62 ± 9
Infarct size (LGE) [% LV]	17.3 ± 7.1
Avg. blood markers	
CK max [U/l]	1806 ± 930
CK-MB max [U/l]	211 ± 124
Troponin T max [U/l]	2.5 ± 1.7
Peak Leukocytes [G/l]	12.8 ± 4.3
Peak Monocytes [G/l]	1.1 ± 0.4

CK creatinine kinase, *LGE* late gadolinium enhancement, *PCI* percutaneous coronary intervention

Mutual comparison of ^{18}F-FDG, ECV and native T1

The total number of sectors after exclusions was 662 for each imaging method, consisting of 32 (mid/basal) or 16 (apical) sectors per patient for each of the 25 subjects. The upper panel of Fig. 2 shows the comparisons of these sector values in a globally pooled fashion. All three comparisons (FDG/ECV, FDG/native T1, ECV/native T1) exhibited similarly significant correlations between subject means (R = 0.60, 0.43, 0.51). The lower panel of Fig. 2 shows the corresponding within-patient correlations, i.e. a linearization of within-slice signal increase for each patient (i.e. each slice) individually. Within-patient analysis yielded much higher correlation factors (R = 0.91, 0.87, 0.88) than the globally pooled comparison.

The underlying inter-patient variability of absolute values at the high end was most clearly discernible for the comparison of FDG/ECV. Consequentially, if only the average of the two maximum sector values from each patient were compared, no significant correlations were observed for FDG/ECV, FDG/native T1 nor ECV/native T1 (Fig. 3). Table 3 shows ranges and averages for maximum and remote values across all patients for each imaging method. While maximum values were determined individually for each imaging method, average distances between sectors containing these were small across modalities, i.e. on average 1.2 sectors between ECV/FDG, 2 sectors between nT_1/FDG and 1.9 sectors between nT_1/ECV.

Comparison of maximum image signals and infarct size

Results for comparing infarct sizes with corresponding maximum values of ECV, ^{18}F-FDG uptake and native T_1 are shown in Fig. 4. Infarct sizes calculated on the basis of LGE images yielded an average infarct size of 17.3 ± 7.1% of LV volume. A highly significant correlation of cellular damage as indicated by maximum ECV with infarct size was observed (p = 0.002). Conversely, no significant correlation between infarct size and either maximum ^{18}F-FDG uptake or maximum native T_1 was observed.

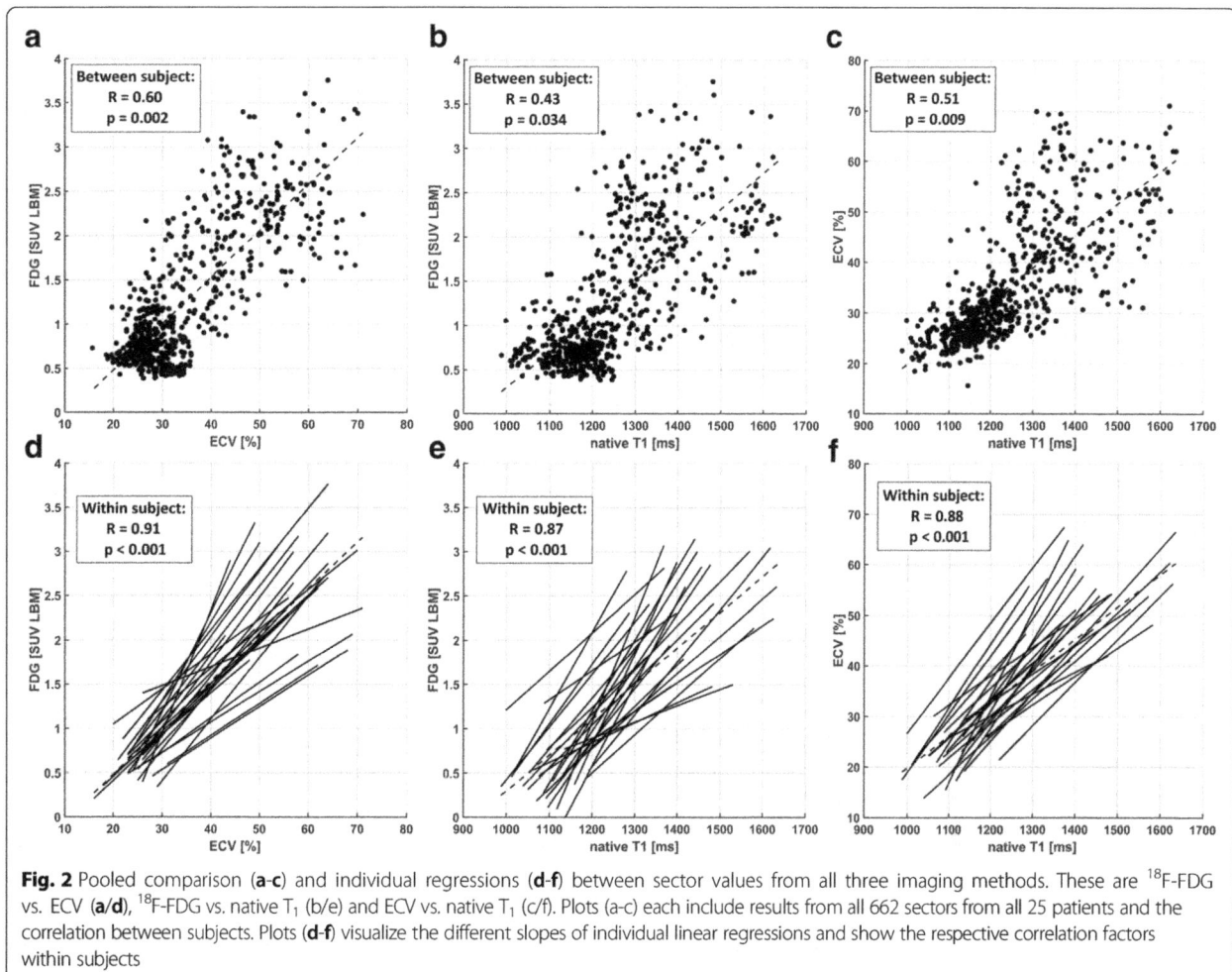

Fig. 2 Pooled comparison (**a-c**) and individual regressions (**d-f**) between sector values from all three imaging methods. These are ^{18}F-FDG vs. ECV (**a/d**), ^{18}F-FDG vs. native T_1 (**b/e**) and ECV vs. native T_1 (**c/f**). Plots (**a-c**) each include results from all 662 sectors from all 25 patients and the correlation between subjects. Plots (**d-f**) visualize the different slopes of individual linear regressions and show the respective correlation factors within subjects

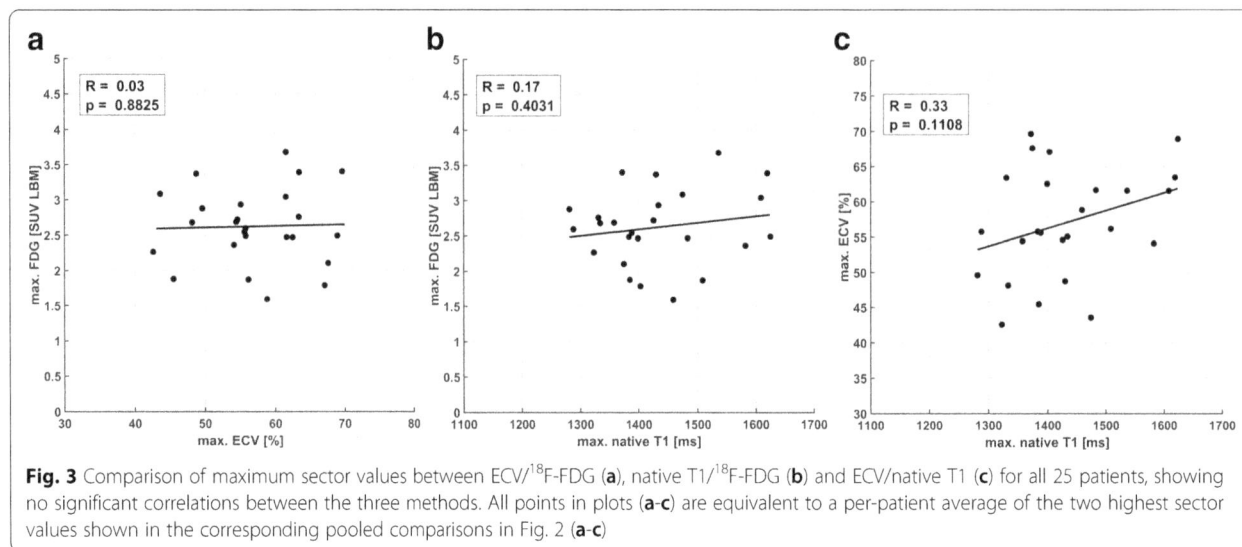

Fig. 3 Comparison of maximum sector values between ECV/^{18}F-FDG (**a**), native T1/^{18}F-FDG (**b**) and ECV/native T1 (**c**) for all 25 patients, showing no significant correlations between the three methods. All points in plots (**a-c**) are equivalent to a per-patient average of the two highest sector values shown in the corresponding pooled comparisons in Fig. 2 (**a-c**)

Comparison of maximum image signals and blood markers

Maximum ECV (Fig. 5), ^{18}F-FDG uptake (absolute (Fig. 6) and TBR) and native T_1 (Fig. 7) were compared to peak values of peripheral blood parameters CK, CK-MB, troponin T as well as peak leukocyte and monocyte counts. Monocyte counts were unavailable for two patients, and were excluded for one additional patient due to splenectomy, resulting in 22 instead of 25 data points for Figs. 5d, 6d, 7d. For maximum ECV, a strong trend towards association with peak CK (p = 0.052) and a significant correlation with peak CK-MB (p = 0.006) were observed, despite no correlation to peak troponin or monocytes. The comparison to peak CK-MB revealed a tight relationship at the low end and a larger variability at the high end of values (Fig. 5b). For absolute ^{18}F-FDG uptake, only a narrowly significant correlation was found with troponin (p = 0.042), and none was found for ^{18}F-FDG TBR normalized to LV blood (see Additional File 1). Maximum native T_1 values did not show significant correlations to CK or CK-MB, but a highly significant correlation (p = 0.

Table 3 Maximum and Remote Values for ECV, native T1 and ^{18}F-FDG

	Mean	SD	Range
Max. ECV [%]	57.0	7.8	42.6–70.0
Maximum native T1 [ms]	1432	101	1281–1624
Max. FDG [SUV LBM]	2.62	0.53	1.62–3.74
Remote ECV [%]	27.8	3.9	20.3–34.7
Remote native T1 [ms]	1163	92	998–1419
Remote FDG [SUV LBM]	0.71	0.22	0.45–1.22

ECV extracellular volume, *FDG* fluorodeoxyglucose, *SUV LBM* standardized uptake values based on lean body mass

005) to peak monocyte counts and a significant correlation with troponin (p = 0.024). The corresponding comparisons to peak leukocyte counts are not shown, yielding a significant trend (p = 0.033) with native T_1.

Discussion

The study at hand has compared absolute measures of ^{18}F-FDG uptake, extracellular volume and native T_1 in patients early after revascularized myocardial infarction using simultaneously acquired PET/CMR data. Quantitative results have been derived for a single, infarct-centric slice position that was co-localized between all three methods, which can be seen as a biopsy-like imaging approach. An effort was made to link the so-obtained image signals to underlying pathophysiological processes using independent measures of infarct size and peripheral blood markers of cardiac damage and inflammatory cell populations. The study did not investigate correlations between image signals and functional recovery post AMI as these have already been given separately for ECV [11], ^{18}F-FDG [15] and native T_1 [9] in quantitative or semi-quantitative fashion.

Comparison of signal localization and magnitude

The first step was the comparison of inter-patient and intra-patient (i.e. intra-slice) signals as shown in Fig. 2. The excellent correlations for the latter suggest a very good co-localization of pathophysiological processes indicated by the three different image signals. While in the vast majority of studies, extents of image signals are compared by global thresholding, e.g. using multiples of standard deviations as binary cutoff values, the intra-patient correlations shown herein are independent of differences in absolute signal increase between patients, i.e. differences seen in the correlation slopes in Fig. 2c-d. Despite the good co-localization of signal increases, the

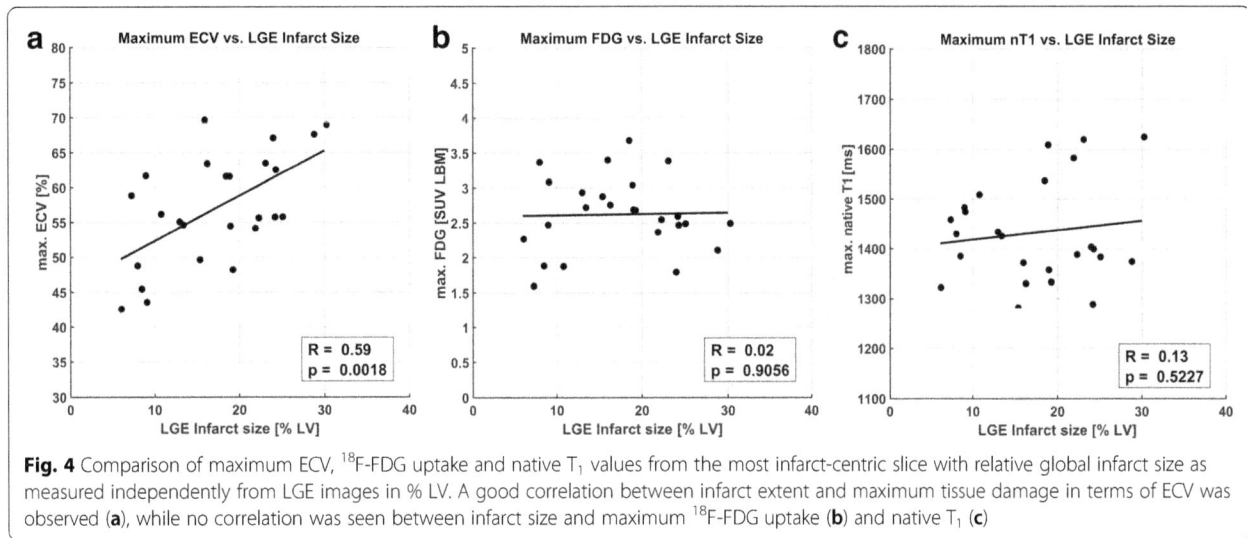

Fig. 4 Comparison of maximum ECV, ^{18}F-FDG uptake and native T_1 values from the most infarct-centric slice with relative global infarct size as measured independently from LGE images in % LV. A good correlation between infarct extent and maximum tissue damage in terms of ECV was observed (**a**), while no correlation was seen between infarct size and maximum ^{18}F-FDG uptake (**b**) and native T_1 (**c**)

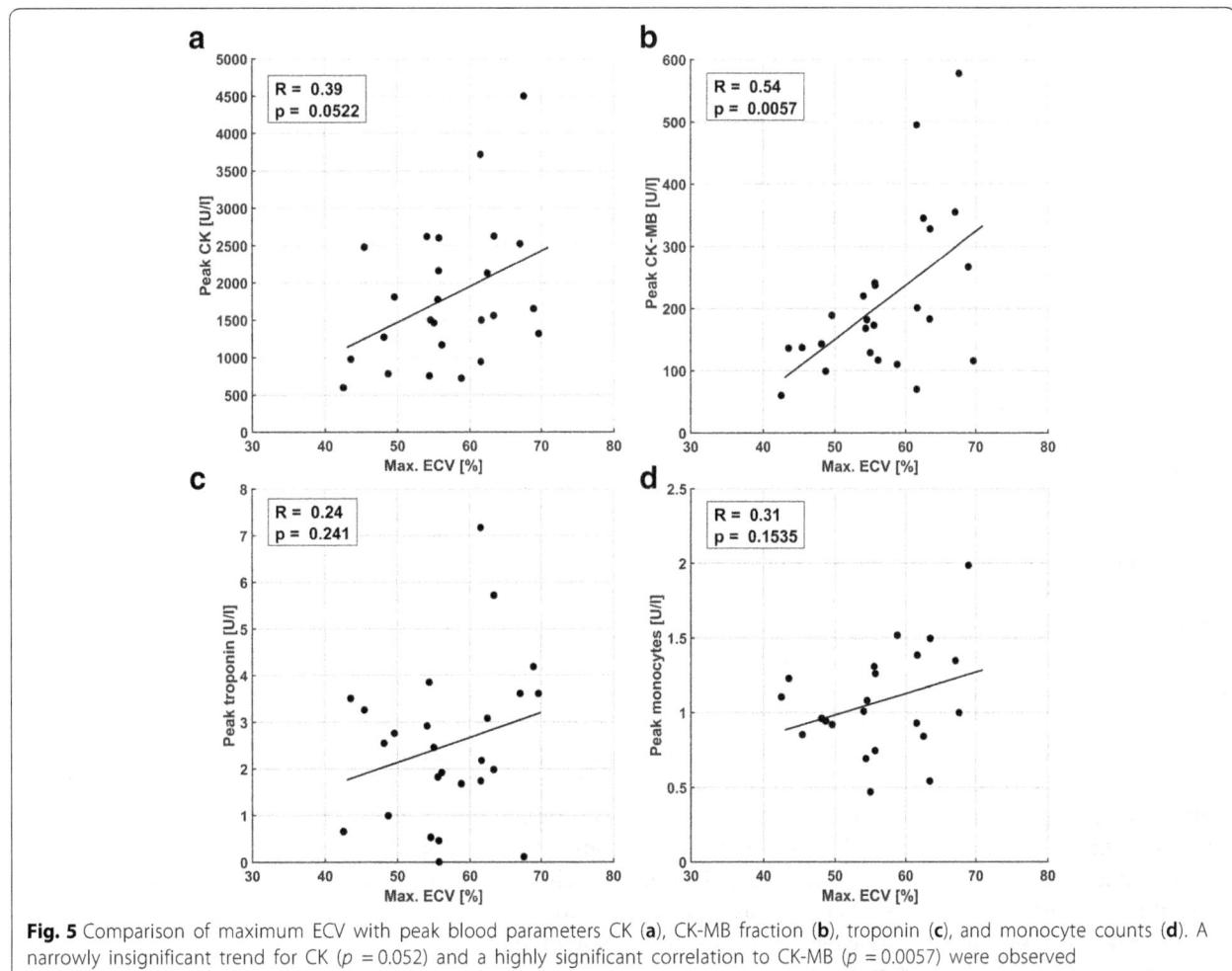

Fig. 5 Comparison of maximum ECV with peak blood parameters CK (**a**), CK-MB fraction (**b**), troponin (**c**), and monocyte counts (**d**). A narrowly insignificant trend for CK ($p = 0.052$) and a highly significant correlation to CK-MB ($p = 0.0057$) were observed

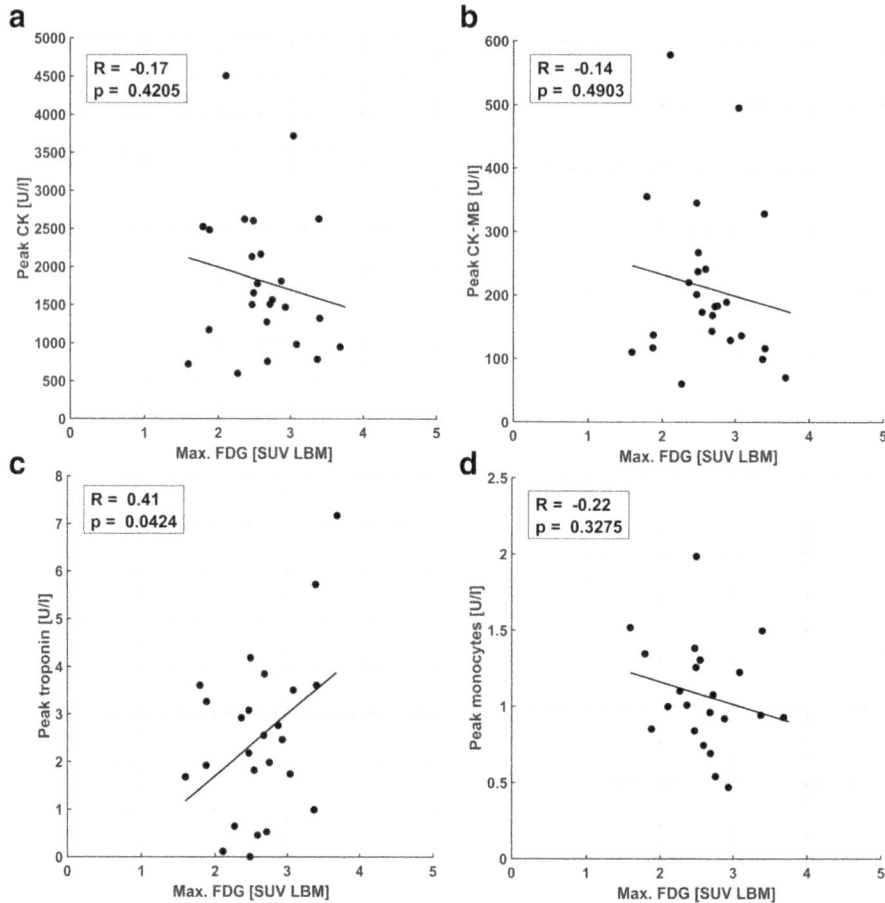

Fig. 6 Comparison of maximum ^{18}F-FDG uptake with peak blood parameters CK (**a**), CK-MB fraction (**b**), troponin (**c**), and monocyte counts (**d**). A narrowly significant trend for troponin ($p = 0.042$) was observed

heterogeneity of these slopes and equivalently the comparison of maximum values in Fig. 3 suggest sensitivities to different underlying tissue properties. Therefore, ECV, ^{18}F-FDG uptake and native T_1 appeared as representing mutually distinct combinations of features with respect to infarct-related pathophysiology, while the respective underlying processes seemed to be largely co-localized.

Comparison of signal magnitudes and external markers

For myocardial ECV, estimates derived from pre- and post-contrast T_1 mapping have been shown to be sensitive to a number of different disease processes [5] and histologically verified to correlate with fibrosis [24]. With respect to AMI, quantitative ECV mapping has only recently been shown to be associated with functional outcome in patients [11] but further investigation of pathophysiological mechanisms are lacking. While significant association of ECV with edema has been documented at day 1 after AMI in pigs [25], the same study reported a disappearance of this association after 7 days, which suggests edema if at all as a minor contributor to ECV estimates from the study

at hand obtained 5 days after AMI. A possible pathophysiological correlate for absolute ECV in this study has been provided in the form of CK/CK-MB blood markers for (myocytic) cellular damage. The significant correlation between peak CK-MB and ECV is in fact remarkable as it reflects the association of a global, peripheral blood parameter with a focal, biopsy-like imaging result. It may however be seen as an epiphenomenon to the additional finding of a highly significant correlation between ECV at the infarct center and infarct size, where peak CK-MB activity is an established marker for the latter [26]. This observed relationship between the extent of the area being subject to ischemic insult and the amount of myocytic damage at its center may be seen as somewhat mechanistically plausible, considering a decrease of the probability for remaining collateralization with distance to the nearest non-infarcted tissue regions. The much smaller significance for the corresponding correlation observed between peak CK and ECV is consistent with a lower specificity of CK to myocardial damage compared to CK-MB.

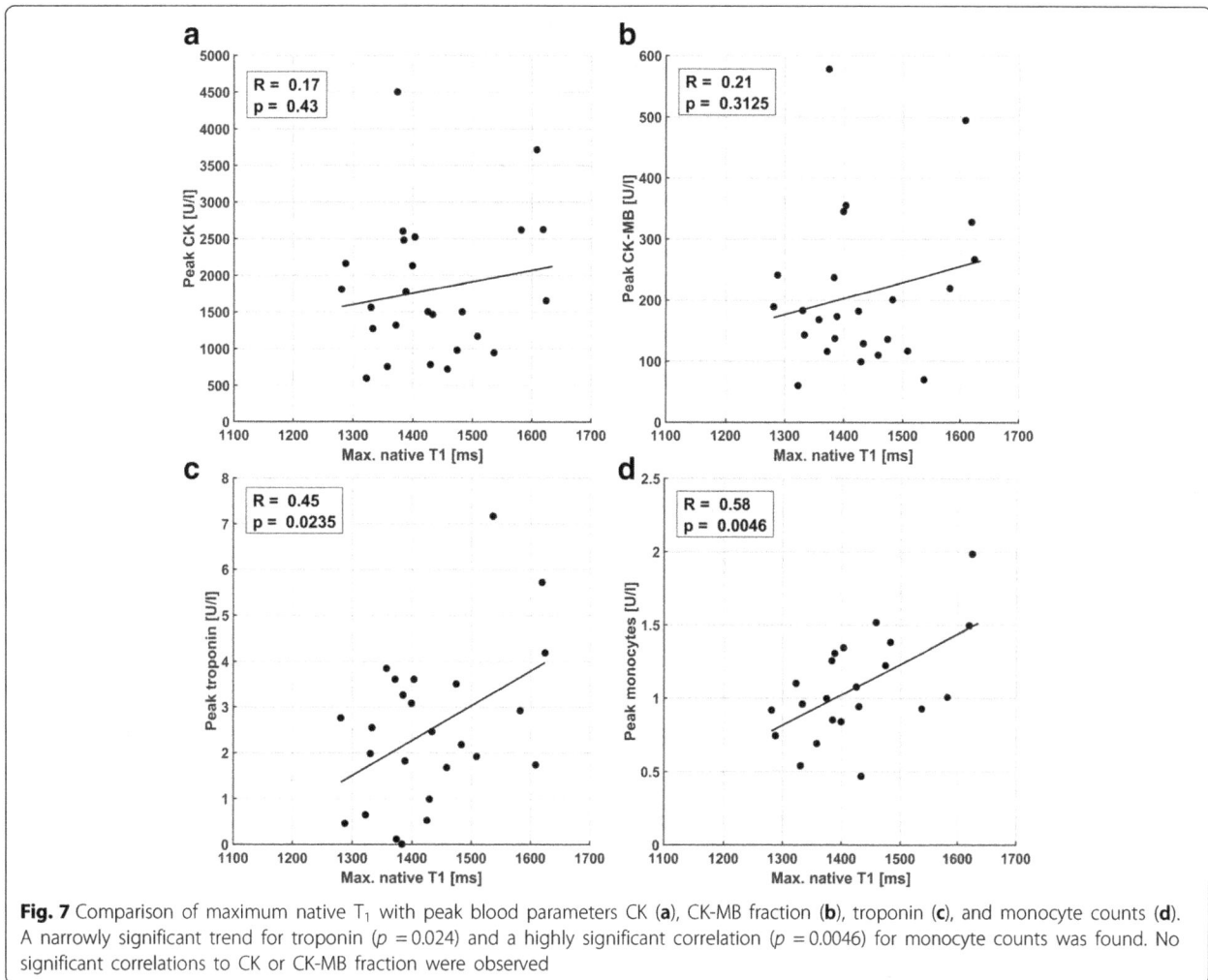

Fig. 7 Comparison of maximum native T_1 with peak blood parameters CK (**a**), CK-MB fraction (**b**), troponin (**c**), and monocyte counts (**d**). A narrowly significant trend for troponin ($p = 0.024$) and a highly significant correlation ($p = 0.0046$) for monocyte counts was found. No significant correlations to CK or CK-MB fraction were observed

With respect to FDG, data from this study suggest no correlation of maximum ^{18}F-FDG uptake at the infarct center with peak monocyte or leukocyte counts or global infarct size. This was irrespective of whether maximum ^{18}F-FDG was evaluated in absolute terms as SUV LBM or normalized to LV blood activity as a TBR. A similar finding [15] has been interpreted as a conceivable disproportionality between systemic/ peripheral inflammatory cell counts and the presence of migrated inflammatory cells within the myocardium begetting the imaging signal. While it is known that ^{18}F-FDG is taken up by inflammatory cell populations [27], the interpretation of a corresponding image signal from the post-ischemic myocardium is challenging due to the concurrent presence of background contributions from myocyte uptake. Despite a somewhat reliable suppression of physiologic FDG metabolism in healthy cardiomyocytes, the potential presence of post-ischemic FDG uptake due to a switch of metabolism from fatty acids towards glucose consumption early after AMI is a major confounder to the interpretation of ^{18}F-FDG uptake as a

purely inflammatory signal [28]. Therefore, ^{18}F-FDG image signals are generally regarded as a mixture of background/blood pool, post-ischemic and inflammatory constituents in this context.

Native myocardial T_1 may reflect a variety of pathologic tissue alterations, but is generally accepted to indicate the edematous increase of free water content early after AMI [8]. The expected increase of infarct-centric native T_1 observed in this study is therefore attributed to an edematous reaction, which, however, did not show a correlation with infarct size as ECV did. With respect to native T_1, the most interesting finding from this study is a highly significant correlation with peak monocyte counts and a weaker but still significant association to peak leukocyte counts, of which monocytes are a subset specific to inflammatory activity. As for ECV, this association of biopsy-like imaging results with peripheral blood markers is remarkable, even more so considering that native T_1 was not found to be related to infarct size. Therefore, the data at hand provides evidence for the fact that myocardial edema and the systemic inflammatory reaction post AMI are quantitatively associated.

Summarizing the comparison of imaging results with peripheral blood parameters, the data at hand suggest ECV as a marker of cellular damage early after reperfused AMI, with maximum values related to infarct size and therefore reflecting most likely a mechanistic property of the respective infarct. Conversely, the missing correlation to infarct size for maximum ^{18}F-FDG uptake and native T_1 suggest their association with a more patient- than infarct-specific reaction to the ischemic insult. This notion is strongly supported by the observed association of native T_1 with peak monocyte counts.

Limitations

An important translational limitation to results from this study is that patients exhibiting MVO post AMI were not amenable to the presented analysis. While there exist propositions on the segmentation of MVO border zones for e.g. ECV mapping [11], the difference in spatial resolution between PET and CMR precluded comparable sub-segmentations of the myocardial wall. For similar reasons, only transmural short-axis sectors were defined for LV myocardium, where especially cardiac motion hampers a meaningful sub-segmentation across the myocardial wall in PET. With respect to segmentation, locations for maximum values were determined individually for each modality because the alternative of having one of the three methods be the reference standard for locating the corresponding sectors would have introduced a bias into the comparison and additionally precluded the translation of conclusions to situations where the reference modality is not available. The small spatial differences introduced by individual determination of reference sectors did not suggest this as a significant limitation to the finding that all three modalities indicate mutually distinct processes within the tissue.

The acquisition scheme (3(3)3(3)6) used in this study for MOLLI T_1 mapping has been shown to be more sensitive to variations in heart rate than other, more recently proposed schemes [29]. However, the fact that resting heart rates in the examined cohort did not vary strongly and that heart rate did not correlate with remote native T_1 ($R = -0.22$, $p = 0.3$) do not suggest this as a major confounder to the presented findings.

Additionally, the practice of using peak values of peripheral blood markers as a surrogate for their summed activity may have introduced additional variability into the reported results. While the described practice is known to be relatively accurate for CK/CK-MB [26], the inflammatory reaction indicated by monocyte counts may behave in a more complex fashion. With respect to statistics, the large number of performed correlation

analyses may have justified the use of a 1% significance level to make type 1 errors less likely. However, the main conclusions presented herein only rely on findings with p-values < 0.01.

Conclusions

Simultaneously acquired PET/CMR data from this study have shown a close spatial concordance of relative signal increase in combination with a divergence of absolute signal magnitudes between ^{18}F-FDG uptake, native T_1 and ECV early after revascularized AMI. A biopsy-like imaging approach has revealed links between CMR-derived ECV estimates and blood markers of muscular damage as well as an association of the edematous response indicated by absolute native T_1 estimates with the systemic inflammatory activity indicated by peripheral monocyte counts.

Abbreviations

AAR: Area at risk; AMI: Acute myocardial infarction; AW-OSEM: Attenuation-weighted ordered-subsets expectation maximization; CK: Creatine kinase; CK-MB: Creatine kinase-MB; CMR: Cardiovascular magnetic resonance; ECV: Extracellular volume; FDG: Fluorodeoxyglucose; Gd-DTPA: Gadopentetic acid; LGE: Late gadolinium enhancement; LV: Left ventricular/left ventricle; MLAA: Maximum likelihood reconstruction of attenuation and activity; MOLLI: Modified Look-Locker inversion recovery; MVO: Microvascular obstruction; PET: Positron emission tomography; SUV LBM: Standardized uptake value based on lean body mass; TBR: Tissue-to-background ratio; TIMI: Thrombolysis in myocardial infarction

Acknowledgements

The authors would like to thank Sylvia Schachoff and Anna Winter for their contributions during the collection of patient data.

Funding

The study was supported by Deutsche Forschungsgemeinschaft (DFG) through DFG grant #8810001759 and the DFG Major Equipment Initiative. Additional Funding was provided by DFG and Technical University of Munich (TUM) in the framework of the Open Access Publishing Program as well as by the European Research Council, ERC grant #294582 MUMI.

Authors' contributions

The study was conceived and patient enrollment was organized by SGN, CR, MS and KL. RJD, HK, FH, CR and TI were responsible for patient recruitment and collection of blood data. KPK and SGN conceived of the retrospective analysis, data analysis and preparation of the manuscript was executed by KPK and CR. All authors read and approved the final manuscript.

Competing interests

SGN and MS receive research support from Siemens Healthcare.

Author details

[1]Nuklearmedizinische Klinik und Poliklinik, Klinikum rechts der Isar, Technische Universität München, Ismaninger Straße 22, 81675 Munich, Germany. [2]Klinik und Poliklinik für Medizin I, Klinikum rechts der Isar, Technische Universität München, Ismaninger Straße 22, 81675 Munich, Germany. [3]DZHK (Deutsches Zentrum für Herz-Kreislauf-Forschung e.V.) partner site Munich Heart Alliance, Munich, Germany.

References

1. Kellman P, Arai AE, Xue H. T1 and extracellular volume mapping in the heart: estimation of error maps and the influence of noise on precision. J Cardiovasc Magn Reson. 2013;15:56.

2. Moon JC, Messroghli DR, Kellman P, Piechnik SK, Robson MD, Ugander M, Gatehouse PD, Arai AE, Friedrich MG, Neubauer S, Schulz-Menger J, Schelbert EB. Myocardial T1 mapping and extracellular volume quantification: a Society for Cardiovascular Magnetic Resonance (SCMR) and CMR working Group of the European Society of cardiology consensus statement. J Cardiovasc Magn Reson. 2013;15:92.

3. White SK, Sado DM, Flett AS, Moon JC. Characterising the myocardial interstitial space: the clinical relevance of non-invasive imaging. Heart. 2012; 98:773–9.

4. Greulich S, Kitterer D, Latus J, Aguor E, Steubing H, Kaesemann P, Patrascu A, Greiser A, Groeninger S, Mayr A, Braun N, Alscher MD, Sechtem U, Mahrholdt H. Comprehensive cardiovascular magnetic resonance assessment in patients with sarcoidosis and preserved left ventricular ejection fraction. Circ Cardiovasc Imaging. 2016;9:e005022.

5. Sado DM, Flett AS, Banypersad SM, White SK, Maestrini V, Quarta G, Lachmann RH, Murphy E, Mehta A, Hughes DA, McKenna WJ, Taylor AM, Hausenloy DJ, Hawkins PN, Elliott PM, Moon JC. Cardiovascular magnetic resonance measurement of myocardial extracellular volume in health and disease. Heart. 2012;98:1436–41.

6. Kellman P, Wilson JR, Xue H, Bandettini WP, Shanbhag SM, Druey KM, Ugander M, Arai AE. Extracellular volume fraction mapping in the myocardium, part 2: initial clinical experience. J Cardiovasc Magn Reson. 2012;14:64.

7. Bulluck H, White SK, Rosmini S, Bhuva A, Treibel TA, Fontana M, Abdel-Gadir A, Herrey A, Manisty C, Wan SMY, Groves A, Menezes L, Moon JC, Hausenloy DJ. T1 mapping and T2 mapping at 3T for quantifying the area-at-risk in reperfused STEMI patients. J Cardiovasc Magn Reson. 2015;17:73.

8. Ugander M, Bagi PS, Oki AJ, Chen B, Hsu LY, Aletras AH, Shah S, Greiser A, Kellman P, Arai AE. Myocardial edema as detected by pre-contrast T1 and T2 CMR delineates area at risk associated with acute myocardial infarction. JACC Cardiovasc Imaging. 2012;5:596–603.

9. Dall'Armellina E, Piechnik SK, Ferreira VM, Si QL, Robson MD, Francis JM, Cuculi F, Kharbanda RK, Banning AP, Choudhury RP, Karamitsos TD, Neubauer S. Cardiovascular magnetic resonance by non contrast T1-mapping allows assessment of severity of injury in acute myocardial infarction. J Cardiovasc Magn Reson. 2012;14:15.

10. Ferreira VM, Piechnik SK, Dall'Armellina E, Karamitsos TD, Francis JM, Choudhury RP, Friedrich MG, Robson MD, Neubauer S. Non-contrast T1-mapping detects acute myocardial edema with high diagnostic accuracy: a comparison to T2-weighted cardiovascular magnetic resonance. J Cardiovasc Magn Reson. 2012;14:42.

11. Kidambi A, Motwani M, Uddin A, Ripley DP, McDiarmid AK, Swoboda PP, Broadbent DA, Musa TA, Erhayiem B, Leader J, Croisille P, Clarysse P, Greenwood JP, Plein S. Myocardial extracellular volume estimation by CMR predicts functional recovery following acute MI. JACC Cardiovasc Imaging. 2017;10:989–99.

12. Carberry J, Carrick D, Haig C, Rauhalammi SM, Ahmed N, Mordi I, McEntegart M, Petrie MC, Eteiba H, Hood S, Watkins S, Lindsay M, Davie A, Mahrous A, Ford I, Sattar N, Welsh P, Radjenovic A, Oldroyd KG, Berry C. Remote zone extracellular volume and left ventricular remodeling in survivors of ST-elevation myocardial infarction. Hypertension. 2016;68:385–91.

13. Treibel TA, Zemrak F, Sado DM, Banypersad SM, White SK, Maestrini V, Barison A, Patel V, Herrey AS, Davies C, Caulfield MJ, Petersen SE, Moon JC. Extracellular volume quantification in isolated hypertension - changes at the detectable limits? J Cardiovasc Magn Reson. 2015;17:74.

14. Messroghli DR, Walters K, Plein S, Sparrow P, Friedrich MG, Ridgway JP, Sivananthan MU. Myocardial T1 mapping: application to patients with acute and chronic myocardial infarction. Magn Reson Med. 2007;58:34–40.

15. Rischpler C, Dirschinger RJ, Nekolla SG, Kossmann H, Nicolosi S, Hanus F, van Marwick S, Kunze KP, Meinicke A, Götze K, Kastrati A, Langwieser N, Ibrahim T, Nahrendorf M, Schwaiger M, Laugwitz KL. Prospective evaluation of 18F-Fluorodeoxyglucose uptake in Postischemic myocardium by

16. simultaneous positron emission tomography/magnetic resonance imaging as a prognostic marker of functional outcome. Circulation Cardiovascular imaging 2016;9:e004316.

16. Wollenweber T, Roentgen P, Schäfer A, Schatka I, Zwadlo C, Brunkhorst T, Berding G, Bauersachs J, Bengel FM. Characterizing the inflammatory tissue response to acute myocardial infarction by clinical multimodality noninvasive imaging. Circ Cardiovasc Imaging. 2014;7:811–8.

17. Rischpler C, Nekolla SG, Kunze KP, Schwaiger M. PET/MRI of the heart. Semin Nucl Med. 2015;45:234–47.

18. Schwaiger M, Kunze K, Rischpler C, Nekolla SG. PET/MR: yet another tesla? J Nucl Cardiol. 2017;24:1019–31.

19. Martinez-Möller A, Souvatzoglou M, Delso G, Bundschuh RA, Chefd'hotel C, Ziegler SI, Navab N, Schwaiger M, Nekolla SG. Tissue classification as a potential approach for attenuation correction in whole-body PET/MRI: evaluation with PET/CT data. J Nucl Med. 2009;50:520–6.

20. Nuyts J, Bal G, Kehren F, Fenchel M, Michel C, Watson C. Completion of a truncated attenuation image from the attenuated PET emission data. IEEE Trans Med Imaging. 2013;32:237–46.

21. Messroghli DR, Radjenovic A, Kozerke S, Higgins DM, Sivananthan MU, Ridgway JP. Modified look-locker inversion recovery (MOLLI) for high-resolution T1 mapping of the heart. Magn Reson Med. 2004;52:141–6.

22. Kunze KP, Rischpler C, Hayes C, Ibrahim T, Laugwitz K-L, Haase A, Schwaiger M, Nekolla SG. Measurement of extracellular volume and transit time heterogeneity using contrast-enhanced myocardial perfusion MRI in patients after acute myocardial infarction. Magn Reson Med. 2017;77:2320–30.

23. Metz S, Ganter C, Lorenzen S, van Marwick S, Herrmann K, Lordick F, Nekolla SG, Rummeny EJ, Wester H-J, Brix G, Schwaiger M, Beer AJ. Phenotyping of tumor biology in patients by multimodality multiparametric imaging: relationship of microcirculation, avb3 expression, and glucose metabolism. J Nucl Med. 2010;51:1691–8.

24. Diao K-Y, Yang Z-G, Xu H-Y, Liu X, Zhang Q, Shi K, Jiang L, Xie L-J, Wen L-Y, Guo Y-K. Histologic validation of myocardial fibrosis measured by T1 mapping: a systematic review and meta-analysis. J Cardiovasc Magn Reson. 2017;18:92.

25. Jablonowski R, Engblom H, Kanski M, Nordlund D, Koul S, Van Der Pals J, Englund E, Heiberg E, Erlinge D, Carlsson M, Arheden H. Contrast-enhanced CMR overestimates early myocardial infarct size: mechanistic insights using ECV measurements on day 1 and day 7. JACC Cardiovasc Imaging. 2015;8:1379–89.

26. Fiolet JW, ter Welle HF, van Capelle FJ, Lie KI. Infarct size estimation from serial CK MB determinations: peak activity and predictability. Br Heart J. 1983;49:373–80.

27. Lee WW, Marinelli B, Van Der Laan AM, Sena BF, Gorbatov R, Leuschner F, Dutta P, Iwamoto Y, Ueno T, Begieneman MPV, Niessen HWM, Piek JJ, Vinegoni C, Pittet MJ, Swirski FK, Tawakol A, Di Carli M, Weissleder R, Nahrendorf M. PET/MRI of inflammation in myocardial infarction. J Am Coll Cardiol. 2012;59:153–63.

28. Schwaiger M, Schelbert HR, Ellison D, Hansen H, Yeatman L, Vinten-Johansen J, Selin C, Barrio J, Phelps ME. Sustained regional abnormalities in cardiac metabolism after transient ischemia in the chronic dog model. J Am Coll Cardiol. 1985;6:336–47.

29. Kellman P, Hansen MS. T1-mapping in the heart: accuracy and precision. J Cardiovasc Magn Reson. 2014;16:2.

5

Right heart catheterization using metallic guidewires and low SAR cardiovascular magnetic resonance fluoroscopy at 1.5 Tesla: first in human experience

Adrienne E. Campbell-Washburn[*†], Toby Rogers[†], Annette M. Stine, Jaffar M. Khan, Rajiv Ramasawmy, William H. Schenke, Delaney R. McGuirt, Jonathan R. Mazal, Laurie P. Grant, Elena K. Grant, Daniel A. Herzka and Robert J. Lederman

Abstract

Background: Cardiovascular magnetic resonance (CMR) fluoroscopy allows for simultaneous measurement of cardiac function, flow and chamber pressure during diagnostic heart catheterization. To date, commercial metallic guidewires were considered contraindicated during CMR fluoroscopy due to concerns over radiofrequency (RF)-induced heating. The inability to use metallic guidewires hampers catheter navigation in patients with challenging anatomy. Here we use low specific absorption rate (SAR) imaging from gradient echo spiral acquisitions and a commercial nitinol guidewire for CMR fluoroscopy right heart catheterization in patients.

Methods: The low-SAR imaging protocol used a reduced flip angle gradient echo acquisition (10° vs 45°) and a longer repetition time (TR) spiral readout (10 ms vs 2.98 ms). Temperature was measured in vitro in the ASTM 2182 gel phantom and post-mortem animal experiments to ensure freedom from heating with the selected guidewire (150 cm × 0.035″ angled-tip nitinol Terumo *Glidewire*). Seven patients underwent CMR fluoroscopy catheterization. Time to enter each chamber (superior vena cava, main pulmonary artery, and each branch pulmonary artery) was recorded and device visibility and confidence in catheter and guidewire position were scored on a Likert-type scale.

Results: Negligible heating (< 0.07°C) was observed under all in vitro conditions using this guidewire and imaging approach. In patients, chamber entry was successful in 100% of attempts with a guidewire compared to 94% without a guidewire, with failures to reach the branch pulmonary arteries. Time-to-enter each chamber was similar (p=NS) for the two approaches. The guidewire imparted useful catheter shaft conspicuity and enabled interactive modification of catheter shaft stiffness, however, the guidewire tip visibility was poor.

Conclusions: Under specific conditions, trained operators can apply low-SAR imaging and using a specific fully-insulated metallic nitinol guidewire (150 cm × 0.035" Terumo *Glidewire*) to augment clinical CMR fluoroscopy right heart catheterization.

Keywords: Interventional MRI catheterization, Right heart catheterization, Guidewire, Cardiac catheters, Medical device heating, Real-time MRI, Invasive hemodynamics, Spiral MRI, Cardiovascular magnetic resonance

* Correspondence: adrienne.campbell@nih.gov
Dr. Graham Wright served as a Guest Editor for this manuscript.
[†]Adrienne E. Campbell-Washburn and Toby Rogers contributed equally to this work.
Cardiovascular Branch, Division of Intramural Research, National Heart, Lung, and Blood Institute, National Institutes of Health, Building 10, Room 2C713, Bethesda, MD 20892-1538, USA

Background

Cardiovascular magnetic resonance (CMR) fluoroscopy catheterization allows simultaneous measurement of chamber pressure and cardiac output, alongside characterization of cardiac tissue, cardiac anatomy and cardiac function in a single procedure [1].

To date, clinical CMR fluoroscopy heart catheterization has relied on polymer catheters that are visualized solely by the contents of distal balloons filled with gas or contrast agents [2–6]. As a result, only catheter tips and not shafts are visible during CMR fluoroscopy, which hampers catheter navigation, especially in patients with challenging anatomy and physiology, such as surgically corrected or uncorrected congenital heart disease, enlarged right sided heart structures and severe valvular regurgitation. Until now, metallic guidewires, an important adjunct for X-ray fluoroscopy catheterization, have not been used during CMR fluoroscopy catheterization out of concern that long conductive structures will heat by coupling electrically with radiofrequency (RF) excitation pulses [7, 8]. Glass and other non-metallic guidewires have been reported for CMR catheterization but suffer insurmountable fragility that will likely preclude wide adoption [9–12]. Non-conductive metallic guidewires have been reported that resist heating during CMR but that are not yet commercially available [13].

We hypothesized that standard commercial metallic guidewires could be safely used in patients by reducing CMR excitation energy (also known as low specific absorption rate (SAR) imaging) [14]. We defined conditions of use for a specific commercial nitinol guidewire having desirable insulation properties, used in combination with reduced excitation energy and prolonged readout times to reduce RF-induced heating. These consisted of reduced flip angle α (to 10° during gradient echo from 45° during balanced steady-state free precession (bSSFP), a long repetition time (TR) spiral readout instead of a short TR rectilinear readout (TR 10 ms vs 2.98 ms), and a specific 150 cm nitinol guidewire having fully-insulated proximal and distal tips (Glidewire 0.035″, Terumo). Using these parameters, we tested guidewire heating under exaggerated geometry conditions in vitro, in situ in post-mortem swine, and finally used this guidewire in consenting research subjects undergoing clinical CMR fluoroscopy catheterization.

Methods

CMR

Procedures were performed in a combined X-ray and CMR fluoroscopy suite (Artis Zee and Aera 1.5 T, Siemens Healthineers, Erlangen, Germany) for both animals and patients. The CMR fluoroscopy room incorporates LCD projectors, wireless sound-suppression communication headsets (IMROC IR, Optoacoustics, Or Yehuda, Israel), and an artifact-suppressing patient physiology interface (PRiME, nhlbi-mr.github.io/PRiME/) [15] for a standard high-fidelity hemodynamic recording system (Sensis, Siemens Healhtineers).

CMR fluoroscopy used one of two possible pulse sequences: **low-SAR with metallic guidewire** (spiral gradient echo (GRE), 16 spiral arms per frame, matrix 128 × 128, TR 10 ms, TE 0.86 ms, flip angle 10°, FOV 400 mm, slice thickness 8 mm, spatial resolution 3.125 mm × 3.125 mm, temporal resolution 160 ms per frame); or **normal-SAR without metallic guidewire** (rectilinear bSSFP, matrix 120 × 160, TR 2.98 ms, TE 1.49 ms, flip angle 45°, field-of-view (FOV) 400 mm, slice thickness 8 mm, GRAPPA acceleration rate 2–4, spatial resolution 3.33 mm × 2.5 mm, temporal resolution 89.4 ms - 178.8 ms per frame). Guidewire heating is proportional to the square of the flip angle and inversely proportional to TR [14] and therefore the parameters used for low-SAR protocol theoretically generated a 67 fold reduction in heating compared to the normal-SAR protocol. A saturation pre-pulse was used to improve visibility of gadolinium filled balloons interactively. The low-SAR sequences used a partial saturation pulse with flip angle 45° [16] and the normal-SAR sequence used a dark blood saturation preparation. Imaging was performed in normal SAR operating mode, limiting time-averaged whole body SAR to 2 W/kg.

Catheter and guidewire devices

We selected a polymer balloon-wedge endhole catheter with a rigid distal curve that in our experience is useful to navigate cardiac chambers (Swan-Ganz Flow-Directed Monitoring Catheter, T-tip, Dual-Lumen including inflation port, Model T111F7, 7Fr × 110 cm, 0.038″ lumen, Edwards Lifesciences, Irvine, California, USA) [2, 3], but had other shapes available on standby (Balloon Wedge Pressure Catheter, Model AI-07127, Arrow-Teleflex, Reading, Pennsylvania, USA). Balloon catheters were filled with gadobutrol (diluted 0.5% from stock) or air.

We selected a specific guidewire for its materials and insulation properties. The guidewire (Glidewire Model GR3506, Terumo Corporation, Tokyo, Japan, 0.035″ × 150 cm, standard stiffness, 3 cm flexible tip, angled tip configuration) has a single nitinol core and is completely insulated with expanded polytetrafluoroethylene (ePTFE) without exposed gaps. By contrast, a popular comparator PTFE-coated nitinol guidewire (Nitrex, Medtronic,Minneapolis, Minnesota, USA, Covidien EV3, for example 0.035″ × 145 cm Model N351452, Medtronic) has exposed and un-insulated tips, which we consider unsafe for use in CMR.

In vitro experiments

Confidence in freedom from heating was established with in vitro experiments using an ASTM 2182 gel phantom. This gel phantom exaggerates heating and in vivo we expect less heating because of blood flow cooling, the central position of the vessels and convective heat dissipation.

Guidewire temperature was evaluated for a range of guidewire configurations, as summarized in Table 1; catheter position relative to guidewire, guidewire looping, guidewire length and guidewire position within the bore were among conditions explored. A fiber optic temperature probes and signal conditioner with ±0.3 °C accuracy were used for temperature measurements (OpSens Solutions Inc., Quebec, Canada). The temperature probe was affixed to the guidewire using a polyimide channel fastened with heat shrink tubing [17], or positioned using a homebuilt modular positioning system that supports both the guidewire and temperature probe in contact.

Animal experiments

Animal experiments were approved by the Institutional Animal Care and Use Committee. Guidewire heating was assessed post-mortem in a 47 kg swine to replicate right-heart catheterization guidewire geometry without blood flow cooling. Temperature was measured at the tip of the selected *Glidewire* extended 1 cm from a 7F catheter (Goodale-Lubin, Medtronic).

Patient catheterization

The clinical research protocol was approved by the Institutional Review Board (NCT03152773). CMR fluoroscopy heart catheterization is a standard medical procedure at our institution. Consecutive patients undergoing medically necessary right heart catheterization between August and November 2017 were invited to participate. All gave written informed consent. Candidates were excluded for

cardiovascular instability, pregnancy or nursing, or ineligibility for CMR. Those with an estimated glomerular filtration rate < 30 mL/min/1.73m^2 were enrolled, but balloon catheters were filled with air rather than dilute gadolinium contrast.

Under moderate sedation, subjects underwent measurement of left ventricular pressure under X-ray guidance, followed by the research CMR fluoroscopy catheterization. Interventional procedures were performed before or after the research study, such as radial artery access or coronary intervention, and heparin anticoagulation was administered at the discretion of the physician. Baseline CMR was performed to assess anatomy, chamber dimensions and biventricular function.

For guidewire CMR fluoroscopy catheterization, time-to-enter each of four targeted chambers (superior vena cava, main pulmonary artery, right and left pulmonary arteries) was recorded. At their discretion, operators interactively retained or extended the guidewire beyond the catheter tip, to probe and enter the target chamber.

The guidewire was introduced following catheter positioning and extended 5-15cm from the catheter tip to engage each target chamber. Alternatively, the guidewire could be kept just inside of the catheter in order to stiffen it to advance the catheter into the chambers. The guidewire was oriented parallel to the z-axis in the cava and was interactively advanced and torqued to engage pulmonary artery branches to guide advancement of the catheter. Each chamber was sampled for hemoglobin oximetry.

As time (and subject patience) allowed, the procedure was repeated without a guidewire under conventional

Table 1 Guidewire configurations tested during in vitro experiments. Experiments were performed in the ASTM-2182 phantom using Terumo *Glidewires* and Medtronic *Nitrex* in a 70 cm bore 1.5 T MRI system (Aera, Siemens, Erlangen, Germany)

Property	Experimental details	Maximum Heating Condition
Catheter insulation	• Heating at guidewire tip and catheter tip were measured simultaneously • Guidewire position relative to catheter: 10 cm, 5 cm, 2 cm, 1 cm (guidewire extended), 0 cm (tips aligned), − 2 cm, − 5 cm (guidewire retracted inside catheter).	• 1 cm guidewire extension; the change in insulation is similar to that of an exposed metallic tip.
Guidewire Length	• Terumo *Glidewires* of lengths 150 cm, 180 cm and 260 cm with catheter insulation (1 cm exposed guidewire)	• 260 cm guidewire for Terumo *Glidewires*
Guidewire position	• The temperature distribution of this phantom with this CMR system has been mapped previously [17]	• Positioned near the edge of the bore (> 12 cm off-isocenter) and near the surface of the gel (> 5 cm depth).
Insertion length	• Insertion lengths 15-65 cm into the ASTM gel phantom were tested for the three lengths of Terumo *Glidewire* with catheter insulation (1 cm exposed guidewire)	• 45 cm–55 cm insertion length for all guidewire lengths.
Looping	• Loops were created in segments of bare wire, as is common in the body, in the coronal plane • Loop diameter = 5 cm and single, double, triple and quadruple loops were compared. • Temperature was measured both at the tip of the guidewire and the contact point of the loops, where a second hotspot is formed.	• Temperature was always higher at the guidewire tip compared to the loop contact point and temperature in both locations increased with increasing number of loops. • Using the bare wire with no catheter insulation, generates lower temperatures and looping was not investigated further

(normal-SAR bSSFP) imaging conditions. Subjects were observed for four hours after research catheterization, after which their research participation concluded.

Absent a safe method, guidewire tip heating was not directly measured in patients. Measures of systemic coagulation (plasma D-dimer immunoassay) and of focal red cell injury (spectrophotometric plasma free hemoglobin, Mayo Labs, Rochester, Minnesota, USA) were collected before and after CMR fluoroscopy catheterization, knowing they may be confounded by clinical conditions. Guidewire tips and catheter effluent were assessed for clot after every chamber sample, knowing that clot formation is common in guidewire catheterization without anticoagulation.

Data analysis

Two independent investigators assigned Likert-type ordinal scales to measure catheter visualization (0 = invisible, 1 = sometimes visible, 2 = most times visible, 3 = all times visible) and confidence in catheter position (0 = uncertain, 1 = probable and requires pressure confirmation, 2 = certain) [5]. Guidewire visibility and confidence in tip position was also scored when the guidewire was extended from the catheter to engage each chamber.

Results are presented as mean ± standard deviation (SD) or median (1st quartile, 3rd quartile) as appropriate and are compared using a Wilcoxon rank sum test. A p value < 0.05 was considered statistically significant.

Results

Guidewire heating

Heating of metallic guidewires was influenced by CMR pulse sequence, guidewire configuration and guidewire physical properties, as summarized in Table 2.

The selected Terumo *Glidewire* was tested under worst-case heating conditions extended 1 cm from catheter tip positioned at the edge of the ASTM 2182 phantom (45 cm insertion, > 5 cm depth, 12.7 cm off-isocenter) in a straight configuration. It generated < 4°C with normal-SAR imaging and < 0.1°C with low-SAR imaging during 2 min of continuous imaging (Fig. 1a). Under identical conditions, the comparator *Nitrex* guidewire generated 15.5°C of heating with normal-SAR imaging and 0.5°C heating with low-SAR imaging during 2 min of continuous imaging (Fig. 1b). The incomplete insulation exposes metal at the tip of the nitinol guidewire concentrates current density and contributes to heating of this guidewire model [8].

Animal post-mortem experiments found maximum heating of 0.3°C with normal-SAR imaging and 0°C with low-SAR imaging during 2 min of continuous scanning. Maximum heating was observed as the guidewire protruded from the femoral sheath into the vasculature.

Patients and clinical findings

Of 13 consecutive patients undergoing right heart catheterization during the study period, 8 consented and 7 underwent the study procedure. One was excluded because of hardware malfunction after vascular access was obtained; the operator felt the patient's discomfort required swift conclusion of the procedure under X-ray. Two were excluded because they required emergency intervention, one declined CMR guidewire catheterization and underwent standard CMR fluoroscopy catheterization without a guidewire, and two required left but not right heart procedures.

Seven patients (46±20 years; 4 (57%) female) underwent guidewire CMR fluoroscopy catheterization. All had normal cardiac anatomy. All had suspected pulmonary hypertension. Underlying illness was sickle cell disease ($n = 3$); atrial septal defect ($n = 2$); cardiomyopathy ($n = 1$); and rheumatologic illness($n = 1$). One had chronic renal failure and underwent catheterization using a gas-filled, instead of gadolinium contrast-filled, balloon catheter. One underwent nitric oxide vasodilator challenge under CMR. One underwent concomitant percutaneous coronary intervention and two underwent atrial sepal defect repair, all under X-ray guidance.

CMR fluoroscopy catheterization took a median of 30 (27, 48) minutes including catheter navigation, repeated procedure steps to measure chamber entry time and conspicuity using up to two imaging pulse sequences (low-SAR with guidewire and normal-SAR without guidewire), CMR flow, and in one case nitric oxide inhalation.

Hemodynamic and CMR findings are summarized in Table 3.

Clinical performance of CMR fluoroscopy catheterization with- and without a guidewire

CMR guidewire fluoroscopy catheterization was successful in entering intended cardiac chambers in 100% of attempts, compared with non-guidewire fluoroscopy catheterization, 94% (p = NS). The failures were exclusively branch pulmonary arteries, both left and right.

Time-to-enter each chamber was not significantly different between the two approaches, low-SAR with guidewire and normal-SAR without guidewire (35 ± 45 s vs 26 ± 38 s, p = NS).

Table 4 shows Likert-type scores of catheter and guidewire tip and shaft visibility compared using the two different imaging techniques. Overall visibility and operator confidence in catheter tip location was comparable among all modalities using saturation pre-pulses. The catheter shaft was rendered slightly more visible by a guidewire susceptibility artifact (Fig. 2), but we observed that catheter shaft visibility was reduced when saturation pre-pulses were applied to confirm contrast-filled balloon position. Guidewire tip visibility was poor

Table 2 Factors that modulate guidewire heating during CMR

Factor	Heating Impact	How to reduce heating
CMR excitation energy		
Radiofrequency excitation, controlled via flip angle α	Heating increases with square of flip angle, α [14]	Reduce α during CMR fluoroscopy
Radiofrequency pulse width duration	Heating decreases linearly with RF pulse width duration	Increase radio frequenchy pulse width duration
Radiofrequency duty cycle	Heating decreases linearly with excitation repetition time (TR)	Prolong TR
Radiofrequency pre-pulses used for CMR magnetization preparation	Heating increases with pre-pulse flip angle and number of RF pulses in preparation, and decreases with RF pulse width duration	Reduce pre-pulses and their SAR characteristics
CMR scanner duty cycle	Additional heat is generated as long as CMR scanning continues	Limit duration of continuous CMR fluoroscopy with a guidewire in place.
Conductive guidewire physical properties		
Guidewire insulation	Insulation gaps, such as at the tip, concentrate current density and increase focal heating [8]	Use guidewires that are fully insulated without gaps
Length of conductive materials	Guidewire length > ¼ wavelength λ of the Larmor frequency in vivo (~ 10 cm at 1.5 T) promotes standing waves and therefore heating [13]	Use guidewires having metallic components shorter than ¼λ (not available commercially)
Guidewire configuration		
Guidewire position with regard to center of CMR bore	Electrical field minimal at the center of scanner bore (in x & y), greatest closer to wall of scanner bore [21]	Keep guidewire close to scanner centerline and away from walls of scanner.
Guidewire position with regard to patient body	Electrical field is greatest at outer (skin) surface of body. Electrical modeling suggests electrical field is greatest at groin and shoulder during CMR	Use in central blood vessels
Guidewire insertion length with regard to vascular access site	Electrical field is highest at outer edges of scanner bore entrance. Guidewire outside of the body is more likely to couple electrically and heat. In other words, minimal guidewire vascular insertion length is associated with maximal heating	Reduce input energy during scanning. Minimize time with guidewire at minimum insertion length.
Guidewire insulation by catheter	The patient is less exposed to guidewire heating when it is covered by insulating catheter	If guidewire is not in active use, retain its position inside catheter or remove from body during CMR.
Guidewire protrusion length from catheter	A change in insulation with minimum guidewire protrusion outside insulating catheters causes concentration of current density and therefore heating	Reduce input energy during scanning.
Guidewire length	Different guidewire lengths are associated with different degrees of heating, in a non-linear fashion, relating to coupling with scanner electrical field [21]	Select guidewire lengths empirically associated with less heating.
Guidewire diameter	Guidewires with smaller diameter generate more heating [8]	Select larger diameter guidewires as appropriate
Guidewire loops overlapping	Guidewire looping can create a second point of heating at wire contact points, which remains less than or equal to guidewire tip heating	Reduce input energy during scanning.
Guidewire heat is dissipated by conduction and convection into surrounding medium	Blood flow cools heated guidewire dramatically. Testing under static conditions, such as ASTM 2182 phantom, maximizes detected heating	Static phantom testing exaggerates heating to provide a margin of safety predicted in vivo, probably by 10-fold.

throughout. Imaging during navigation from inferior to superior vena cava is shown in Additional file 1: Video 1 available online. As expected, GRE imaging (low-SAR pulse sequence) provided inferior blood-myocardium contrast compared to bSSFP imaging (normal-SAR pulse sequence) (comparison images provided in Fig. 3).

Safety
There were no adverse events in this small cohort.

To test for subclinical sequelae of guidewire heating, and out of caution, we measured baseline and follow-up markers of coagulation (plasma D-dimer) and of erythrocyte destruction (plasma free hemoglobin). These were all unchanged except for one patient who had undergone percutaneous coronary stenting using heparin anticoagulation, in whom plasma free hemoglobin rose from 6.4 to 15.2 mg/dL, which is the upper limit of normal.

We also inspected guidewires and catheter aspirates for thrombus formation after use. Clot was observed on the

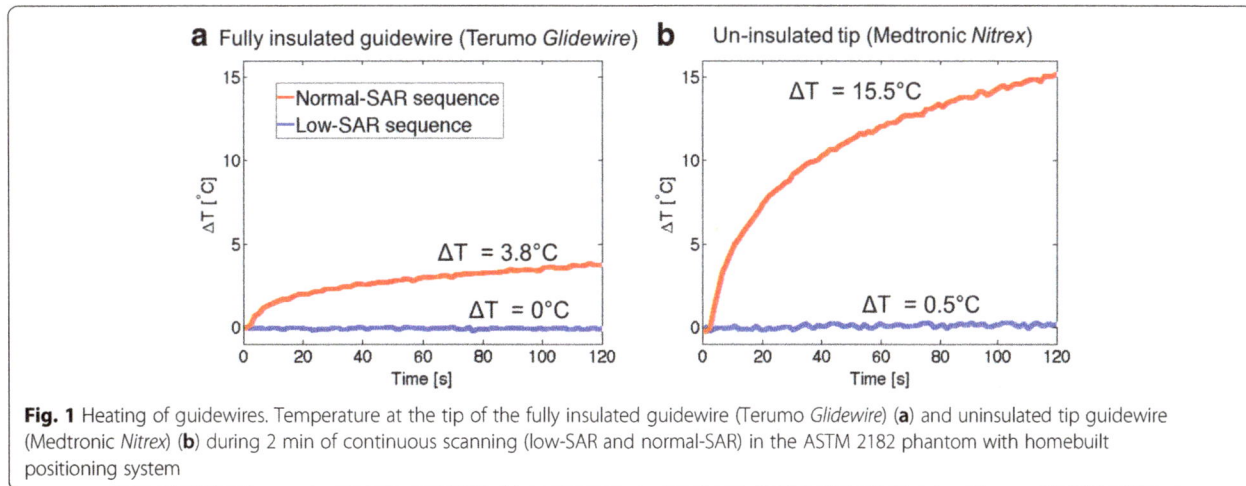

Fig. 1 Heating of guidewires. Temperature at the tip of the fully insulated guidewire (Terumo *Glidewire*) (**a**) and uninsulated tip guidewire (Medtronic *Nitrex*) (**b**) during 2 min of continuous scanning (low-SAR and normal-SAR) in the ASTM 2182 phantom with homebuilt positioning system

guidewire or catheter aspirate in 15% of guidewire specimens versus 11% of non-guidewire specimens (p = NS), and none among subjects who received heparin anticoagulation (one for percutaneous coronary stenting, two for left atrial catheterization).

Discussion

Adoption of CMR fluoroscopy catheterization has been hampered by the unavailability of safe CMR-compatible clinical devices, especially guidewires. Metallic guidewires by definition are conductive and therefore prone to heating in the conditions required for CMR fluoroscopy catheterization in adults. Certain steps in right heart catheterization are difficult or impossible without a guidewire in some patients [2, 3, 5], especially selecting branch pulmonary arteries. The mechanical properties

Table 3 CMR Catheterization Findings

Measurement	Value
Heart rate (bpm)	71 ± 10
Right atrial pressure (mm Hg)	9 ± 2
Right ventricular pressure (mm Hg)	42 ± 14 / 10 ± 5
Pulmonary artery mean / wedge pressure (mm Hg)	25 ± 9 / 12 ± 7
Aorta systolic/diastolic/mean pressure (mm Hg)	124 ± 19 / 67 ± 7 / 87 ± 9
Right atrium volume index (mL/m^2)	14 ± 5
Right ventricular end-diastolic volume index / end-systolic (mL/m^2) / ejection fraction	87 ± 37 / 35 ± 15 / 59 ± 5
Left atrial volume index (mL/m^2)	40 ± 11
Left ventricular end-diastolic volume index / end-systolic (mL/m^2) / ejection fraction	69 ± 6 / 26 ± 4 / 62 ± 6
Left ventricular mass index	54 ± 36
Q_P / Q_S / Ratio	3.6 ± 1.2 / 2.9 ± 0.9 / 1.3 ± .5

of commercial metallic guidewires are superior to non-metallic guidewires and we are not aware of any non-metallic guidewires with satisfactory mechanical properties for catheterization. To address concerns of metallic guidewire heating, we comprehensively tested and confirmed the safety of CMR catheterization using a specific guidewire under specific low-SAR imaging conditions, both in vitro and in animals before translating into human patients. Post-mortem animal experiments were chosen to exaggerate potential heating with no blood flow cooling. Heating of the selected guidewire with the low-SAR pulse sequence was negligible (< 0.07 °C) and less than the equipment accuracy of ±0.3 °C for all conditions tested in vitro.

This is the first in human report of CMR fluoroscopy cardiac catheterization with a standard commercially available metallic guidewire. The main findings of this study are that (1) a specific nitinol guidewire (*Glidewire* 0.035″ 150 cm angled-tip) can be used under specific low-SAR conditions to facilitate CMR fluoroscopy right heart catheterization at 1.5 T; (2) the guidewire imparts conspicuity to the shaft of otherwise-invisible polymer balloon-tipped catheters; (3) the incremental stiffness imparted to the polymer catheter facilitates procedure success under CMR fluoroscopy; (4) systemic measurements of coagulation (D-dimer) and erythrocyte injury (plasma free hemoglobin), although of unknown sensitivity, were not significantly perturbed using the guidewire; (5) clot accumulated on the guidewire and on guidewire-free catheters in patients undergoing CMR fluoroscopy when not anticoagulated, a known phenomenon under X-ray of unclear significance under these conditions; (6) Despite the reduced contrast-to-noise ratio, the low-SAR imaging mode was adequate to guide catheter navigation for CMR fluoroscopy right heart catheterization; and, (7) the visual performance of the specific nitinol guidewire used under CMR fluoroscopy is grossly inferior to X-ray in that the tip is not conspicuous,

Table 4 Likert-type scoring of device visibility and confidence in catheter and guidewire position. Only catheter shaft visibility reached statistical significance ($p = 0.001$)

Imaging test	Guidewire low-SAR spiral GRE	No guidewire normal-SAR rectilinear bSSFP
Tip visibility of balloon catheter with saturation pre-pulse(scale 0–3)	3.0 ± 0.2	2.9 ± 0.3
Shaft visibility of balloon catheter (scale 0–3)	1.1 ± 1.2	0.0 ± 0.0
Confidence that balloon catheter tip is at the intended location (scale 0–2)	2.0 ± 0.0	2.0 ± 0.0
Tip visibility of guidewire (scale 0–3)	0.5 ± 0.8	N/A
Shaft visibility of guidewire (scale 0–3)	1.6 ± 1.1	N/A
Confidence that guidewire tip is at the intended location (scale 0–2)	0.4 ± 0.6	N/A

which is a common problem for passive devices in CMR [18] that must be considered carefully by operators.

Ours is not the first human interventional CMR procedure using a Terumo guidewire device. Paetzel et al. reported femoropopliteal balloon angioplasty in 15 patients under real-time CMR guidance at 1.5 T in 2005 [19]. They used low-SAR gradient echo pulse sequences and assured adequate insertion length and proximity to isocenter before CMR, and found no heating related events. The authors did not report on guidewire visibility, which presumably was as poor as in our experience.

Recommended workflow
Our approach would be simple to replicate at other medical centers. We describe a procedure for nitinol guidewire-assisted CMR fluoroscopy right heart catheterization using specific conditions at 1.5 T. We believe this approach should be only undertaken by expert catheter operators familiar with this operating environment to avoid (1) inadvertent guidewire scanning using normal-SAR conditions (high flip angle, short TR), (2) tissue injury or myocardial perforation caused by inadequate guidewire tip visualization despite tactile cues, (3) selection of an alternative commercial guidewire with unsafe heating properties.

Based on this experience, we intend to employ guidewires (with low-SAR CMR fluoroscopy) catheterization only when needed, much as they are employed during X-ray fluoroscopy catheterization. We recommend other sites adopt a workflow that clearly assures low-SAR imaging modes during guidewire steps, such as explicit team communications, checklists, and visual warnings on imaging displays. We also recommend routine low-dose anticoagulation which is widely employed by pediatric but not by most adult catheterization programs, in light of the low but appreciable incidence of clots recognized in all arms of this study.

We performed this work in a combined X-Ray/CMR suite, although this procedure would also be feasible in a standard 1.5 T CMR suite with an appropriate evacuation plan in case of emergency. A CMR compatible defibrillator [20] might be helpful for complex CMR-guided procedures.

Limitations
We have not yet tested CMR fluoroscopy guidewire catheterization during retrograde left heart catheterization in patients, and we caution against such procedure absent assurance about guidewire tip visualization during CMR fluoroscopy. We also warn against the likely danger of

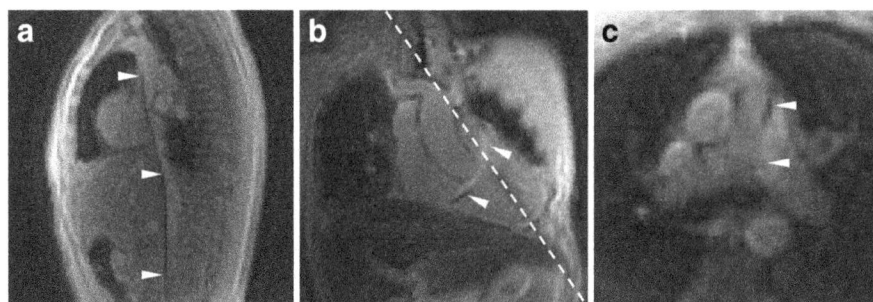

Fig. 2 Catheter shaft conspicuity imparted by guidewire. Example low-SAR spiral GRE images, with catheter and guidewire (arrowheads) positioned in the superior vena cava (**a**), main pulmonary artery (**b**) and left pulmonary artery (**c**); the guidewire imparts both hypo- and hyper-intense signal along the shaft. The dotted line indicates signal saturation caused by an orthogonal slice plane interleaved during imaging

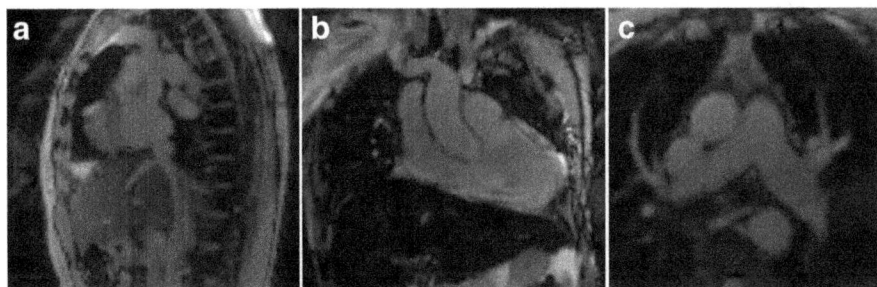

Fig. 3 Comparator rectilinear bSSFP images. Image orientation comparable to Fig. 2 showing improved blood-tissue contrast with bSSFP rectilinear images (normal-SAR imaging mode) for inferior/superior vena cava view (**a**), main pulmonary artery view (**b**) and branched pulmonary arteries view (**c**). No devices were present during imaging

using guidewires other than the specific device described unless carefully examined for heating. The specific device has insulation and length properties and we were able to demonstrate freedom from heating under the conditions of use.

Visualization of commercial nitinol guidewires remains a challenging, though work in positive contrast imaging methods may improve the visibility at the expense of temporal resolution [14]. We chose an 8 mm slice thickness to avoid out-of-plane guidewire motion, but thinner slices could be explored to improve visualization of the signal void.

Conclusion

Metallic guidewires are an important adjunct for catheterization as they interactively control shaft stiffness, and help to select and enter target chambers. By lowering SAR (through reduced RF excitation flip angle and increased repetition time, implemented as spiral gradient echo CMR), and by selecting a specific fully-insulated nitinol guidewire, we safely employed a metallic guidewire during CMR fluoroscopy catheterization. The guidewire also improved shaft conspicuity, which we believe facilitated procedure success. These findings should not be applied to other nitinol guidewire devices or similar devices having different lengths without specific testing to assure freedom from heating. Though the guidewire visual performance is inferior to X-ray in that the tip is not conspicuous, the ability to safely use a metallic guidewire during CMR fluoroscopy could enable new and more complex CMR-guided procedures.

Abbreviations
bSSFP: Balanced steady state free precession; CMR: Cardiovascular magnetic resonance; FOV: Field-of-view; GRE: Gradient recalled echo; LV: Left ventricle; NS: Non-significant; PTFE: Polytetrafluoroethylene; RF: Radiofrequency; RHC: Right heart catheterization; RV: Right ventricle; SAR: Specific absorption rate; TR: Repetition time; α: Flip angle; λ: Wavelength

Acknowledgements
The authors acknowledge Burcu Basar for her assistance with guidewire heating experiments.

Funding
This work was supported by the Division of Intramural Research, National Heart, Lung, and Blood Institute, National Institutes of Health, USA (Z01-HL005062, Z01-HL006061, Z1A-HL006213).

Authors' contributions
ACW, TR, RJL Designed, executed, analyzed experiments including CMR interpretation and drafted the manuscript. JMK, RR, DAH Executed and analyzed experiments including CMR interpretation and revised the manuscript. AMS, WHS, DRM, JRM, LPG, EKG Executed experiments and revised the manuscript. All authors read and approved the final manuscript

Competing interests
NIH and Siemens Medical Systems have a collaborative research and development agreement for interventional cardiovascular MRI.

References
1. Rogers T, Ratnayaka K, Lederman RJ. MRI catheterization in cardiopulmonary disease. Chest. 2014;145:30–6.
2. Rogers T, Ratnayaka K, Khan JM, Stine A, Schenke WH, Grant LP, Mazal JR, Grant EK, Campbell-Washburn A, Hansen MS, et al. CMR fluoroscopy right heart catheterization for cardiac output and pulmonary vascular resistance: results in 102 patients. J Cardiovasc Magn Reson. 2017;19:54.

3. Ratnayaka K, Kanter JP, Faranesh AZ, Grant EK, Olivieri LJ, Cross RR, Cronin IF, Hamann KS, Campbell-Washburn AE, O'Brien KJ, et al. Radiation-free CMR diagnostic heart catheterization in children. J Cardiovasc Magn Reson. 2017;19:65.

4. Pushparajah K, Tzifa A, Bell A, Wong JK, Hussain T, Valverde I, Bellsham-Revell HR, Greil G, Simpson JM, Schaeffter T, Razavi R. Cardiovascular magnetic resonance catheterization derived pulmonary vascular resistance and medium-term outcomes in congenital heart disease. J Cardiovasc Magn Reson. 2015;17:28.

5. Ratnayaka K, Faranesh AZ, Hansen MS, Stine AM, Halabi M, Barbash IM, Schenke WH, Wright VJ, Grant LP, Kellman P, et al. Real-time MRI-guided right heart catheterization in adults using passive catheters. Eur Heart J. 2013;34:380–9.

6. Razavi R, Hill DL, Keevil SF, Miquel ME, Muthurangu V, Hegde S, Rhode K, Barnett M, van Vaals J, Hawkes DJ, Baker E. Cardiac catheterisation guided by MRI in children and adults with congenital heart disease. Lancet. 2003; 362:1877–82.

7. Konings MK, Bartels LW, Smits HF, Bakker CJ. Heating around intravascular guidewires by resonating RF waves. J Magn Reson Imaging. 2000;12:79–85.

8. Yeung CJ, Susil RC, Atalar E. RF safety of wires in interventional MRI: using a safety index. Magn Reson Med. 2002;47:187–93.

9. Massmann A, Buecker A, Schneider GK. Glass-Fiber-based MR-safe guidewire for MR imaging-guided endovascular interventions: in vitro and preclinical in vivo feasibility study. Radiology. 2017;284:541–51.

10. Tzifa A, Krombach GA, Krämer N, Krüger S, Schütte A, von Walter M, Schaeffter T, Qureshi S, Krasemann T, Rosenthal E, et al. Magnetic resonance-guided cardiac interventions using magnetic resonance-compatible devices: a preclinical study and first-in-man congenital interventions. Circ Cardiovasc Interv. 2010;3:585–92.

11. Buecker A, Spuentrup E, Schmitz-Rode T, Kinzel S, Pfeffer J, Hohl C, van Vaals JJ, Gunther RW. Use of a nonmetallic guide wire for magnetic resonance-guided coronary artery catheterization. Investig Radiol. 2004;39:656–60.

12. Brecher C, Emonts M, Brack A, Wasiak C, Schutte A, Kramer N, Bruhn R. New concepts and materials for the manufacturing of MR-compatible guide wires. Biomed Tech (Berl). 2014;59:147–51.

13. Basar B, Rogers T, Ratnayaka K, Campbell-Washburn AE, Mazal JR, Schenke WH, Sonmez M, Faranesh AZ, Lederman RJ, Kocaturk O. Segmented nitinol guidewires with stiffness-matched connectors for cardiovascular magnetic resonance catheterization: preserved mechanical performance and freedom from heating. J Cardiovasc Magn Reson. 2015;17:105.

14. Campbell-Washburn AE, Rogers T, Basar B, Sonmez M, Kocaturk O, Lederman RJ, Hansen MS, Faranesh AZ. Positive contrast spiral imaging for visualization of commercial nitinol guidewires with reduced heating. J Cardiovasc Magn Reson. 2015;17:114.

15. Kakareka JW, Faranesh AZ, Pursley RH, Campbell-Washburn AE, Herzka DA, Rogers T, Kanter J, Ratnayaka K, Lederman RJ and Pohida TJ. Physiological Recording in the MRI Environment (PRiME): MRI-compatible hemodynamic recording system. IEEE Journal of Translational Engineering in Health and Medicine 2018;6:4100112.

16. Velasco Forte MN, Pushparajah K, Schaeffter T, Valverde Perez I, Rhode K, Ruijsink B, Alhrishy M, Byrne N, Chiribiri A, Ismail T, et al. Improved passive catheter tracking with positive contrast for CMR-guided cardiac catheterization using partial saturation (pSAT). J Cardiovasc Magn Reson. 2017;19:60.

17. Sonmez M, Saikus CE, Bell JA, Franson DN, Halabi M, Faranesh AZ, Ozturk C, Lederman RJ, Kocaturk O. MRI active guidewire with an embedded temperature probe and providing a distinct tip signal to enhance clinical safety. J Cardiovasc Magn Reson. 2012;14:38.

18. Campbell-Washburn AE, Tavallaei MA, Pop M, Grant EK, Chubb H, Rhode K, Wright GA. Real-time MRI guidance of cardiac interventions. J Magn Reson Imaging. 2017;46:935–50.

19. Paetzel C, Zorger N, Bachthaler M, Hamer OW, Stehr A, Feuerbach S, Lenhart M, Volk M, Herold T, Kasprzak P, Nitz WR. Magnetic resonance-guided percutaneous angioplasty of femoral and popliteal artery stenoses using real-time imaging and intra-arterial contrast-enhanced magnetic resonance angiography. Investig Radiol. 2005;40:257–62.

20. Schmidt EJ, Watkins RD, Zviman MM, Guttman MA, Wang W, Halperin HA, Magnetic Resonance A. Imaging-conditional external cardiac defibrillator for resuscitation within the magnetic resonance imaging scanner bore. Circ Cardiovasc Imaging. 2016;9

21. Yeung CJ, Karmarkar P, McVeigh ER. Minimizing RF heating of conducting wires in MRI. Magn Reson Med. 2007;58:1028–34.

6

Cardiovascular magnetic resonance guided ablation and intra-procedural visualization of evolving radiofrequency lesions in the left ventricle

Philippa R. P. Krahn[1,2]*, Sheldon M. Singh[3,4,5], Venkat Ramanan[2], Labonny Biswas[2], Nicolas Yak[2], Kevan J. T. Anderson[2], Jennifer Barry[2], Mihaela Pop[1,2,3] and Graham A. Wright[1,2,3]

Abstract

Background: Radiofrequency (RF) ablation has become a mainstay of treatment for ventricular tachycardia, yet adequate lesion formation remains challenging. This study aims to comprehensively describe the composition and evolution of acute left ventricular (LV) lesions using native-contrast cardiovascular magnetic resonance (CMR) during CMR-guided ablation procedures.

Methods: RF ablation was performed using an actively-tracked CMR-enabled catheter guided into the LV of 12 healthy swine to create 14 RF ablation lesions. T_2 maps were acquired immediately post-ablation to visualize myocardial edema at the ablation sites and T_1-weighted inversion recovery prepared balanced steady-state free precession (IR-SSFP) imaging was used to visualize the lesions. These sequences were repeated concurrently to assess the physiological response following ablation for up to approximately 3 h. Multi-contrast late enhancement (MCLE) imaging was performed to confirm the final pattern of ablation, which was then validated using gross pathology and histology.

Results: Edema at the ablation site was detected in T_2 maps acquired as early as 3 min post-ablation. Acute T_2-derived edematous regions consistently encompassed the T_1-derived lesions, and expanded significantly throughout the 3-h period post-ablation to 1.7 ± 0.2 times their baseline volumes (mean $\pm$ SE, estimated using a linear mixed model determined from $n = 13$ lesions). T_1-derived lesions remained approximately stable in volume throughout the same time frame, decreasing to 0.9 ± 0.1 times the baseline volume (mean $\pm$ SE, estimated using a linear mixed model, $n = 9$ lesions).

Conclusions: Combining native T_1- and T_2-based imaging showed that distinctive regions of ablation injury are reflected by these contrast mechanisms, and these regions evolve separately throughout the time period of an intervention. An integrated description of the T_1-derived lesion and T_2-derived edema provides a detailed picture of acute lesion composition that would be most clinically useful during an ablation case.

Keywords: Image-guided intervention, Catheter ablation, Tissue characterization, Arrhythmias

* Correspondence: philippa.krahn@mail.utoronto.ca
[1]Department of Medical Biophysics, University of Toronto, Toronto, ON, Canada
[2]Sunnybrook Research Institute, Toronto, ON, Canada
Full list of author information is available at the end of the article

Background

Ventricular tachycardia (VT) ablation is now frequently performed, with the rate of use of these procedures increasing substantially in the last decade [1]. Recurrence of VT after a single ablation procedure remains high, with 35% of patients who receive initially successful ablation treatment later experiencing VT recurrence during 6–23 month follow-up periods [2]. VT recurrence after an ablation procedure is complex and may be related to the inability to localize the critical circuit, or, when the circuit is defined, inability to obliterate the critical channels [3]. Once the critical isthmus of a VT circuit is isolated, radiofrequency (RF) ablation is performed with the hope of creating a necrotic lesion (permanent injury) at the putative isthmus, rendering VT non-inducible. The insult of ablation also leads to edema (reversible injury) surrounding the ablation site [4–8]. This reversible injury is thought to result in transient conduction block, with conduction recovering once the edema has resorbed [9–11], potentially leading to late arrhythmia recurrence. The ability to detect whether the arrhythmogenic substrate has been permanently destroyed, as evidenced by the presence of a lesion at a critical ablation site, may be invaluable and provide an additional intra-procedural endpoint to gauge long-term procedural success.

Cardiovascular magnetic resonance (CMR)-based identification of the critical isthmus sites may be used to guide ablation toward these targets [12], and the therapeutic lesions themselves can be directly visualized using native (non-contrast enhanced) CMR [4–8, 10, 13–16].

Ablation lesions visualized using native T_1 reflect injury that is associated with lethal heating [17], that persists at least for 3 weeks [13], and that correlates to chronic lesions [6], therefore likely represents permanent injury. Conversely, myocardial edema is visualized with native T_2 [18] and is transient, largely resolved within 3 months as seen in follow-up T_2-weighted imaging after atrial ablation [8]. The T_1-derived lesion and T_2-derived edema are individually significant in clinical ablations as the distributions of these injured regions could determine whether electrical block will remain permanently or resolve after healing (leading to recurrent VT). To evaluate these regions, this study includes concurrent native T_1- and T_2-based imaging to compare their relative extents and to construct a comprehensive understanding of the acute lesion composition.

A major potential value of intra-procedural CMR imaging lies in the ability to directly visualize and interpret the functional effect of therapeutic ablation lesions during the period when intra-procedural modification is possible. It is therefore important to identify how different aspects of CMR information evolve in this time window and how this information might be related to conventional electrophysiology (EP) endpoints. This study aims to characterize the evolution of lesions, as previously suggested to take place [16], but using concurrent imaging of both the T_2-derived edema and T_1-derived lesion to provide volumetric measurements of each. We hypothesize that the acute ablation-induced T_2-derived edema evolves during the acute time frame while the T_1-derived lesion remains at a consistent size. Furthermore, adding T_2 mapping to this imaging framework provides unambiguous quantification of edema severity. These techniques to study the acute lesion composition build upon prior work studying lesion characteristics via the surrogate measure of gadolinium kinetics [19]. This study aims to show temporal characteristics of the native T_1-derived lesion and T_2-derived edema within a time frame of particular relevance to direct CMR guidance of ablative therapies, extending the current understanding of lesion evolution previously established using native-contrast CMR [5] to an earlier time frame. Insights from lesion evolution could be applied to both CMR-guided and traditional ablation cases.

Methods
Animal preparation
CMR-guided RF ablation was performed in vivo in 12 healthy Yorkshire swine (58 ± 18 kg). The Animal Care Committee of Sunnybrook Research Institute approved all protocols. All animals received an intramuscular injection of ketamine (33 mg/kg) and atropine (0.05 mg/kg) pre-anaesthesia, followed by isoflurane gas (1–5%) continuously delivered via mechanical ventilation to maintain the surgical stage of anaesthesia. A sheath in one carotid artery acted as a port for catheter introduction. To mitigate arrhythmia, a bolus of amiodarone (75 mg) was given prior to the intervention, in addition to lidocaine (20 mg) as needed.

CMR-guided intervention
The entire intervention was performed within a 1.5 T wide-bore scanner (MR450w, General Electric Healthcare Waukesha, Wisconsin, USA). Figure 1 illustrates the interventional workflow and timing of data collection throughout. A 4-channel anterior cardiac array coil was used for all imaging, and was connected to the scanner bed separately from the catheter tip tracking coils. The CMR-enabled EP hardware configuration has been described previously [20].

Pre-procedure scans included short- and long-axis stacks of 2D balanced steady-state free-precession (bSSFP; CINE) images to serve as anatomical roadmaps (20 cardiac phases across 1 R-R interval, TR/TE = 5.2/1.9 ms, resolution = 1.25 × 1.5 mm, slice thickness = 6 mm). Both orientations were acquired at a rate of 1 breath-hold (approximately 14 s) per slice over 8 ± 3 min in total.

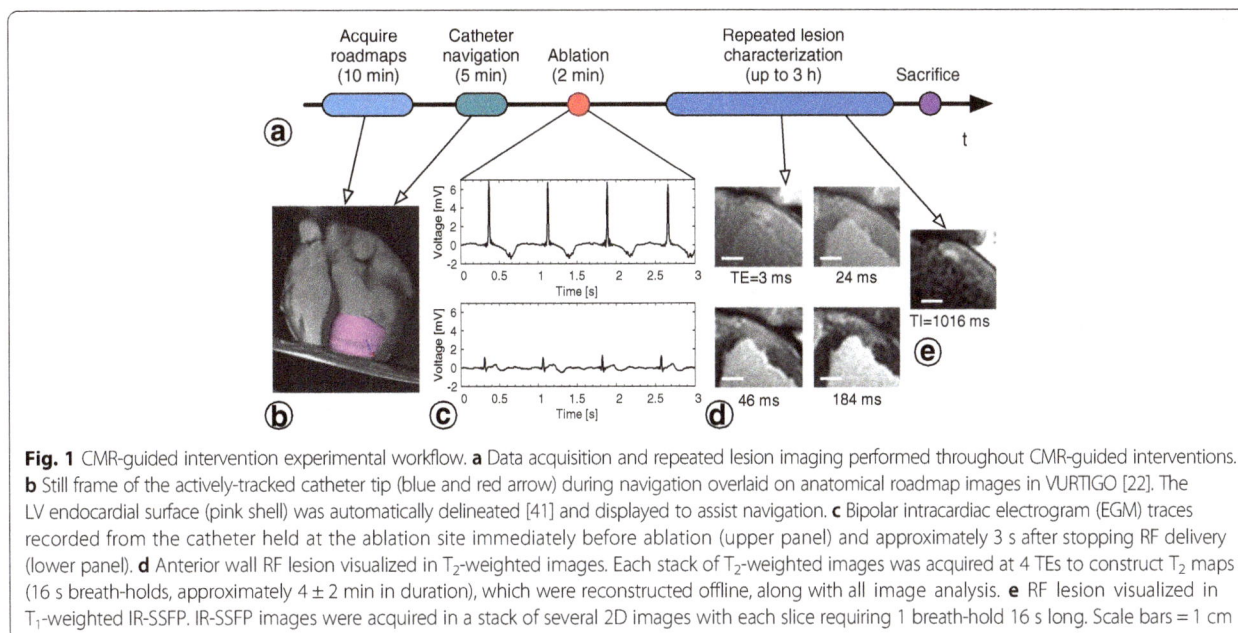

Fig. 1 CMR-guided intervention experimental workflow. **a** Data acquisition and repeated lesion imaging performed throughout CMR-guided interventions. **b** Still frame of the actively-tracked catheter tip (blue and red arrow) during navigation overlaid on anatomical roadmap images in VURTIGO [22]. The LV endocardial surface (pink shell) was automatically delineated [41] and displayed to assist navigation. **c** Bipolar intracardiac electrogram (EGM) traces recorded from the catheter held at the ablation site immediately before ablation (upper panel) and approximately 3 s after stopping RF delivery (lower panel). **d** Anterior wall RF lesion visualized in T_2-weighted images. Each stack of T_2-weighted images was acquired at 4 TEs to construct T_2 maps (16 s breath-holds, approximately 4 ± 2 min in duration), which were reconstructed offline, along with all image analysis. **e** RF lesion visualized in T_1-weighted IR-SSFP. IR-SSFP images were acquired in a stack of several 2D images with each slice requiring 1 breath-hold 16 s long. Scale bars = 1 cm

A 9 F CMR-enabled catheter (Imricor Medical Systems, Burnsville, Minnesota, USA) equipped with 2 micro-receive coils and 2 electrodes (3.7-mm tip electrode and 3.5-mm inter-electrode spacing) was used for the entire intervention. Active catheter tracking using a projection sequence [21] (FOV = 60 cm, flip angle = 5°, TR = 14.3 ms, tracking rate = 23 fps) was implemented in RTHawk software (HeartVista Inc., Menlo Park, California, USA). The catheter tip position was updated in real time and visualized overlaid on static anatomical roadmap images (Fig. 1b) simultaneously in VURTIGO, 4D visualization software for cardiovascular interventional guidance (Sunnybrook Research Institute, Toronto, Ontario, Canada) [22]. Bipolar intracardiac electrogram (EGM; Fig. 1c) traces from the catheter tip's electrodes were recorded by the Advantage-MR system (Imricor Medical Systems). EP traces and VURTIGO catheter navigation visualization were displayed on monitors in the CMR control room and on CMR-compatible monitors near the scanner bed to assist the interventionalist. Once the catheter was inserted into the heart to access the LV via the aortic valve, ablations were delivered from the catheter's distal electrode (1500 T14 generator, St Jude Medical, St. Paul, Minnesota, USA) with 17 mL/min irrigation and with the dispersive electrode placed on the animal's back. Ablations were delivered endocardially, in accordance with the more common clinical ablation approach (details given in Table 1). Conservative ablation parameters were chosen to avoid inducing arrhythmia during ablation. Ablation was generally performed in similar locations for consistency, but targeting accuracy was not directly evaluated as no specific targeting was used for lesion placement. Vital signs including electrocardiogram

(ECG), end-tidal CO_2, and peripheral capillary oxygen saturation were monitored using the Expression CMR Patient Monitor (Invivo Corp., Gainesville, Florida, USA). Peripheral pulse sensing from each animal's foot was sufficient for robust cardiac gating, and respiratory motion was frozen during imaging by pausing mechanical ventilation.

CMR imaging protocol

Imaging began immediately after catheter withdrawal (as early as 3 min after the start of ablation) to visualize the lesion near the catheter contact point. The two primary native contrast (non-contrast enhanced) imaging sequences used were alternated regularly at consistent slice locations to evaluate RF lesion temporal evolution.

T_2 mapping was performed using a previously validated T_2-prepared spiral sequence to detect regional T_2 changes near the ablation site reflecting inflamed edematous tissue (4 TEs between 3 and 184 ms, TR = 2 R-R intervals, 10 interleaves, 3072 points, FOV = 240 mm, readout bandwidth = 125 kHz, effective resolution = 1.3×1.3 mm, slice thickness = 6 mm). Images at one TE were acquired per breath-hold (approximately 16 s), and complete maps were acquired in 4 ± 2 min.

An IR-SSFP sequence generated images with various inversion times at 40 cardiac phases across 2 R-R intervals [23]. Typical acquisition parameters were: views/segment = 16, flip angle = 45°, TR/TE = 5.6/2.0 ms, readout bandwidth = 62.5 kHz, FOV = 240 mm, matrix = 192×160, and slice thickness = 6 mm. Although SSFP sequences yield best quality with shorter TRs (e.g., TR = 2.7–4 ms at 1.5 T [7, 23]), this TR was longer than ideal in this wide-bore system with lower gradient specifications. This was the shortest achievable TR while maintaining other sequence

Table 1 Summary of ablation details and imaging data

Lesion #	Location	RF power / Duration	T_2 map time span [min]	IR-SSFP time span [min]	MCLE	Gross pathology lesion diameter [mm]	Subject mode of death
1	Anterolateral wall	30 W/60 s	40–60	*	+	8.0	Arrhythmia
2	Anteroseptal wall	30 W/60 s	19–56	*	+	6.8	Euthanasia
3	Anterior wall	30 W/60 s	13–73	24–81	+	10.1	Euthanasia
4	Anterolateral wall	30 W/60 s	8–68	*	+	10.3	Euthanasia
5	Anterior wall	30 W/90 s	Not used due to artifact	33–55	–	11.8	Arrhythmia
6	Anteroseptal wall, apical	30 W/90 s	10–224	36–246	+	8.1	Arrhythmia
7	Anterolateral wall, apical	30 W/70 s	8–64	*	+	9.1	Arrhythmia
8	Anterior wall	30 W/100 s	3–172	20–184	–	11.9	Arrhythmia
9	Anterior wall	30 W/120 s	11–71	*	–	4.3	Arrhythmia
10	Anterior wall	35 W/120 s	11–127	18–132	–	7.9	Arrhythmia
11	Anterior wall	35 W/120 s	6–109	23–114	+	8.7	Euthanasia
12	Anterior wall	35 W/120 s	6–98	15–107	+	12.1	Arrhythmia
13	Anterior wall	30 W/90 s	9–171	19–184	+	7.1	Euthanasia
14	Anteroseptal wall	35 W/120 s	21–250	13–245	+	7.4	Euthanasia

Abbreviations: *IR-SSFP* inversion recovery balanced steady-state free precession, *MCLE* multi-contrast late enhancement, *RF* radiofrequency
T_2 map and IR-SSFP time spans indicate the first and last acquisitions of each type (* = lesion not clearly apparent, likely due to partial-volume effects, +/− = acquired/ not acquired). Lesions 3 and 4 were created in the same individual, likewise for lesions 6 and 7

parameters. Local shimming was performed to mitigate any off-resonance effects, and dark-band artifacts were not observed in the regions of interest.

RF ablation lesions were hyper-enhanced in IR-SSFP images due to shorter T_1 compared to the healthy myocardium [7, 24]. TIs longer than approximately 700 ms (yielding optimal contrast for lesion core visualization [7, 13, 25]) were set to occur within diastole. Image acquisition was performed at 1 slice per breath-hold (each approximately 16 s), such that 5 slices with 2 rest breaths between each slice could be acquired within 2 min. Sequence parameters were adjusted slightly to accommodate animal size and heart rate (typically 75–95 bpm).

Native-contrast imaging was repeated up to approximately 3 h post-ablation. At the end of the CMR study a bolus of Gd-DTPA (0.2 mmol/kg, Magnevist, Bayer Healthcare Pharmaceuticals, Berlin, Germany) was injected for contrast-enhanced imaging to confirm the pattern of ablation. The IR-SSFP sequence was repeated after contrast agent injection (referred to as MCLE [23]), acquired at 1 slice per breath-hold, at 6 ± 5 min post-injection. Four of 12 animals succumbed to arrhythmia before the end of the imaging study when MCLE images were to be acquired. Animals were not moved during the CMR study; therefore, all images were well aligned post-ablation (confirmed via anatomical landmarks in corresponding images).

Ex vivo examination

After the imaging study (within hours of ablation), animals were euthanized and the hearts explanted immediately, then preserved in a 10% formalin solution. Hearts were embedded in dental alginate gel and sliced to 4-mm blocks aligned to the imaging plane for gross examination and measurement of lesion dimensions. Tissue blocks were sliced to 4-μm sections and stained with Hematoxylin and Eosin (H&E) and Masson's trichrome (MT) to emphasize tissue morphological changes and viability, respectively. Slides were scanned under light microscopy (Leica SCN400 F, Leica Microsystems, Wetzlar, Germany) at 20× magnification (0.5 μm resolution) to observe features of healthy tissue, the lesion, and peripheral regions around the ablation site. Edema extent was not assessed *ex vivo* given the challenge of determining associated borders in tissue sections. CMR images were taken as a more accurate representation of the extent of edema in vivo. Observations from histopathology were qualitative in support of the image-based observations of ablation injury patterns.

Data analysis & statistics

All analysis was performed offline in MATLAB (MathWorks, Inc., Natick, Massachusetts, USA). Images were interpolated to a 256 × 256 matrix (DICOM format) before processing. T_2 maps were generated using a previously-validated 3-parameter model [26] (approximately 15 s per map using non-optimized code). Regions of edematous tissue exhibiting increased T_2 were segmented semi-automatically by applying a threshold of 3 standard deviations (SDs) above mean T_2 in healthy tissue (similarly to the approach used in a prior ablation study [27]). Morphological operations were applied to this mask to remove noise and other erroneous pixels (MATLAB Image Processing Toolbox), identify edema as contiguous regions of segmented pixels, and fill these regions while preserving borders. This semi-automatic approach was implemented to yield reproducible volumes despite the often-diffuse quality of edema, and could be performed within approximately 2 min per slice.

IR-SSFP images acquired at TIs longer than approximately 700 ms were selected for lesion segmentation, with matching contrast in subsequent acquisitions. The T_1-derived lesion volumes were segmented semi-automatically using a threshold of 2 SD above adjacent healthy myocardial signal intensity (SI), and correlated well with an expert viewer's manual delineation of lesion volumes (Pearson's $r = 0.95$, intercept $= -0.078$, slope $= 1.2$, $p < < 0.0001$; 2 SD segmented volumes larger by 0.0017 ± 0.10 mL overall; 95% limits of agreement $[-0.030, 0.033]$). Segmentation required approximately 3 min per slice.

All native T_1-weighted images and T_2 maps included in analysis were acquired in vivo. To assess temporal changes in the T_1-derived lesions and T_2-derived edema, CMR-based volume measurements were normalized to those from the initial imaging time point post-ablation. We report all post-ablation times with respect to the start of ablation, as lesion formation commences at this point. Lesion volume temporal evolution was evaluated using a linear mixed model (LMM) to account for clustering by animal and baseline differences (MATLAB Statistics Toolbox). The ratio of T_2-derived edema and T_1-derived lesion volumes was calculated to provide a direct comparison of these volumes across individual ablations at different time intervals, assessed using analysis of variance (ANOVA). T_2 evolution was assessed in three key ROIs: healthy tissue; T_1-derived lesions; and edematous regions (the largest edematous ROIs for each ablation, to examine changes in a consistent tissue region). LV wall thickness and lesion transmurality (lesion depth divided by wall thickness) were also compared at different time points.

Lesion diameters measured manually from the final in vivo IR-SSFP images acquired were compared to those from morphologically matched gross tissue slices (the gold standard for lesion formation). Lesions in MCLE images were segmented manually to compare lesion volumes derived from native-contrast and contrast-enhanced images. Both comparisons were performed using Bland-Altman analysis. All measurements are reported as the mean $\pm$ SD unless indicated otherwise, and $p < 0.05$ was considered statistically significant.

Results
RF lesion temporal evolution

The native T_1-derived lesion and T_2-derived edema were clearly visualized and reflected the characteristic teardrop shape of RF lesions observed in corresponding contrast-enhanced images, gross pathology, and histopathology (Fig. 2). Elevated T_2 indicating edema surrounding the ablation site was evident in the first T_2 maps acquired as early as 3 min after the start of ablation. T_2 maps were analyzed across 13 ablations visualized in 1–3 adjacent imaging slices in 11 animals. Each T_2-derived edematous region was visualized at 5 ± 3 (median 4) time points following ablation. These regions tended to initially appear more focal and localized to the lesion border, assuming a more diffuse appearance by later time points (Fig. 3).

The volume of T_2-derived edema was 0.77 ± 0.55 mL ($n = 13$) at the baseline measurements from the earliest T_2 maps acquired (median 10 min post-ablation). The development of edema is shown in Fig. 4, illustrating the overall increase in volume compared to baseline. Normalized edema volume increased significantly beyond baseline (LMM slope $= 0.003 \pm 0.001$, mean $\pm$ SE, $p = 0.009$, intercept $= 1.20 \pm 0.01$, $p < 0.0001$). Using this model, T_2-derived edema expanded to an estimated 1.7 ± 0.2 (mean $\pm$ SE) times the baseline volume by 180 min post-ablation. Although the overall trend indicated increasing volume, in 6/13 of T_2-derived edematous regions the volume increased then later dropped (while still remaining 1.3 ± 0.6 times larger than baseline). The maximum T_2-derived edema volume estimated across all lesions was 1.5 ± 1.0 mL. T_2-derived edema did not consistently develop concentrically around the catheter contact point.

The TIs used for T_1-derived lesion visualization using IR-SSFP were TI $= 831 \pm 150$ ms. These lesion volumes were measured in 9 lesions in 9 animals, each visualized in 1–3 adjacent imaging slices at 5 ± 2 (median 4) time points post-ablation (summarized in Fig. 5). The mean volume from the baseline IR-SSFP images was 0.48 ± 0.23 mL ($n = 9$, median 20 min post-ablation). Cumulatively, a small trend towards decreasing normalized T_1-derived lesion volume was detected up to 180 min post-ablation (LMM slope $= -0.0006 \pm 0.0003$, mean $\pm$ SE, $p = 0.09$, intercept $= 1.01 \pm 0.04$, $p < 0.0001$). Using this model, T_1-derived lesion volumes reached an estimated 0.9 ± 0.1 (mean $\pm$ SE) times the baseline volume by 180 min post-ablation.

The T_2-derived edema consistently encompassed T_1-derived lesions at individual ablation sites (Fig. 6), further supporting the distinctive tissue regions identified with each imaging contrast. The edema-lesion volume ratio was initially 2.1 ± 1.0 (0–25 min post-ablation, 95% CI [1.1, 3.0]). This ratio increased to 3.6 ± 1.1 (60–80 min; 95% CI [2.5, 4.8]), and reached 4.4 ± 3.2 (95% CI [1.1, 7.8]) by the final time interval at 80–185 min post-ablation. Although differences between intervals were not statistically significant ($p = 0.2$, ANOVA), volume ratios were greater than 1 within each interval ($p < 0.05$). The RF energy delivered did not correlate to the maximum measured T_1-derived lesion or T_2-derived edema volumes ($r = -0.2$, 0.4; $p = 0.7$, 0.2, Spearman's rho test); however, true energy

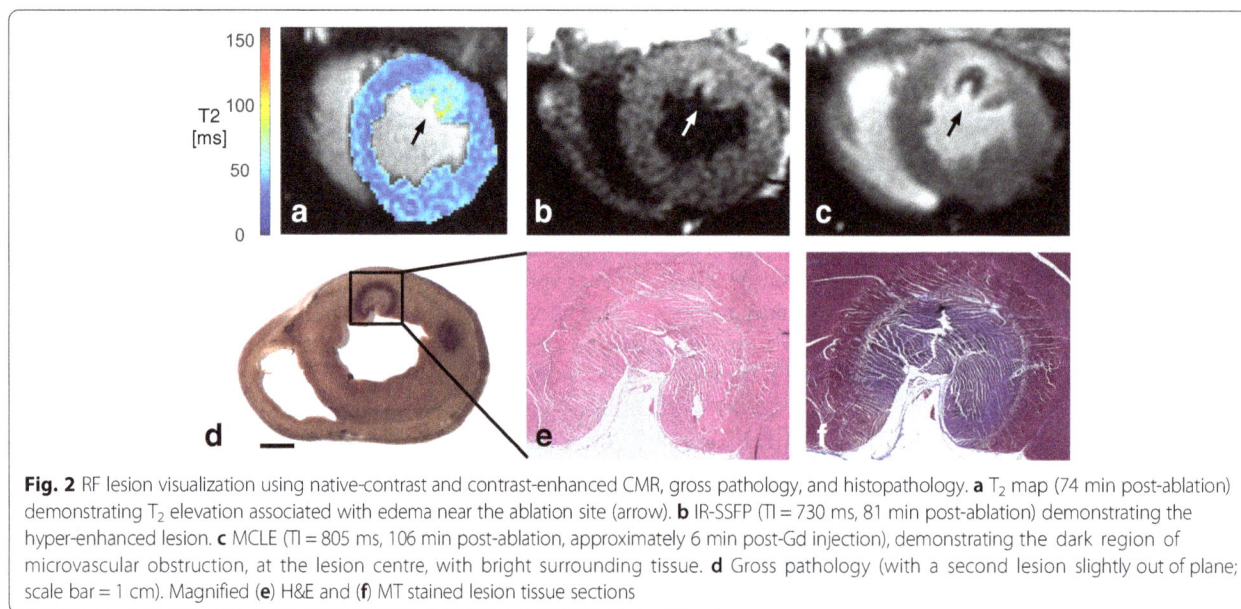

Fig. 2 RF lesion visualization using native-contrast and contrast-enhanced CMR, gross pathology, and histopathology. **a** T_2 map (74 min post-ablation) demonstrating T_2 elevation associated with edema near the ablation site (arrow). **b** IR-SSFP (TI = 730 ms, 81 min post-ablation) demonstrating the hyper-enhanced lesion. **c** MCLE (TI = 805 ms, 106 min post-ablation, approximately 6 min post-Gd injection), demonstrating the dark region of microvascular obstruction, at the lesion centre, with bright surrounding tissue. **d** Gross pathology (with a second lesion slightly out of plane; scale bar = 1 cm). Magnified (**e**) H&E and (**f**) MT stained lesion tissue sections

deposition likely varied with catheter contact force, orientation, and blood flow.

T_2 was evaluated in 3 critical regions: the T_1-derived lesion; maximum T_2-derived edematous region; and healthy tissue (Fig. 7). T_2 within the T_1-derived lesion ROIs increased between 0 and 25 min (53 ± 10 ms) and 60–80 min post-ablation (55 ± 8 ms, $p = 0.04$), then returned to the initial T_2 at 80–185 min (53 ± 7 ms, $p = 0.08$). T_2 within the largest edematous regions was significantly higher than in the T_1-derived lesions overall ($p < 0.001$) and initially increased between 0 and 25 min (53 ± 15 ms) and 60–80 min post-ablation (58 ± 13 ms, $p < 0.001$), then decreased at 80–185 min, still remaining significantly higher than baseline (56 ± 15 ms, $p < 0.001$). T_2 within both T_1-derived lesions and largest edematous

regions were significantly higher than in healthy tissue (39 ± 5 ms, $p < 0.001$), and T_2 in healthy tissue did not change significantly during corresponding time intervals ($p = 0.2$, ANOVA).

The lesions were not generally transmural. T_2-derived edema was 76 ± 18% transmural at baseline (15 ± 10 min post-ablation), reaching 79 ± 22% at final measurement (120 ± 67 min; $p = 0.9$). Similarly, transmurality of the T_1-derived lesion did not change significantly from initial measurements of 52 ± 10% (21 ± 7 min post-ablation) to 50 ± 11% (162 ± 63 min; $p = 0.3$). LV wall swelling occurred at the ablation sites between pre-ablation (8 ± 2 mm) and baseline post-ablation measurements (11 ± 2 mm; $p = 0.01$), but further swelling through to the end of the studies was not substantial (12 ± 2 mm; $p = 0.2$). Wall

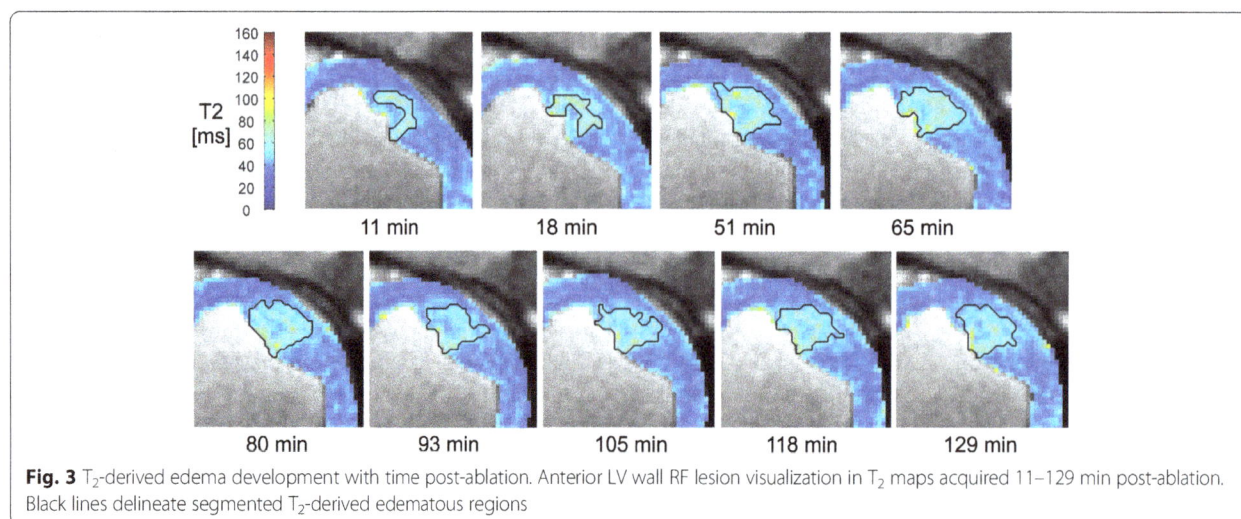

Fig. 3 T_2-derived edema development with time post-ablation. Anterior LV wall RF lesion visualization in T_2 maps acquired 11–129 min post-ablation. Black lines delineate segmented T_2-derived edematous regions

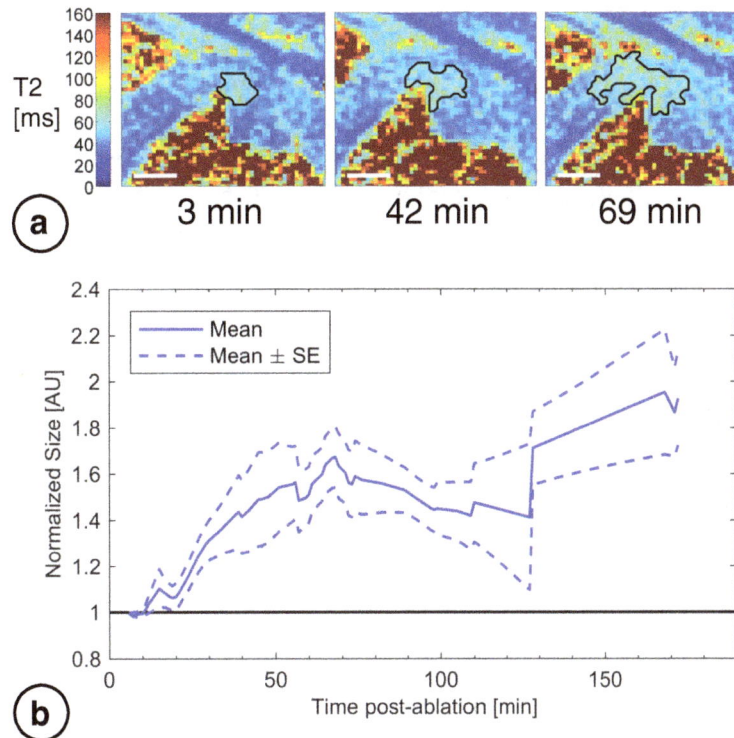

Fig. 4 Evolution in volumes of acute T_2-derived edema post-ablation. **a** Anterior wall RF lesion visualized in T_2 maps with T_2-derived edema delineated (black lines; scale bars = 1 cm). **b** Cumulative volume of T_2-derived edema normalized to baseline (the first image acquisition), with time after ablation. Interpolated data from 13 lesions were used to calculate mean and SE curves. All acquired data were used; the mean curve is shown only out to 172 min due to insufficient data beyond this point to create error bars

thickness at remote sites remained consistent with pre-ablation measurements of 9 ± 2 mm, reaching 8 ± 2 mm initially post-ablation ($p = 0.5$) and 9 ± 2 mm ($p = 0.9$) at the end of the studies.

Final pattern of ablation

MCLE validation imaging reflected the lesion geometry consistently observed in corresponding intra-procedural images (Fig. 2). The MCLE-derived lesion volumes were 0.75 ± 0.39 mL ($n = 9$), significantly larger than those measured in the corresponding final IR-SSFP acquisitions ($n = 6$; bias = 0.41 ± 0.31 mL, $p = 0.03$; 95% limits of agreement [0.08, 0.74]), and smaller than the corresponding final T_2-derived edema volumes ($n = 9$; bias = 0.45 ± 0.79 mL, $p = 0.2$; 95% limits of agreement [−0.16, 1.1]).

Lesion diameters observed in gross pathology slices and in the final IR-SSFP acquisition were well correlated ($n = 9$ lesions, Pearson's $r = 0.87$, slope = 0.9, $p = 0.003$), with a relatively small bias of 0.4 ± 1.0 mm (gross lesion diameter = 9.7 ± 2.0 mm, T_1-derived lesion diameter = 10.1 ± 2.0 mm; 95% limits of agreement [−0.41, 1.2]).

Histological characteristics of RF lesions

RF lesions exhibited the characteristic pale pink core of thermal injury bordered by a dark rim in gross pathology (Fig. 2d), also reflected in histological sections (Fig. 2e-f). Morphologic changes were emphasized using H&E (cytoplasm and extracellular matrix are stained pink, nuclei stained purple), and viability emphasized using MT (ischemic or necrotic tissue is stained purple, healthy viable myocytes red, and connective tissue blue).

The lesion core in H&E sections (Fig. 8a-b) exhibited disrupted cellular architecture consistent with thermal coagulation [28, 29] and the purple colour of the corresponding MT section (Fig. 8f) suggested non-viability of this tissue. The surrounding rim (Fig. 8c) was also distinguished by altered cellular architecture, and contained extravasated red blood cells, evidence of hemorrhage. The purple-to-red colour gradient outward from the lesion rim (Fig. 8g) suggested an increasing proportion of viable myocytes with distance from the catheter contact point. Interstitial space was increased conspicuously throughout the lesion (Fig. 8b-c) and extending beyond the lesion rim (compared to healthy tissue; Fig. 8d), consistent with observations of broad T_2-derived edematous regions.

Discussion
Main findings

Native-contrast CMR was used to construct a comprehensive description of RF lesion composition and temporal

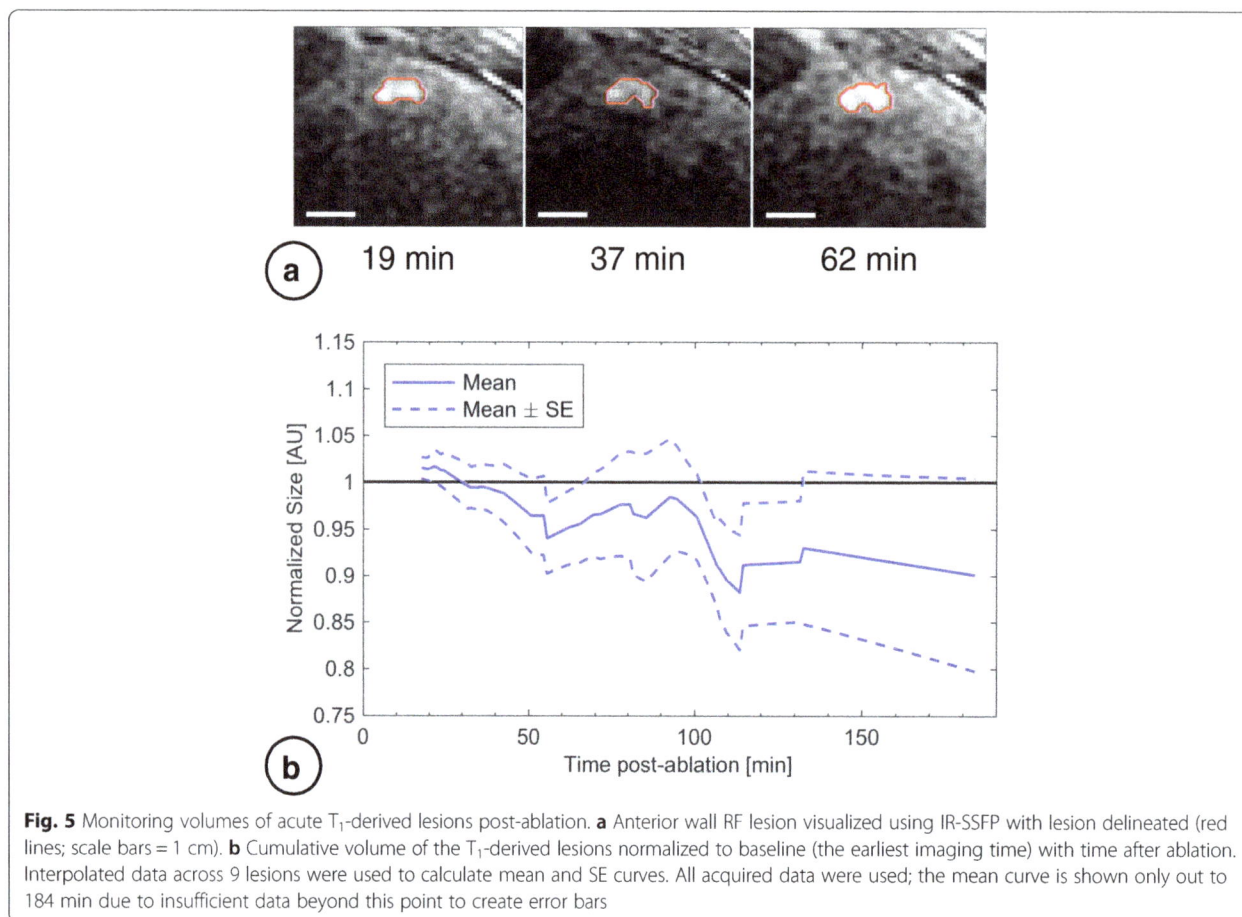

Fig. 5 Monitoring volumes of acute T_1-derived lesions post-ablation. **a** Anterior wall RF lesion visualized using IR-SSFP with lesion delineated (red lines; scale bars = 1 cm). **b** Cumulative volume of the T_1-derived lesions normalized to baseline (the earliest imaging time) with time after ablation. Interpolated data across 9 lesions were used to calculate mean and SE curves. All acquired data were used; the mean curve is shown only out to 184 min due to insufficient data beyond this point to create error bars

evolution in the LV. Intra-procedural T_1- and T_2-based imaging performed concurrently each reflect a distinctive region of tissue injury, evolving separately throughout the time period of an intervention. Acute T_1-derived lesions (thought to represent the permanent lesion) remained at a relatively stable size whereas the broader T_2-derived edema (likely transient injury) was dynamic, tended to expand over time, and consistently extended beyond T_1-derived lesions.

Lesion visualization immediately post-ablation
By performing ablation under CMR guidance, intra-procedural visualization of the T_1-derived lesions and T_2-derived edema was achieved within minutes after ablation. T_1 contrast after ablation is believed to originate from oxidation of ferrous (Fe^{2+}) to ferric (Fe^{3+}) iron associated with the transformation of hemoglobin to paramagnetic methemoglobin occurring at 55–65 °C [7, 30], and a recent study using real-time CMR thermometry during ablation showed that native T_1 contrast reflects tissue which received a lethal thermal dose [17].

The acute lesions appeared desiccated in the central core, from T_2 maps showing a zone of shorter T_2 than

the surrounding tissue (Fig. 3). Ablation-induced injury may be explained by comparison to general descriptions of thermal injury and edema pathogenesis [28, 31]. A sub-lethal thermal dose in tissue surrounding the lesion core is likely the cause of edema formation there. Microvessel permeability may be initially increased around the lesion core due to the release of biochemical factors such as histamine into injured tissue, leading to accumulation of fluid (edema).

Acute lesion evolution minutes to hours post-ablation
Native-contrast CMR facilitated repeated measurement of both the T_1-derived lesion and the T_2-derived edema to assess their acute evolution throughout the interventional procedure. The evolution of native CMR contrast is of particular importance since lesion measurements can be repeated easily at different points in the procedure, while gadolinium-enhanced studies are limited to a single injection of contrast.

The acute T_1-derived lesions appeared largely stable in volume, corroborating and extending existing studies that showed T_1-derived lesions visualized acutely had a consistent extent which corresponded well to lesions

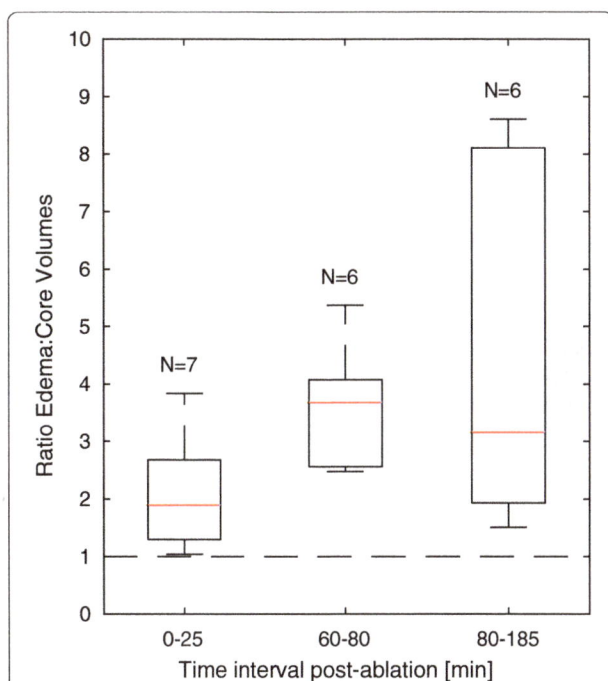

Fig. 6 Ratio of T_2-derived edema volumes to T_1-derived lesion volumes post-ablation. T_2-derived edema volume compared to T_1-derived lesion volume at corresponding time points within 3 time intervals: initial lesion measurements within 0–25 min post-ablation; lesion progression within 60–80 min; and towards the end of CMR studies within 80–185 min post-ablation

visualized hours, weeks, and months post-ablation [5, 6, 13, 17]. By combining the results from this study with the existing data on T_1-derived lesions, we suggest that the spatial extent of these lesions is established immediately after ablation, with damaged tissue later replaced by fibrotic scar. The subtle trend seen in this study toward decreasing T_1-derived lesion size with time could be explained by passive edema diffusion toward the initially

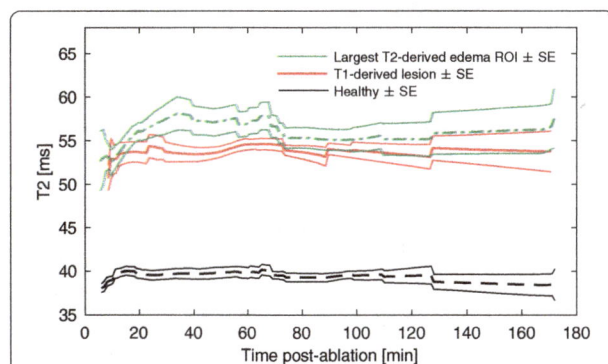

Fig. 7 Longitudinal T_2 post-ablation in healthy tissue, T_2-derived edematous regions, and T_1-derived lesions. Time course of: T_2 in healthy tissue ($n = 13$ volumes); T_2-derived edematous regions ($n = 13$); and T_1-derived lesions ($n = 8$). Traces are shown for the time course corresponding to that shown in Figs. 4 and 5

desiccated centre of the lesion, driven by reduced interstitial pressure there. Interstitial pressure changes in burned tissue are generally driven by the release of particles which drive osmotic pressure, drawing fluid into the interstitium [31]. Increasing water content would elevate local T_1, opposing the reduction of T_1 due to iron transformation.

The interstitium in thermally injured tissue tends to become more compliant, perpetuating fluid accumulation, with damage to matrix molecules such as collagen and hyaluronic acid. Increased permeability of injured microvessels leads to continued fluid leakage into the interstitial space [31]. Microvascular injury has previously been detected up to 6 mm beyond the pathological RF lesion core [29, 32], and the resulting ischemic effects likely contributed to the continuing increase in T_2-derived edematous volumes and the increasing T_2 within these regions up to approximately 60 min post-ablation (Fig. 7). The edema likely reached a stable extent once opposing interstitial and vascular pressures equalized, then later a more homogeneous fluid distribution with passive diffusion, consistent with the decreasing then stable T_2 after the initial peak seen in edematous tissue towards the end of the CMR studies.

Non-concentric edema development of the T_2-derived edema, and stable transmurality, could reflect preferential fluid spread occurring along cleavage planes between myocardial sheets, in line with LV muscle fibres that primarily run circumferentially. Beyond 120 min post-ablation, edematous regions appeared to have more diffuse borders (e.g., Fig. 3). Variable volume measurements at later time points could result from cases in which T_2 elevation at the ablation site dropped below the 3 SD threshold; intensity-based segmentation is less robust to this diffuse pattern. Despite volume variability, the T_2-derived edema volumes were still larger than immediate post-ablation dimensions (Fig. 4) and the corresponding T_1-derived lesion volumes (Fig. 6).

Prior studies using T_2-weighted CMR showed little change in edematous area beyond 3 min post-ablation [16] and that the maximum lesion SI occurred at approximately 12 min post-ablation in the right ventricle (RV) [4]. In the current study, elevated T_2 in the maximum T_2-derived edema ROIs reached a maximum at approximately 60 min post-ablation, possibly arising from a greater capacity for edema development in the LV (compared to thin-walled RV and atria), or the approach used to delineate the edema.

Study limitations & future work

The earliest T_2 map acquisition in this study was 3 min after the start of RF energy delivery, and delays typically included catheter withdrawal and waiting for any ablation-induced arrhythmia to settle. T_1-weighted image acquisition was performed at 13 min at the earliest; therefore any

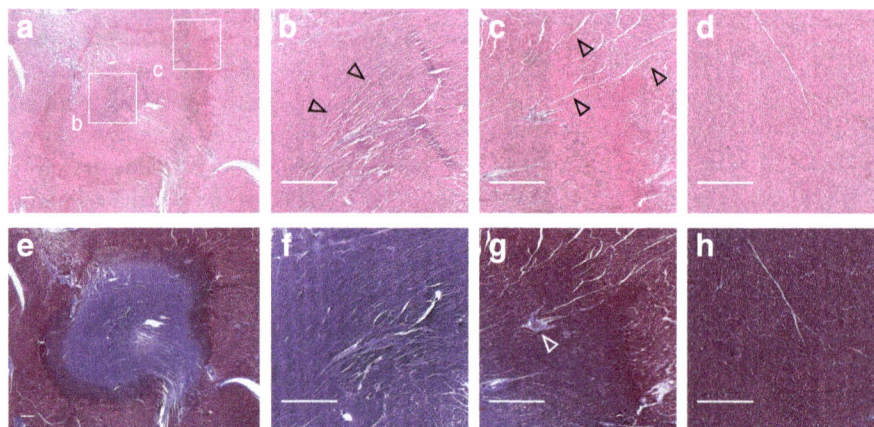

Fig. 8 Histological sections of ablated tissue. Full extent of the lesion is shown in (**a**) stained with H&E, which highlights morphologic changes. **e** Full extent of the lesion stained with MT. **b** Magnified H&E section from the lesion core, showing cells exhibiting redistribution of extra/intracellular fluids due to thermal coagulation (resulting in the darker appearance of tissue). **c** Magnified H&E section from the lesion rim. Wide interstitium (black arrowheads) is evident relative to (**d**), healthy remote tissue. **f-h** Magnified MT sections from tissue zones corresponding to the H&E panels above. In the lesion rim, panels (**c**) and (**g**), extravasated red blood cells (RBCs) and vessels containing thrombosed RBCs (white arrowhead), blocking blood flow, are evident. All scale bars = 1 mm

earlier changes among T_1-derived lesions were missed. Nevertheless, these lesions appeared consistently smaller than the T_2-derived edema, and were stable or shrinking instead of expanding for time points beyond 13 min post-ablation.

The 2D imaging sequences used in this study were appropriate to maintain relatively short scan times for concurrent imaging of the T_1-derived lesion and T_2-derived edema. We anticipate the use of 3D MCLE, a novel sequence using compressed sensing to acquire images of isotropic resolution in a single breath-hold developed for infarct characterization, in future procedures for rapid lesion assessment [33]. Moving towards a future clinical workflow, high-resolution imaging would likely be necessary for pre-ablation targeting–the importance of fine detail to describe complex re-entry circuits is well established in both interventional EP and imaging communities [34, 35]–as well as benefiting lesion assessment, as seen recently [13].

The pro-arrhythmic potential of tissue containing mixed viable and non-viable myocytes and potentially microvascular injury near the periphery of RF lesions was not investigated. However, prior work showed chronic lesions resembling well-circumscribed scar [6], a pattern associated with lower arrhythmogenic potential than heterogeneous scar. The potential for pro-arrhythmia is likely greater in healthy tissue, as was the case in the healthy swine model used for this study. Practically, in the presence of infarcted tissue (as is typical for VT in structural heart disease), lesion pro-arrhythmia may have a small effect since areas ablated are likely to be already ischemic and surrounded by chronic fibrotic tissue. Investigating the properties of ablations on or adjacent to infarcted tissue would build on promising recent results [13] and is an important direction for future studies. In ongoing CMR-based lesion assessment studies, we are also investigating the effect of ablation on the functional properties of local myocardial tissue [36], extending previous studies of infarcted tissue [37].

CMR-based intra-procedural lesion assessment
Native-contrast CMR imaging reflects ablation-induced tissue changes and facilitates consistent lesion assessment throughout MR-guided ablation. Considering the complexity of the arrhythmogenic substrate, lesion assessment should be repeatable when convenient for the interventionalist, supporting an iterative treatment approach.

Patients undergoing ablation for structural heart disease often exhibit multiple arrhythmia morphologies, suggestive of multiple re-entry circuits. CMR-based lesion assessment could be performed after delivering several ablations towards blocking a target re-entry circuit. Intermittent imaging exams and analysis would require 10–20 min to perform using the techniques employed in the current study (with segmentation not fully optimized for speed).

One proposed workflow for future clinical cases could involve identifying re-entry circuits in prior CMR-derived maps of scar and EP mapping, then delivering several ablations at a re-entry circuit while relying on EP data. T_1-weighted CMR could be used to visualize a series of lesions created at the re-entry circuit. We suggest that ablation while incorporating this feedback should aim to produce lesions which appear continuous using T_1-weighted imaging. Based on these T_1-weighted images, remaining gaps identified at the re-entry circuit would clearly indicate that further ablation is needed, potentially constituting an additional procedural endpoint. T_2 mapping could be used to interpret possibly discordant EP measures of procedural success, but should not be used alone for lesion assessment as the T_2-derived edema likely reflects transient injury not contributing to long-term procedural success.

RF lesions could be visualized with the catheter held in place if lesions extend beyond the minimal artifact at the catheter tip, and others have proposed imaging and hardware based solutions for interventions [38, 39]. Catheter withdrawal before imaging (as in this study) may introduce challenges by causing the interventionalist to lose the catheter's position at the ablation site such that it would need to be directed back precisely for further ablations.

Conscious patients under light sedation may be able to perform breath-holds during intra-procedural CMR imaging, but for those unable, existing respiratory-navigated or real-time sequences could be adapted for lesion imaging [40]. Rapid intra-procedural registration of lesion images to prior scar maps would be needed to provide useful feedback to the interventionalist.

Finally, contrast-enhanced imaging should be reserved to confirm the pattern of ablation at the true completion of the procedure. An alternative sequence recently proposed visualizes both scar and RF lesions with native T_1 contrast [13]. For either approach, high-resolution coverage of an extended region of the heart, after ablating multiple re-entry circuits, would require a respiratory-navigated acquisition of about 10–20 min. The timing of this acquisition after contrast-agent injection should also be chosen carefully given known contrast agent kinetics.

Clinical implications

Comprehensive understanding of acute lesion composition and evolution could be applied to both CMR-guided and non-CMR-guided ablation cases. In general, operators should be cognizant of the dynamic nature of edema, which could cause the acute appearance of a successful ablation procedure. The evolving, broad extent of T_2-derived edema may mask the smaller T_1-derived lesions (specifically indicated by the ratio of these volumes) which are thought to reflect true procedural success. T_1-based imaging could potentially constitute an additional procedural endpoint. CMR-based lesion assessment could make a critical difference in scenarios where re-entry circuits appear to be blocked, for instance with more transmural T_2-derived edema injuring deep epicardial re-entry circuits not reached by the T_1-derived lesion. These findings may be used to help explain mechanisms of arrhythmia recurrence after acutely successful appearing procedures.

Conclusions

Native T_1- and T_2-based imaging performed concurrently throughout CMR-guided ablations demonstrated

that acute T_1-derived lesions remained at a stable size while the T_2-derived edema was dynamic, expanded over time, and consistently extended beyond the T_1-derived lesion. T_2 quantification provides an unambiguous measure of edema development and severity near ablation sites. Lesion evolution is important for comparing CMR lesion visualization and EP-based endpoints, data which may be acquired at disparate time points. Integrated information on the T_1-derived lesion and T_2-derived edema provides a description of acute lesion composition that could be most useful during ablation procedures.

Abbreviations
ANOVA: Analysis of variance; bpm: Beats per minute; bSSFP: balanced steady state free precession; CMR: cardiovascular magnetic resonance; DSC: dice similarity coefficient; EGM: electrogram; EP: electrophysiology; FOV: field of view; fps: frames per second; H&E: Hematoxylin and Eosin; IR-SSFP: Inversion-recovery balanced steady-state free precession; LMM: linear mixed model; LV: left ventricle/left ventricular; MCLE: multi-contrast late enhancement; MT: Masson's Trichrome; ROI: region of interest; RV: right ventricle/right ventricular; SD: standard deviation; SE: standard error; SI: signal intensity; TE: echo time; TI: inversion time; TR: repetition time; VT: ventricular tachycardia

Acknowledgements
The authors sincerely thank Dr. Nilesh Ghugre for insights on image analysis and relaxometry, Sebastian Ferguson for assistance in CMR-guided ablation studies, Dr. Alex Kiss for helpful discussions on statistical methods, and Adebayo Adeeko and Taha Rashed for histopathology processing.

Funding
Funding provided by Ontario Graduate Scholarships, Imricor Medical Systems, the Federal Development Agency of Canada, and the Canadian Institute of Health Research (grant MOP-93531) are gratefully acknowledged.

Authors' contributions
PRPK: CMR-guided ablation, data analysis, drafted manuscript. SMS: critically reviewed the manuscript. VR: CMR protocol development, image acquisition, and interpretation. LB: image processing for guidance during interventions. NY: managed hardware. KA: managed hardware and device tracking sequences. JB: prepared and monitored animals, performed catheter manipulation. MP: guided study design, data interpretation, critically reviewed the manuscript. GAW: guided study design, data analysis and interpretation, critically reviewed the manuscript. All authors have read and approved the final manuscript.

Competing interests
This work was supported in part by Imricor Medical Systems and the authors report a pending patent related to RF lesion characterization using T_1-weighted CMR imaging. The authors declare no other competing interests.

Author details
[1]Department of Medical Biophysics, University of Toronto, Toronto, ON, Canada. [2]Sunnybrook Research Institute, Toronto, ON, Canada. [3]Schulich Heart Research Program, Sunnybrook Research Institute, Toronto, ON, Canada. [4]Division of Cardiology, Schulich Heart Centre, Sunnybrook Health Sciences Centre, Toronto, ON, Canada. [5]Faculty of Medicine, University of Toronto, Toronto, ON, Canada.

References

1. Palaniswamy C, Kolte D, Harikrishnan P, Khera S, Aronow WS, Mujib M, et al. Catheter ablation of postinfarction ventricular tachycardia: ten-year trends in utilization, in-hospital complications, and in-hospital mortality in the United States. Heart Rhythm. 2014;11:2056–63.
2. Mallidi J, Nadkarni GN, Berger RD, Calkins H, Nazarian S. Meta-analysis of catheter ablation as an adjunct to medical therapy for treatment of ventricular tachycardia in patients with structural heart disease. Heart Rhythm. 2011;8:503–10.
3. D'Avila A, Singh SM. Ventricular tachycardia ablation: are we winning the battle but losing the war? J Am Coll Cardiol. 2016;67:684–6.
4. Lardo AC, McVeigh ER, Jumrussirikul P, Berger RD, Calkins H, Lima J, et al. Visualization and temporal/spatial characterization of cardiac radiofrequency ablation lesions using magnetic resonance imaging. Circulation. 2000;102:698–705.
5. Dickfeld T, Kato R, Zviman M, Nazarian S, Dong J, Ashikaga H, et al. Characterization of acute and subacute radiofrequency ablation lesions with non-enhanced magnetic resonance imaging. Heart Rhythm. 2007;4:208–14.
6. Kholmovski EG, Ranjan R, Vijayakumar S, Silvernagel JM, Marrouche NF. Acute Assessment of Radiofrequency Ablation Cardiac Lesions by Non-Contrast MRI. In: Proc. ISMRM, 22nd Annual Meeting. Milan; 2014.
7. Celik H, Ramanan V, Barry J, Ghate S, Leber V, Oduneye S, et al. Intrinsic contrast for characterization of acute radiofrequency ablation lesions. Circ Arrhythmia Electrophysiol. 2014;7:718–27.
8. Arujuna A, Karim R, Caulfield D, Knowles B, Rhode K, Schaeffter T, et al. Acute pulmonary vein isolation is achieved by a combination of reversible and irreversible atrial injury after catheter ablation. Circ Arrhythmia Electrophysiol. 2012;5:691–700.
9. Yamada T, Murakami Y, Okada T, Okamoto M, Shimizu T, Toyama J, et al. Incidence, location, and cause of recovery of electrical connections between the pulmonary veins and the left atrium after pulmonary vein isolation. Europace. 2006;8:182–8.
10. Knowles BR, Caulfield D, Cooklin M, Rinaldi CA, Gill J, Bostock J, et al. 3-D visualization of acute RF ablation lesions using MRI for the simultaneous determination of the patterns of necrosis and edema. IEEE TBME. 2010;57:1467–75.
11. Ranjan R, Kato R, Zviman MM, Dickfeld TM, Roguin A, Berger RD, et al. Gaps in the ablation line as a potential cause of recovery from electrical isolation and their visualization using MRI. Circ Arrhythm Electrophysiol. 2011;4:279–86.
12. Piers SRD, Tao Q, De Riva Silva M, Siebelink HM, Schalij MJ, Van Der Geest RJ, et al. CMR-based identification of critical isthmus sites of ischemic and nonischemic ventricular tachycardia. JACC Cardiovasc Imaging. 2014;7:774–84.
13. Guttman MA, Tao S, Fink S, Kolandaivelu A, Halperin HR, Herzka DA. Non-contrast-enhanced T1-weighted MRI of myocardial radiofrequency ablation lesions. Magn Reson Med. 2017;0:1–11.
14. Rassa AC, Kholmovski E, Suksaranjit P, Wilson BD, Akoum N, Marrouche N, et al. Dynamic T2 signal changes on MRI after radiofrequency ablation injury to the atrial myocardium. J Clin Trials Cardiol. 2015;2:1–5.
15. Vergara GR, Vijayakumar S, Kholmovski EG, Blauer JJE, Guttman MA, Gloschat C, et al. Real-time magnetic resonance imaging-guided radiofrequency atrial ablation and visualization of lesion formation at 3 tesla. Heart Rhythm. 2011;8:295–303.
16. Nordbeck P, Hiller KH, Fidler F, Warmuth M, Burkard N, Nahrendorf M, et al. Feasibility of contrast-enhanced and nonenhanced MRI for intraprocedural and postprocedural lesion visualization in interventional electrophysiology: animal studies and early delineation of isthmus ablation lesions in patients with typical atrial flutter. Circ Cardiovasc Imaging. 2011;4:282–94.
17. Toupin S, Bour P, Lepetit-Coiffé M, Ozenne V, Denis de Senneville B, Schneider R, et al. Feasibility of real-time MR thermal dose mapping for predicting radiofrequency ablation outcome in the myocardium in vivo. J Cardiovasc Magn Reson. 2017;19:14.
18. Higgins CB, Herfkens R, Lipton MJ, Sievers R, Sheldon P, Kaufman L, et al. Nuclear magnetic resonance imaging of acute myocardial infarction in dogs: alterations in magnetic relaxation times. Am J Cardiol. 1983;52:184–8.
19. Dickfeld T, Kato R, Zviman M, Lai S, Meininger G, Lardo AC, et al. Characterization of radiofrequency ablation lesions with gadolinium-enhanced cardiovascular magnetic resonance imaging. J Am Coll Cardiol. 2006;47:370–8.
20. Oduneye SO, Biswas L, Ghate S, Ramanan V, Barry J, Laish-FarKash A, et al. The feasibility of endocardial propagation mapping using magnetic resonance guidance in a swine model, and comparison with standard electroanatomic mapping. IEEE TMI. 2012;31:977–83.
21. Dumoulin CL, Souza SP, Darrow RD. Real-time position monitoring of invasive devices using magnetic resonance. Magn Reson Med. 1993;29:411–5.
22. Radau PE, Pintilie S, Flor R, Biswas L, Oduneye SO, Ramanan V, et al. VURTIGO: visualization platform for real-time, MRI-guided cardiac Electroanatomic mapping. Lect Notes Comput Sci. 2012;7085:244–53.
23. Detsky JS, Stainsby JA, Vijayaraghavan R, Graham JJ, Dick AJ, Wright GA. Inversion-recovery-prepared SSFP for cardiac-phase-resolved delayed-enhancement MRI. Magn Reson Med. 2007;58:365–72.
24. Herzka DA, Tao S, Fink S, Kolandaivelu A, Guttman MA, Halperin H. Assessment of RF ablation lesions with T1 mapping. In: 20th annual SCMR scientific sessions; 2017. p. 203.
25. Krahn P, Ramanan V, Biswas L, Yak N, Anderson K, Barry J, et al. Intrinsic MR visualization of RF lesions after RF ablation for ventricular arrhythmia. In: Proc. ISMRM, 24th Annual Meeting. Singapore; 2016.
26. Ghugre NR, Enriquez CM, Gonzalez I, Nelson MD, Coates TD, Wood JC. MRI detects myocardial iron in the human heart. Magn Reson Med. 2006;56:681–6.
27. Chubb H, Harrison JL, Weiss S, Krueger S, Koken P, Bloch LØ, et al. Development, pre-clinical validation, and clinical translation of a cardiac magnetic resonance-electrophysiology system with active catheter tracking for ablation of cardiac arrhythmia. JACC Clin Electrophysiol. 2017;3:89–103.
28. Thomsen S. Mapping of thermal injury in biologic tissues using quantitative pathologic techniques. In: proceedings of thermal treatment of tissue with image guidance. San Jose, California: SPIE; 1999. p. 82–95.
29. Nath S, Redick JA, Whayne JG, Haines DE. Ultrastructural observations in the myocardium beyond the region of acute coagulation necrosis following radiofrequency catheter ablation. J Cardiovasc Electrophysiol. 1994;5:838–45.
30. Farahani K, Saxton RE, Yoon H-C, De Salles AAF, Black KL, Lufkin RB. MRI of thermally denatured blood: methemoglobin formation and relaxation effects. Magn Reson Imaging. 1999;17:1489–94.
31. Demling RH. The burn edema process: current concepts. J Burn Care Rehabil. 2005;26:207–27.
32. Nath S, Whayne JG, Kaul S, Goodman NC, Jayaweera a R, Haines DE. Effects of radiofrequency catheter ablation on regional myocardial blood flow. Possible mechanism for late electrophysiological outcome. Circulation. 1994;89:2667–72.
33. Zhang L, Athavale P, Pop M, Wright GA. Multicontrast reconstruction using compressed sensing with low rank and spatially varying edge-preserving constraints for high-resolution MR characterization of myocardial infarction. Magn Reson Med. 2017;78:598–610.
34. Pop M, Ramanan V, Yang F, Zhang L, Newbigging S, Ghugre NR, et al. High-resolution 3-D T1*-mapping and quantitative image analysis of GRAY ZONE in chronic fibrosis. IEEE TBME. 2014;61:2930–8.
35. Ashikaga H, Sasano T, Dong J, Zviman MM, Evers R, Hopenfeld B, et al. Magnetic resonance-based anatomical analysis of scar-related ventricular tachycardia: implications for catheter ablation. Circ Res. 2007;101:939–47.
36. Krahn P, Ramanan V, Biswas L, Yak N, Anderson K, Barry J, et al. MRI-based myocardial ablation lesion extent relates to area of voltage reduction in MR-guided electroanatomical voltage maps. In: Proc. ISMRM, 25th Annual Meeting. Honolulu; 2017.
37. Oduneye SO, Pop M, Shurrab M, Biswas L, Ramanan V, Barry J, et al. Distribution of abnormal potentials in chronic myocardial infarction using a real time magnetic resonance guided electrophysiology system. J Cardiovasc Magn Reson. 2015;17:1–9.
38. Daniel BL, Butts K. The use of view angle tilting to reduce distortions in magnetic resonance imaging of cryosurgery. Magn Reson Imaging. 2000;18:281–6.
39. Dominguez-Viqueira W, Karimi H, Lam WW, Cunningham CH. A controllable susceptibility marker for passive device tracking. Magn Reson Med. 2014;72:269–75.
40. Detsky JS, Graham JJ, Vijayaraghavan R, Biswas L, Stainsby JA, Guttman MA, et al. Free-breathing, nongated real-time enhancement MRI of myocardial infarcts: a comparison with conventional delayed enhancement. J Magn Reson Imaging. 2008;28:621–5.
41. Lu Y, Radau P, Connelly K, Dick A, Wright GA. Segmentation of left ventricle in cardiac Cine MRI: an automatic image-driven method. Lect Notes Comput Sci. 2009;5528:339–47.

7

Prognostic value of myocardial strain and late gadolinium enhancement on cardiovascular magnetic resonance imaging in patients with idiopathic dilated cardiomyopathy with moderate to severely reduced ejection fraction

Seung-Hoon Pi[1†], Sung Mok Kim[2†], Jin-Oh Choi[1*] ⓘ, Eun Kyoung Kim[1], Sung-A Chang[1], Yeon Hyeon Choe[2], Sang-Chol Lee[1] and Eun-Seok Jeon[1]

Abstract

Background: It has been reported that left ventricular (LV) myocardial strain and late gadolinium enhancement (LGE) on cardiovascular magnetic resonance (CMR) imaging have prognostic value in patients with heart failure (HF). However, previous studies included patients with various systolic functions. This study aimed to investigate the prognostic value of LV myocardial strain and LGE on CMR imaging in patients with idiopathic dilated cardiomyopathy (DCM) with reduced ejection fraction (EF < 40%).

Methods: From a prospectively followed cohort who underwent CMR between November 2008 and December 2015, subjects with LV EF < 40% and a diagnosis of idiopathic DCM were eligible for this study. The CMR images were analyzed for LV and right ventricular (RV) function, presence and extent of LGE, and LV myocardial strain. The primary outcome was a composite of all-cause death and heart transplantation. The secondary outcome was hospitalization for HF.

Results: A total of 172 patients were included, in whom mean LV EF was 23.7 ± 7.9% (EF 30–40% n = 47; EF < 30% n = 125). During a median follow-up of 47 months, the primary outcome occurred in 43 patients (16 heart transplantations, 29 all-cause deaths), and there were 41 hospitalizations for HF. Univariate Cox proportional hazard regression analysis showed that mean arterial pressure, serum sodium concentration, log of plasma NT-proBNP level, and presence of LGE (HR 2.277, 95% CI: 1.221–4.246) were significantly associated with the primary outcome. However, LV strain had no significant association (HR 1.048, 95% CI: 0.945–1.163). Multivariable analysis showed that presence of LGE (HR 4.73, 95% CI: 1.11–20.12) and serum sodium (HR 0.823, 95% CI: 0.762–0.887) were independently associated with the primary outcome.

(Continued on next page)

* Correspondence: choijean5@gmail.com
†Seung-Hoon Pi and Sung Mok Kim contributed equally to this work.
[1]Department of Internal Medicine, Heart Vascular Stroke Institute, Samsung Medical Center, Sungkyunkwan University School of Medicine, 81 Irwon-ro, Gangnam-gu, Seoul 06351, Republic of Korea
Full list of author information is available at the end of the article

(Continued from previous page)

Conclusions: LGE in CMR imaging was a good predictor of adverse outcomes for patients with idiopathic DCM and reduced EF. Identification of LGE could thus improve risk stratification in high-risk patients. LV strain had no significant prognostic value in patients with moderate to severe systolic dysfunction.

Keywords: Cardiovascular magnetic resonance imaging, Myocardial strain, Prognosis, Late gadolinium enhancement, Idiopathic dilated cardiomyopathy

Background

Idiopathic dilated cardiomyopathy (DCM) accounts for a substantial proportion of heart failure (HF) cases [1, 2]. It is associated with significant morbidity and mortality due to HF and sudden cardiac death [3–5]. Although several factors in patients with HF [6–15] are associated with an adverse prognosis, risk stratification remains challenging. Therefore, better tools are needed for risk stratification in order to guide individualized treatment strategies and patient surveillance.

Cardiovascular magnetic resonance (CMR) imaging has become recognized as the gold standard for assessment of cardiac function and mass [16, 17], and it can be used to distinguish the etiology of HF [18, 19]. Additionally, it has been reported that the appearance of late gadolinium enhancement (LGE) [20–23] and left ventricular (LV) myocardial strain in CMR imaging [24] have prognostic value in patients with non-ischemic DCM. However, those studies included patients with various systolic functions.

Therefore, we investigated the prognostic value of LV myocardial strain and LGE in the CMR images of patients with idiopathic DCM with reduced ejection fraction (EF).

Methods

Study population

From a prospectively followed cohort who underwent CMR at Samsung Medical Center, Seoul, Korea, between November 2008 and December 2015, subjects whose LV EF was less than 40% were eligible for this study (n = 441). Medical records were reviewed, and those from patients with an LV EF less than 40% who had been diagnosed previously with idiopathic DCM were evaluated. The diagnosis of DCM was made according to the criteria of the World Health Organization/International Society and Federation of Cardiology [25]. Patients had to exhibit dilatation and impaired contraction of the LV or both ventricles in the absence of valvular disease, hypertensive heart disease, and congenital abnormalities. The possibility of ischemic heart disease was excluded by invasive x-ray coronary angiography or non-invasive testing such as coronary computed tomography angiography (defined as ≥50% luminal stenosis) [24] or CMR itself (subendocardial or transmural pattern of LGE

suggestive of previous myocardial infarction) [18], according to each physician's clinical decision.

Of all potentially eligible patients (n = 441), pediatric patients (n = 20) and 154 patients with ischemic heart disease, constrictive pericarditis, tachycardia-induced cardiomyopathy, cardiomyopathy due to endocrine dysfunction, cardiomyopathy due to infection with the human immunodeficiency virus, stress induced cardiomyopathy, infiltrative myocardial disease, hypertensive heart disease, cardiomyopathy due to systemic auto-immune disease, alcoholic cardiomyopathy, cardiomyopathy related to chemotherapeutic agents, restrictive cardiomyopathy, significant organic valvular disease, or hypertrophic cardiomyopathy were excluded. Of 267 patients with a diagnosis of idiopathic DCM, we excluded 95 because their CMR images were inappropriate for strain measurement, resulting in a final sample size of 172 patients (Fig. 1). This study and all of its analyses were approved by the Institutional Review Board of Samsung Medical Center which waived written informed consent.

CMR image acquisition

All subjects underwent CMR in a 1.5 T scanner (Magnetom Avanto, Syngo MR B17 version; Siemens Healthineers, Erlangen, Germany) with a 32-channel phased-array receiver coil. CMR scans consisted of localizing images (axial, coronal, and sagittal), cine scans, and LGE scans. After localization, cine images of the LV were acquired using a balanced steady-state free-precession sequence in the 4-, 3-, and 2-chamber and short axis views to obtain contiguous slices that included the entire LV, with a 6-mm slice thickness and 4-mm intersection gaps. At each level, cine images were composed of 30 phases per cardiac cycle. Cine images were obtained during multiple breath-holds. LGE imaging was acquired using a phase-sensitive inversion recovery technique 10 min after injection of 0.2 mmol/kg gadobutrol (Gadovist; Bayer Healthcare, Berlin, Germany) at a rate of 3 ml/ sec, followed by a 30-ml saline flush. Contiguous short-axis image acquisition of 10–12 slices was used, with 6 mm thickness and a 4-mm interslice gap. Inversion delay times were typically 280–360 msec.

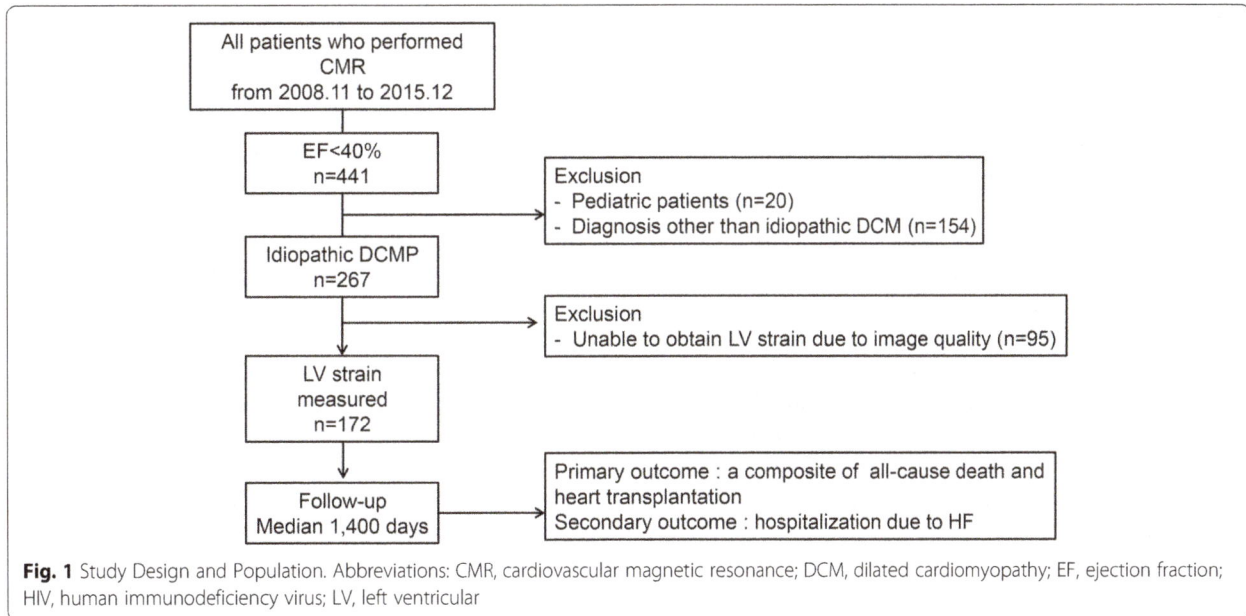

Fig. 1 Study Design and Population. Abbreviations: CMR, cardiovascular magnetic resonance; DCM, dilated cardiomyopathy; EF, ejection fraction; HIV, human immunodeficiency virus; LV, left ventricular

LV myocardial strain analysis

CMR tissue tracking analyses were performed using commercially available software (cvi42 version 5, Circle Cardiovascular Imaging Inc., Calgary, Alberta, Canada). Two-, three-, and four-chamber and short axis images were uploaded into the software, which reconstructs a 3D model that we used to analyze 2D-radial, circumferential, and longitudinal LV strain. The preferred images were loaded into the analysis/viewer frame of the software and analyzed in random order by two investigators (SHP with 1 year and JWH with 3 years of CMR experience) who were independently blinded to the clinical findings. Tissue tracking analysis was manually performed by drawing the endo- and epicardial surfaces in end-diastolic phase (reference phase) using short axis stacked slices (Fig. 2). A short axis reference point was manually delineated at the right ventricle (RV) upper and lower septal insertion of the LV for regional and global analysis of strain and the generation of polar map views. Next, the software automatically drew the contour and traced its myocardium voxel points throughout the remainder of the cardiac cycle. The algorithm

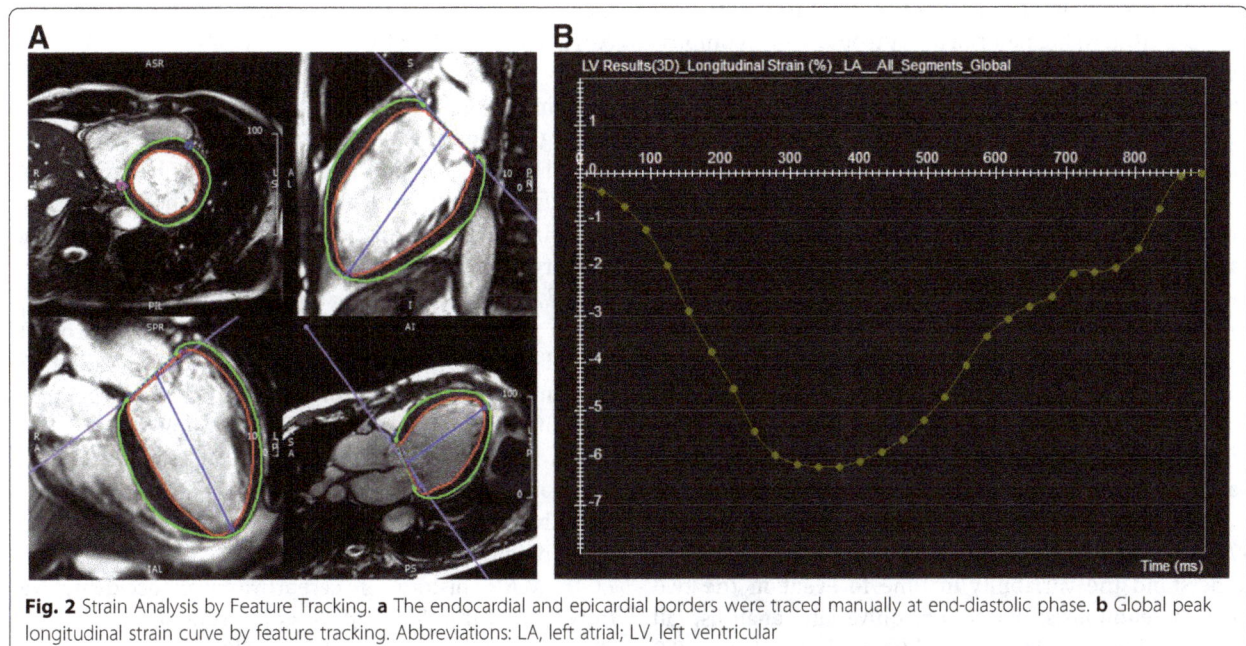

Fig. 2 Strain Analysis by Feature Tracking. **a** The endocardial and epicardial borders were traced manually at end-diastolic phase. **b** Global peak longitudinal strain curve by feature tracking. Abbreviations: LA, left atrial; LV, left ventricular

determined and depicted the left borders of the LV myo-cardium in the following phases of a cardiac cycle based on the endo- and epicardial contours of the reference phase. The software automatically performed 2D strain analyses of all slices.

The routine cine images of 172 patients included for strain analysis consist of 30 images per cardiac cycle. Those images were acquired using retrospective (electro-cardiogram (ECG)-gated, multi-breathhold technique. The patients excluded from the analyses for strain underwent different scan technique using single-breathhold method for obtaining cine images be-cause of arrhythmia or lack of breath-hold. Because of this, the number of image frames was variable (10~24 images), so the temporal resolution was also different and we could not perform the analysis of LV strain.

LGE measurement

The presence and extent of LGE were evaluated by one observer experienced in LGE-CMR, who was blinded to clinical data and outcomes. For quantification of fibrosis, LGE was defined as areas with a signal intensity >6SD [26, 27] above the mean signal intensity of remote myo-cardium in the same short-axis slice using commercial software (CAAS MRV version 1.0, Pie Medical Imaging B.V., Maastricht, The Netherlands). Areas are expressed as mass and percentage of myocardial mass.

Follow-up and endpoints

All patients were followed by medical record review. Vital status was cross-checked in all of the patients using National Insurance data from the Korean government, which contain unique identifiers for the patients [28]. The median follow-up duration was 1400 days (Q1–Q3: 770 to 2210 days). The primary outcome was a compos-ite of all-cause death and heart transplantation. The sec-ondary outcome was first hospitalization due to HF.

Statistical analysis

Categorical variables are presented as numbers and relative frequencies (percentages), and continuous variables as means and standard deviations or medians with interquartile ranges (Q1–Q3), according to their distribution, which was checked using the Kolmogorov-Smirnov test. Categorical variables were compared using chi-square tests, and continuous vari-ables were compared using Student's t-test or analysis of variance. Cumulative events rates were calculated based on Kaplan-Meier censoring estimates, and the log-rank test was used to compare survival curves. We proceeded with multiple Cox regression model to understand the variability in time to event in the two primary endpoints. Based on univariate analysis, all demographic or clinical variables with p-values < 0.2

were initially considered to enter the model. Then, we eliminated insignificant variables ($p > 0.05$) one by one to obtain a robust and parsimonious model for prediction. We verified the model assumption of pro-portional hazards via Schoenfeld residuals. When the assumption fails, we attempted accommodating time-dependent covariates and stratified analyses. As a measure of goodness of the prediction model, we obtained the Harrel's c-index. Pearson correlation coeffi-cient was calculated to assess the correlation between LVEF and LV myocardial strains. Inter- and intra-observer variabilities for strain values were assessed by the repeated analysis of 30 randomly selected patients. Statistical analyses were performed using SAS version 9.3 (SAS Institute, Cary, North Carolina, USA), and SPSS (version 19.0, International Business Machines, Armonk, New York, USA). P-values < 0.05 (2-sided) were considered statistically significant.

Results

Baseline characteristics

The baseline clinical characteristics and CMR variables of all 172 patients are summarized in Tables 1 and 2. Also these data of those who were excluded from and included in the strain analysis was presented in the Additional file 1: Tables S1 and S2. There was no signifi-cant difference between 95 excluded and 172 included patients except gender, presence of LBBB, LV myocardial mass. There was no difference in the presence of LGE between the two groups. Mean LV EF of the study sub-jects was 23.7 ± 7.9% (EF 30–40% $n = 47$; EF < 30% $n = 125$) and LGE was observed in 66 (38.2%) patients. The Pearson correlation coefficients between LV EF and GLS, GCS, and GRS were – 0.733 ($P < 0.01$), – 0.780 ($P < 0.01$), and 0.739 ($P < 0.01$).

Outcomes

During the follow-up period, the primary outcome oc-curred in 43 patients (16 heart transplantations, 29 all-cause deaths), and there were 41 hospitalizations for HF. Between patients with and without the primary outcome, significant differences were ob-served in terms of mean arterial pressure (MAP), serum sodium (sNa), log transformed NT-proBNP [ln(NT-proBNP)], and presence of LGE. Regarding LV myocardial strain, none of the systolic strain parame-ters differed significantly between groups.

Survival analysis

By univariate analysis, the following clinical parameters were predictors of the primary outcome: presence of LGE, MAP, history of cerebrovascular accident, Na, ln(NT-proBNP), RV end-diastolic volume (EDV), and RV end-systolic volume (ESV). The presence of LGE,

Table 1 Baseline characteristics and CMR parameters for patients with and without the primary outcome

Parameters	All patients (n = 172)	Patients without the primary outcome (n = 129)	Patients with the primary outcome (n = 43)	P value
Age (years)	56.4 ± 14.3	57.0 ± 14.6	54.8 ± 13.5	0.398
Male gender, n (%)	116 (67.4)	85 (65.9)	31 (72.1)	0.452
Mean arterial pressure (mmHg)	84 ± 13	86 ± 13	80 ± 12	0.015
Hypertension, n (%)	58 (33.7)	44 (34.1)	14 (32.6)	0.852
Diabetes mellitus, n (%)	36 (20.9)	25 (19.4)	11 (25.6)	0.387
Dyslipidemia, n (%)	11 (6.4)	8 (6.2)	3 (7.0)	0.857
Current smoker, n (%)	49 (28.5)	37 (28.7)	12 (27.9)	0.734
Chronic kidney disease[a], n (%)	31 (18.0)	21 (16.3)	10 (23.3)	0.303
Previous CVA, n (%)	4 (2.3)	1 (0.8)	3 (7.0)	0.049
Body mass index (kg/m^2)	24.0 ± 4.5	24.2 ± 4.5	23.5 ± 4.4	0.347
ECG at baseline				
Heart rate (bpm)	83 ± 20	84 ± 19	83 ± 22	0.883
Left bundle-branch block, n (%)	31 (18.0)	23 (17.8)	8 (19.0)	0.859
QRS duration (ms)	113 ± 29	112 ± 30	117 ± 29	0.305
Laboratory data				
Serum creatinine (mg/dl)	0.97 ± 0.27	0.96 ± 0.25	1.01 ± 0.31	0.247
Na (mmol/l)	139.6 ± 3.3	140.2 ± 2.8	137.6 ± 3.8	< 0.001
ln(NT-proBNP) (pg/ml)	7.22 ± 1.27	7.08 ± 1.29	7.60 ± 1.16	0.022
Cardiac medications				
Beta-blockers, n (%)	120 (69.8)	87 (67.4)	33 (76.7)	0.250
ACE-inhibitors/ARB, n(%)	134 (77.9)	104 (80.6)	39 (90.7)	0.126
Spironolactone, n (%)	101 (58.7)	74 (57.4)	27 (62.8)	0.531
Diuretics, n (%)	125 (72.7)	93 (72.1)	32 (74.4)	0.767
Digoxin, n (%)	33 (19.2)	21 (16.3)	12 (27.9)	0.094

Primary outcome: all-cause death, heart transplantation during follow-up. Values are mean ± SD, n(%)
[a]Chronic kidney disease was defined as eGFR < 60 ml/min/1.73m^2, calculated using the 4-component MDRD study equation
Abbreviations: *ACE* angiotensin-converting-enzyme, *ARB* angiotensin II receptor blockers, *BNP* B-type natriuretic peptide, *CVA* cerebrovascular accident
ECG electrocardiography

MAP, sNa, ln(NT-proBNP), LV ESV, RV EF, RV ESV, and LV mass were all predictors of the secondary outcome. LV myocardial strain had no significant association with either the primary or secondary outcome (Table 3). Kaplan-Meier curves for the clinical outcomes according to presence of LGE and global longitudinal strain (GLS) are shown in Fig. 3. In Fig. 3c, d, patients were divided into two groups by the median GLS of the total population (– 6.8%).

Multivariable analysis showed that presence of LGE and sNa were independently associated with the primary outcome and presence of LGE, sNa, myocardial mass and ln(NT-proBNP) were independent predictors for secondary outcome. However, the effect of LGE did not satisfy the proportional hazard assumption for the primary outcome, and as stated in the Statistical methods section, we accommodate the LGE effects as time-dependent. The best model indicated that the effect

of LGE was significant and dramatically apparent after about 6 months (Table 4).

Reliability

Intra- and inter-observer reliability values were excellent. Intra- and inter-observer intraclass correlation coefficients were 0.993 (95% CI: 0.985–0.997) and 0.944 (95% CI: 0.875–0.975), respectively, for GLS; 0.993 (95% CI: 0.985–0.997) and 0.962 (95% CI: 0.915–0.983), respectively, for global circumferential strain (GCS); and 0.986 (95% CI: 0.971–0.993) and 0.955 (95% CI: 0.899–0.980), respectively, for global radial strain (GRS).

Discussion

In this study, we evaluated the clinical outcomes of idiopathic DCM patients with moderate to severe LV systolic dysfunction according to CMR-derived LV strain and

Table 2 Baseline standard CMR-data and myocardial deformation parameters of patients with and without the primary outcome

Parameters	All patients (n = 172)	Patients without the primary outcome (n = 129)	Patients with the primary outcome (n = 43)	P value
LV EF (%)	23.7 ± 7.9	23.6 ± 8.0	24.1 ± 7.5	0.675
LV EDV (ml)	284.3 ± 91.4	279.2 ± 81.5	299.9 ± 116.0	0.199
LV ESV (ml)	219.9 ± 85.7	215.5 ± 76.4	233.2 ± 109.0	0.242
Cardiac output (L/min)	5.04 ± 1.53	4.95 ± 1.51	5.32 ± 1.57	0.166
Cardiac index (L/min/m^2)	2.95 ± 0.84	2.89 ± 0.82	3.12 ± 0.88	0.114
RV EF (%)	41.2 ± 17.0	42.3 ± 18.0	37.7 ± 12.8	0.129
RV EDV (ml)	145.6 ± 60.7	140.7 ± 56.3	160.3 ± 70.9	0.066
RV ESV (ml)	91.6 ± 56.7	87.1 ± 53.8	105.1 ± 63.3	0.071
RV cardiac output (L/min)	4.21 ± 1.33	4.14 ± 1.23	4.43 ± 1.59	0.227
Presence of LGE, n (%)	66 (38.4)	42 (33.1)	24 (58.5)	0.004
Myocardial mass (g)	142.2 ± 41.1	144.1 ± 43.6	136.5 ± 31.9	0.232
Quantitative LGE mass (g)	6.8 ± 14.5	5.6 ± 13.3	10.6 ± 17.2	0.093
LGE mass/LV myocardial mass (%)	4.7 ± 9.5	3.8 ± 8.6	7.4 ± 11.5	0.073
Global radial strain (%)	12.3 ± 5.6	12.5 ± 5.6	11.9 ± 5.8	0.563
Global circumferential strain (%)	−7.3 ± 3.1	−7.3 ± 3.1	−7.2 ± 3.2	0.869
Global longitudinal strain (%)	−7.1 ± 2.9	−7.2 ± 2.9	−6.9 ± 2.7	0.613

Primary outcome: all-cause death, heart transplantation. Values are mean ± SD, n(%)
Abbreviations: *CMR* cardiovascular magnetic resonance, *EDV* end-diastolic volume, *EF*, ejection fraction, *ESV* end-systolic volume, *LGE* late gadolinium enhancement, *LV* left ventricle, *RV* right ventricle

LGE. Our major finding was that LV strain had no significant prognostic value in these high-risk patients while the presence of LGE was a significant predictor of adverse outcomes.

Differential prognosis according to LV strain

To the best of our knowledge, a study published by Buss et al. has been the only other study that evaluated the prognostic value of CMR-derived LV strain in the DCM population [24]. In contrast to our study, they found that CMR-derived LV longitudinal strain was an independent predictor of survival in DCM that offered incremental information for risk stratification beyond clinical parameters, biomarkers, and standard CMR. However, they included patients with various systolic functions, and the LV EF of their study population was 36.1 ± 13.8%, much higher than that in our study (23.7 ± 7.9%).

LV myocardial strain is inevitably related to LV EF, and it has been reported that LV EF is determined by global myocardial strain and myocardial thickness [29]. In our study, the Pearson correlation coefficients between LV EF and GLS, GCS, and GRS were − 0.733 (P < 0.01), − 0.780 (P < 0.01), and 0.739 (P < 0.01), respectively. LV EF was not associated with the outcomes in our study, as expected because all of our study patients had severely depressed LV EF. Likewise, it is not

surprising that LV strain could not predict adverse outcomes because it is so closely related to LV EF.

Differential prognosis according to LGE

Regarding the differential clinical outcomes according to LGE, previous studies have well demonstrated this correlation in patients with DCM. It has been reported that presence of LGE was associated with adverse clinical outcomes such as cardiovascular death, hospitalization due to HF, and sudden death [20–23, 30]. This study showed results similar to those of previous studies: the presence of LGE was the strong independent predictor for adverse outcomes. We also considered the quantitative extent of LGE, but the extent of LGE was not significantly related to clinical outcomes. The presence of LGE might thus be more important than the extent of LGE when predicting adverse outcomes.

Limitations

This study has some important limitations. First, there are inherent limitations in non-randomized comparisons, such as allocation bias, uneven distribution of risk factors, and the possibility of unmeasured confounders. Second, data regarding the cause of death such as cardiovascular death including pump failure and sudden cardiac death was not available. Third, the follow-up duration varied by individual

Table 3 Univariate analysis of primary and secondary outcomes

	Primary outcome			Secondary outcome		
	HR	95% CI	P value	HR	95% CI	P value
Age (years)	0.993	0.973–1.013	0.487	0.991	0.970–1.011	0.373
Male gender	1.350	0.693–2.631	0.378	0.726	0.388–1.361	0.318
Mean arterial pressure (mmHg)	0.971	0.945–0.997	0.028	0.959	0.931–0.986	0.004
Hypertension	1.257	0.663–2.384	0.483	0.896	0.449–1.789	0.756
Diabetes mellitus	1.417	0.712–2.818	0.321	1.387	0.679–2.833	0.369
Dyslipidemia	1.521	0.469–4.936	0.485	0.945	0.228–3.917	0.938
Current smoker	0.978	0.474–2.017	0.951	0.853	0.403–1.807	0.678
Chronic kidney disease[a]	1.660	0.813–3.389	0.164	1.709	0.837–3.492	0.141
Previous CVA	3.501	1.079–11.362	0.037	2.265	0.545–9.418	0.261
Body mass index, kg/m^2	0.960	0.888–1.037	0.298	0.936	0.858–1.021	0.134
ECG at baseline						
Heart rate (bpm)	1.000	0.984–1.015	0.972	1.013	0.997–1.029	0.109
Left bundle-branch block	1.122	0.519–2.426	0.770	1.580	0.774–3.224	0.209
QRS duration (ms)	1.005	0.995–1.015	0.353	1.003	0.993–1.013	0.598
Laboratory data						
Serum creatinine (mg/dl)	2.249	0.784–6.455	0.132	0.950	0.271–3.334	0.950
Na (mmol/l)	0.810	0.751–0.875	< 0.001	0.860	0.794–0.931	< 0.001
ln(NT-proBNP) (pg/ml)	1.376	1.083–1.748	0.009	1.519	1.190–1.939	0.001
Cardiac medications						
Beta-blockers	1.148	0.564–2.334	0.704	0.767	0.396–1.486	0.432
ACE-inhibitors/ARB	1.492	0.531–4.192	0.447	2.171	0.669–7.050	0.197
Spironolactone	1.100	0.588–2.056	0.766	1.380	0.724–2.632	0.328
Diuretics	0.921	0.463–1.832	0.814	1.732	0.767–3.914	0.187
Digoxin	1.658	0.847–3.242	0.140	1.662	0.847–3.258	0.140
LV EF (%)	1.006	0.969–1.044	0.759	0.970	0.933–1.009	0.132
LV EDV (ml)	1.003	1.000–1.006	0.093	1.003	1.000–1.006	0.090
LV ESV (ml)	1.003	0.999–1.006	0.108	1.004	1.000–1.007	0.041
Cardiac output (L/min)	1.092	0.908–1.314	0.349	0.961	0.784–1.177	0.699
Cardiac index (L/min/m^2)	1.228	0.868–1.738	0.245	1.024	0.708–1.481	0.901
RV EF (%)	0.984	0.964–1.005	0.124	0.976	0.955–0.998	0.033
RV EDV (ml)	1.005	1.000–1.009	0.041	1.004	0.999–1.009	0.080
RV ESV (ml)	1.005	1.000–1.009	0.049	1.005	1.000–1.010	0.045
RV stroke volume (ml)	1.007	0.991–1.024	0.376	0.995	0.977–1.012	0.556
RV cardiac output (L/min)	1.122	0.894–1.407	0.320	0.962	0.759–1.220	0.751
Presence of LGE	2.277	1.221–4.246	0.010	2.023	1.066–3.839	0.031
Myocardial mass (g)	0.997	0.990–1.005	0.510	0.987	0.978–0.997	0.008
Quantitative LGE mass (g)	1.014	0.998–1.031	0.086	1.009	0.990–1.028	0.370
LGE mass/LV myocardial mass (%)	1.024	0.998–1.051	0.068	1.018	0.989–1.047	0.232
Global radial strain (%)	0.974	0.921–1.030	0.363	0.955	0.901–1.013	0.129
Global circumferential strain (%)	1.030	0.934–1.136	0.554	1.062	0.963–1.172	0.229
Global longitudinal strain (%)	1.048	0.945–1.163	0.375	1.066	0.955–1.191	0.254

[a]Chronic kidney disease was defined as eGFR < 60 ml/min/1.73m^2, calculated using the 4-component MDRD study equation

Abbreviations: *ACE* angiotensin-converting-enzyme, *ARB* angiotensin II receptor blockers, *BNP* B-type natriuretic peptide, *CI* confidence interval, *CVA* cerebrovascular accident, *ECG*, electrocardiography, *EDV* end-diastolic volume, EF, ejection fraction, *ESV*, end-systolic volume, *HR*, hazard ratio, *LGE* late gadolinium enhancement, *LV*, left ventricle, *RV*, right ventricle

patient. Next limitation was that those with several forms of reversible cardiomyopathies such as tachycardia induced cardiomyopathy or hypertensive heart failure were excluded. Furthermore, many patients were excluded from the analysis of LV strain. Since this might have resulted in selection bias, so the

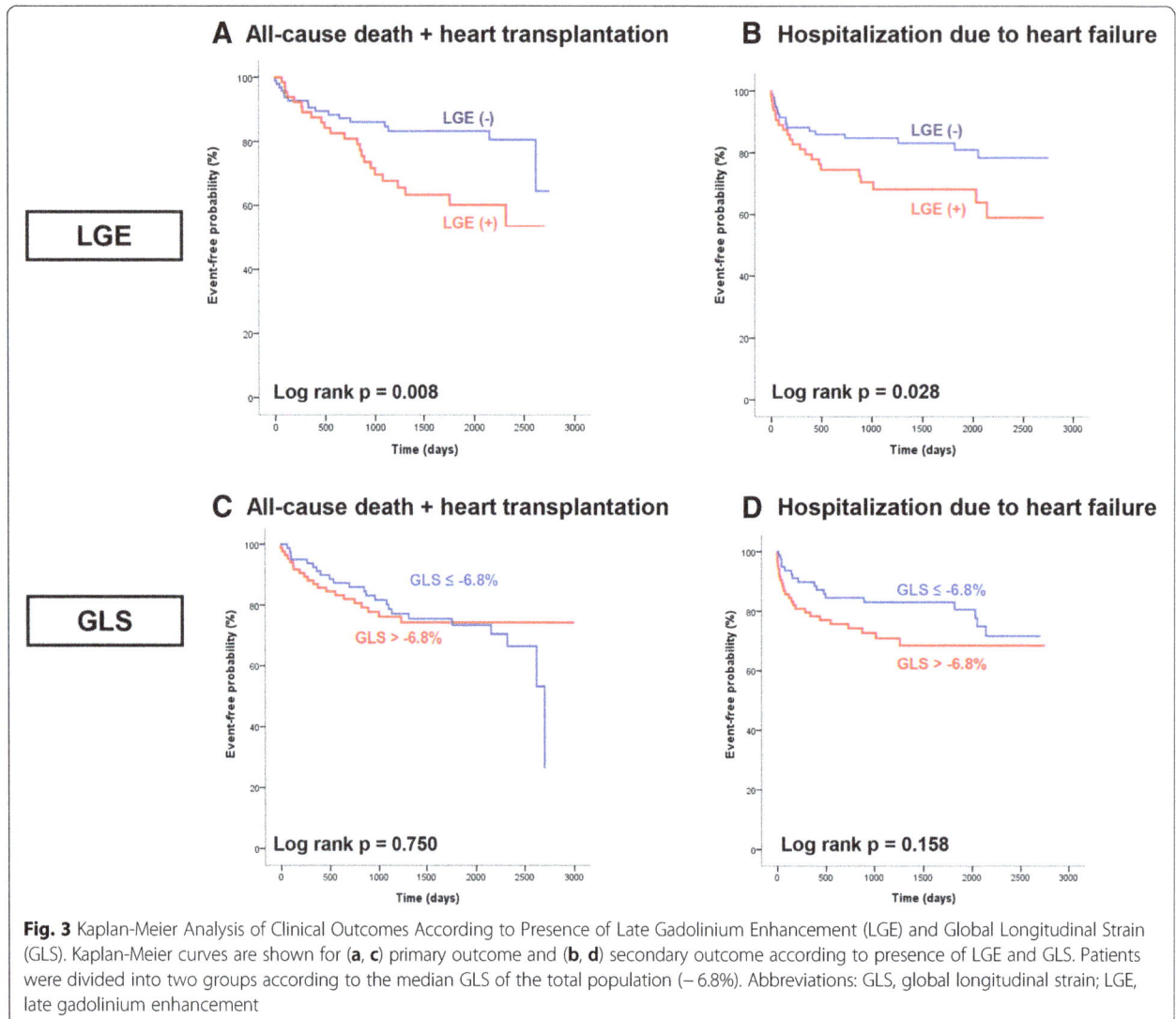

Fig. 3 Kaplan-Meier Analysis of Clinical Outcomes According to Presence of Late Gadolinium Enhancement (LGE) and Global Longitudinal Strain (GLS). Kaplan-Meier curves are shown for (**a**, **c**) primary outcome and (**b**, **d**) secondary outcome according to presence of LGE and GLS. Patients were divided into two groups according to the median GLS of the total population (− 6.8%). Abbreviations: GLS, global longitudinal strain; LGE, late gadolinium enhancement

findings of our study would not be generalizable to the entire HF with reduced EF population. However, there was no difference in the presence of LGE which was one of main CMR variable between those who were included in the strain analysis and excluded patients. Thus the overall finding might be not affected. Lastly, HF management was not controlled; thus, our conclusions should not be extrapolated to all patients with idiopathic DCM. A further study with a prospective and multicenter design is required.

Table 4 Multivariable proportional-hazard model of primary and secondary outcomes

	Primary outcome[a]			Secondary outcome		
	HR	95% CI	P value	HR	95% CI	P value
Na (mmol/l)	0.821	0.761–0.885	< 0.001	0.896	0.817–0.982	0.019
Presence of LGE	4.729	1.111–20.121	0.0355	2.358	1.229–4.523	0.010
Myocardial mass				0.986	0.975–0.996	0.009
lnNT-proBNP				1.352	1.031–1.771	0.029

[a]Based on a multivariable Cox model with time-dependent covariates at 6 months. Before 6 months, the HR was 0.71 (p-value = 0.58, 95% CI: 0.206, 2.415), while after 6 months, the HR is as given in the Table
The Harrell's c-index of multivariable Cox proportional hazards model were 0.727 (95% CI: 0.616 to 0.838) and 0.744 (95% CI: 0.648 to 0.839) for primary and secondary outcomes, respectively
Abbreviations: NT-proBNP, N-terminal pro-B-type natriuretic peptide; CI confidence interval, HR hazard ratio, LGE late gadolinium enhancement

Conclusions

In idiopathic DCM patients with reduced EF, CMR LGE is a good predictor of adverse outcomes. LV strain, however, had no significant prognostic value in patients with moderate to severe systolic dysfunction. As our study was analyzed retrospectively and selection bias could not be excluded, further studies with prospective design are warranted to support our findings.

Abbreviations

ACE: Angiotensin converting enzyme inhibitor; ARB: Angiotensin receptor blocker; CMR: Cardiovascular magnetic resonance; DCM: Dilated cardiomyopathy; EDV: End diastolic volume; EF: Ejection fraction; ESV: End-systolic volume; GCS: Global circumferential strain; GLS: Global longitudinal strain; GRS: Global radial strain; HF: Heart failure; HR: Hazard ratio; LGE: Late gadolinium enhancement; LV: Left ventricle/Left ventricular; MAP: Mean arterial pressure; RV: Right ventricle/Right ventricular; SD: Standard deviation; sNA: Serum sodium

Acknowledgements

The authors thank Prof. Keumhee Carriere (Research Professor, Samsung Medical Center, and Professor of Statistics, Department of Mathematical and Statistical Sciences, University of Alberta, Canada) for providing statistical consultation.

Authors' contributions

Each author contributed significantly to the submitted work: SHP and SMK contributed to data acquisition, analysis, and interpretation and drafted the manuscript. EKK, SAC, YHC, SCL, ESJ contributed to the data interpretation and edited the manuscript. JOC designed and coordinated the study, contributed to the data interpretation, and edited the manuscript. All authors read and approved the final manuscript.

Competing interests

The authors declare that they have no competing interests.

Author details

[1]Department of Internal Medicine, Heart Vascular Stroke Institute, Samsung Medical Center, Sungkyunkwan University School of Medicine, 81 Irwon-ro, Gangnam-gu, Seoul 06351, Republic of Korea. [2]Department of Radiology, Cardiovascular Imaging Center, Samsung Medical Center, Sungkyunkwan University School of Medicine, Seoul, Republic of Korea.

References

1. Felker GM, Thompson RE, Hare JM, Hruban RH, Clemetson DE, Howard DL, et al. Underlying causes and long-term survival in patients with initially unexplained cardiomyopathy. N Engl J Med. 2000;342:1077–84.
2. Choi DJ, Han S, Jeon ES, Cho MC, Kim JJ, Yoo BS, et al. Characteristics, outcomes and predictors of long-term mortality for patients hospitalized for acute heart failure: a report from the korean heart failure registry. Korean Circ J. 2011;41:363–71.
3. Fuster V, Gersh BJ, Giuliani ER, Tajik AJ, Brandenburg RO, Frye RL. The natural history of idiopathic dilated cardiomyopathy. Am J Cardiol. 1981;47: 525–31.
4. Juilliere Y, Danchin N, Briancon S, Khalife K, Ethevenot G, Balaud A, et al. Dilated cardiomyopathy: long-term follow-up and predictors of survival. Int J Cardiol. 1988;21:269–77.
5. Maron BJ, Towbin JA, Thiene G, Antzelevitch C, Corrado D, Arnett D, et al. Contemporary definitions and classification of the cardiomyopathies: an American Heart Association scientific statement from the council on clinical cardiology, heart failure and transplantation committee; quality of care and outcomes research and functional genomics and translational biology interdisciplinary working groups; and council on epidemiology and prevention. Circulation. 2006;113:1807–16.
6. Curtis JP, Sokol SI, Wang Y, Rathore SS, Ko DT, Jadbabaie F, et al. The association of left ventricular ejection fraction, mortality, and cause of death in stable outpatients with heart failure. J Am Coll Cardiol. 2003;42:736–42.
7. Wang NC, Maggioni AP, Konstam MA, Zannad F, Krasa HB, Burnett JC Jr, et al. Clinical implications of QRS duration in patients hospitalized with worsening heart failure and reduced left ventricular ejection fraction. JAMA. 2008;299:2656–66.
8. Anand IS, Fisher LD, Chiang YT, Latini R, Masson S, Maggioni AP, et al. Changes in brain natriuretic peptide and norepinephrine over time and mortality and morbidity in the valsartan heart failure trial (Val-HeFT). Circulation. 2003;107:1278–83.
9. Miller WL, Hartman KA, Burritt MF, Grill DE, Rodeheffer RJ, Burnett JC Jr, et al. Serial biomarker measurements in ambulatory patients with chronic heart failure: the importance of change over time. Circulation. 2007;116:249–57.
10. Yusuf S, Pitt B, Davis CE, Hood WB, Cohn JN. Effect of enalapril on survival in patients with reduced left ventricular ejection fractions and congestive heart failure. N Engl J Med. 1991;325:293–302.
11. Yusuf S, Pitt B, Davis CE, Hood WB Jr, Cohn JN. Effect of enalapril on mortality and the development of heart failure in asymptomatic patients with reduced left ventricular ejection fractions. N Engl J Med. 1992;327:685–91.
12. Grayburn PA, Appleton CP, DeMaria AN, Greenberg B, Lowes B, Oh J, et al. Echocardiographic predictors of morbidity and mortality in patients with advanced heart failure. the Beta-blocker Evaluation of Survival Trial (BEST) J Am Coll Cardiol. 2005;45:1064–71.
13. Lee WH, Packer M. Prognostic importance of serum sodium concentration and its modification by converting-enzyme inhibition in patients with severe chronic heart failure. Circulation. 1986;73:257–67.
14. Adams KF Jr, Dunlap SH, Sueta CA, Clarke SW, Patterson JH, Blauwet MB, et al. Relation between gender, etiology and survival in patients with symptomatic heart failure. J Am Coll Cardiol. 1996;28:1781–8.
15. Oh C, Chang HJ, Sung JM, Kim JY, Yang W, Shim J, et al. Prognostic estimation of advanced heart failure with low left ventricular ejection fraction and wide QRS interval. Korean Circ J. 2012;42:659–67.
16. Karamitsos TD, Francis JM, Myerson S, Selvanayagam JB, Neubauer S. The role of cardiovascular magnetic resonance imaging in heart failure. J Am Coll Cardiol. 2009;54:1407–24.
17. Gonzalez JA, Kramer CM. Role of imaging techniques for diagnosis, prognosis and Management of Heart Failure Patients: cardiac magnetic resonance. Curr Heart Fail Rep. 2015;12:276–83.
18. McCrohon JA, Moon JC, Prasad SK, McKenna WJ, Lorenz CH, Coats AJ, et al. Differentiation of heart failure related to dilated cardiomyopathy and coronary artery disease using gadolinium-enhanced cardiovascular magnetic resonance. Circulation. 2003;108:54–9.
19. Krittayaphong R, Boonyasirinant T, Saiviroonporn P, Udompunturak S. Late gadolinium enhancement from cardiac magnetic resonance in ischemic and non-ischemic cardiomyopathy. J Med Assoc Thail. 2011;94(Suppl 1):S33–8.
20. Kuruvilla S, Adenaw N, Katwal AB, Lipinski MJ, Kramer CM, Salerno M. Late gadolinium enhancement on cardiac magnetic resonance predicts adverse cardiovascular outcomes in nonischemic cardiomyopathy: a systematic review and meta-analysis. Circ Cardiovasc Imaging. 2014;7:250–8.
21. Gulati A, Jabbour A, Ismail TF, Guha K, Khwaja J, Raza S, et al. Association of fibrosis with mortality and sudden cardiac death in patients with nonischemic dilated cardiomyopathy. JAMA. 2013;309:896–908.
22. Lehrke S, Lossnitzer D, Schob M, Steen H, Merten C, Kemmling H, et al. Use of cardiovascular magnetic resonance for risk stratification in chronic heart failure: prognostic value of late gadolinium enhancement in patients with non-ischaemic dilated cardiomyopathy. Heart. 2011;97:727–32.
23. Wu KC, Weiss RG, Thiemann DR, Kitagawa K, Schmidt A, Dalal D, et al. Late gadolinium enhancement by cardiovascular magnetic resonance heralds an adverse prognosis in nonischemic cardiomyopathy. J Am Coll Cardiol. 2008;51:2414–21.

24. Buss SJ, Breuninger K, Lehrke S, Voss A, Galuschky C, Lossnitzer D, et al. Assessment of myocardial deformation with cardiac magnetic resonance strain imaging improves risk stratification in patients with dilated cardiomyopathy. Eur Heart J Cardiovasc Imaging. 2015;16:307–15.

25. Richardson P, McKenna W, Bristow M, Maisch B, Mautner B, O'Connell J, et al. Report of the 1995 World Health Organization/international society and Federation of Cardiology Task Force on the definition and classification of cardiomyopathies. Circulation. 1996;93:841–2.

26. Liu T, Ma X, Liu W, Ling S, Zhao L, Xu L, et al. Late gadolinium enhancement amount as an independent risk factor for the incidence of adverse cardiovascular events in patients with stage C or D heart failure. Front Physiol. 2016;7:484.

27. Maron MS. Contrast-enhanced CMR in HCM: what lies behind the bright light of LGE and why it now matters. JACC Cardiovasc Imaging. 2013;6:597–9.

28. Lee JM, Rhee TM, Hahn JY, Hwang D, Park J, Park KW, et al. Comparison of outcomes after treatment of in-stent restenosis using newer generation drug-eluting stents versus drug-eluting balloon: patient-level pooled analysis of Korean multicenter in-stent restenosis registry. Int J Cardiol. 2017;230:181–90.

29. MacIver DH, Adeniran I, Zhang H. Left ventricular ejection fraction is determined by both global myocardial strain and wall thickness. IJC Heart & Vasculature. 2015;7:113–8.

30. Assomull RG, Prasad SK, Lyne J, Smith G, Burman ED, Khan M, et al. Cardiovascular magnetic resonance, fibrosis, and prognosis in dilated cardiomyopathy. J Am Coll Cardiol. 2006;48:1977–85.

8

Age-related changes of right atrial morphology and inflow pattern assessed using 4D flow cardiovascular magnetic resonance: results of a population-based study

Thomas Wehrum[1]* (iD), Thomas Lodemann[1], Paul Hagenlocher[1], Judith Stuplich[2], Ba Thanh Truc Ngo[2], Sebastian Grundmann[2], Anja Hennemuth[3], Jürgen Hennig[4] and Andreas Harloff[1]

Abstract

Background: To assess age-related changes of blood flow and geometry of the caval veins and right atrium (RA) using 4D flow cardiovascular magnetic resonance (CMR) data obtained in a population-based study.

Methods: An age-stratified sample ($n = 126$) of the population of the city of Freiburg, Germany, underwent transthoracic echocardiography and electrocardiogram-triggered and navigator-gated 4D flow CMR at 3 Tesla covering the caval veins and right heart. Study participants were divided into three age groups (1:20–39; 2:40–59; and 3:60–80 years of age). Analysis planes were placed in the superior and inferior caval vein. Subsequently, RA morphology and three-dimensional blood inflow pattern was assessed.

Results: Blood flow of the RA showed a clockwise rotating helix without signs of turbulence in younger subjects. By contrast, such rotation was absent in 12 subjects of group 3 and turbulences were significantly more frequent ($p < 0.001$). We observed an age-related shift of the caval vein axis. While the outlets of the superior and inferior caval veins were facing each other in group 1, lateralization occurred in older subjects ($p < 0.001$). A convergence of axes was observed from lateral view with facing axes in older subjects ($p = 0.004$). Finally, mean and peak systolic blood flow in the caval veins decreased with age (group $3 < 2 < 1$).

Conclusions: We have provided reference values of 4D CMR blood flow for different age groups and demonstrated the significant impact of age on hemodynamics of the RA inflow tract. This effect of aging should be taken into account when assessing pathologic conditions of the heart in the future.

Keywords: Aging, Heart failure, Pulmonary hypertension, Magnetic resonance imaging (MRI)

Background

Impaired venous return and right-heart function can be caused by a variety of pathologic conditions such as heart-failure, pulmonary hypertension, tricuspid valve disease, arrhythmogenic right ventricular (RV) cardiomyopathy and congenital heart disease [1–3]. However,

the likelihood of development of right heart failure is increased in elderly patients independent of the underlying disease [4]. The specific reasons for this age dependency remain unknown so far. The main diagnostic method used for monitoring right-heart pressures is the pulmonary floatation catheter [5]. However, this technique is an invasive procedure which requires a central venous access and can lead to complications such as pneumothorax and hemothorax, arterial laceration, cardiac arrhythmias, valvular damage, pulmonary artery perforation, false aneurysms, and catheter knotting in the case

* Correspondence: thomas.wehrum@uniklinik-freiburg.de
[1]Department of Neurology and Neuroscience, Medical Center - University of Freiburg, Faculty of Medicine, University of Freiburg, Breisacher Straße 64, 79106 Freiburg, Germany
Full list of author information is available at the end of the article

of right-heart catheterization [6]. A non-invasive alternative for assessment of morphological and functional aspects of the caval veins and right heart is 2D transthoracic echocardiography (TTE). Unfortunately, TTE accuracy is limited by the complex crescent shaped RV geometry and by its location behind the sternum [7]. While 3D-TTE can overcome some of these restraints, its applicability is often limited by suboptimal acoustic windows. This limitation can be overcome by using 3D imaging techniques such as 3D cardiovascular magnetic resonance (CMR) which can improve assessment of morphological features [8]. Furthermore, application of flow-sensitive 3D phase-contrast CMR (4D flow CMR) allows in-vivo visualization of blood flow from the caval veins through the right atrium (RA) into the RV [9]. 4D flow CMR was already used to highlight the role of vortex formation in healthy individuals as a driving force of RA filling [10]. Furthermore, it can be used to evaluate indices of RV systolic function from volume segmentation [11]. Despite its inherent potential to comprehensively assess right heart filling and associated pathologic conditions, most applications of cardiac 4D flow CMR, however, have focused on the left heart [12, 13] or the pulmonary arteries [11, 14].

One major reason for this may be the lack of age stratified reference data for 4D flow CMR, which hamper interpretation of hemodynamic findings. Therefore, it was our aim to assess age-related morphological and functional changes of the RV inflow tract using 4D flow CMR data obtained in an age-stratified population and to provide reference values for future clinical applications.

Methods
Study population
We performed a cross-sectional observational study of an age-stratified sample of the population of the city of Freiburg, Germany (for details see [14]). The cohort was established on the basis of data obtained from the German Civil Registration System. We used six blocks of 20 subjects (ten female and ten male) with the following age-intervals: 20–29, 30–39, 40–49, 50–59, 60–69, and 70–80 years. Starting in October 2012, 3500 age-stratified and randomly selected registered residents of Freiburg were contacted by mail, asked to participate in our study, and provided with details on how to contact the study team. Three hundred eight subjects responded to our mail and were contacted by phone on the basis of first-come, first-served. One hundred forty-seven were excluded because of known CMR contraindications, too many participants in this group of age, or because of scheduling difficulties. One hundred sixty-one subjects were finally scheduled for CMR. In 23 subjects the CMR protocol was not completed for

technical reasons, 11 were absent on the appointed day, 11 aborted the CMR examination because of claustrophobia, and five were not suitable for CMR due to contraindications. Because of insufficient response within the group of 20–29 year olds, the study was advertised on the University Hospital Freiburg intranet and persons within this age-interval were invited to participate. The first 16 persons who contacted the study team by email were included. One person had to be excluded for technical difficulties during CMR and one subject was absent on the appointed day. Finally, datasets of 126 subjects were available for data analysis. Cardiovascular risk factors and demographics were determined by interview. The study was approved by the University of Freiburg ethics committee (IRB number 227/14) and written informed consent was obtained from all participants.

Transthoracic echocardiography
All participants underwent additional TTE using a Toshiba Artida system (4.8-2MHz PST-30BT transducer; Toshiba Medical Systems Corporation, Tokyo, Japan) based on the recommendations and standards of the American Society of Echocardiography [15]. Median time between CMR and TTE was 0 days (inter quartile range: 0–1).

4D flow CMR imaging
CMR examinations were conducted on a routine clinical 3 Tesla CMR system (TIM Trio, Siemens Healthineers, Erlangen, Germany), using a standard 12-element body coil. 4D flow CMR was acquired to obtain time-resolved and three-dimensional blood flow parameters of the caval veins, the RA, and the RV. All experiments were electrocardiogram (ECG)-synchronized as well as respiration-controlled and used navigator-gating to allow free breathing [16]. All datasets were acquired in end-expiration with the navigator placed on the liver dome in order to minimize motion artefacts induced by respiration. Parameters of 4D flow CMR were: echo time/repetition time = 2.6/5.1 ms, flip angle = 7°, temporal resolution = 20.4 ms, matrix size = $320 \times 240 \times 58$, bandwidth = 450 Hz/pixel, spatial resolution = $2.1 \times 2.1 \times 2.5$ mm^3, velocity sensitivity along all three directions = 150 cm/s, and parallel imaging (PEAK-GRAPPA) along the phase encoding direction (y) with an acceleration factor of $R = 5$ (20 reference lines).

CMR data analysis
CMR data were analysed using MEVISFlow software (Fraunhofer MEVIS, Bremen, Germany) (for technical details see [17]). After corrections for eddy-currents and phase-wraps, and vessel-segmentation, analysis planes were positioned perpendicular to the vessel

lumen in the superior vena cava vein (SVC), the inferior vena cava (IVC), and in the ascending aorta to measure cardiac stroke volume. The SVC and IVC planes were located with a distance of 1 cm from the entry to the RA to account for flow turbulences in this area (see Fig. 1). For each analysis plane, a lumen contour surrounding the lumen had to be defined manually while the contour was adapted automatically to all time points [17] and flow was visualized simultaneously in the SVC and IVC plane. Flow analysis comprised the following parts:

1) The visual pattern of RA inflow was studied based on movies of individual 3D blood flow (Additional file 1: Video S1) that could be contemplated from different views. A blinded observer with experience in 4D flow CMR data analysis of 6 years performed the assessment of the data. The right-heart was analyzed from a lateral and a frontal point-of-view and the appearance of RV inflow was graded as 1: appearance of vortex with clockwise rotation, 2: appearance of vortex with counter-clockwise rotation, and 3: no visible rotation.
2) Furthermore, the geometry of the RV inflow tract was analyzed on 3D vessel segmentations obtained during 4D flow CMR. Two axes through the centers of the SVC and IVC lumen were manually defined and the shift of axes was measured in sagittal and frontal view in cm (see Fig. 2). Measurements were made to the nearest whole centimetre.
3) Flow volumes in the SVC, IVC, and ascending aorta analysis plane were quantified for every time step.

Measurement of individual right atrial volume

One investigator who was blinded to patient data performed area measurements of the RA in four-chamber view and right-sided two-chamber view utilizing retrospectively gated 3D phase contrast CMR images which were acquired in end-expiration. Impax software (Agfa Healthcare, Bonn, Germany) was used for area measurements. The RA appendage was not included in the measurements. The equation (RA volume = 3.08 * (2C area) + 3.36 * (4C area) − 44.4) [18] was previously used to calculate right atrial volume. All areas derived from 2D images were measured in the phase at which the RA size was at a maximum, i.e. during ventricular systole. Body surface area (BSA) was calculated according to the Mosteller formula [19]. RA volume was indexed to BSA to obtain the right atrial volume indexed to BSA (RAVI).

Statistical analysis

Data are presented as mean ± standard deviations (SD) or median (interquartile range) for continuous, absolute, and relative frequencies for categorical variables. Patients were categorized according to their age into three groups which were used for comparisons of planar blood flow, inflow visualization, and geometry of the inflow tract: group 1 (20–39 years), group 2 (40–59 years), and group 3 (60–80 years). The TTE parameter dPmax RVRA which represents the maximum pressure gradient between the RV and the RA was used as a surrogate of pulmonary arterial (PA) systolic pressure and was used to test for an association between elevated PA pressure and occurrence of morphological changes and changes of the RA inflow pattern. Furthermore, we tested whether presence of tricuspid regurgitation influences the studied parameters. Departures from normality were

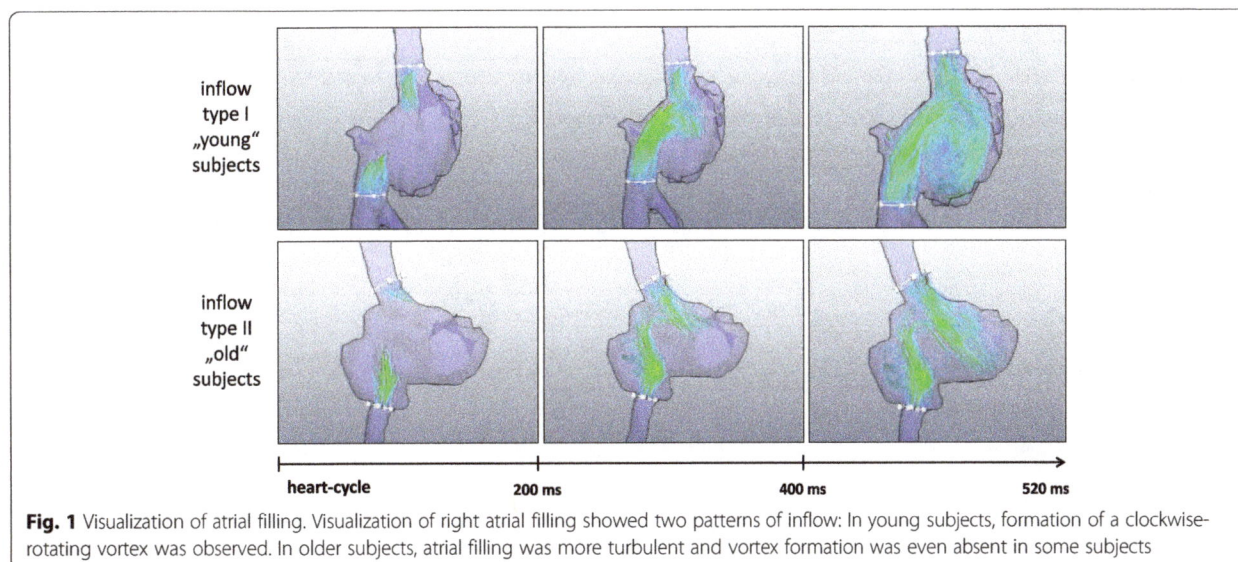

Fig. 1 Visualization of atrial filling. Visualization of right atrial filling showed two patterns of inflow: In young subjects, formation of a clockwise-rotating vortex was observed. In older subjects, atrial filling was more turbulent and vortex formation was even absent in some subjects

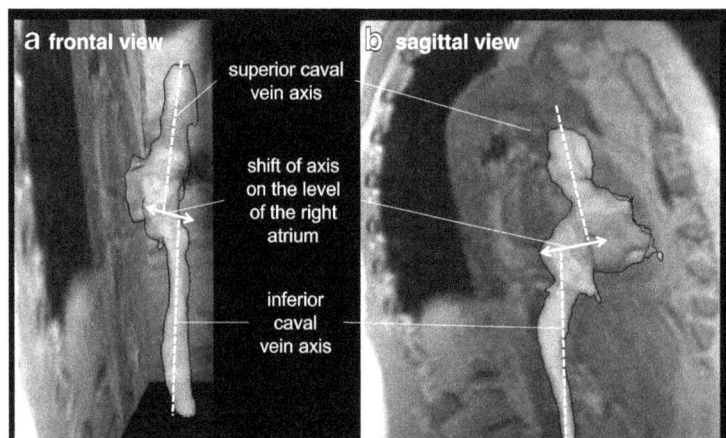

Fig. 2 Measurement of axis-shift. Measurement of axis-shift of the superior and inferior caval vein in (**a**) frontal and (**b**) lateral view. Two axes through the centers of the superior vena cava (SVC) and inferior vena cava (IVVC) lumen were manually defined and the shift of axes was measured in sagittal and frontal view in cm

detected with the Shapiro-Wilk statistic. Homogeneity of variance was assessed using Levene's test. Differences between patient groups were evaluated using Fisher's exact test and one-way ANOVA with Tukey's HSD post-hoc test. All tests were two-sided with 0.05 as the level of statistical significance. Statistical analyses were performed using SPSS (Statistics version 19.0.1. International Business Machines, Armonk, New York, USA)

Results

Patient characteristics

Cardiovascular disease risk factors and patient demographics are presented in Table 1. Hypertension and

hypercholesterolemia occurred more often in older subjects (group 3 > 2 > 1) while no differences between groups were observed regarding other risk factors. Only few subjects had diabetes ($n = 2$), prior stroke ($n = 2$), coronary-artery-disease ($n = 2$), and none of the subjects suffered from peripheral vascular disease.

Transthoracic echocardiography (TTE)

Results of TTE are displayed in Table 2. None of the subjects had significant tricuspid and/or pulmonary valve pathologies (regurgitation grade III or IV) and/or reduced ejection fraction. We observed a small trend towards a higher prevalence of the presence of tricuspid valve regurgitation grade I or II in the elder study group

Table 1 Demographics and cardiovascular risk factors of study participants

Characteristics of patients	Group 1 (20–39 years) $n = 43$	Group 2 (40–59 years) $n = 44$	Group 3 (60–80 years) $n = 39$	p-value
Age, years ± SD	30.1 ± 5.4	50.4 ± 5.5	68.9 ± 5.2	< 0.001*
Female, n (%)	19 (44.2)	24 (54.6)	21 (53.9)	0.564
Hypertension, n (%)	1 (2.3)	7 (16.3)	13 (33.3)	< 0.001*
Hypercholesterolemia, n (%)	1 (2.3)	9 (20.5)	11 (28.2)	0.005*
Diabetes, n (%)	0 (0.0)	1 (2.3)	1 (2.6)	0.587
Smoker, n (%)	11 (25.6)	6 (13.6)	5 (12.8)	0.223
Body mass index, 1 ± SD	24.0 ± 4.0	26.0 ± 4.4	24.31 ± 3.8	0.051
Prior stroke, n (%)	0 (0.0)	2 (4.6)	0 (0.0)	0.151
Coronary arterydisease, n (%)	0 (0.0)	0 (0.0)	2 (5.1)	0.104
Peripheral arterial disease, n (%)	0 (0.0)	0 (0.0)	0 (0.0)	–
Mean systolic blood pressure, mmHg ± SD	120.6 ± 11.1	126 ± 15.7	133.8 ± 19.2	< 0.001*
Mean diastolic blood pressure, mmHg ± SD	76.5 ± 7.0	81.9 ± 8.3	81.1 ± 11.4	0.014*
Heart rate, bpm ± SD	67.2 ± 7.9	65.6 ± 7.7	66.1 ± 9.1	0.655

Values are given as absolute values (percentage) or ± SD = standard deviation, *bpm* beats per minute; *Significant

Table 2 Results from transthoracic echocardiography of study participants

Characteristics of patients	Group 1 (20–39 years) n = 43	Group 2 (40–59 years) n = 44	Group 3 (60–80 years) n = 39	p-value
Ejection fraction, % ± SD	56.6 ± 20.7	57.6 ± 19.2	53.6 ± 22.5	0.669
IVC collapse not complete, n (%)	1 (2.3)	1 (2.3)	0 (0.0)	0.595
PR grade I or II, n (%)	3 (7.1)	1 (2.3)	1 (2.6)	0.246
PR grade III or IV, n (%)	0 (0.0)	0 (0.0)	0 (0.0)	n/a
TR grade I or II, n (%)	6 (13.9)	4 (9.1)	13 (33.3)	0.019*
TR grade III or IV, n (%)	0 (0.0)	0 (0.0)	0 (0.0)	n/a
TAPSE, cm ± SD	22.9 ± 4.1	22.6 ± 3.3	23.1 ± 3.7	0.821
TVS', cm/s ± SD	15.5 ± 2.9	15.53 ± 1.8	15.8 ± 1.8	0.847
dPmax MV, mmHg ± SD	3.5 ± 1.8	3.5 ± 1.3	3.6 ± 1.4	0.864
dPmax RVRA, mmHg ± SD	15.8 ± 2.4	18.2 ± 4.8	22.1 ± 5.7	< 0.001*

EF ejection fraction, *IVC* inferior vena cava, *PR* pulmonary egurgitation, *TR* tricuspid regurgitation, *TAPSE* tricuspid annular plane systolic excursion, *TVS'* tissue Doppler derived right ventricular systolic excursion velocity, *dPmax MV* maximum pressure gradient at the level of the mitral valve in diastole, *dPmax RVRA* maximum pressure at the level of the right ventricle/right atrium; *Significant

(group 3: $n = 13$ (33.3%) vs. group 2: $n = 4$ (9.1%) vs. group 1: $n = 6$ (13.9%); $p = 0.019$). Furthermore, maximum pressure difference between the RV and RA increased significantly from group 1 = 15.8 ± 2.4, group 2 = 18.2 ± 4.8, to group 3 = 22.1 ± 5.7 ($p < 0.001$). However, no significant trends were observed regarding other RA TTE parameters.

Visualization of right atrial flow

In three datasets visualisation of flow was not possible due to technical reasons; those datasets were omitted in the following analysis. Pathline visualization of RA inflow showed a clockwise rotating helix without signs of turbulence in younger patients. Subjects in the group of 60–80 year olds had no visible rotation in 12 cases as compared to four and three participants in group 1 and 2, respectively (see Table 3.). The degree of visually observed

turbulence was significantly higher in older subjects ($p < 0.001$).

Geometry of the right ventricular inflow tract

Interestingly, an age related shift of the caval vein axis was observed (Fig. 1). Median (inter quartile range) frontal axis shift was 0 (0–0) cm for group 1, 1 (0–1) cm for group 2, 1 (0–2) cm for group 3, and lateral axis shift was 1 (1–2) cm for group 1, 1 (1–2) cm for group 2, and 1 (0–2) cm for group 3. While the outlets of the SVC and IVC were directly facing each other on frontal view in most young subjects, a lateralization was observed in older subjects which was most prominent in the group of 60–80 year olds ($p < 0.001$) (see Table 4.). Furthermore, a convergence of axes was observed from a lateral view and older subjects tended to have facing lateral axes ($p = 0.004$).

Table 3 Prevalence of patterns of inflow and flow turbulence

	Group 1 (20–39 years) n = 43	Group 2 (40–59 years) n = 44	Group 3 (60–80 years) n = 39	All n = 126
Inflow-morphology				
Clockwise	38 (88.4)	36 (81.8)	17 (43.6)	91 (72.2)
Counter-clockwise	1 (2.3)	4 (9.1)	8 (20.5)	13 (10.3)
No rotation	4 (9.3)	3 (6.8)	12 (30.8)	19 (15.1)
Flow turbulence				
No	37 (86.1)	17 (38.6)	7 (17.9)	61 (48.4)
Weak	2 (4.7)	8 (18.2)	5 (12.8)	15 (11.9)
Medium	1 (2.3)	12 (4.6)	9 (23.1)	22 (17.5)
Strong	3 (6.9)	6 (13.6)	16 (41.0)	25 (19.8)

Table 4 Degree of frontal and lateral axis shift in study participants

	Group 1 (20–39 years) $n = 43$	Group 2 (40–59 years) $n = 44$	Group 3 (60–80 years) $n = 39$	All $n = 126$
Frontal axis shift, n (%)				
0 cm	38 (88.4)	20 (45.5)	14 (35.9)	72 (57.1)
1 cm	2 (4.7)	19 (43.2)	14 (35.9)	35 (27.8)
2 cm	3 (6.9)	4 (9.1)	9 (23.1)	16 (12.7)
Lateral axis shift, n (%)				
0 cm	2 (4.7)	6 (13.6)	12 (30.8)	20 (15.9)
1 cm	28 (65.1)	25 (56.8)	11 (28.2)	64 (50.8)
2 cm	13 (30.2)	12 (27.3)	12 (30.8)	37 (29.4)
3 cm	0 (0.0)	0 (0.0)	2 (5.1)	2 (1.6)

Age related change of caval flow

Parameters of planar flow in the SVC and IVC are given in Table 5. RV inflow from the caval veins was lower in older patients (group $3 < 2 < 1$), while the relative contribution of the single SVC and IVC to overall inflow remained constant (46–52%; $p = 0.43$). This finding is consistent with the change of stroke volume, which was also lower in older patients as measured in a standardized analysis plane of the ascending aorta (group $3 < 2 < 1$), see Fig. 3. We did not detect differences between male and female subjects after adjustment for age and body-mass-index. The flow profile in the SVC and IVC showed flow peaks in systole and diastole (Fig. 3). Furthermore, blood flow reversal occurred in some subjects at the end of the heart cycle, which represented atrial systole. Peak systolic flow volumes were greater in younger patients in the SVC (group $1 > 2 > 3$) and IVC (group $1 > 2 > 3$), which was also true for peak diastolic flow in the ICV (group $1 > 2 > 3$) but not in the SVC where no significant difference was observed (see Table 5).

Right atrium volume

RAVI was 25.2 ± 6.3 ml/m^2 for group 1, 30.8 ± 9.4 ml/m^2 for group 2, and 37.6 ± 9.4 ml/m^2 for group 3. Thus, RAVI increased with age ($p < 0.05$ level for the three conditions [$F(2,117) = 1509.7, p < 0.001$]). In addition, we detected a trend of lower RAVI in subjects with a more shifted lateral caval vein axis [$F(4,115) = 3.7, p = 0.007$], and a higher RAVI in subjects with occurrence of RA turbulences [$F(4,115) = 4.8, p = 0.001$]. However, no association was visible for RAVI and the caval flow volumes, frontal axis shift, and flow morphology.

Table 5 Planar flow volumes as measured in the superior (SCV), inferior (ICV), and both caval veins (CV)

	Group 1 (20–39 years) $n = 43$	Group 2 (40–59 years) $n = 44$	Group 3 (60–80 years) $n = 39$	F(2,375)	p-value
$Q_{antegrade}$, mL $\pm$ SD					
SVC	24.2 ± 6.4	24.5 ± 7.6	22.0 ± 6.8	1.6	0.210
IVC	57.2 ± 21.0	51.3 ± 18.4	45.8 ± 1.6	3.8	0.025*
CV	81.4 ± 23.3	75.9 ± 21.9	67.8 ± 17.8	4.2	0.017*
$Q_{retrograde}$, mL $\pm$ SD					
SVC	0.5 ± 0.6	0.2 ± 0.3	0.2 ± 0.4	4.3	0.015*
IVC	0.4 ± 0.6	0.1 ± 0.3	0.1 ± 0.3	4.2	0.017*
CV	0.8 ± 1.1	0.4 ± 0.5	0.4 ± 0.5	5.9	0.004*
$Q_{ratio\ (SCV/ICV)}$	0.5 ± 0.2	0.5 ± 0.2	0.5 ± 0.3	0.9	0.427
SV, mL/cycle ± SD					
AAo	82.2 ± 20.9	73.4 ± 15.6	66.5 ± 13.9	8.7	< 0.001*
CO, L/min ± SD	5.3 ± 1.6	4.8 ± 0.9	4.4 ± 1.1	6.1	0.003*
Qmax systole					
SVC	74.2 ± 24.2	68.8 ± 20.7	59.9 ± 23.4	4.1	0.02*
IVC	151.1 ± 55.3	119.8 ± 49.6	100.5 ± 40.7	3.7	0.02*
Qmax diastole					
SVC	36.4 ± 18.8	37.5 ± 12.3	31.5 ± 15.7	11.2	< 0.001*
IVC	109.1 ± 45.9	90.0 ± 31.2	71.3 ± 30.8	10.8	< 0.001*

Qantegrade flow rate (ml/min) in antegrade direction, *Qretrograde* flow rate (ml/min) in retrograde direction, *Qratio* ratio of total flow in SVC and IVC, *SV* stroke volume, *CO* cardiac output, *Qmax systole* maximum flow in systole, *Qmax diastole* maximum flow in diastole; *Significant

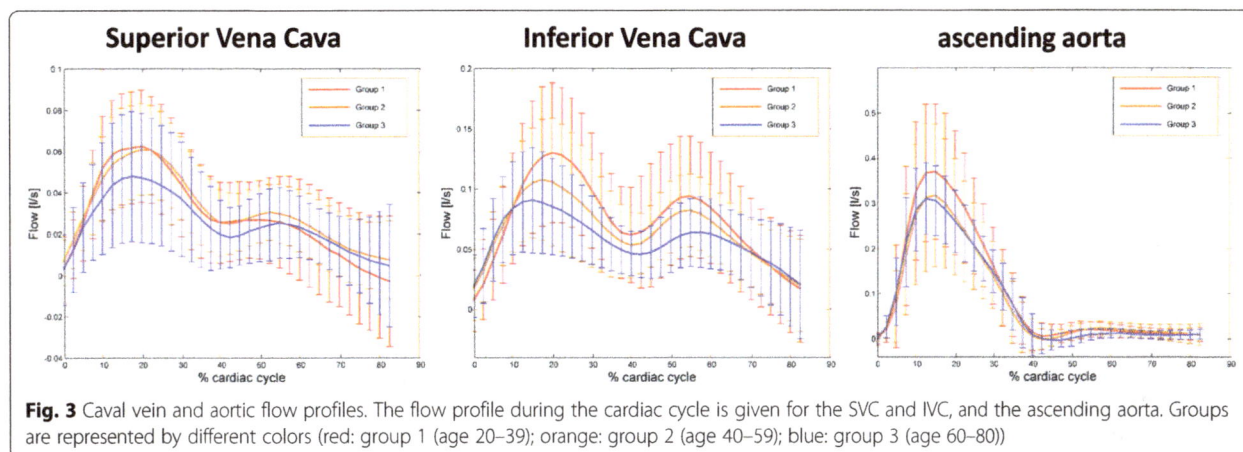

Fig. 3 Caval vein and aortic flow profiles. The flow profile during the cardiac cycle is given for the SVC and IVC, and the ascending aorta. Groups are represented by different colors (red: group 1 (age 20–39); orange: group 2 (age 40–59); blue: group 3 (age 60–80))

Influence of pulmonary arterial pressure and tricuspid insufficiency

We did not detect significant differences of dPmax RVRA between patients with different inflow morphology ($p = 0.181$), turbulences ($p = 0.089$), and frontal axis shift ($p = 0.145$). However, dPmax RVRA was significantly lower in subjects with larger lateral caval vein axis shift [$F(3,50) = 2.8$, $p = 0.047$]: 0 cm: 22.7 ± 4.7 mmHg, 1 cm: 17.2 ± 4.5 mmHg, 2 cm: 18.5 ± 5.4 mmHg. When comparing the presence of tricuspid regurgitation with our studied parameters we did not find a significant association of the inflow morphology ($p = 0.49$), the occurrence of turbulences ($p = 0.50$), lateral axis shift ($p = 0.78$), frontal axis shift ($p = 0.55$).

Discussion

We performed 4D flow CMR of the RA inflow tract and the SVC and IVC in an age-stratified sample of 126 subjects of the population of a medium sized city in southern Germany. This is the first study investigating morphological and functional changes of the RA inflow tract in a large sample of the general population, systematically covering all age groups. Our results indicate that blood flow to the heart decreases with age. This effect may be a result of declining cardiac output which in turn leads to decreased venous return to the heart. One recent study quantified RA filling in 12 healthy subjects (8 male; 40 ± 13 years) using 4D flow CMR. They found similar combined stroke volumes of the RA inflow tract with a total stroke volume of 76.6 ± 21.4 ml (SVC 18.1 ± 7.1 ml; IVC 58.9 ± 19.6 ml) [10], compared to 75.9 ± 21.9 ml (SVC 24.5 ± 7.63 ml, IVC 51.3 ± 18.35 ml) in the group of 40–59 year old subjects in our study. The same was true for one study examining 10 healthy subjects (6 male; mean age 30 years) in which median flow at end inspiration was 31.0 ml in the SVC and 56.1 ml in the IVC [20], as compared to 24.2 ± 6.39 ml for the SVC and 57.2 ± 21.01 ml for the IVC in the group of 20–39 year

old subjects in our study. A further study investigating SVC and IVC blood flow in atrio-pulmonary anastomosis did show higher stroke volumes in the SVC (70.0 ± 30.0 ml) and IVC (180.0 ± 40.0 ml) [21]. However, the SVC to IVC ratio ($\sim 1{:}2$) was similar to our and the aforementioned studies [10, 21]. Interestingly, the ratio between SVC and IVC did not differ between different age groups in our study.

Our results indicate that morphological and functional changes of RA venous filling take place in the aging heart. Many studies have focussed on the effects of aging on left ventricular and left atrial morphology and the occurrence of cardiac hypertrophy and atrial fibrillation. However, our study is the first to systematically investigate morphological changes of the RA inflow tract during aging in a large sample of the general population. One recent study (13 healthy subjects [6 male, mean age 40 years] and 13 subjects [6 male, 40 years] with cryptogenic stroke and patent foramen ovale) also assessed the position of the caval veins by comparing the points at which the centerlines of the respective caval vein flows intersected with the orthogonal planes placed at the junction with the RA, and found positions of the caval veins to be constant in the antero-posterior direction but significantly variable in the right-left direction [22]. In the right-left plane the separation between the IVC and the SVC was greater in the group of subjects with patent foramen ovale compared to controls (10 ± 5 mm versus 3 ± 3 mm, $p = 0.002$) [22], as compared to 8.6 mm in the group of 60–80 year olds in our study.

RA volume was larger in older patients in our study and may explain the phenomena reported in our study in particular given the fact, that the occurrence of turbulences and the lateral axis shift was associated with changes in atrial volume. Our results regarding RAVI are lower than reported in the literature (54 mL/m2 [95% CI: 34, 75]) [18]. All diameters and areas derived from 2D images in the literature [18] and in our study were measured in the phase at which the RA size and volume measurements were at a maximum, i.e. ventricular systole. In the literature, measurements of RA volumes [18] were performed using retrospectively ECG triggered balanced steady-state free precession imaging end-expiratory breath-hold cines which were acquired in the two (left and right chambers) and four chamber views, with subsequent contiguous short-axis cines from the atrioventricular ring to the base of the atria. This sequence was not included in our current study protocol and our measurements were based on a combination of the extracted vessel surface based on 3D phase contrast CMR datasets and a volume rendering of the magnitude image. This may have resulted in underestimation of the absolute RA volumes, however as this effect applies to all our study subjects it should not have influence on the association of RA volumes and the flow phenomena reported in this study.

We only detected a significant association between lateral caval vein axis shift and higher PA pressure with the parameter dPmax RVRA. However, our data demonstrate a trend that patients with elevated PA pressure also had more turbulent RA inflow, although the statistical level of significance was missed ($p = 0.089$) potentially due to the limited sample size. Furthermore, no subjects with pulmonary artery hypertension were included in our population based study. Accordingly, studying morphological and functional parameters of RA inflow using 4D flow CMR would be interesting in future studies investigating changes in patients with pulmonary artery hypertension.

Cardiac looping during embryonic development leads to asymmetries and curvatures which have potential fluidic and dynamic advantages [23]. This is expressed by the uniform clockwise rotating helix of blood flow in healthy subjects comprising 80% of ventricular inflow volume as shown in a previous study [10]. This mechanism allows the momentum of inflowing streams to be redirected towards atrio-ventricular valves. Interference with ventricular ejection flow may be minimized by the change in direction at the ventricular level which can enhance ventriculo-atrial coupling and may minimize dissipative interaction between entering, recirculating and outflowing streams [23]. These factors might combine to improve hemodynamics when heart rate and output increase during exercise. However, this mechanism may be weakened by morphological changes of the aging heart such as divergence of the frontal axis of the caval veins and convergence of the lateral axis. As a result, the convergence of inflowing streams of blood from the IVC and SVC occurs at a different angle, which impedes formation of a clockwise rotating helix and makes room for turbulences to occur. These turbulences and the loss of fluidic and dynamic advantages lead to diminished inflow and may

further increase susceptibility for right heart failure in elderly patients. Furthermore, one recent study showed that absence of the 'standard' vortex during systole and diastole was more common in 13 subjects with patent foramen ovale and cryptogenic stroke compared to age-matched controls [22]. Hence, future large scale studies on cryptogenic stroke may be a potential application of vortex analysis using 4D flow CMR in the RA.

Respiratory activity affects venous return through changes in RA pressure and changes of the volume of the caval veins (e.g. vena cava compression) and cardiac chambers (e.g. changing cardiac preload). During expiration the chest wall collapses and the diaphragm ascends which makes the intrapleural pressure become more positive resulting in reduction of cardiac chamber and caval vein size. All datasets were acquired in end-expiration in this study. Accordingly, absolute flow values and volumes presented here may be smaller compared with data acquisition in end-inspiration. However, as all datasets were acquired similarly this has no influence on the analysis of age-related changes of RA morphology and filling.

Potential limitations of our study were the relative small sample size and the amount of initial nonresponse to our study invitation. When compared with registry data [24] and data from another German population-based study [25] the subjects under investigation less often had hypertension, hypercholesterolemia, diabetes, were less often smokers, obese, and only few patients suffered from a cardiovascular disease. This was probably due to the recruitment modality which required participants to actively contact the study team and to visit the University Medical Center without receiving a reimbursement. Accordingly, particularly healthier or health-conscious residents were probably interested in collaborating in this study. Inclusion of sufficient number of young (20–29 years of age) males is a common problem in cohorts like ours. Accordingly, 14 included subjects were recruited from the personnel of our institution ($n = 922$ male 20–29 years of age) on the basis of first-come, first-served to minimize bias.

Conclusions

In conclusion, we have shown that 4D flow CMR can be used to visualize and assess flow in the caval veins and in the RA inflow tract. Furthermore, we provided reference values for 4D flow CMR based flow quantification in the caval veins. We demonstrated that age has a significant impact on caval blood flow and RV hemodynamics. This effect of aging should be taken into account when assessing pathologic conditions of the heart in future studies using 4D flow CMR. Findings of this population-based study are highly valuable for comparison with those in patients with manifest cardiac diseases.

Abbreviations
BP: Blood pressure; BSA: Body surface area; CMR: Cardiovascular magnetic resonance; dPmax RVRA: maximum pressure at the level of the right ventricle/right atrium; ECG: Electrocardiogram; GRAPPA: Generalized Autocalibrating Partially Parallel Acquisitions; IVC: Inferior vena cava; PA: Pulmonary artery; PR: Pulmonary regurgitation; RA: Right atrium/right atrial; RAVI: Right atrial volume index; RV: Right ventricle/right ventricular; SVC: Superior vena cava; TR: Tricuspid regurgitation; TTE: Transthoracic echocardiography

Acknowledgements
The authors thank Adriana Komancsek for performing CMR examinations and Dr. Konrad Whittaker for proofreading the final manuscript.

Funding
Prof. Dr. Andreas Harloff and Dr. Thomas Wehrum received funding from the German Research Foundation (DFG) grant #HA5399/3-1. The article processing charge was funded by the German Research Foundation (DFG) and the Albert Ludwigs University Freiburg in the funding program Open Access Publishing.

Authors' contributions
Each author contributed significantly to the submitted work: TW was involved in the design of the study, performed data analysis, interpreted the data and drafted the manuscript. TL and PH recruited participants, performed CMR examinations and were involved in drafting the manuscript. JS and BN performed transthoracic echocardiography and revised the manuscript. SG helped with the design of the study and revised the manuscript. AHe developed our 4D flow CMR-data analysis software and revised the manuscript. JH helped with the design of the study regarding the 4D flow CMR-sequence and revised the manuscript. AHa designed the study, interpreted data and revised the manuscript. All authors read and approved the manuscript.

Competing interests
The authors declare that they have no competing interests.

Author details
[1]Department of Neurology and Neuroscience, Medical Center - University of Freiburg, Faculty of Medicine, University of Freiburg, Breisacher Straße 64, 79106 Freiburg, Germany. [2]Department of Cardiology, University Heart Center Freiburg, Faculty of Medicine, University of Freiburg, Freiburg, Germany. [3]Charité – Universitätsmedizin Berlin, Institute for Imaging Science and Computational Modelling in Cardiovascular Medicine, Berlin, Germany. [4]Department of Diagnostic Radiology – Medical Physics, Medical Center, University of Freiburg, Faculty of Medicine, University of Freiburg, Freiburg, Germany.

References
1. Haddad F, Doyle R, Murphy DJ, Hunt SA. Right ventricular function in cardiovascular disease, part II: pathophysiology, clinical importance, and management of right ventricular failure. Circulation. 2008;117:1717–31.
2. Simon MA. Assessment and treatment of right ventricular failure. Nat Rev Cardiol. 2013;10:204–18.
3. Funk DJ, Jacobsohn E, Kumar A. Role of the venous return in critical illness and shock: part II-shock and mechanical ventilation. Crit Care Med. 2013;41:573–9.
4. Strait JB, Lakatta EG. Aging-associated cardiovascular changes and their relationship to heart failure. Heart Fail Clin. 2012;8:143–64.
5. Rapoport J. Patient characteristics and ICU organizational factors that influence frequency of pulmonary artery catheterization. J Am Med Assoc. 2000;283(19):2559–67.
6. Layon AJ. The pulmonary artery catheter: nonexistential entity or occasionally useful tool? Chest. 1999;115:859–62.
7. Jurcut R, Giusca S, La Gerche A, Vasile S, Ginghina C, Voigt JU. The echocardiographic assessment of the right ventricle: what to do in 2010? Eur J Echocardiogr. 2010;11:81–96.
8. Haddad F, Hunt SA, Rosenthal DN, Murphy DJ. Right ventricular function in cardiovascular disease, part I: anatomy, physiology, aging, and functional assessment of the right ventricle. Circulation. 2008;117(11):1436–48.
9. Fredriksson A, Zajac J, Eriksson J, Dyverfeldt P, Bolger A, Ebbers T, et al. 4-D blood flow in the human right ventricle. Am J Phys. 2011;301:H2344–50.
10. Callaghan FM, Arnott C, Figtree GA, Kutty S, Celermajer DS, Grieve SM. Quantifying right atrial filling and emptying: a 4D-flow MRI study. J Magn Reson Imaging. 2017;45:1046–54.
11. Reiter U, Reiter G, Kovacs G, Stalder AF, Gulsun MA, Greiser A, et al. Evaluation of elevated mean pulmonary arterial pressure based on magnetic resonance 4D velocity mapping: comparison of visualization techniques. PLoS One. 2013;8:e82212.
12. Fyrenius A, Wigström L, Ebbers T, Karlsson M, Engvall J, Bolger AF. Three dimensional flow in the human left atrium. Heart. 2001;86:448–55.
13. Dyverfeldt P, Kvitting JPE, Carlhäll CJ, Boano G, Sigfridsson A, Hermansson U, et al. Hemodynamic aspects of mitral regurgitation assessed by generalized phase-contrast MRI. J Magn Reson Imaging. 2011;33:582–8.
14. Wehrum T, Hagenlocher P, Lodemann T, Vach W, Dragonu I, Hennemuth A, et al. Age dependence of pulmonary artery blood flow measured by 4D flow cardiovascular magnetic resonance: results of a population-based study. J Cardiovasc Magn Reson. 2016;18:31.
15. Lang RM, Badano LP, Mor-Avi V, Afilalo J, Armstrong A, Ernande L, et al. Recommendations for cardiac chamber quantification by echocardiography in adults: an update from the American Society of Echocardiography and the European Association of Cardiovascular Imaging. J Am Soc Echocardiogr. 2015;28:1–39.e14.
16. Markl M, Harloff A, Bley TA, Zaitsev M, Jung B, Weigang E, et al. Time-resolved 3D MR velocity mapping at 3T: improved navigator-gated assessment of vascular anatomy and blood flow. J Magn Reson Imaging. 2007;25:824–31.
17. Wehrum T, Kams M, Schroeder L, Drexl J, Hennemuth A, Harloff A. Accelerated analysis of three-dimensional blood flow of the thoracic aorta in stroke patients. Int J Cardiovasc Imaging. 2014;30:1571–7.
18. Maceira AM, Cosín-Sales J, Roughton M, Prasad SK, Pennell DJ. Reference right atrial dimensions and volume estimation by steady state free precession cardiovascular magnetic resonance. J Cardiovasc Magn Reson. 2013;15:29.
19. Mosteller RD. Simplified calculation of body-surface area. N Engl J Med. 1987;317:1098.
20. Kuzo RS, Pooley RA, Crook JE, Heckman MG, Gerber TC. Measurement of caval blood flow with MRI during respiratory maneuvers: implications for vascular contrast opacification on pulmonary CT angiographic studies. Am J Roentgenol. 2007;188:839–42.
21. Klimes K, Abdul-Khaliq H, Ovroutski S, Hui W, Alexi-Meskishvili V, Spors B, et al. Pulmonary and caval blood flow patterns in patients with intracardiac and extracardiac Fontan: a magnetic resonance study. Clin Res Cardiol. 2007;96:160–7.
22. Parikh JD, Kakarla J, Keavney B, O'Sullivan JJ, Ford GA, Blamire AM, et al. 4D flow MRI assessment of right atrial flow patterns in the normal heart – influence of caval vein arrangement and implications for the patent foramen ovale. PLoS One. 2017;12:e0173046.
23. Kilner PJ, Yang GZ, Wilkes AJ, Mohiaddin RH, Firmin DN, Yacoub MH. Asymmetric redirection of flow through the heart. Nature. 2000;404:759–61.
24. Health in Germany. Robert Koch Institute, Federal Statistical Office of Germany. Berlin; 2008. https://www.rki.de/EN/Content/Health_Monitoring/Health_Reporting/HealthInGermany/health_germany_node.html. Accessed 21 Aug 2017.
25. Lorenz MW, Von Kegler S, Steinmetz H, Markus HS, Sitzer M. Carotid intima-media thickening indicates a higher vascular risk across a wide age range: prospective data from the Carotid Atherosclerosis Progression Study (CAPS). Stroke. 2006;37:87–92.

9

Two-center clinical validation and quantitative assessment of respiratory triggered retrospectively cardiac gated balanced-SSFP cine cardiovascular magnetic resonance imaging in adults

Amol S Pednekar[1][*] (iD), Hui Wang[2], Scott Flamm[3], Benjamin Y. Cheong[4] and Raja Muthupillai[4]

Abstract

Background: Breath-hold (BH) requirement remains the limiting factor on the spatio-temporal resolution and coverage of the cine balanced steady-state free precession (bSSFP) cardiovascular magnetic resonance (CMR) imaging. In this prospective two-center clinical trial, we validated the performance of a respiratory triggered (RT) bSSFP cine sequence for evaluation of biventricular function.

Methods: Our study included 23 asymptomatic healthy subjects and 60 consecutive patients from Institute A ($n = 39$) and Institute B ($n = 21$) referred for a clinically indicated CMR study. We implemented a RT sequence with a respiratory synchronized drive to steady state (SS) of bSSFP signal, before the commencement of image data acquisition with prospective cardiac arrhythmia rejection and retrospectively cardiac gated reconstruction in real-time. Left (LV) and right (RV) ventricular function and LV mass were evaluated by using RT-bSSFP and conventional BH-bSSFP sequences with one cardiac cycle for SS preparation keeping all the imaging parameters identical. The performance of the sequences was evaluated by using quantitative and semi-quantitative metrics.

Results: Global LV and RV functional parameters and LV mass obtained from the RT-bSSFP and BH-bSSFP sequences were in good agreement. Quantitative metrics designed to capture fluctuation in SS signal intensity showed no significant difference between sequences. In addition, blood-to-myocardial contrast was nearly identical between sequences. The combined clinical score for image quality was excellent or good for 100% of cases with the BH-bSSFP and 83% of cases with the RT-bSSFP sequence. The de facto image acquisition time for RT-bSSFP was statistically significantly longer than that for conventional BH-bSSFP (7.9 ± 3.4 min vs. 5.1 ± 2.6 min).

Conclusions: Cine RT-bSSFP is an alternative for evaluating global biventricular function with contrast and spatio-temporal resolutions that are similar to those attained by using the BH-bSSFP sequence, albeit with a modest time penalty and a small reduction in image quality.

Keywords: Cardiovascular magnetic resonance, Left ventricular function, Free breathing respiratory-triggered cine

* Correspondence: vedamol@gmail.com
[1]Department of Radiology, Texas Children's Hospital, 6701 Fannin Street, Suite D470.09, Houston, TX 77030-2399, USA
Full list of author information is available at the end of the article

Background

In patients with cardiovascular disease, ventricular volume, mass, and ejection fraction (EF) are powerful predictors of prognosis [1–5]. In several studies of individuals with normal and abnormal ventricles, cardiovascular magnetic resonance (CMR) has been used to evaluate biventricular volume, mass, and EF with high accuracy and low inter- and intra-observer variability [6–9]. For the accurate measurement of ventricular functional indices in CMR, it is necessary to have: a) sufficient and consistent blood-to-myocardium contrast throughout the cardiac cycle to reliably define endocardial contour, b) adequate spatio-temporal resolution to accurately capture end-diastole and end-systole, and c) immunity to cardiorespiratory motion and pulsatile blood flow. In routine clinical CMR practice, cine balanced steady-state free precession (bSSFP) is a sequence of choice for evaluation of ventricular function [10] as it offers the highest signal-to-noise ratio (SNR) per unit time of all other CMR imaging sequences along with a T_2/T_1-weighted image contrast [11]. In order to obtain diagnostic image quality, the bSSFP sequence mandates the shortest possible repetition time (TR) to minimize banding artifacts [11], high flip angle for adequate blood to myocardial contrast [12], and uninterrupted radiofrequency (RF) excitations to maintain the magnetization at steady-state (SS) to elude contrast variability [13] and artifacts [14, 15]. In addition, cine bSSFP acquisition employs retrospective cardiac gating to obtain the entire cardiac cycle along with prospective arrhythmia rejection. In clinical practice breath-holds (BH) are used to mitigate respiratory motion artifacts. Respiratory suspension for sufficient duration is not feasible in sedated patients and patients with impaired breath-holding capacity. Therefore, it would be of clinical interest to obtain cine bSSFP images without the constraint of breath holding while retaining the necessary features described above.

Approaches to combat artifacts introduced by respiratory motion in cine CMR imaging fall in three broad categories: (1) rapid imaging with data undersampling [16–18]; (2) respiratory motion synchronized data acquisition using signals from an external respiratory bellows or RF navigator positioned over the lung-diaphragm interface [19–23]; and (3) self-gated motion compensation methods [24–26]. Combinations of data undersampling and self-gating are being explored for respiratory motion-state cine imaging [27]. Some of these approaches require contrast administration [18, 24, 28], or prospective cardiac gating [16, 17] and undersampling methods may require considerably longer reconstruction times and/or advanced hardware capabilities [16, 18, 24, 25, 27]. The dual RF navigator gated approach was limited to partial acquisition of the cardiac cycle [19]. In contrast, respiratory synchronized acquisition methods using bellows or diaphragmatic RF navigators permit retrospective cardiac gating and real-time reconstruction of bSSFP cine sequences, which are used in clinical practice without imposing any hardware or reconstruction burden [20–23]. Furthermore, these respiratory motion synchronized techniques allow the flexibility to be seamlessly combined with undersampling strategies such as compressed sensing that may become clinically available in the future.

We have previously demonstrated respiratory synchronized bSSFP cine acquisitions using both respiratory bellows and diaphragmatic RF navigator, in a healthy cohort study [20]. These implementations require SS to be reached before the acquisition of cardiac gated cine data to ensure uniform signal and contrast throughout the cardiac cycle. The bellows based respiratory triggered (RT) implementation was validated in a pediatric population [22]. Similar approaches using respiratory bellows and diaphragmatic RF navigator for respiratory synchronized bSSFP cine acquisition have also been reported [21, 23]. However, these implementations use the available time between the respiratory trigger and the subsequent R-top for SS preparation. This can cause artifacts because the variable time interval may not be long enough to attain SS in certain respiratory cycles [21]. In this manuscript we describe a two-center clinical validation of a bellows based RT-bSSFP in an adult population with rigorous quantitative assessment of the temporal stability of the myocardial signal as well as blood-to-myocardial contrast.

Methods

Numerical simulation

Numerical simulations were performed in MATLAB (The MathWorks™ Inc., Natick, Massachusetts, USA), to determine the minimum number of RF excitations required for myocardial tissue to reach SS in a bSSFP sequence starting with an $\alpha/2$ preparation pulse, followed after a time period of TR/2 by successively alternating $\pm\alpha$ excitation pulses every TR. Temporal evolution of myocardial magnetization from the unperturbed state to SS with uninterrupted RF excitations, characteristic of the bSSFP sequence, was numerically simulated with the following parameters: magnetic field strength, 1.5 T ± 3 ppm; TR/TE/flip angle, 3 ms/1.5 ms/65°; T_1, 950 ms; T_2, 50 ms. The steady state magnetization (M_{SS}) was defined as magnetization where the rate of change of magnetization was close to zero (< 0.5%).

Cine bSSFP CMR with respiratory triggering (RT)

A commercially available BH cine bSSFP sequence with retrospective cardiac gating and prospective arrhythmia rejection was modified to implement a free-breathing RT sequence on clinical scanner (Achieva, Philips

Healthcare, Best, the Netherlands). A schematic showing the building blocks of this technique, described previously [22], is shown in Fig. 1. In the RT sequence, the RF excitations started immediately after the trigger signal (could be set to an arbitrary delay from inspiration or expiration trigger point) derived from the respiratory bellows unmodified from the commercial implementation on the scanner. The data acquisition corresponding to the initial RF excitations were discarded (dummy excitations), for a minimum user-prescribed time (τ), to drive to M_{SS}. The subsequent arrival of the first cardiac R-top (at time point after the trigger > τ) was used as a cardiac synchronization point to accept data acquisition of the segment of phase-encoding steps in k-space in a multi-phase manner during that cardiac cycle. Upon arrival of the subsequent R-top, RF excitations were terminated, and the commercially available real-time arrhythmia rejection algorithm either accepted or rejected the data. In the case of rejection, the same phase-encoding segment was re-acquired. This process was repeated until the entire k-space was acquired, after which the retrospective cardiac gating reconstruction algorithm performed the required nonlinear stretching of variable R-R intervals to reconstruct cine images.

Two-center clinical validation

The prospective clinical validation studies were performed at Institute A and Institute B in patients referred for a clinical CMR for various indications. Institute A

implemented the RT sequence and Institute B, located 2000 km away from Institute A, used this investigational sequence without supervision from Institute A. Institute A recruited 23 asymptomatic subjects (10 men). The mean age of these healthy subjects was 44 years (range, 24–60 years). At Institute A, 39 consecutive patients (21 men) were enrolled in the study. The mean age of these patients was 50 years (range, 19–82 years). At Institute B, 21 consecutive patients (12 men) were enrolled in the study. The mean age of these patients was 47 years (range, 23–86 years). All patients underwent biventricular function evaluation as a part of routine clinical protocol to evaluate the following conditions: left and right ventricular (LV, RV) cardiomyopathies (31), myocardial viability (12), valvular function (9), pericarditis (7), and congenital heart disease (1). This study was approved by the Institutional Ethics Committee of Catholic Health Initiative's Institute for Research and Innovation under evolution MRI techniques protocol and complied with the Health Insurance Portability and Accountability Act of 1996. All subjects gave written informed consent before being enrolled in the study. All healthy subject and patient imaging was performed at 1.5 T CMR scanner (Achieva, Philips Healthcare, Best, the Netherlands) with a 5-element or 32-element phased-array surface coil for signal reception and vector-cardiographic (VCG) gating, with respiratory bellows placed at mediastinum. Authors employed by

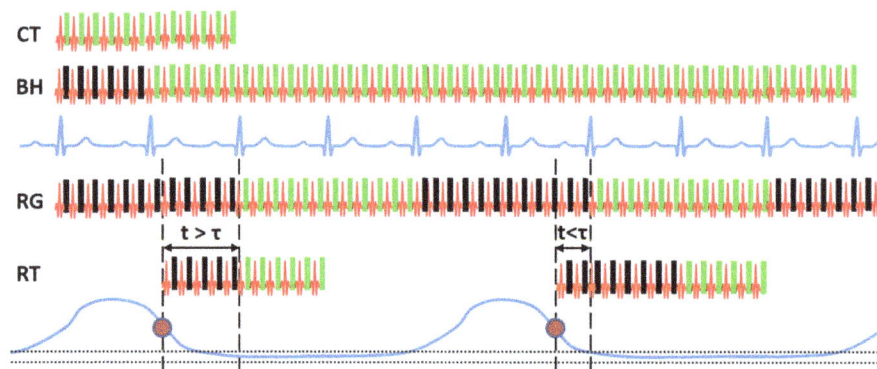

Fig. 1 Steady-state (SS) magnetization preparation methods for cardiac-gated balanced steady-state free precession (bSSFP) cine. CT: In simple cardiac-triggered (CT) acquisition with no SS preparation, all data acquired after the detection of a valid cardiac trigger are accepted for image formation (green boxes). BH: In conventional breath-hold (BH) SS preparation, data acquired during the first RR interval are discarded (black boxes). All subsequent data acquired with cardiac gating during suspended respiration are used for image formation. RG: In the respiratory-gated (RG) method, uninterrupted radiofrequency (RF) excitations applied throughout the acquisition act as the means for SS retention, and only those cardiac-gated data that are acquired when the respiratory bellows signal falls within the user-defined threshold (horizontal dotted lines) are accepted for image formation. RT: In the respiratory-triggered (RT) approach proposed in this paper, RF excitation commences after the detection of a respiratory trigger (e.g., inspiration or expiration), and only data acquired during an RR interval that lags the respiratory trigger point by at least a predefined duration of τ is used for image formation. Unlike RG, RF excitation ceases after the RR interval in which image data are acquired. Electrical signals from the cardiac leads and respiratory bellows are shown in blue. Note that this algorithm is fully compatible and is implemented with prospective rejection of cardiac arrhythmias and retrospective cardiac gating. Phase-encoding steps for the multi-phase segmented k-space acquisition are changed only after successful acceptance of the data. Red dot, expiration trigger; RF, radio frequency; black rectangle, data are discarded; green rectangle, data are accepted for further processing; t, time after respiratory trigger; τ, time to attain steady state; dotted line, respiratory acceptance window

the CMR scanner manufacturer were not part of the clinical patient data acquisition and image quality assessment.

Cardiovascular magnetic resonance imaging protocol

In all 83 study participants, scout images of the thoracic cavity were obtained along the three orthogonal planes by using a non-VCG-gated bSSFP technique. With these single-phase scout scans, a series of VCG-gated cine images were acquired during suspended respiration (BH technique) in the following order: a two-chamber view, a four-chamber view, and a series of 12 to 14 contiguous short-axis slices covering the entire LV from the apex to the base (the level of the mitral valve annulus). Identical imaging parameters and short-axis slice prescription were used with the RT acquisition. Patients were completely blinded to the imaging sequences and were not given any special instructions for breathing during RT technique.

The imaging parameters for both BH and RT cine bSSFP techniques were as follows: TR/TE/flip angle = 2.5–2.7 ms/1.25–1.35 ms/65°; acquired voxel size = 1.7–2.0×1.6–2.0×8 mm^3; SENSitivity Encoding (SENSE) acceleration factor = 1.3–1.9; temporal resolution = 40-50 ms. In the case of BH, each cine slice was acquired during suspended respiration (6–8 R-R intervals/slice, 10–16 heartbeats brath hold time for 2 slices). In the case of RT, a user controllable parameter, minimum time (τ) to drive SSFP signal to M_{SS}, was kept fixed at the default value of 450 ms for all the subjects. For the purpose of evaluating the impact of signal evolution during approach to SS on image quality, additional single-shot cardiac-triggered cine bSSFP (Fig. 1) images without preparation for SS were also acquired in 10 volunteers in a mid-ventricular slice with other imaging parameters identical to those used for BH and RT sequences.

Image analysis

All data were anonymized, randomized, and transferred to a commercial post processing workstation (Extended-WorkSpace, Philips Healthcare).

Quantitative assessment of signal variation

For 23 healthy subjects, regions of interest (ROI) were drawn in the liver, myocardium, and blood pool at mid-ventricular level and were propagated across all cardiac phases in all cine bSSFP sequences. A histogram-based analysis was used to define two quantitative metrics designed to capture the extent of signal intensity (SI) variation across the cardiac cycle, as well as the percent duration of the cardiac cycle (PCC) during which tissue magnetization was close to the theoretically predicted M_{SS}. The signal intensity of ROIs was normalized to the minimum SI across the cardiac cycle. To construct a histogram, normalized signal

intensity values were plotted against the PCC spent at that normalized intensity level. Cumulative density function of normalized signal intensity of myocardial ROI over the cardiac cycle was computed for all healthy subjects. The ratio of the normalized signal intensity values at 95 and 5% of cumulative density function was computed as a metric to characterize the extent of signal intensity variation during the cardiac cycle. A normalized signal intensity of 1.25, which corresponded to M_{SS} based on the simulations, was used to compute the PCC spent in SS. The blood-myocardial contrast (BMC) was normalized to myocardial signal intensity. Box plots were used to evaluate the signal intenisty variation (SIV), the PCC spent in SS by the liver and myocardium, and BMC; in these plots, non-overlapping notches indicate that the medians of the two groups differed at the 5% significance level. In addition, paired two-sided Student's t-statistics for SIV, PCC, and BMC were used to compare among cardiac triggered, BH, and RT sequences.

Quantitative assessment of ventricular measurements

Two independent CMR readers, each with at least a decade of experience in clinical CMR, independently drew the ventricular contours necessary to compute LV and RV volumetric indices (end-diastolic volume, end-systolic volume, and EF) and LV mass. Descriptive statistics of each of these parameters for 60 patients using BH and RT are reported as mean ± standard deviation in absolute values and percentages. Bland-Altman analysis [29] and paired two-sided Student's t-statistics were used to compare each of these parameters computed using the BH sequence with those computed using the RT sequence in 60 patients. Inter-observer variability for each of these parameters was assessed using Bland-Altman analysis in both BH and RT acquisitions in 60 patients.

Image quality assessment

For 60 patients, an independent expert with 12 years of experience in CMR who was blinded to the study design reviewed the stack of short-axis images. The image quality between the two techniques was compared by using the clinical scores, which were based on three parameters: BMC, endocardial-edge definition, and motion artifact. Each parameter was graded on a scale from 1 (non-diagnostic) to 5 (excellent) on review of all the images in the short-axis stack. In cases where all but one or two of the slices were of high quality, the clinical score was lowered for the entire stack. Details of the scoring criteria are provided in Table 1. For each of the three scoring criteria considered in the study, the percentage of clinical subjects that received a range of clinical scores was plotted as a bar graph. In addition, a similar bar graph was constructed with the combined score, computed as the equal weight average of the three

Table 1 Clinical score criteria

Score	Blood-to-myocardial contrast	Endocardial edge definition	Motion artifact
5 - Excellent	Blood pool is hyper intense with excellent contrast against the myocardium; myocardium is uniformly bright throughout the cardiac cycle with little evidence of flashing.	Papillary and endocardial trabeculae are clearly visible in the bright backdrop of the blood pool.	Image is nearly artifact free.
4 - Good	Blood pool is significantly brighter than the myocardium, or myocardial signal intensity is fairly uniform throughout the cardiac cycle.	Papillary and endocardial trabeculae are visible but somewhat blurred during the cardiac cycle.	Some motion artifact is present but does not affect overall image quality.
3 - Moderate	Image is of diagnostic quality but features significant loss of blood to myocardial contrast or noticeable variation in myocardial signal throughout the cardiac cycle.	Myocardial walls are barely distinguishable from endocardial trabeculae.	Motion artifacts are visible, but image is still of diagnostic quality.
2 - Poor	Blood-to-myocardial contrast is poor, but the image is still of diagnostic quality.	Myocardial walls and endocardial trabeculae are significantly blurred.	Images are nearly nondiagnostic with significant artifacts.
1 - Nondiagnostic	Blood-to-myocardial contrast is poor; image was deemed nondiagnostic.	Blood-to-myocardial edge definition is poor; image was deemed nondiagnostic.	Image is of nondiagnostic quality.

scores, to underscore the overall performance of the technique on the basis of all three criteria. One-sided Wilcoxon signed rank tests were performed on clinical scores assigned to the BH and RT techniques.

Results

Numerical simulation

Numerical simulations showed that the signal intensity for the myocardium could be 6 to 8 times that of the M_{SS} after the first few RF excitations, and as many as 140 continuous RF excitations (with a flip angle of 65° at a repetition time of 3 ms) were required to reach myocardial M_{SS}. After the rate of change of myocardial magnetization fell below 0.5%, the magnetization corresponded to 125% of the M_{SS} predicted by the analytical

expression for the steady state signal (Fig. 2a). For healthy subject 3, liver and myocardial signal intensity curves with cardiac triggering (no dummy excitations) confirmed the requirement of continuous RF excitation for 350 ms and 450 ms (at TR interval of 3 ms), respectively, for the liver and myocardium (Fig. 2b) to attain steady signal intensity levels. Liver and myocardial signal intensity curves obtained with the RT sequence (dummy excitations for a duration of 450 ms) matched closely with those obtained using the BH sequence (dummy excitations for a duration of one R-R interval), confirming the attainment of M_{SS} after 140 continuous RF pulses, as indicated by the numerical simulation (Fig. 2). Representative clinical images from healthy subject 3 are shown for all three techniques in Fig. 3.

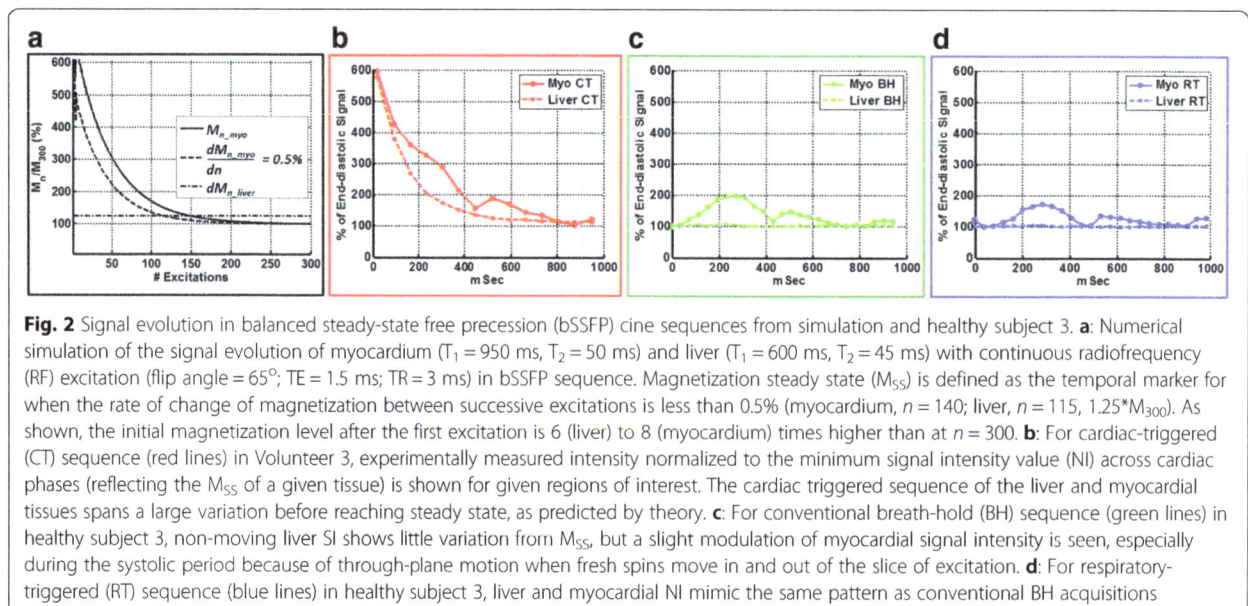

Fig. 2 Signal evolution in balanced steady-state free precession (bSSFP) cine sequences from simulation and healthy subject 3. **a**: Numerical simulation of the signal evolution of myocardium ($T_1 = 950$ ms, $T_2 = 50$ ms) and liver ($T_1 = 600$ ms, $T_2 = 45$ ms) with continuous radiofrequency (RF) excitation (flip angle = 65°; TE = 1.5 ms; TR = 3 ms) in bSSFP sequence. Magnetization steady state (M_{SS}) is defined as the temporal marker for when the rate of change of magnetization between successive excitations is less than 0.5% (myocardium, $n = 140$; liver, $n = 115$, $1.25*M_{300}$). As shown, the initial magnetization level after the first excitation is 6 (liver) to 8 (myocardium) times higher than at $n = 300$. **b**: For cardiac-triggered (CT) sequence (red lines) in Volunteer 3, experimentally measured intensity normalized to the minimum signal intensity value (NI) across cardiac phases (reflecting the M_{SS} of a given tissue) is shown for given regions of interest. The cardiac triggered sequence of the liver and myocardial tissues spans a large variation before reaching steady state, as predicted by theory. **c**: For conventional breath-hold (BH) sequence (green lines) in healthy subject 3, non-moving liver SI shows little variation from M_{SS}, but a slight modulation of myocardial signal intensity is seen, especially during the systolic period because of through-plane motion when fresh spins move in and out of the slice of excitation. **d**: For respiratory-triggered (RT) sequence (blue lines) in healthy subject 3, liver and myocardial NI mimic the same pattern as conventional BH acquisitions

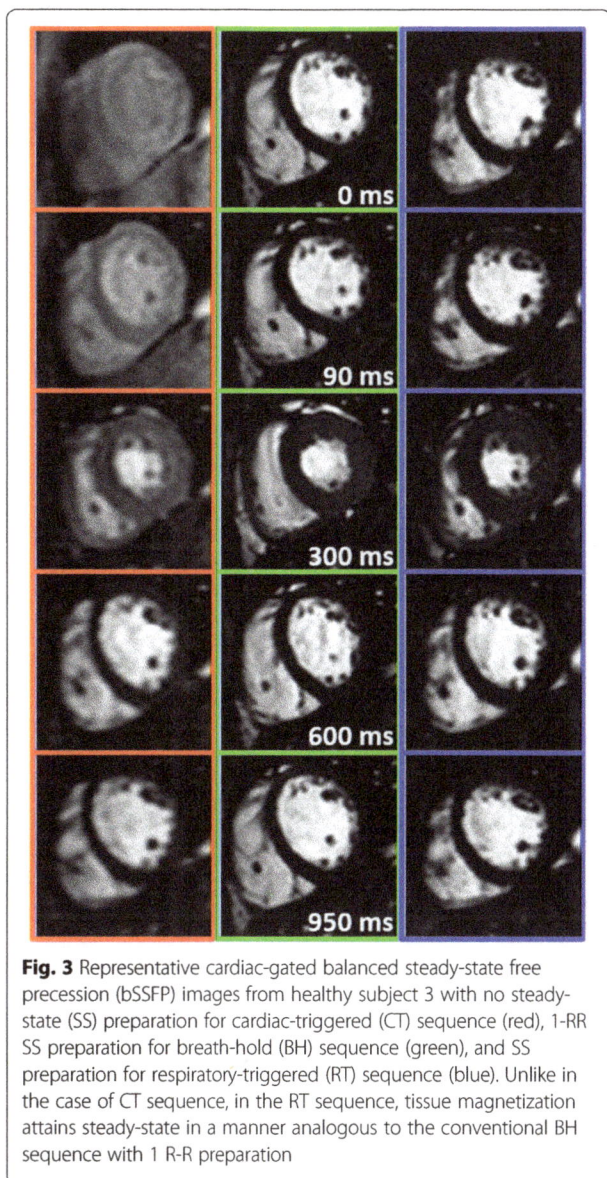

Fig. 3 Representative cardiac-gated balanced steady-state free precession (bSSFP) images from healthy subject 3 with no steady-state (SS) preparation for cardiac-triggered (CT) sequence (red), 1-RR SS preparation for breath-hold (BH) sequence (green), and SS preparation for respiratory-triggered (RT) sequence (blue). Unlike in the case of CT sequence, in the RT sequence, tissue magnetization attains steady-state in a manner analogous to the conventional BH sequence with 1 R-R preparation

Quantitative assessment of signal variation

Using histogram analysis, we showed the mean normalized signal intensity among all 23 healthy subjects for liver and myocardial ROIs for the BH and RT sequences, and among 10 healthy subjects for cardiac triggered sequences (Fig. 4a-b). When compared to the histogram mode of normalized signal intensity of liver tissue, the histogram mode of normalized signal intensity of the myocardium occupied a much smaller fraction of the cardiac cycle for all three techniques. The cumulative density function of myocardial normalized signal intensity indicated that, on average, the BH and RT techniques spent more than 95% of the cardiac cycle below a normalized signal intensity of 2, whereas for cardiac triggering, that value was 4 (Fig. 4d). Notably, the quantitative metrics of SIV, BMC, and PCC spent in SS for the

cardiac triggered technique were significantly different from those for the BH and RT techniques ($p < 0.001$) (Fig. 5). In contrast, the difference in SIV and PCC spent in SS by myocardium was not statistically significant between the BH and RT techniques (Fig. 5a, b). Similarly, BMC was also not statistically different between the BH and RT techniques (Fig. 5c). The differences in SIV and the PCC between the liver and myocardium were statistically significant ($p < 0.001$) for both the BH and RT techniques because of through-plane motion of the myocardium (Fig. 5a, b).

Quantitative assessment of ventricular measurements

The RT sequence ran successfully in all 60 patients. The mean heart rate was 74 bpm (range 43–116), and the mean respiratory rate was 18 bpm (range 12–20). Total image acquisition time for RT was significantly longer than that for conventional BH (7.9 ± 3.4 min vs. 5.1 ± 2.6 min) ($p < 0.001$). In two cases, RT scan time was three times longer than that of the BH sequence because of specific breathing patterns. Table 2 provides descriptive statistics of the LV and RV volumetric indices and LV mass computed using BH and RT sequences in the 60 patients. Figure 6 depicts Bland-Altman plots comparing each of these parameters between BH and RT in 60 patients. Inter-observer variability for each of these parameters in both BH and RT acquisitions in 60 patients is reported in Table 3. For all the parameters the bias and limits of agreement between BH and RT sequences are in good agreement with inter-observer variability in both BH and RT sequences.

Image quality assessment

The combined clinical score was excellent (87%) to good (13%) for BH and excellent (38%) to good (45%) to moderate (17%) for RT (Fig. 6 H). In 17% of cases, the scores were equal, whereas the difference in combined clinical score was less than 0.5 in 48% and less than 1 in 82% of cases. In only one patient, edge definition and motion artifact were scored as poor for the RT sequence. The difference between clinical scores for the BH and RT sequences was statistically significant ($p < 0.0001$). Figure 7 shows representative BH and RT images from patients with a good to excellent clinical score for BH.

Discussion

The results from the two-center clinical study show that RT-bSSFP yielded diagnostic image quality cine images in all 60 patients encompassing a wide range of heart rates (43–116 bpm), respiratory rates (12–20 bpm), and ventricular indices (LV end-diastolic volume 84–397 mL, LV end-systolic volume 35–325 mL, LVEF 18–71%) with spatial, temporal, and contrast resolutions that were comparable to BH-bSSFP. To the best of our

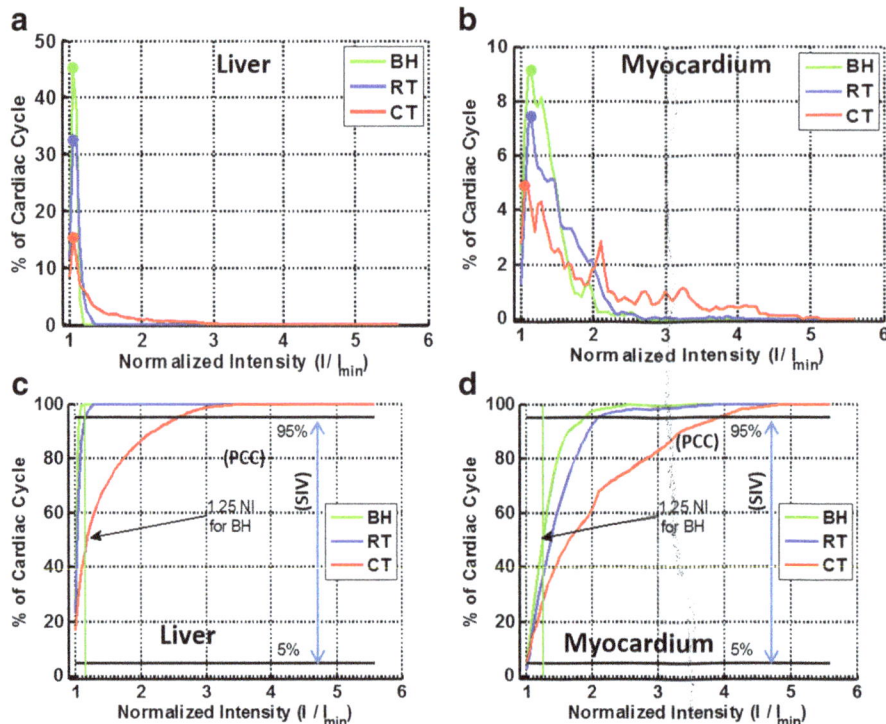

Fig. 4 Extraction of quantitative metrics from histogram analysis of liver and myocardial normalized intensity (NI, mean of all subjects) across the cardiac cycle for three steady state (SS) preparations. To generate a histogram, the normalized signal intensity of liver **a** and myocardial **b** signal intensity (SI) is plotted against the fraction of the cardiac cycle occupied by that normalized signal intensity level. When data are plotted in this manner, the mode of the histogram (circles) indicates the in vivo steady state normalized signal intensity level for each of the SS preparation methods. **c**, **d**: Cumulative density functions of histograms plotted in A and B are used to calculate the percentage of cardiac cycle spent below a specific normalized signal intensity level. Total percentage of cardiac cycle (PCC) spent close to steady-state level is defined as cumulative density function at 1.25*normalized signal intensity (vertical line) level (refer to legend in Fig. 2). Temporal signal intensity variation (SIV) is defined as the ratio of normalized signal intensity values at 95 and 5% (horizontal lines) of cumulative density function

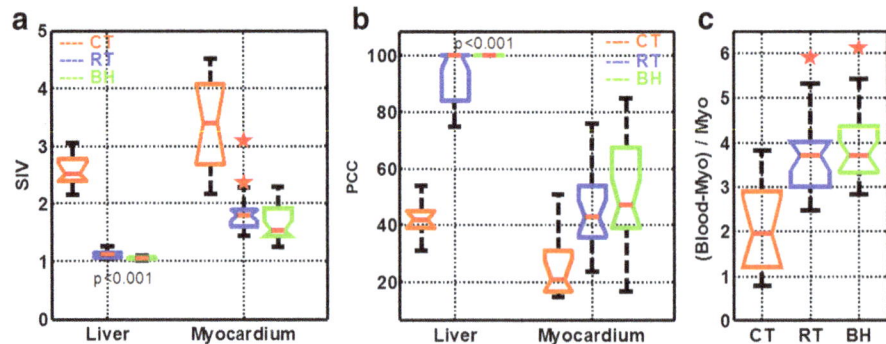

Fig. 5 Box-plot analyses of normalized intensity (NI) variation over a cardiac cycle. **a**: Signal intensity variation (SIV) of myocardium was similar between breath-hold (BH) and respiratory-triggered (RT) techniques in study participants (p = nonsignificant [NS]), but SIV of myocardium and liver was significantly higher for the CT technique than for either the BH or RT technique ($p < 0.001$); **b**: Percentage of cardiac cycle (PCC) of myocardium was similar between BH and RT techniques (p = NS), but the PCC of myocardium and liver was significantly lower for the cardiac triggered technique than for either the BH or RT technique ($p < 0.001$); **c**: The blood-to-myocardial contrast (BMC) of the BH and RT techniques were similar (p = NS), but the BMC of the cardiac triggered technique was lower than that of either the BH or RT technique ($p < 0.001$). Although the liver and myocardium have similar tissue relaxation parameters, SIV and PCC were significantly different ($p < 0.001$) between the two tissues for both BH and RT because of through-plane motion of the myocardium. Non-overlapping notches indicate that the medians of the two groups differ at the 5% significance level. Outliers beyond 1.5 times the interquartile distance are indicated with five-point stars in red. P-values derived from paired t-test are labeled next to box plots where non-overlapping notches are unclear

Table 2 Left and right ventricular volumetric indices and LV mass and difference in their values between breath-hold sequence and respiratory-triggered sequence in patients

	LV EDV (ml)	LV ESV (ml)	LV EF (%)	LV Mass (g)	RV EDV (ml)	RV ESV (ml)	RV EF (%)
BH	177.5 ± 65.8	86.7 ± 56.7	53.9 ± 11.5	126.6 ± 49.9	147.3 ± 45.9	70.2 ± 29.5	53.1 ± 7.6
RT	174.8 ± 65.1	84.6 ± 55.3	54.3 ± 11.8	126.4 ± 49.6	149.8 ± 45.0	73.0 ± 30.3	52.2 ± 7.0
BH-RT	2.8 ± 10.6	2.1 ± 6.8	-0.4 ± 4.1	0.2 ± 7.7	-2.5 ± 7.8	-2.7 ± 5.7	0.9 ± 4.0
BH-RT / BH (%)	1.4 ± 6.5	2.2 ± 9.5	-0.9 ± 7.7	-0.2 ± 6.2	-2.1 ± 5.2	-4.5 ± 7.2	1.72 ± 8.9
BH-RT (p)	0.047	0.022	0.450	0.822	0.105	< 0.001	0.072

All values from observer 1

BH breath-hold, *EDV* end-diastolic volume, *EF* ejection fraction, *ESV* end-systolic volume, *LV* left ventricle, *p* p value from paired t-test, *RT* respiratory triggered, *RV* right ventricle

knowledge, this is the first study that has performed clinical validation of the free breathing cine bSSFP imaging in a large cohort of adult patients. The bias and limits of agreement between RT and BH sequences for LV and RV volumetric indices and LV mass were comparable to inter-observer variability in both RT and BH sequences. An interesting observation was that while the LV volumes were slightly overestimated (mean bias of 2–3 mL) with BH sequence compared to RT sequence, RV volumes were slightly underestimated (mean bias of 2–3 mL). Although such small differences in ventricular volumes may not be clinically significant, it may be worth investigating if the intra-thoracic pressure differences between respiratory suspended state and free breathing could be a contributing factor.

There are several key findings from the study that are worth noting. Firstly, conventional respiratory triggering methods for circumventing the breath-holding in bSSFP imaging that do not account for signal intensity modulation during the approach to SS can introduce significant artifacts as demonstrated in this study. Interestingly, even in BH bSSFP acquisitions, through-plane motion of the base toward the apex of the ventricle during systole introduces quantifiable temporal signal heterogeneity in the myocardium. Compared to other previously published respiratory triggered bSSFP cine CMR implementations [21, 23], RT sequence implementation [20, 22] mandates attainment of M_{ss} prior to cardiac gated data acquisition. Metrics to quantify the temporal stability of the signal demonstrated that the RT sequence attained SS in synchrony with the physiologic cycle that is comparable to BH bSSFP. Importantly, the proposed acquisition technique and image quality evaluation metric have the potential to be used more broadly in other clinical applications. Also, it is worth noting that RT-bSSFP cine sequence is inherently compatible with prospective

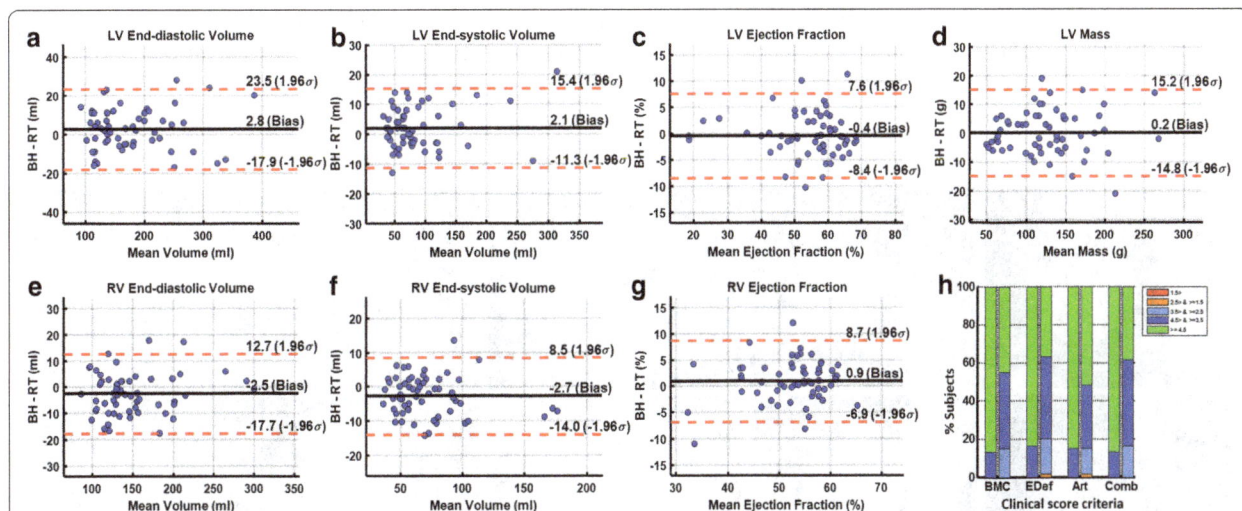

Fig. 6 Bland-Altman plots (**a-g**) comparing left and right ventricular (LV, RV) volumetric indices and LV mass between BH and RT, and bar-plot analysis (**h**) for combined clinical scores for criteria defined Table 1 (For each criteria, scores for BH are plotted on the left, and RT are plotted on the right). H: Percentage of patients that had clinical scores of excellent, good, moderate, or poor for criteria related to blood-to-myocardial contrast (BMC), endocardial edge definition (Edef), and artifacts (Art). The combined clinical score is the equal-weights average of the three scores, which underscores the overall performance of the technique. **BH**: breath-hold (BH), with a dummy excitation duration of one R-R interval; **RT**: prospectively respiratory-triggered (RT) with dummy excitation duration of 450 ms

Table 3 Inter-observer agreement for left and right ventricular volumetric indices and LV mass obtained with breath-hold sequence and respiratory-triggered sequence in patients

	LV EDV (ml)	LV ESV (ml)	LV EF (%)	LV Mass (g)	RV EDV (ml)	RV ESV (ml)	RV EF (%)
BH (O_1-O_2)	0.3 ± 10.4	1.3 ± 9.8	−0.7 ± 6.2	1.6 ± 8.3	4.6 ± 6.7	0.4 ± 5.8	1.4 ± 2.8
RT (O_1-O_2)	−0.1 ± 11.4	−2.0 ± 8.5	1.9 ± 5.0	− 0.2 ± 8.9	2.7 ± 7.7	1.0 ± 5.6	0.4 ± 3.1
BH (O_1-O_2)/ O_1 (%)	−0.8 ± 8.1	−0.7 ± 16.0	−2.4 ± 12.3	− 0.1 ± 8.4	3.1 ± 4.5	0.2 ± 7.2	2.4 ± 5.5
RT (O_1-O_2)/ O_1 (%)	−0.2 ± 7.3	−6.1 ± 16.3	2.7 ± 8.4	−1.9 ± 9.7	1.6 ± 4.9	0.7 ± 6.5	0.5 ± 6.6

BH breath-hold, *EDV* end-diastolic volume, *EF* ejection fraction, *ESV* end-systolic volume, *LV* left ventricle, O_1 observer 1, O_2 observer 2, *RT* respiratory triggered, *RV* right ventricle

arrhythmia rejection and retrospective cardiac gating that are typically used with BH techniques, allowing the acquisition of a complete cardiac cycle. Furthermore, the cardio-respiratory synchronization approach can be seamlessly combined with other techniques such as non-cartesian sampling, sparse sampling, and self-navigation.

Secondly, bSSFP cine acquisition is feasible with both respiratory triggering using bellows and respiratory triggering with slice tracking using diaphragmatic RF navigators [20]. One advantage of using diaphragmatic RF navigators is the ability to track slice location in real time from the navigator information. However, the relatively long duration (at least one RR interval) between the slice position measurement from RF navigators and the completion of cine data acquisition may diminish this potential benefit. Furthermore, the quality of RF navigators may be compromised in patients with significant iron overload [23]. In contrast to RF navigators, respiratory bellows do not provide a direct measure of the lung-diaphragmatic interface. However, respiratory bellows provide the ability to monitor respiratory motion continuously and independent of CMR data acquisition without incurring additional RF dose.

Thirdly, respiratory triggered cine bSSFP sequences have several strengths. In contrast to continuous multi-NSA sequences which are often used to obtain cine bSSFP images in sedated patients or those with compromised respiratory function [22], the RF duty cycle in these sequences remains at about 50%, mitigating the specific energy deposition concerns and permits data acquisition over a longer scan duration. Freedom from the breath-hold constraint further allows one to attain bSSFP cine images with higher spatial resolution, temporal resolution, or coverage. Therefore, this technique has the potential to broaden the scope of clinical applications for cine bSSFP sequences, such as assessing diastolic function by obtaining a high temporal resolution dataset.

Another advantage of the RT bSSFP cine sequence is that it would reduce the potential for errors in estimation of ventricular chamber volumes due to inconsistent breath-holds. Although CMR is considered the gold standard for the estimation of ventricular chamber volumes, inconsistencies in the level of the diaphragm across breath-holds for each slice can result in under and/or over sampling of the myocardium in the direction of the ventricular long axis. This too may lead to variability in calculated volumes and EF, especially sampling-dependent inclusion or exclusion of the basal slice in end-systole [30]. This problem would be significantly diminished with free-breathing acquisitions [19].

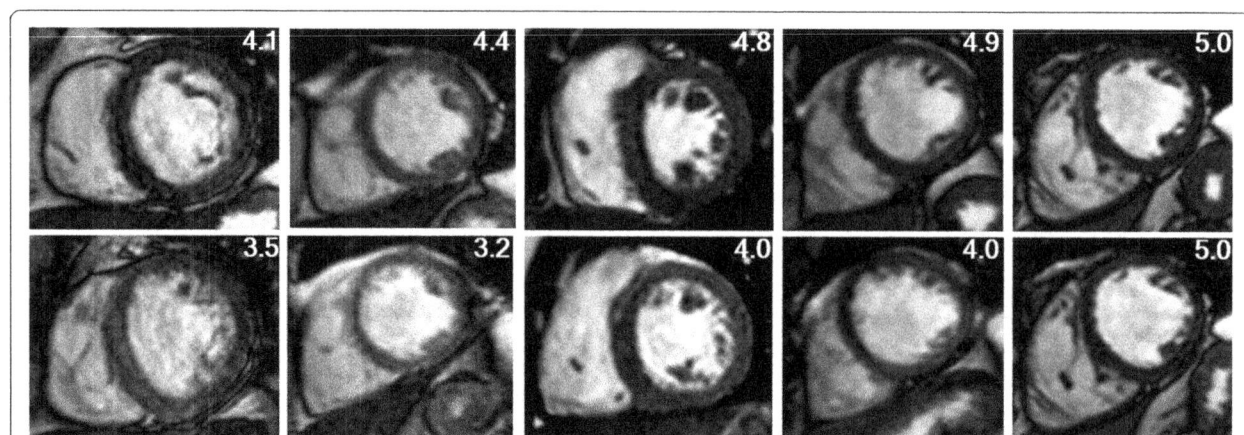

Fig. 7 A panel of representative breath-hold (BH) (top) and respiratory-triggered (RT) (bottom) cardiac balanced steady-state free precession (bSSFP) images from patients with a combined clinical score for BH images ranging from 4.1 (good) to 5 (excellent) and a combined clinical score for corresponding RT images ranging from 3.2 (moderate) to 5 (excellent)

Although we made no attempt to include only patients with compromised respiratory function, our clinical results suggest that the reduction in image quality of RT bSSFP was only small compared to the image quality attainable with the BH bSSFP technique. Notably, in our previous study, the image quality obtained with the RT-SSFP technique was better than that obtained with the multiple signal averaging that is routinely used in sedated pediatric patients [22]. In this two-center study in adults, our findings with respect to LV mass and ventricular volumetric results obtained with the RT and BH sequences are in line with the inter-observer variability.

The current implementation of RT-SSFP cine sequence has two key limitations. First, image quality of RT-bSSFP, while good, was inferior to that of the BH-bSSFP sequence. In 10/60 subjects, RT-SSFP image quality scores were moderate (still diagnostic) and we speculate that this reduction in image quality may be partly because of inconsistent respiratory patterns, such as when a patient starts inspiration before data acquisition from the expiratory trigger has completed, or respiratory drift over the course of an examination. The extent of the image quality degradation is dependent on the location of the acquisition segment with respect to center of the k-space. The image quality of the RT sequence could be improved by imposing an additional prospective constraint for rejecting data that were acquired during such respiratory inconsistencies at the cost of increasing scan time. A second limitation of the RT-bSSFP sequence is that it takes on an average 55% more time than the conventional cine BH-bSSFP sequence. For a cardiac cine bSSFP technique that requires n shots for a complete data acquisition, the RT-bSSFP sequence takes the time required for n respiratory cycles, whereas the BH-bSSFP sequence takes the time required for n + 1 heartbeats (1 extra beat to drive to M_{SS}). This is because the RT sequence, in its current implementation, acquires data for a single cardiac cycle after each respiratory trigger. Often, the expiratory phase of the respiratory cycle is longer than one cardiac cycle and may permit data acquisition for several cardiac cycles, which would reduce the acquisition time of the RT sequence. Although this was not considered in this study, data acquisition over consecutive cardiac cycles during expiration with prospective constraint for rejecting the data are an important area of future investigation [31] as respiratory bellows permits continuous and simultaneous tracking of the respiratory motion.

Conclusion

In conclusion, we have shown that the RT sequence is a robust, free-breathing alternative to BH-bSSFP for evaluating ventricular function in patients with impaired breath-holding capacity and/or arrhythmia. The RT sequence yields cine images with contrast and spatio-temporal resolutions that are identical to those attained by using the BH sequence, albeit with a modest time penalty and a small reduction in image quality. We believe that the elimination of the BH constraint on a cine bSSFP sequence has the potential to improve the evaluation of ventricular function in subjects with compromised respiratory capacity with small reduction in image quality. Moreover, this would allow one to acquire high temporal resolution cine images necessary for the assessment of transient phenomena, such as isovolumic relaxation time, as well as the ability to acquire multi-phase, high-resolution anatomic images, such as coronary MR angiography.

Abbreviations
M: magnetization; SS: Steady state; BA: Bland-Altman analysis; BH: Breathhold; BMC: Blood-myocardial contrast; bSSFP: Balanced steady-state free precession; CMR: Cardiovascular magnetic resonance; EDV: End-diastolic volume; EF: Ejection fraction; ESV: End-systolic volume; LV: Left ventricle/left ventricular; NI: Normalized signal intensity; PCC: Percent duration of the cardiac cycle; RF: Radio frequency; RG: Respiratory gated; ROI: Region of interest; RT: Respiratory triggered; RV: Right ventricle/right ventricular; SENSE: Snesitivity encoding; SI: Signal intensity; SIV: Signal intensity variation; SNR: Signal-to-noise ratio; ss: Steady state; TE: Echo time; TR: Time; VCG: Vector electrocardiogram

Acknowledgements
We gratefully acknowledge Janie Swaab, RT, Sharon Berry, RT, Kathy Kohut, RT, Debra Dees, RN, and Melissa Andrews, RN for their help in data collection.

Authors' contributions
AP: performed numerical simulation, performed CMR pulse sequence design and implementation, performed statistical analysis, drafted the manuscript. HW: participated in data collection, helped drafting the manuscript. SF: participated in data collection and data analysis. BC: participated in data collection, data analysis, and drafting the manuscript. RM: participated in CMR pulse sequence design, designed the study, helped in statistical analysis and equal contribution in drafting the manuscript. All authors read and approved the final manuscript.

Competing interests
AP: employee of Philips Healthcare until January 2017.
HW: employee of Philips Healthcare.
Authors employed by the CMR scanner manufacturer were not part of the clinical patient data acquisition and image quality assessment.

Author details
[1]Department of Radiology, Texas Children's Hospital, 6701 Fannin Street, Suite D470.09, Houston, TX 77030-2399, USA. [2]Philips Healthcare, Gainesville, FL, USA. [3]Department of Diagnostic Radiology, Cleveland Clinic, Cleveland, OH, USA. [4]Department of Radiology, Baylor St. Luke's Medical Center, Houston, TX, USA.

References

1. Dodge HT, Baxley WA. Left ventricular volume and mass and their significance in heart disease. Am J Cardiol. 1969;23:528–37.
2. Levy D, Garrison RJ, Savage DD, Kannel WB, Castelli WP. Prognostic implications of Echocardiographically determined left ventricular mass in the Framingham heart study. N Engl J Med. 1990;322:1561–6.
3. Anavekar N, Skali H, McMurray J, Swedberg K, Yusus S, Granger C, et al. Influence of ejection fraction on cardiovascular outcomes in a broad Spectrum of heart failure patients. Circulation. 2005;112:3738–44.
4. Taniguchi K, Nakano S, Hirose H, Matsuda H, Shirakura R, Sakai K, et al. Preoperative left ventricular function: minimal requirement for successful late results of valve replacement for aortic regurgitation. J Am Coll Cardiol. 1987;10:510–8.
5. White HD, Norris RM, Brown MA, Brandt PW, Whitlock RM, Wild CJ. Left ventricular end-systolic volume as the major determinant of survival after recovery from myocardial infarction. Circulation. 1987;76:44–51.
6. Bellenger NG, Davies LC, Francis JM, Coats AJ, Pennell DJ. Reduction in sample size for studies of remodeling in heart failure by the use of cardiovascular magnetic resonance. J Cardiovasc Magn Reson Off J Soc Cardiovasc Magn Reson. 2000;2:271–8.
7. Bottini PB, Carr AA, Prisant LM, Flickinger FW, Allison JD, Gottdiener JS. Magnetic resonance imaging compared to echocardiography to assess left ventricular mass in the hypertensive patient. Am J Hypertens. 1995;8:221–8.
8. Grothues F, Smith GC, Moon JCC, Bellenger NG, Collins P, Klein HU, et al. Comparison of interstudy reproducibility of cardiovascular magnetic resonance with two-dimensional echocardiography in normal subjects and in patients with heart failure or left ventricular hypertrophy. Am J Cardiol. 2002;90:29–34.
9. Pennell DJ, Sechtem UP, Higgins CB, Manning WJ, Pohost GM, Rademakers FE, et al. Clinical indications for cardiovascular magnetic resonance (CMR): consensus panel report. Eur Heart J. 2004;25:1940–65.
10. Finn JP, Nael K, Deshpande V, Ratib O, Laub G. Cardiac MR imaging: state of the technology. Radiology. 2006;241:338–54.
11. Scheffler K, Lehnhardt S. Principles and applications of balanced SSFP techniques. Eur Radiol. 2003;13:2409–18.
12. Srinivasan S, Ennis DB. Optimal flip angle for high contrast balanced SSFP cardiac cine imaging. Magn Reson Med. 2015;73:1095–103.
13. Scheffler K. On the transient phase of balanced SSFP sequences. Magn Reson Med. 2003;49:781–3.
14. Hargreaves BA, Vasanawala SS, Pauly JM, Nishimura DG. Characterization and reduction of the transient response in steady-state MR imaging. Magn Reson Med. 2001;46:149–58.
15. Markl M, Alley MT, Elkins CJ, Pelc NJ. Flow effects in balanced steady state free precession imaging. Magn Reson Med. 2003;50:892–903.
16. Sudarski S, Henzler T, Haubenreisser H, Dösch C, Zenge MO, Schmidt M, et al. Free-breathing sparse sampling cine MR imaging with iterative reconstruction for the assessment of left ventricular function and mass at 3. 0 T Radiology. 2016;282:74–83.
17. Vincenti G, Monney P, Chaptinel J, Rutz T, Coppo S, Zenge MO, et al. Compressed sensing single-breath-hold CMR for fast quantification of LV function, volumes, and mass. JACC Cardiovasc Imaging. 2014;7:882–92.
18. Zhou Z, Han F, Rapacchi S, Nguyen K-L, Brunengraber DZ, G-HJ K, et al. Accelerated ferumoxytol-enhanced 4D multiphase, steady-state imaging with contrast enhancement (MUSIC) cardiovascular MRI: validation in pediatric congenital heart disease. NMR Biomed. 2017;30
19. Peters DC, Nezafat R, Eggers H, Stehning C, Manning WJ. 2D free-breathing dual navigator-gated cardiac function validated against the 2D breath-hold acquisition. J Magn Reson Imaging. 2008;28:773–7.
20. Pednekar A, Krishnamurthy R, Arena C, Muthupillai R, Cheong B, Dees D. Respiratory triggered retrospectively cardiac gated cine steady-state free precession (SSFP) imaging. In: 20th proc. Intl. Soc. mag. Reson. Med. Melbourne; 2012. p. 3938.
21. Henningsson M, Chan R, Goddu B, Goepfert LA, Razavi R, Botnar RM, et al. Contrast-enhanced specific absorption rate-efficient 3D cardiac cine with respiratory-triggered radiofrequency gating. J Magn Reson Imaging. 2013;37:986–92.
22. Krishnamurthy R, Pednekar A, Atweh LA, Vogelius E, Chu ZD, Zhang W, et al. Clinical validation of free breathing respiratory triggered retrospectively cardiac gated cine balanced steady-state free precession cardiovascular magnetic resonance in sedated children. J Cardiovasc Magn Reson. 2015;17 https://doi.org/10.1186/s12968-014-0101-1.
23. Moghari MH, Komarlu R, Annese D, Geva T, Powell AJ. Free-breathing steady-state free precession cine cardiac magnetic resonance with respiratory navigator gating. Magn Reson Med. 2015;73:1555–61.
24. Han F, Zhou Z, Han E, Gao Y, Nguyen K-L, Finn JP, et al. Self-gated 4D multiphase, steady-state imaging with contrast enhancement (MUSIC) using rotating cartesian K-space (ROCK): validation in children with congenital heart disease. Magn Reson Med. 2016;
25. Sayin O, Saybasili H, Zviman MM, Griswold M, Halperin H, Seiberlich N, et al. Real-time free-breathing cardiac imaging with self-calibrated through-time radial GRAPPA. Magn Reson Med. 2017;77:250–64.
26. Yerly J, Ginami G, Nordio G, Coristine AJ, Coppo S, Monney P, et al. Coronary endothelial function assessment using self-gated cardiac cine MRI and k-t sparse SENSE. Magn Reson Med. 2016;76:1443–54.
27. Feng L, Axel L, Chandarana H, Block KT, Sodickson DK, Otazo R. XD-GRASP: golden-angle radial MRI with reconstruction of extra motion-state dimensions using compressed sensing. Magn Reson Med. 2016;75:775–88.
28. Han F, Rapacchi S, Khan S, Ayad I, Salusky I, Gabriel S, et al. Four-dimensional, multiphase, steady-state imaging with contrast enhancement (MUSIC) in the heart: a feasibility study in children. Magn Reson Med. 2015;74:1042–9.
29. Bland JM, Altman DG. Statistical methods for assessing agreement between two methods of clinical measurement. Lancet. 1986;1:307–10.
30. Karamitsos TD, Hudsmith LE, Selvanayagam JB, Neubauer S, Francis JM. Operator induced variability in left ventricular measurements with cardiovascular magnetic resonance is improved after training. J Cardiovasc Magn Reson. 2007;9:777–83.
31. Pednekar A. Clinical Validation of Free Breathing CArdioREspiratory Synchronized (CARESynch) Balanced Steady-State Free Precession (bSSFP) Cine Imaging. In: 20th Annual SCMR Scientific Sessions Abstract Supplement. Washington, DC; 2017.

10

Aortic flow patterns and wall shear stress maps by 4D-flow cardiovascular magnetic resonance in the assessment of aortic dilatation in bicuspid aortic valve disease

José Fernando Rodríguez-Palomares[1][*][†], Lydia Dux-Santoy[1][†], Andrea Guala[1], Raquel Kale[1], Giuliana Maldonado[1], Gisela Teixidó-Turà[1], Laura Galian[1], Marina Huguet[2], Filipa Valente[1], Laura Gutiérrez[1], Teresa González-Alujas[1], Kevin M. Johnson[3], Oliver Wieben[3], David García-Dorado[1] and Arturo Evangelista[1]

Abstract

Background: In patients with bicuspid valve (BAV), ascending aorta (AAo) dilatation may be caused by altered flow patterns and wall shear stress (WSS). These differences may explain different aortic dilatation morphotypes. Using 4D-flow cardiovascular magnetic resonance (CMR), we aimed to analyze differences in flow patterns and regional axial and circumferential WSS maps between BAV phenotypes and their correlation with ascending aorta dilatation morphotype.

Methods: One hundred and one BAV patients (aortic diameter ≤ 45 mm, no severe valvular disease) and 20 healthy subjects were studied by 4D-flow CMR. Peak velocity, flow jet angle, flow displacement, in-plane rotational flow (IRF) and systolic flow reversal ratio (SFRR) were assessed at different levels of the AAo. Peak-systolic axial and circumferential regional WSS maps were also estimated. Unadjusted and multivariable adjusted linear regression analyses were used to identify independent correlates of aortic root or ascending dilatation. Age, sex, valve morphotype, body surface area, flow derived variables and WSS components were included in the multivariable models.

Results: The AAo was non-dilated in 24 BAV patients and dilated in 77 (root morphotype in 11 and ascending in 66). BAV phenotype was right-left (RL-) in 78 patients and right-non-coronary (RN-) in 23. Both BAV phenotypes presented different outflow jet direction and velocity profiles that matched the location of maximum systolic axial WSS. RL-BAV velocity profiles and maximum axial WSS were homogeneously distributed right-anteriorly, however, RN-BAV showed higher variable profiles with a main proximal-posterior distribution shifting anteriorly at mid-distal AAo. Compared to controls, BAV patients presented similar WSS magnitude at proximal, mid and distal AAo ($p = 0.764$, 0.516 and 0.053, respectively) but lower axial and higher circumferential WSS components ($p < 0.001$ for both, at all aortic levels). Among BAV patients, RN-BAV presented higher IRF at all levels ($p = 0.024$ proximal, 0.046 mid and 0.002 distal AAo) and higher circumferential WSS at mid and distal AAo ($p = 0.038$ and 0.046, respectively) than RL-BAV. However, axial WSS was higher in RL-BAV compared to RN-BAV at proximal and mid AAo ($p = 0.046$, 0.019, respectively). Displacement and axial WSS were independently associated with the root-morphotype, and circumferential WSS and SFRR with the ascending-morphotype.

(Continued on next page)

* Correspondence: jfrodriguezpalomares@gmail.com; jfrodrig@vhebron.net
[†]Equal contributors
[1]Hospital Universitari Vall d'Hebron, Department of Cardiology. Vall d'Hebron Institut de Recerca (VHIR), Universitat Autònoma de Barcelona, Paseo Vall d'Hebron 119-129, 08035 Barcelona, Spain
Full list of author information is available at the end of the article

(Continued from previous page)

Conclusions: Different BAV-phenotypes present different flow patterns with an anterior distribution in RL-BAV, whereas, RN-BAV patients present a predominant posterior outflow jet at the sinotubular junction that shifts to anterior or right anterior in mid and distal AAo. Thus, RL-BAV patients present a higher axial WSS at the aortic root while RN-BAV present a higher circumferential WSS in mid and distal AAo. These results may explain different AAo dilatation morphotypes in the BAV population.

Keywords: Bicuspid aortic valve, 4D flow cardiovascular magnetic resonance (4D flow CMR), Wall shear stress, Ascending aorta, Aorta hemodynamics, Aortic dilatation

Background

Bicuspid aortic valve (BAV) is the most common congenital valvular abnormality, occurring in 1–2% of the general population [1]. Between 60 and 80% BAV patients develop aortic dilatation that is associated with an increased risk of aortic dissection and rupture [2, 3]. Aortic diameter alone has proved to be largely ineffective to predict these complications [4–6].

The most common BAV fusion phenotype involves the right and left cusps (RL-BAV) and is associated with dilatation of the tubular ascending aorta (AAo) and aortic root primarily along the convexity of the aorta. While the fusion of the right and non-coronary cusps (RN-BAV) induces arch dilatation with involvement of the tubular ascending aorta, with relative sparing of the root [3]. However, not all patients with the same BAV phenotype have the same pattern of aortopathy and, furthermore, 26–35% of BAV present a non-dilated aorta [2]. Therefore, other factors beyond valve phenotype may be related to aortic dilatation. Although controversy exists regarding the influence of hemodynamic [7, 8] and genetic factors in aortic dilatation [9], different studies have provided significant evidence that altered outflow pattern is related to aortic morphology [7, 10].

In recent years, time-resolved three-dimensional phase-contrast cardiovascular magnetic resonance (CMR 4D-flow) has emerged as a potential tool to provide comprehensive information on aortic hemodynamics with 3D visualization of blood-flow patterns [11, 12]. Using 4D-flow, several studies have analyzed flow and wall shear stress (WSS) on specific analysis planes in the ascending aorta [7, 11, 13, 14], and their relation to aortic dilatation [7]. Although some studies have analyzed WSS components [11, 13], their eventual association to different dilatation morphotype has not been investigated [11]. Only one study analyzed a BAV population differentiating between dilatation morphotype, but the computed WSS was not referenced to local direction [7]. Additionally, it has recently been shown that regions with increased WSS correspond to extracellular matrix dysregulation and elastic fiber degeneration in the ascending aorta and contribute to the development of aortopathy [8, 15, 16]. Thus, a more detailed 3D representation of WSS components [12, 17] may help to explain the

different aortic dilatation morphotypes. However, there is not yet sufficient evidence to include these variables for clinical management [7, 11].

The aim of our study was to assess the relation between aortic flow patterns and axial and circumferential WSS by 4D flow CMR through the entire ascending aorta in a large BAV population, and to establish their association with aortic dilatation and morphotype.

Methods
Study population

Patients with RL- or RN-BAV phenotype, aortic root and AAo diameters ≤45 mm and no severe valvular disease (aortic regurgitation ≤ Grade III; aortic velocity < 3 m/s) by echo were consecutively and prospectively recruited. Inclusion criteria were: age > 18 years, no cardiovascular disease, sinus rhythm, no hypertension, no connective tissue disorders, no aortic coarctation or other congenital heart diseases and no contraindication for CMR. Also, 20 healthy subjects matched with the BAV population in age and aortic diameters were studied. The study was approved by the local ethics committee and informed consent was obtained from all participants.

Cardiovascular magnetic resonance protocol

CMR studies were performed on a 1.5 T scanner (Signa, General Electric Healthcare, Waukesha, Wisconsin, USA). The protocol included 2D balanced steady-state free-precession (bSSFP) cine imaging which was used to assess BAV phenotype and aortic diameters (using the double-oblique multiplanar reconstruction), and a 4D-flow acquisition with retrospective electrocardiogram (ECG)-gating during free-breathing. Endovenous contrast was not given.

For 4D-flow CMR, phase-contrast (PC) VIPR sequence [18], a radially undersampled acquisition with 5-point balanced velocity encoding was used [19]. The acquisition volume was set to include the entire thoracic aorta. Acquisitions were made with an eight-channel cardiac coil (HD Cardiac, GE Healthcare) using the following parameters: velocity encoding (VENC) 200 cm/s, field of view (FOV) 400x400x400 mm, scan matrix 160 × 160 × 160 (voxel size of 2.5 × 2.5 × 2.5 mm^3), flip angle 8°, repetition time 4.2–6.4 ms and echo time 1.9–3.7 ms.

This data set was reconstructed the nominal temporal resolution of each patient and was (5xTR) 21 ms–32 ms. Reconstructions were performed offline with corrections for background phase from concomitant gradients and eddy currents, and trajectory errors of the 3D radial acquired k-space [19, 20].

Data analysis: 4D flow data processing
Eight double-oblique analysis planes were equally distributed in the AAo between the sinotubular junction and the origin of the brachiocephalic trunk (see red and blue lines on the left side of Fig. 1b). The vessel lumen was manually segmented in every analysis plane for all systolic phases using an angiogram derived from the 4D-flow data using complex difference processing [21]. Mass Research Software (Leiden University Medical Center, Leiden, the Netherlands) was used for the location of the analysis planes and lumen segmentation. Lumen contour points and 3D velocity data for each plane were exported for calculations to be made using custom Matlab software (MathWorks Inc., Natick, Massachusetts, USA).

Flow parameters
Peak velocity, flow jet angle, normalized flow displacement, and in-plane rotational flow were calculated at 3 different levels at the proximal, mid and distal AAo (blue lines on Fig. 1b). Flow parameters were averaged using 1 time-frame before and 2 frames after peak systole to mitigate noise.

Flow jet angle and normalized flow displacement were obtained as described by Sigovan et al. [22]. In-plane rotational flow was quantified as the through-plane component (Γ_T) of circulation (Γ), which is a parameter used in fluid dynamics to quantify rotation of flow within a plane. To this aim, vorticity (ω) was computed in each double-oblique analysis plane and circulation (Γ) was obtained as the integral of vorticity with respect to cross-sectional area, $\Gamma = \iint \omega \, dS$ [23].

Flow volumes were calculated as the time-integral over systolic phases of forward and backward through-plane flow rate curves, and used for the calculation of systolic flow reversal ratio (SFRR) [24] at mid and distal AAo (Figs. 1 and 2).

$$SFRR(\%) = \frac{\int_0^{T_s} v_{SBF}(t)dt}{\int_0^{T_s} v_{SFF}(t)dt} \cdot 100$$

Where v_{SFF} and v_{SBF} represent the forward and backward flow rates, respectively, and T_s is systolic time interval.

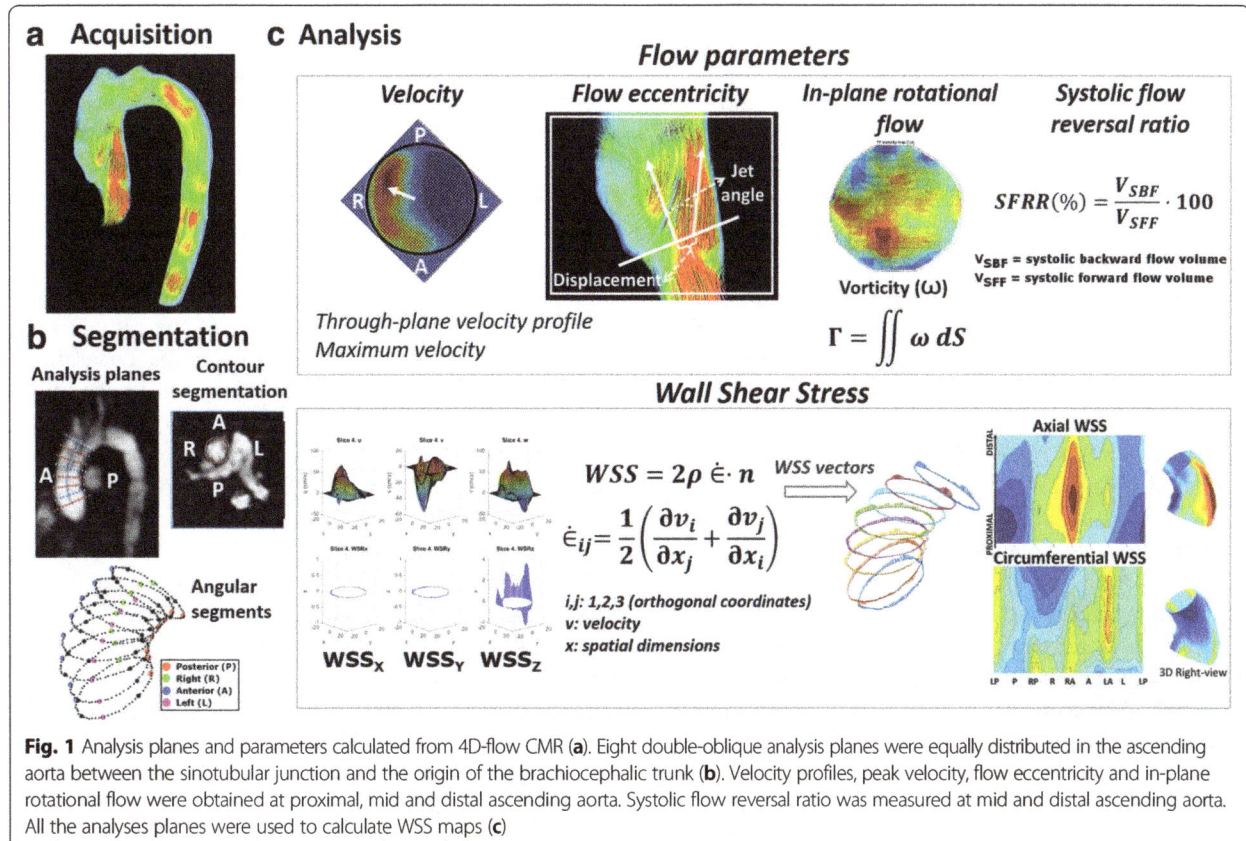

Fig. 1 Analysis planes and parameters calculated from 4D-flow CMR (**a**). Eight double-oblique analysis planes were equally distributed in the ascending aorta between the sinotubular junction and the origin of the brachiocephalic trunk (**b**). Velocity profiles, peak velocity, flow eccentricity and in-plane rotational flow were obtained at proximal, mid and distal ascending aorta. Systolic flow reversal ratio was measured at mid and distal ascending aorta. All the analyses planes were used to calculate WSS maps (**c**)

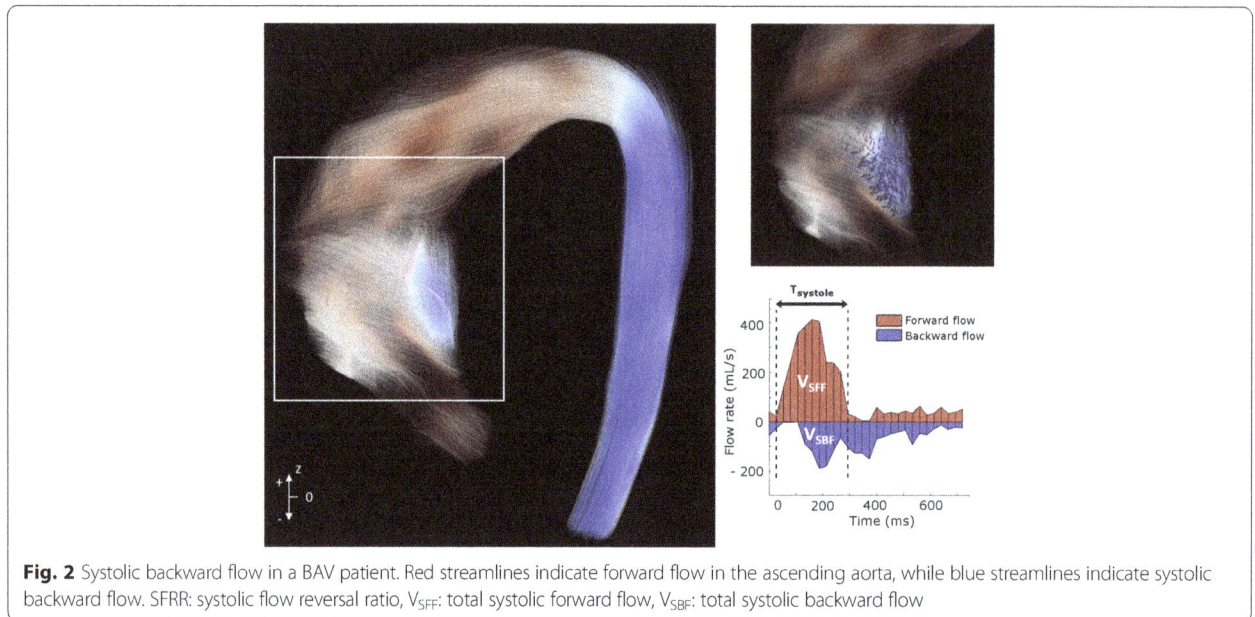

Fig. 2 Systolic backward flow in a BAV patient. Red streamlines indicate forward flow in the ascending aorta, while blue streamlines indicate systolic backward flow. SFRR: systolic flow reversal ratio, V_{SFF}: total systolic forward flow, V_{SBF}: total systolic backward flow

Wall shear stress

Peak-systolic WSS vectors (averaged from 1-time frame before, and 2-time frames after peak) were calculated at 64 points equally distributed along the aortic lumen for the 8 cross sectional analysis planes by fitting the 3D velocity data with B-spline surfaces and computing velocity derivatives on the segmented vessel lumen [25]. WSS vectors were decomposed in their through-plane (axial) and in-plane (circumferential) components.

Contour-averaged magnitude ($WSS_{mag,avg}$) and WSS components ($WSS_{ax,avg}$ and $WSS_{circ,avg}$) were calculated at proximal, mid and distal AAo.

Averaged WSS maps were obtained for each BAV phenotype and dilatation morphotype (Figs. 1c, 6 and 8). To this aim, the 64 points of the lumen contour per cross-sectional plane were aligned for all patients using the inner aortic curvature as a reference. Averaged WSS maps were calculated by computing point-to-point WSS means for all the 8 sections analyzed. Finally, statistical significance maps of axial and circumferential WSS were calculated for the mean WSS value for 8 standardized angular segments [14] of the aortic wall. Averaged WSS maps and statistical significance maps were visualized using bilinear interpolation.

Dilatation morphotypes

In order to determine the presence of aortic root or ascending dilatation, aortic diameters were adjusted with a logarithm transformation to set the z-score for both sinuses (zsinus) and ascending aorta (zAscAo) accounting for sex, age and body surface area (BSA) as described by Campens et al. [26]. Using a z-score cutoff for aortic dilatation of 2 standard error of estimate, patients were

categorized according to the tract predominantly or exclusively involved in dilatation according to Della Corte's classification [2]. Thus, patients were classified as non-dilated (zsinus≤2 and zAscAo≤2), root-morphotype (zsinus> 2 and zsinus>zAscAo) or ascending-morphotype (zAscAo> 2 and zAscAo>zsinus).

Statistical analysis

Continuous demographic variables were expressed as mean ± standard deviation. The Kolmogorov-Smirnov test was used to evaluate the normality distribution of variables. Differences between groups for continuous parameters were assessed by Student's t-test if they presented a normal distribution or ANOVA with Bonferroni correction for multiple comparisons, and Mann-Whitney U test if they did not present a normal distribution. For categorical variables, general characteristics of the sample were assessed by percentages (chi-square test). Logarithmic transformation (ln) was performed for variables with both positive and negative values (such as circulation and WSS) to preserve the distinction between negative, zero and positive values as described by Whittaker et al. [27].

Multivariable logistic regression analyses with a forward selection procedure were used to evaluate specific relations between demographic and flow variables and aortic root or ascending dilatation. Variables were entered into the model if $P < 0.25$ in univariate analyses. The aortic root morphotype was compared to the rest of groups (non-dilated and ascending), whereas, the ascending group was compared to non-dilated and root morphotype as described elsewhere [28]. To avoid multicollinearity, variables were excluded from the multivariable logistic regression if the tolerance test was < 0.1 or the variation inflation factor > 5. This is the case of the same flow variables computed at different locations. The variables entered the multivariable model were chosen as those demonstrating better predictive value, i.e. those having higher AUC in the Receiver operating characteristic (ROC) curve, as compared to the same variable computed at another location. ROC curves were performed to assess the relationship between variables obtained in the multivariable analysis and aortic morphotypes.

A two-tailed P value < 0.05 was considered statistically significant. SPSS (version 19.0, International Business Machines, Armonk, New York, USA) was used for the analysis.

Results

One hundred and one BAV patients (78 RL- and 23 RN-phenotype) and 20 healthy subjects completed the study protocol. Demographic characteristics and aortic diameters among groups are shown in Table 1. Demographics did not significantly differ among the three groups (controls, RN-BAV, RL-BAV). Although aortic diameters were larger in BAV compared to controls, no statistically-significant differences were observed. However, z-scores

were higher in the RL-BAV phenotype at the sinuses of Valsalva and at the AAo in the RN-BAV.

In the RL-BAV group ($n = 78$), 20 patients (25.6%) presented a non-dilated, 10 (12.8%) a root- and 48 (61.5%) an ascending-morphotype aorta. In the RN-BAV group ($n = 23$), 4 patients (17.4%) presented a non-dilated, 1 (4.3%) a root- and 18 (78.3%) an ascending-morphotype. Only three of the patients with root-morphotype did not present ascending aorta dilatation (zAscAo< 2). These root-only dilated patients were all men (mean age 40 years), RL-BAV and presented different degrees of aortic regurgitation and no aortic stenosis.

Peak velocity and flow eccentricity

Through-plane and magnitude velocity, jet angle and normalized displacement at proximal, mid and distal AAo are shown in Table 2. Compared to healthy control subjects, BAV patients presented higher through-plane velocity values at proximal AAo, and higher velocity magnitude, jet angle and flow displacement at the proximal and mid AAo but not in the distal part (Fig. 3). Also, RN- compared to RL-BAV presented

Table 1 Demographics and aortic dimensions in controls and bicuspid aortic valve patients

	Healthy Controls	RL-BAV	RN-BAV	p-value
N	20	78	23	
Age (years)	50.04 ± 16.39	48.43 ± 13.15	46.97 ± 16.00	0.659
Men (%)	73.30	62.80	65.20	0.736
Weight (kg)	78.57 ± 9.24	76.17 ± 10.38	76.17 ± 10.38	0.270
Height (cm)	169.42 ± 7.73	170.00 ± 10.66	172.00 ± 9.91	0.433
Body Surface Area (m²)	1.89 ± 0.13	1.83 ± 0.21	1.88 ± 0.16	0.278
Degree of Aortic Regurgitation (%)				0.240
0	–	26.8	35.3	
1	–	21.1	5.9	
2	–	49.3	47.0	
3	–	2.8	11.8	
Degree of Aortic Stenosis (%)				0.695
Absent	–	92.9	90	
Mild	–	5.7	10	
Moderate	–	1.4	0	
Maximum aortic velocity (m/s)	97.34 ± 19.0	111.15 ± 24.35	119.32 ± 21.22	0.067
Mean pressure gradient (mm Hg)	3.24 ± 1.21	4.9 ± 1.13	5.69 ± 1.71	0.074
Systolic Arterial Pressure (mm Hg)	136.26 ± 19.47	134.18 ± 17.32	142 ± 17.76	0.064
Diastolic Arterial Pressure (mm Hg)	76.73 ± 8.85	75.72 ± 9.06	79.69 ± 9.11	0.133
Sinus of Valsalva Diameter (mm)	32.77 ± 3.44	36.68 ± 5.10	34.78 ± 2.69	0.796
Ascending Aorta Diameter (mm)	35.58 ± 2.96	39.86 ± 7.51	40.30 ± 6.10	0.070
z-score sinus of Valsalva diameter	0.01 ± 0.84	1.41 ± 1.29	0.82 ± 1.11	0.001
z-score ascending aorta diameter	0.02 ± 0.71	2.87 ± 1.71	3.03 ± 1.4	< 0.001

P-values reported are the result of ANOVA comparison between 3 groups: controls, RL-BAV and RN-BAV in continuous variables and Chi-square test for categorical variables

Table 2 Flow dynamics in controls and BAV patients depending on BAV phenotype and dilatation morphotype

Plane	Measurements	Total population			BAV phenotype				Ascending aorta morphotype (only BAV)			
		CONTROLS (n = 20)	BAV (n = 101)	p	RL-BAV (n = 78)	p	RN-BAV (n = 23)	p	Non-dilated (n = 24)	Root (n = 11)	Ascending (n = 66)	p
Prox	Peak velocity magnitude (cm/s)	111.7 ± 21.9	133.9 ± 28.3	0.004	128.5 ± 27.7	0.001	152.4 ± 22.2		122.6 ± 26.8	134.0 ± 23.9	138.0 ± 28.8	0.073
	Peak TP velocity (cm/s)	97.3 ± 19	113.0 ± 23.8	0.020	111.2 ± 24.4	0.112	119.3 ± 21.2		106.8 ± 26.1	113.4 ± 22.0	115.2 ± 23.2	0.343
	Jet angle (°)	24.3 ± 6.2	25.7 ± 12.1	0.666	23.3 ± 11.3	< 0.0001	33.8 ± 11.8		21.1 ± 14.0	24.2 ± 13.8	27.7 ± 10.8	0.042
	Normalized displacement	0.04 ± 0.02	0.15 ± 0.07	< 0.001	0.15 ± 0.06	0.045	0.12 ± 0.06		0.10 ± 0.06	0.12 ± 0.05	0.16 ± 0.05	< 0.0001
	IRF (cm²/s)	−22.9 ± 65.9	139.1 ± 143.5	< 0.001	123.0 ± 128.4	0.024	193.4 ± 178.3		54.2 ± 124.3	162.3 ± 162.4	166.1 ± 136.5	0.001
	WSS$_{mag,avg}$ (N/m²)	0.52 ± 0.09	0.56 ± 0.16	0.764	0.55 ± 0.15	0.789	0.57 ± 0.17		0.53 ± 0.14	0.55 ± 0.18	0.56 ± 0.15	0.608
	WSS$_{ax,avg}$ (N/m²)	0.41 ± 0.11	0.18 ± 0.12	< 0.001	0.19 ± 0.11	0.046	0.13 ± 0.09		0.26 ± 0.14	0.21 ± 0.11	0.14 ± 0.08	0.001
	WSS$_{circ,avg}$ (N/m²)	−0.03 ± 0.11	0.30 ± 0.20	< 0.001	0.29 ± 0.18	0.590	0.31 ± 0.35		0.18 ± 0.22	0.32 ± 0.20	0.33 ± 0.18	0.007
Mid	Peak velocity magnitude (cm/s)	93.1 ± 24.3	118.8 ± 31.1	0.002	116.8 ± 32.3	0.232	125.8 ± 26.0		110.4 ± 22.7	114.5 ± 30.1	122.6 ± 33.5	0.282
	Peak TP velocity (cm/s)	89.7 ± 24.3	100.7 ± 27.7	0.060	101.0 ± 30.3	0.833	99.5 ± 16.5		99.0 ± 22.7	95.8 ± 22.8	102.0 ± 30.1	0.877
	Jet angle (°)	10.2 ± 5.9	28.7 ± 11.4	< 0.001	28.3 ± 12.0	0.384	30.1 ± 8.8		23.0 ± 10.6	25.4 ± 10.3	31.4 ± 11.0	0.001
	Normalized displacement	0.03 ± 0.01	0.09 ± 0.06	< 0.001	0.09 ± 0.06	0.639	0.09 ± 0.04		0.07 ± 0.06	0.06 ± 0.04	0.11 ± 0.06	0.001
	IRF (cm²/s)	35.1 ± 50.7	199.6 ± 190.3	< 0.001	186.2 ± 177.4	0.046	245.0 ± 227.4		101.1 ± 94.4	190.8 ± 200.2	236.9 ± 203.5	0.003
	WSS$_{mag,avg}$ (N/m²)	0.54 ± 0.15	0.58 ± 0.21	0.516	0.57 ± 0.21	0.907	0.59 ± 0.22		0.55 ± 0.16	0.56 ± 0.21	0.59 ± 0.23	0.888
	WSS$_{ax,avg}$ (N/m²)	0.46 ± 0.14	0.29 ± 0.14	< 0.001	0.30 ± 0.13	0.019	0.23 ± 0.11		0.37 ± 0.17	0.30 ± 0.12	0.25 ± 0.10	0.010
	WSS$_{circ,avg}$ (N/m²)	0.06 ± 0.07	0.29 ± 0.22	< 0.001	0.27 ± 0.20	0.038	0.34 ± 0.26		0.17 ± 0.17	0.28 ± 0.24	0.33 ± 0.21	0.004
	SFRR (%)	3.99 ± 3.74	20.9 ± 13.5	< 0.001	21.4 ± 14.6	0.777	19.2 ± 8.7		12.3 ± 12.7	15.0 ± 11.7	25.0 ± 12.3	< 0.0001
Dist	Peak velocity magnitude (cm/s)	96.3 ± 21.6	106.1 ± 30.0	0.195	105.0 ± 30.2	0.439	109.8 ± 29.4		105.7 ± 20.4	107.5 ± 30.7	106.0 ± 33.0	0.991
	Peak TP velocity (cm/s)	87.4 ± 18.1	85.6 ± 23.6	0.886	86.7 ± 23.3	0.388	81.8 ± 24.7		91.1 ± 19.0	88.3 ± 22.4	83.1 ± 25.1	0.374
	Jet angle (°)	23.0 ± 9.0	24.0 ± 10.6	0.690	25.1 ± 10.8	0.138	20.4 ± 9.5		19.5 ± 6.6	24.1 ± 9.1	25.6 ± 11.6	0.051
	Normalized displacement	0.03 ± 0.01	0.06 ± 0.04	0.027	0.06 ± 0.04	0.749	0.05 ± 0.03		0.05 ± 0.03	0.06 ± 0.05	0.06 ± 0.04	0.813
	IRF (cm²/s)	36.6 ± 35.3	120.9 ± 140.0	0.013	96.2 ± 117.8	0.002	204.7 ± 176.1		60.7 ± 70.8	106.1 ± 178.3	145.2 ± 146.7	0.005
	WSS$_{mag,avg}$ (N/m²)	0.58 ± 0.13	0.50 ± 0.18	0.053	0.48 ± 0.16	0.333	0.53 ± 0.20		0.48 ± 0.15	0.53 ± 0.18	0.49 ± 0.18	0.767
	WSS$_{ax,avg}$ (N/m²)	0.36 ± 0.13	0.24 ± 0.12	0.001	0.25 ± 0.12	0.356	0.22 ± 0.10		0.28 ± 0.16	0.27 ± 0.11	0.22 ± 0.09	0.082
	WSS$_{circ,avg}$ (N/m²)	0.07 ± 0.05	0.22 ± 0.19	< 0.001	0.19 ± 0.17	0.046	0.29 ± 0.22		0.13 ± 0.13	0.19 ± 0.24	0.25 ± 0.19	0.020
	SFRR (%)	2.63 ± 3.47	10.9 ± 9.0	< 0.001	11.5 ± 9.6	0.469	9.1 ± 5.8		9.3 ± 11.6	8.3 ± 5.5	11.9 ± 8.3	0.026

Values are mean ± SD

TP through-plane, BAV bicuspid aortic valve, RL right-left, RN right-non coronary, IRF in-plane rotational flow, WSS wall shear stress, WSSmag, avg. contour-averaged WSS magnitude, WSSax, avg. contour-averaged axial WSS, WSScirc, avg. contour-averaged circumferential WSS, SFRR systolic flow reversal ratio

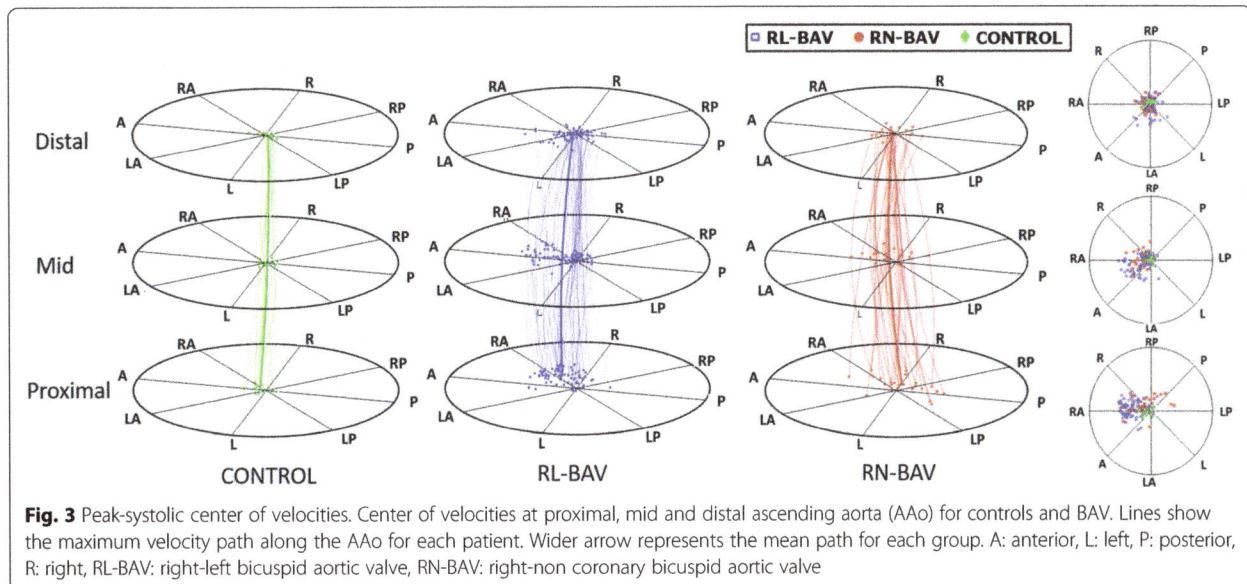

Fig. 3 Peak-systolic center of velocities. Center of velocities at proximal, mid and distal ascending aorta (AAo) for controls and BAV. Lines show the maximum velocity path along the AAo for each patient. Wider arrow represents the mean path for each group. A: anterior, L: left, P: posterior, R: right, RL-BAV: right-left bicuspid aortic valve, RN-BAV: right-non coronary bicuspid aortic valve

significant differences in peak velocity and eccentricity at proximal AAo.

When the aortic morphotype was considered in BAV, the ascending and root-morphotypes (dilated morphotype) compared to the non-dilated presented higher jet angles and displacement at the proximal and mid AAo ($P < 0.05$). However, the ascending versus the root-morphotypes did not present differences (Table 2).

When the location of the center of velocities and flow direction were analyzed in BAV, RL-BAV presented a consistent pattern (Fig. 3), showing a right (28% cases) to right-anterior position (55% cases) in the proximal aorta, with a similar profile in the mid segment and an axisymmetric profile at the distal AAo (Fig. 4a and additional movie file [Additional file 1]). However, RN-BAV presented a higher variability in their flow pattern (Fig. 3) with a predominant posterior to right-posterior outflow jet (78% cases) in the proximal aorta that shifted to the anterior segments (55% right-anterior and 20% anterior) in the mid and distal AAo (Fig. 4b and additional movie file [Additional file 2]). Control patients presented non-eccentric and predominantly laminar flow (see additional movie file [Additional file 3]).

In-plane rotational flow and systolic flow reversal ratio
In-plane rotational flow (IRF) was significantly higher in RN- compared to RL-phenotype at all aortic levels. Although a trend for higher SFRR was observed in RL-BAV compared to RN-BAV, these differences did not reach statistical significance (Table 2).

Dilated BAV presented higher values of IRF and SFRR compared to healthy controls or non-dilated morphotype (Table 2, Fig. 5). IRF was mostly right-handed (98%) in all aortic morphotypes with no statistically-significant

differences. However, patients with the ascending-morphotype presented higher IRF and SFRR than the root-morphotype at all aortic levels (Table 2) (Fig. 5).

WSS and regional WSS maps
Compared to controls, BAV presented similar magnitude ($WSS_{mag,avg}$) ($P > 0.05$) but lower axial ($WSS_{ax,avg}$) and higher circumferential WSS ($WSS_{circ,avg}$) at all levels ($P < 0.001$) (Table 2).

According to the valve phenotype, RL- compared to RN-BAV presented higher $WSS_{ax,avg}$ in proximal and mid AAo ($P < 0.05$), whereas $WSS_{circ,avg}$ was higher in RN-phenotype in mid and distal AAo (Table 2). These differences were also observed in regional WSS maps (Figs. 6 and 7).

Based on the aortic morphotype, non-dilated BAV presented similar $WSS_{mag\ avg}$ and $WSS_{ax,avg}$ but higher $WSS_{circ,avg}$ compared to controls at all levels ($P < 0.05$). In BAV patients, the $WSS_{mag,avg}$ was similar among the different aortic morphotypes. However, $WSS_{ax,avg}$ was significantly higher in the root-morphotype and $WSS_{circ,avg}$ was higher in the ascending-morphotype at all levels (Table 2). Regional differences ($p < 0.05$) between morphotypes were more pronounced for circumferential than axial WSS, and were associated with regions of systolic flow reversal for axial WSS (Figs. 8 and 9).

The outflow jet direction matched the location of maximum systolic axial WSS in the aortic wall (Figs. 3 and 6). Thus, in RN-BAV, maximum systolic axial WSS extends from posterior to right-posterior proximally towards anterior to right-anterior in mid and distal AAo. However, in RL-BAV, maximum systolic axial WSS extends from right to right-anterior at all aortic levels (Figs. 6 and 7).

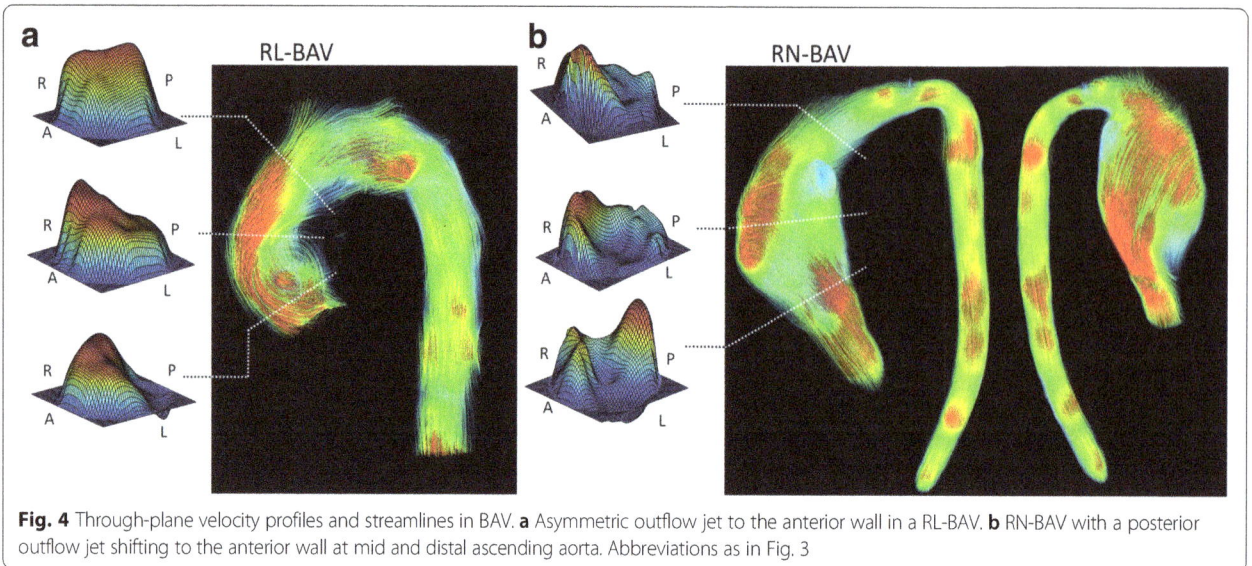

Fig. 4 Through-plane velocity profiles and streamlines in BAV. **a** Asymmetric outflow jet to the anterior wall in a RL-BAV. **b** RN-BAV with a posterior outflow jet shifting to the anterior wall at mid and distal ascending aorta. Abbreviations as in Fig. 3

Correlates of root or ascending-morphotypes

Significant bivariable (unadjusted) and multivariable adjusted correlates of aortic dilatation (> 2 z-score) [26] in BAV are listed in Table 3 (variables selected from the 4D-flow-derived variables listed in Table 2 and including sex, age and body surface area). Displacement, IRF and WSS were transformed to their natural logarithms.

On multivariable analysis, only sex (male), natural logarithms of displacement and $WSS_{ax,avg}$ were related to the presence of the root-morphotype with an AUC: 0.91 ($P < 0.001$) (Fig. 10). However, RN-phenotype, SFRR and $WSS_{circ,avg}$ in the mid AAo were related to

the presence of the ascending- morphotype with an AUC: 0.89 ($P < 0.001$) (Table 3) (Fig. 10).

Discussion

In our study, we assessed the relation between aortic flow patterns and regional WSS components (magnitude, axial and circumferential) through the entire ascending aorta in a large BAV population. In order to avoid the effect of changes in flow dynamics and WSS secondary to aortic dilatation [29] or severe valvular disease, only BAV patients with non-severe valvular dysfunction and aortic diameters ≤45 mm were included.

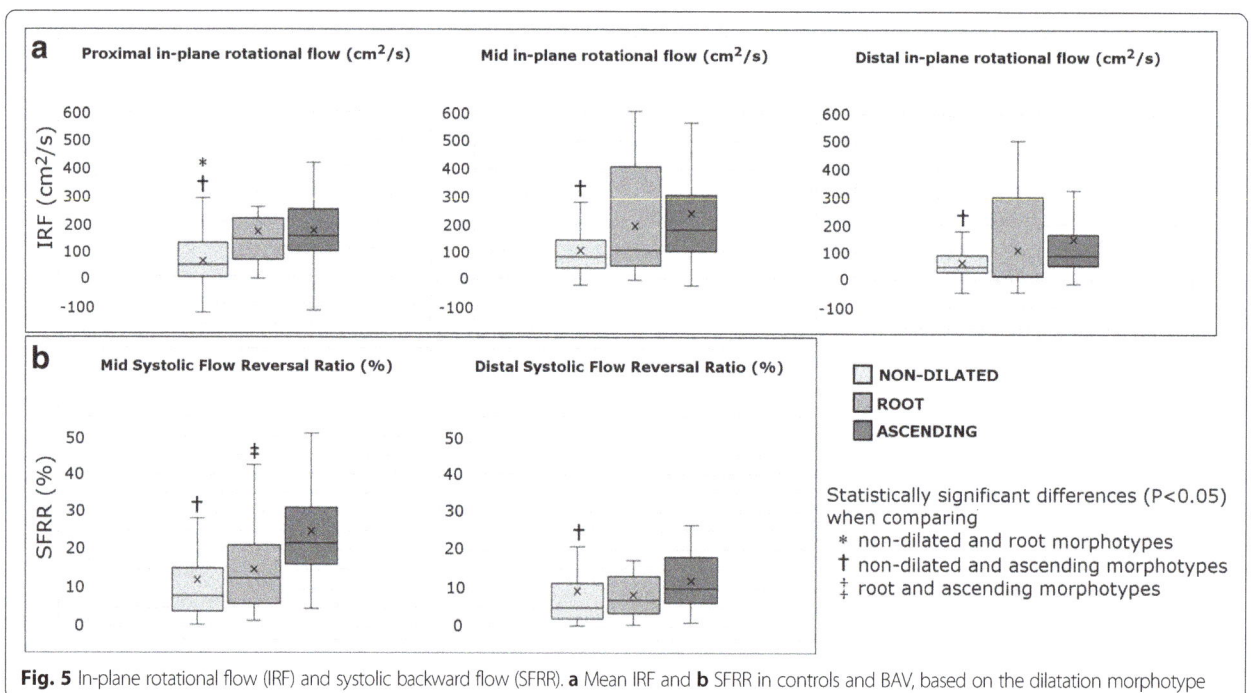

Fig. 5 In-plane rotational flow (IRF) and systolic backward flow (SFRR). **a** Mean IRF and **b** SFRR in controls and BAV, based on the dilatation morphotype

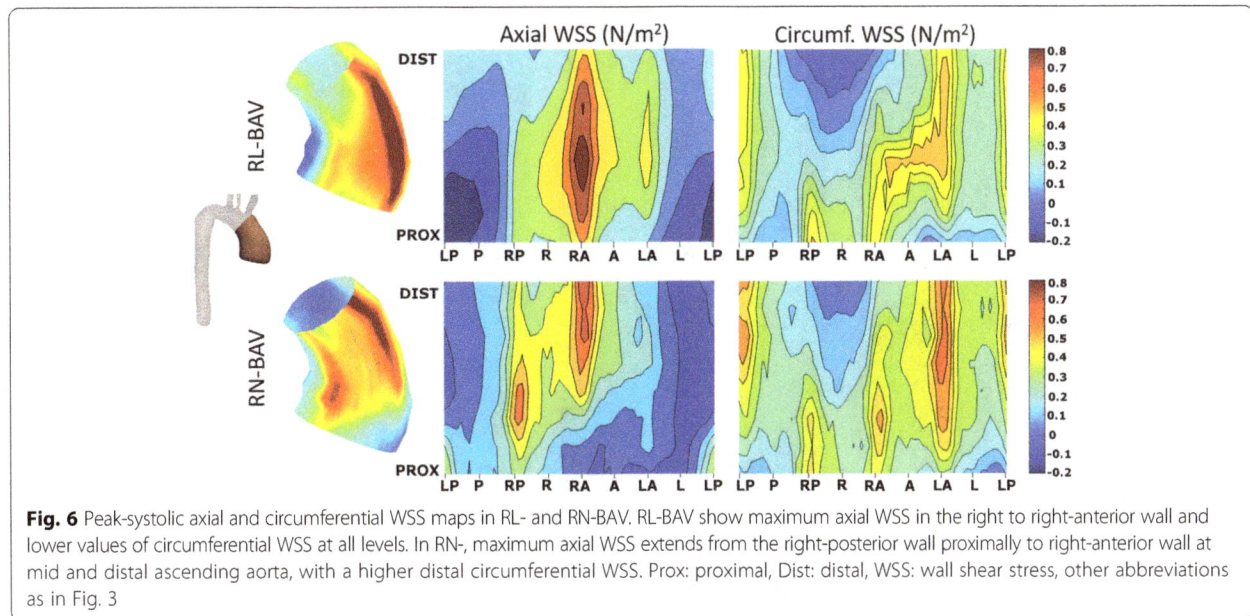

Fig. 6 Peak-systolic axial and circumferential WSS maps in RL- and RN-BAV. RL-BAV show maximum axial WSS in the right to right-anterior wall and lower values of circumferential WSS at all levels. In RN-, maximum axial WSS extends from the right-posterior wall proximally to right-anterior wall at mid and distal ascending aorta, with a higher distal circumferential WSS. Prox: proximal, Dist: distal, WSS: wall shear stress, other abbreviations as in Fig. 3

Also, the specific role of flow parameters and WSS components in the ascending aorta dilatation and morphotype was assessed by unadjusted and multivariable adjusted analysis.

The main findings of our study were that: 1) RL-BAV patients present a sustained flow towards the anterior and right-anterior aortic walls, whereas, RN-BAV present a predominantly posterior output flow that shifts towards the right and right-anterior walls in the mid and distal AAo inducing an increase in the IRF. This flow distribution reflects into regional WSS patterns. 2) Sex (male), normalized displacement and axial WSS in the proximal AAo are the main factors associated with the root-morphotype, whereas RN-phenotype, SFRR and circumferential WSS are the main factors related to the ascending-morphotype.

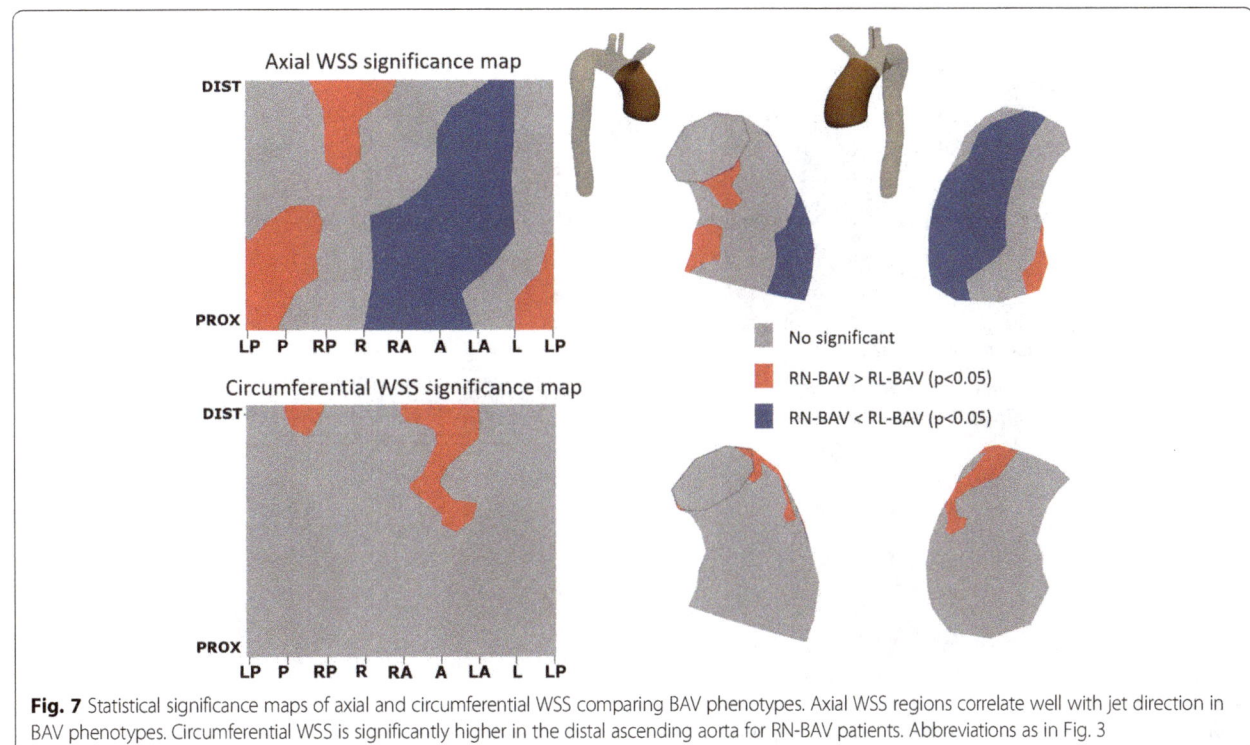

Fig. 7 Statistical significance maps of axial and circumferential WSS comparing BAV phenotypes. Axial WSS regions correlate well with jet direction in BAV phenotypes. Circumferential WSS is significantly higher in the distal ascending aorta for RN-BAV patients. Abbreviations as in Fig. 3

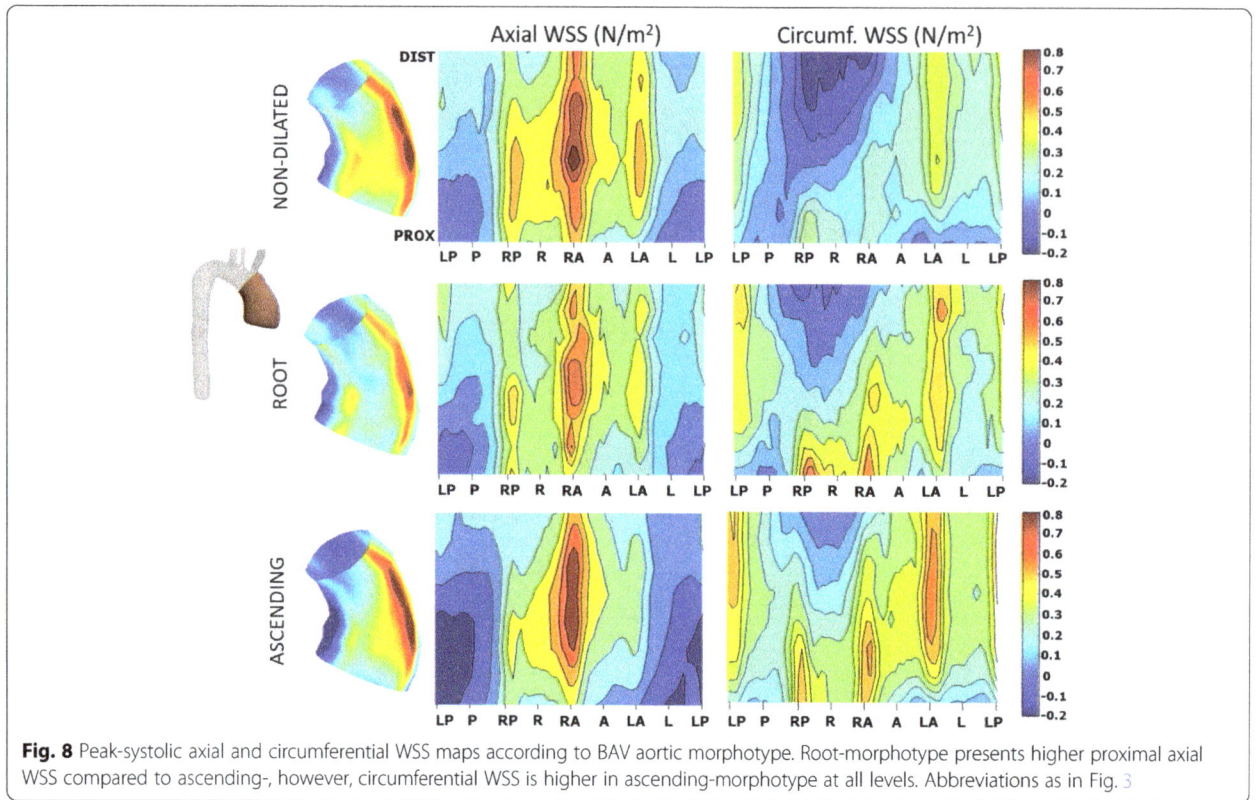

Fig. 8 Peak-systolic axial and circumferential WSS maps according to BAV aortic morphotype. Root-morphotype presents higher proximal axial WSS compared to ascending-, however, circumferential WSS is higher in ascending-morphotype at all levels. Abbreviations as in Fig. 3

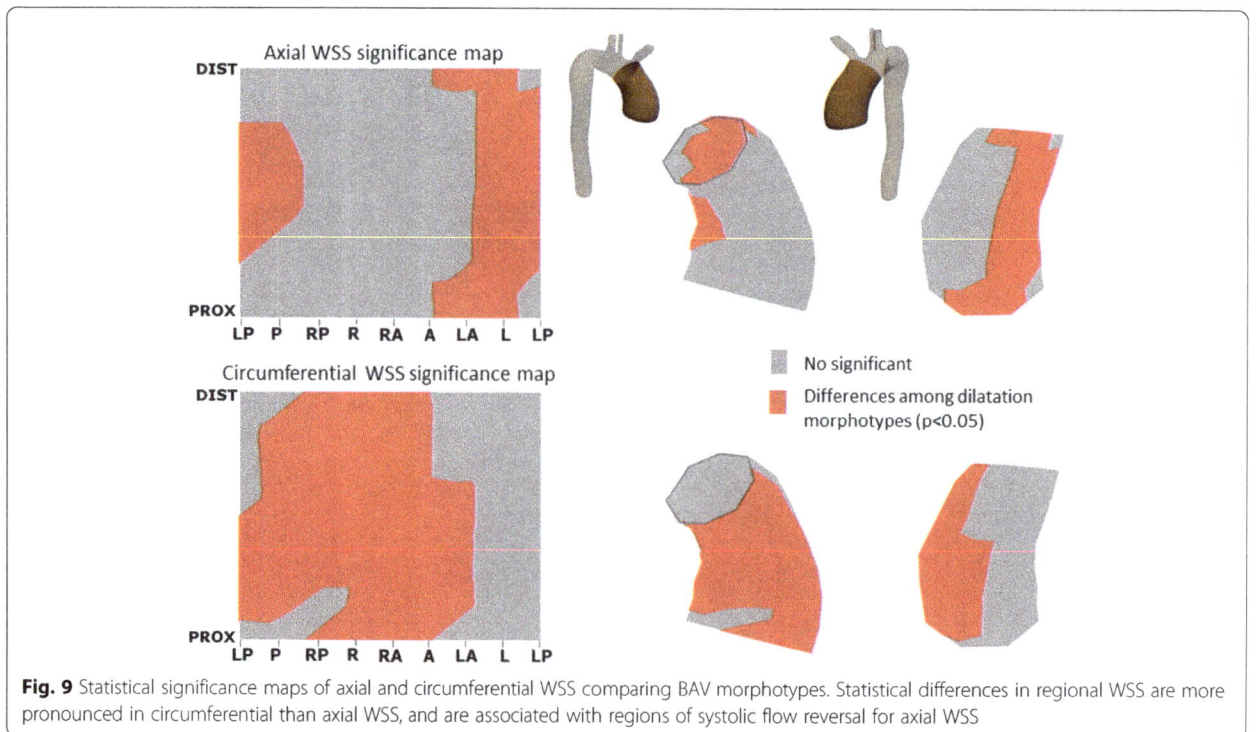

Fig. 9 Statistical significance maps of axial and circumferential WSS comparing BAV morphotypes. Statistical differences in regional WSS are more pronounced in circumferential than axial WSS, and are associated with regions of systolic flow reversal for axial WSS

Aortic flow patterns and wall shear stress maps by 4D-flow cardiovascular magnetic resonance...

105

Table 3 Unadjusted and adjusted relationship of demographic and flow variables to root (top) and ascending (bottom) morphotypes

Root morphotype	Univariate adjusted correlates of root morphotype		Multivariable adjusted correlates of root morphotype	
	OR	p-value	OR	p-value
Age	0.99 (0.96–1.02)	0.530		
BSA	0.17 (0.02–1.45)	0.104	0.08	0.291
BAV phenotype (RN vs RL)	1.41 (1.17–2.28)	0.005	1.35	0.998
Sex (male)	1.59 (1.32–1.95)	0.050	1.25	0.011
Proximal peak velocity magnitude (cm/s)	1.01 (0.98–1.22)	0.719		
Proximal jet angle (°)	1.03 (0.95–1.51)	0.490		
Ln Proximal normalized displacement	1.98 (1.01–2.93)	0.040	1.1	0.009
Ln Proximal IRF (cm^2/s)	1.22 (1.02–1.45)	0.002	0.79	0.940
Ln Proximal WSS$_{mag,avg}$ (N/m^2)	1.54 (0.09–4.52)	0.761		
Ln Proximal WSS$_{ax,avg}$ (N/m^2)	1.621 (0.93–2.95)	0.081	1.13	0.003
Ln Proximal WSS$_{circ,avg}$ (N/m^2)	2.76 (0.41–4.71)	0.243	0.02	0.673
Ascending morphotype	Univariate adjusted correlates of ascending morphotype		Multivariable adjusted correlates of ascending morphotype	
	OR	p-value	OR	p-value
Age	0.99 (0.96–1.03)	0.917		
BSA	2.51 (0.30–2.17)	0.398		
BAV phenotype (RN vs RL)	1.99 (1.61–3.48)	0.026	1.73	0.04
Sex (male)	0.82 (0.32–2.10)	0.678		
Mid jet angle (°)	1.09 (1.03–1.14)	0.001	1.025	0.353
Ln Mid normalized displacement	2.85 (1.56–5.23)	0.001	1.510	0.270
Ln Mid IRF (cm^2/s)	2.98 (1.54–5.78)	0.001	1.195	0.802
Ln Mid WSS$_{ax,avg}$ (N/m^2)	0.14 (0.04–0.48)	0.221	0.960	0.950
Ln Mid WSS$_{circ,avg}$ (N/m^2)	1.51 (1.16–3.68)	0.002	1.61	0.011
Mid SFRR (%)	1.12 (1.06–1.19)	0.001	1.11	0.001

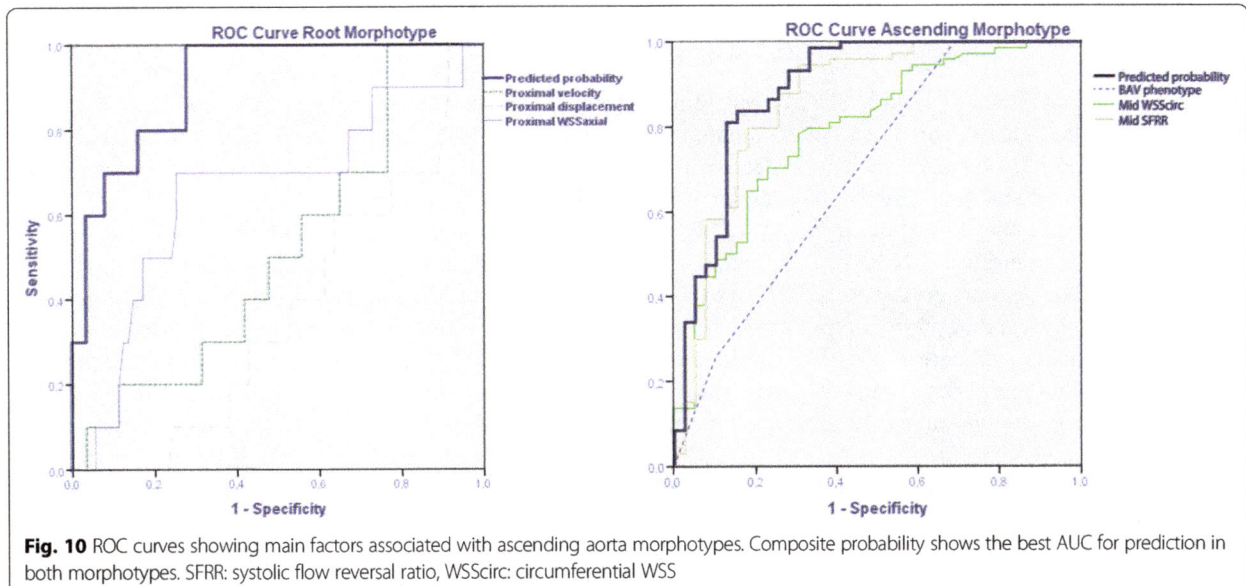

Fig. 10 ROC curves showing main factors associated with ascending aorta morphotypes. Composite probability shows the best AUC for prediction in both morphotypes. SFRR: systolic flow reversal ratio, WSScirc: circumferential WSS

To our knowledge, this is the first large study conducted in BAV patients in which different patterns of axial and circumferential regional WSS maps were used to explain variations in the AAo dilatation morphotype. Previous studies have emphasized differences in flow variables and WSS between the RN- and RL-BAV [7, 10, 11, 13, 14] with little or no correlation with the aortic dilatation morphotype [7, 11]. In this regard, Mahadevia et al. [7] did not analyze rotational flow or WSS components when studying BAV aortopathy, while Bissell et al. [11] only showed an increased rotational flow at larger aortic diameters suggesting a potential causative role. Thus, it is of great interest to ascertain the main factors associated with aortic dilatation since aortic diameter and structural changes in the aortic wall are related to clinical events regardless of valve phenotype [6, 8].

Flow patterns

Owing to the asymmetric valve opening, there is an increase in the jet angle and in the displacement of the center of velocities with respect to the center of the lumen that induces an asymmetric distribution of the WSS pattern as previously described [7, 11, 13, 14]. Similar to those of Mahadevia et al. [7], our results confirm that the jet angle is wider in RN-phenotype, whereas normalized displacement is greater in the RL-phenotype. Also, we demonstrated that these variables are greater at the proximal aorta with a progressive reduction at the distal AAo that suggests that flow tends to be more symmetric in the distal AAo. Our results differ from those of Mahadevia et al. [7] since they reported flow angle and displacement to be the main factors involved in AAo dilatation. However, they determined the absolute value of the displacement, whereas we report this value normalized by aortic diameter as suggested elsewhere [22].

In-plane rotational flow and SFRR

Similar to previous studies [11, 13, 30, 31], we found that BAV presented greater rotational flow compared to controls, with the RN-phenotype being greater than in RL- at the mid and distal AAo. This finding can be justified by the fact that the flow shifts from posterior towards anterior segments in RN-BAV. This rotational flow is not only significantly greater in RN-BAV but also in those with the ascending-morphotype. An increased rotational flow induces an increase in the circumferential WSS which justifies that both parameters were statistically significant in the ascending-morphotype on univariable analysis.

In our population, most of the BAV patients presented right-handed flow (98%). The lack of left handed helical flow seen in our study could be a sign of left handed helical flow being associated with severe/late disease process [11], and therefore, not seen in the benign aortopathy population (≤ 45 mm) included in our study.

The presence of retrograde flow at systole has been reported in patients with greater aortic diameters [29, 32, 33]. We found that higher values of SFRR are associated with the ascending-morphotype and not with the root-morphotype. An increase in the SFRR may induce an asymmetric increase and directional variations in the WSS contributing to dilatation. It is not clear whether this parameter is the cause or consequence of aortic dilatation; however, we observed that this craniocaudal flow also exists in BAV with normal aortic diameters. This finding suggests that this flow may act as a causal agent of aortic dilatation and would increase as the aorta dilates, thereby perpetuating this process.

WSS and aortic dilatation

Our study is consistent with previous publications [7, 13] which suggest that the magnitude of WSS lacks significance since its value is similar in controls and BAV. However, controls present increased axial WSS because of predominant laminar flow, while helical flow in BAV increases circumferential WSS [13]. Thus, the different WSS components (axial and circumferential) constitute an interesting parameter in the assessment of aortic dilatation [11].

A detailed analysis of WSS permitted us to use a 3D representation of axial and circumferential WSS maps along the AAo, showing asymmetrical patterns that may contribute to structural changes in the aortic wall (elastin and metalloproteinases) related to aortic dilatation [8]. Furthermore, the presence of eccentric but uniform flow along the anterior AAo in the RL-phenotype determines that the axial component of WSS is greater in this subgroup of patients; however, the eccentric but helical flow in the RN-phenotype determines that the circumferential component of WSS is greater in this subgroup. This variation in WSS components may also influence the aortic morphotype. Thus, patients with a greater axial component exhibit more dilatation at the aortic root; however, greater circumferential WSS is associated with dilatation in the AAo.

Despite the correlations found here and elsewhere, the causative role of the observed flow disturbances need to be assessed in longitudinal studies. In particular, it has been mainly discussed in root only dilatation in BAV, which is thought to be a predominantly genetic form of BAV disease [9]. Our data confirmed the previously found association between root (only) dilatation and male sex [2].

The association of male sex, normalized displacement, and axial WSS in the proximal aorta discriminated the root-morphotype with an AUC of 0.91. However, the combination of an RN-phenotype, circumferential WSS and SFRR discriminated the ascending-morphotype with an AUC of 0.89. Thus, we believe these parameters should be considered in the evaluation of BAV beyond aortic diameters. This additional information could identify patients at higher risk of aortopathy that may require a closer follow-up.

Limitations

The prospective nature of our study determined the inclusion of more patients with the RL-phenotype than RN-; however, our cohort reflects the distribution of fusion phenotypes in the general BAV population.

Healthy subjects were recruited to match BAV patients for age and aortic diameters. Although aortic diameters were slightly larger in BAV, these differences were not statistically significant.

Owing to the limited spatial and temporal resolution of 4D-flow, WSS is known to be underestimated [25, 34, 35]. However, all acquisitions were made with the same imaging parameters and analyzed with the same methodology and previous work highlighted that regions of high/low WSS are matched despite different spatial and temporal resolutions [35]. Additionally, manual segmentation causes intra- and inter-observer variability. Nevertheless, the robustness of WSS measurements employed in this study and their reproducibility has been previously demonstrated [36].

WSS estimation was limited to 8 slices in the AAo at peak systole. Thus, very localized regions of altered WSS may have been lost and temporal variations were not assessed. The use of a volumetric WSS method [37, 38], would allow a more detailed analysis.

Despite flow variables are likely to vary during the ejection phase, our measurements of jet angle, flow displacement, IRF and WSS were performed only at peak systole. Moreover, these measurements were performed averaging the results obtained at four successive time instants to reduce noise. Despite this approach has been used by several authors [7, 11, 13], and have proved high reproducibility [38], it may imply the loss of possible information contained in other systolic phases.

We conducted a cross-sectional study to evaluate the impact of flow dynamics in aortic dilatation in BAV. However, the real influence of these parameters on the concurrence of aortic dilatation needs to be determined in further longitudinal studies.

Conclusions

BAV patients present altered flow patterns that vary depending on their valvular phenotype. RL-BAV patients present an anterior distribution, whereas, RN-BAV present a predominant posterior outflow jet at the sinotubular junction that shifts to anterior or right anterior in mid and distal AAo. This flow distribution induces an increase in the $WSS_{ax\ avg}$ in the anterior aortic wall in RL-BAV patients, while, an increase in the in-plane rotational flow and $WSS_{circ\ avg}$ in the mid and distal AAo in RN-BAV patients. These results may explain different AAo dilatation morphotypes in the BAV population. Thus, in addition to aortic diameters, the assessment of the different WSS components (axial and circumferential) and derived flow parameters may contribute to identify more completely, and precisely which patients have a higher risk of aortic dilatation. The follow-up of our series will permit validation of our results.

Abbreviations

4D-flow: Time-resolved three-dimensional phase-contrast magnetic resonance imaging; AAo: Ascending aorta; BAV: Bicuspid aortic valve; bSSFP: Balanced steady state free precession; CMR: Cardiovascular magnetic resonance; ECG: Electrocardiogram; FOV: Field of view; IRF: In-plane rotational flow; PC: Phase contrast; RL-BAV: Bicuspid aortic valve with fusion of the right and left coronary cusps; RN-BAV: Bicuspid aortic valve with fusion of the right coronary cusp and the non-coronary cusp; ROC: Region of interest; SFRR: Systolic flow reversal ratio; VENC: Velocity encoding; WSS: Wall shear stress; $WSS_{ax\ avg}$: Circumferentially-averaged axial WSS; $WSS_{circ\ avg}$: Circumferentially-averaged circumferential WSS; $WSS_{mag\ avg}$: Circumferentially-averaged magnitude WSS

Acknowledgements

We would like to thank Christopher François (University of Wisconsin-Madison) and Rob van der Geest (Leiden University Medical Center) for advice on 4D-flow sequences, and Roberto García Álvarez (GE Healthcare) for technical support. We are also grateful to Augusto Sao Avilés for statistical analysis and Christine O'Hara for English revisions.

Funding

This study has been funded by Instituto de Salud Carlos III through the project PI11/01081, La Marató de TV3 (project number 20151330), and by Ministerio de Economía y Competitividad through Retos-Colaboración 2016 (RTC-2016-5152-1). Guala A. has received funding from the European Union Seventh Framework Programme FP7/People under grant agreement n° 267128.

Authors' contributions

JFR and LD: conception and design, analysis and interpretation of data, drafting the manuscript. RK, GT, LG, AG: analysis and interpretation of data. GM, FV: data collection, analysis and interpretation of data. MH: data collection. LGu, TG: selection of patients based on echo criteria, analysis and interpretation of data. KJ and OW: provided and maintained the 4D flow sequence, analysis and interpretation of data. DG: conception and design. AE: conception and design, analysis and interpretation of data. All authors critically reviewed the manuscript and approved the final version.

Competing interests

The authors declare that they have no competing interests.

Author details

[1]Hospital Universitari Vall d'Hebron, Department of Cardiology. Vall d'Hebron Institut de Recerca (VHIR), Universitat Autònoma de Barcelona, Paseo Vall d'Hebron 119-129, 08035 Barcelona, Spain. [2]Cardiac Imaging Department, CETIR-ERESA, Clínica del Pilar-Sant Jordi, Barcelona, Spain. [3]Departments of Medical Physics & Radiology, University of Wisconsin – Madison, Madison, WI, USA.

References

1. Tzemos N, Therrien J, Thanassoulis G, et al. With bicuspid aortic valves. World Health. 2013;300(11):1317–25.

2. Della Corte A, Bancone C, Dialetto G, et al. The ascending aorta with bicuspid aortic valve: a phenotypic classification with potential prognostic significance. Eur J Cardio-Thoracic Surg. 2014;46(2):240–7. https://doi.org/10.1093/ejcts/ezt621.

3. Verma S, Siu SC. Aortic dilatation in patients with bicuspid aortic valve. N Engl J Med. 2014;370(20):1920–9. https://doi.org/10.1056/NEJMra1207059.

4. Elefteriades JA, Farkas EA. Thoracic aortic aneurysm. Clinically pertinent controversies and uncertainties. J Am Coll Cardiol. 2010;55(9):841–57. https://doi.org/10.1016/j.jacc.2009.08.084.

5. Pape LA, Tsai TT, Isselbacher EM, et al. Aortic diameter > 5.5 cm is not a good predictor of type a aortic dissection observations from the International Registry of Acute Aortic Dissection (IRAD). Circulation. 2007; 116:1120–7. https://doi.org/10.1161/CIRCULATIONAHA.107.702720.

6. Michelena HI, Khanna AD, Mahoney D, et al. Incidence of aortic complications in patients with bicuspid aortic valves. JAMA. 2011;306(10): 1104–12. https://doi.org/10.1001/jama.2011.1286306/10/1104 [pii].

7. Mahadevia R, Barker AJ, Schnell S, et al. Bicuspid aortic cusp fusion morphology alters aortic three-dimensional outflow patterns, wall shear stress, and expression of aortopathy. Circulation. 2014;129(6):673–82. https://doi.org/10.1161/CIRCULATIONAHA.113.003026.

8. Guzzardi DG, Barker AJ, Van Ooij P, et al. Valve-related hemodynamics mediate human bicuspid aortopathy: insights from wall shear stress mapping. J Am Coll Cardiol. 2015;66(8):892–900. https://doi.org/10.1016/j.jacc.2015.06.1310.

9. Girdauskas E, Borger MA, Secknus M-A, Girdauskas G, Kuntze T. Is aortopathy in bicuspid aortic valve disease a congenital defect or a result of abnormal hemodynamics? A critical reappraisal of a one-sided argument. Eur J Cardio-Thoracic Surg. 2011;39(6):809–14. https://doi.org/10.1016/j.ejcts.2011.01.001.

10. Hope MD, Hope TA, Meadows AK, et al. Bicuspid aortic valve : four-dimensional MR evaluation of ascending aortic systolic methods : results. Radiology. 2010;255(1):53–61.

11. Bissell MM, Hess AT, Biasiolli L, et al. Aortic dilation in bicuspid aortic valve disease: flow pattern is a major contributor and differs with valve fusion type. Circ Cardiovasc Imaging. 2013;6(4):499–507. https://doi.org/10.1161/CIRCIMAGING.113.000528.

12. Bieging ET, Frydrychowicz A, Wentland AL, et al. In vivo three-dimensional mr wall shear stress estimation in ascending aortic dilatation. J Magn Reson Imaging. 2011;33(3):589–97. https://doi.org/10.1002/jmri.22485.

13. Meierhofer C, Schneider EP, Lyko C, et al. Wall shear stress and flow patterns in the ascending aorta in patients with bicuspid aortic valves differ significantly from tricuspid aortic valves: a prospective study. Eur Heart J Cardiovasc Imaging. 2013;14:797–804. https://doi.org/10.1093/ehjci/jes273.

14. Barker AJ, Markl M, Bürk J, et al. Bicuspid aortic valve is associated with altered wall shear stress in the ascending aorta. Circ Cardiovasc Imaging. 2012;5(4):457–66. https://doi.org/10.1161/CIRCIMAGING.112.973370.

15. Malek AM, Alper SL, Izumo S. Hemodynamic shear stress and its role in atherosclerosis. JAMA. 1999;282(21):2035–42. https://doi.org/10.1001/jama.282.21.2035.

16. Ruddy JM, Jones JA, Stroud RE, Mukherjee R, Spinale FG, Ikonomidis JS. Differential effect of wall tension on matrix metalloproteinase promoter activation in the thoracic aorta. J Surg Res. 2010;160(2):333–9. https://doi.org/10.1016/j.jss.2008.12.033S0022-4804(08)01590-4 [pii].

17. van Ooij P, Potters WV, Collins J, et al. Characterization of abnormal wall shear stress using 4D flow MRI in human bicuspid aortopathy. Ann Biomed Eng. 2015;43(6):1385–97. https://doi.org/10.1007/s10439-014-1092-7.

18. Gu T, Korosec FR, Block WF, et al. PC VIPR: a high-speed 3D phase-contrast method for flow quantification and high-resolution angiography. AJNR Am J Neuroradiol. 2005;26(4):743–9.

19. Johnson KM, Markl M. Improved SNR in phase contrast velocimetry with five-point balanced flow encoding. Magn Reson Med. 2010;63:349–55. https://doi.org/10.1002/mrm.22202.

20. Johnson KM, Lum DP, Turski PA, Block WF, Mistretta CA, Wieben O. Improved 3D phase contrast MRI with off-resonance corrected dual Echo VIPR. Magn Reson Med. 2009;60(6):1329–36. https://doi.org/10.1002/mrm.21763.Improved.

21. Markl M, Frydrychowicz A, Kozerke S, Hope MD, Wieben O. 4D flow MRI. J Magn Reson Imaging. 2012;36(5):1015–36. https://doi.org/10.1002/jmri.23632.

22. Sigovan M, Hope MD, Dyverfeldt P, Saloner D. Comparison of four-dimensional flow parameters for quantification of flow eccentricity in the ascending aorta. J Magn Reson Imaging. 2011;34(5):1226–30. https://doi.org/10.1002/jmri.22800.

23. Hess AT, Bissell MM, Glaze SJ, et al. Evaluation of circulation, Γ, as a quantifying metric in 4D flow MRI. J Cardiovasc Magn Reson. 2013;15(Suppl 1):E36. https://doi.org/10.1186/1532-429X-15-S1-E36.

24. Bensalah MZ, Bollache E, Kachenoura N, et al. Geometry is a major determinant of flow parameters in proximal aorta. Am J Physiol Heart Circ Physiol. 2014;306:1408–16. https://doi.org/10.1152/ajpheart.00647.2013.

25. Stalder AF, Russe MF, Frydrychowicz A, Bock J, Hennig J, Markl M. Quantitative 2D and 3D phase contrast MRI: optimized analysis of blood flow and vessel wall parameters. Magn Reson Med. 2008;60(5):1218–31. https://doi.org/10.1002/mrm.21778.

26. Campens L, Demulier L, De Groote K, et al. Reference values for echocardiographic assessment of the diameter of the aortic root and ascending aorta spanning all age categories. Am J Cardiol. 2014;114(6):914–20. https://doi.org/10.1016/j.amjcard.2014.06.024.

27. Whittaker J, Somers M, Whitehead C. The netlog transformation and quantile regression for the analysis of a large credit scoring database. Journal R Stat Soc Ser C. 2005;54(5):863–78. https://doi.org/10.1111/j.1467-9876.2005.00520.x.

28. Evangelista A, Gallego P, Calvo-Iglesias F, et al. Anatomical and clinical predictors of valve dysfunction and aortic dilation in bicuspid aortic valve disease. Heart. 2017; https://doi.org/10.1136/heartjnl-2017-311560.

29. Bürk J, Blanke P, Stankovic Z, et al. Evaluation of 3D blood flow patterns and wall shear stress in the normal and dilated thoracic aorta using flow-sensitive 4D CMR. J Cardiovasc Magn Reson. 2012;14(1):84. https://doi.org/10.1186/1532-429X-14-84.

30. Lorenz R, Bock J, Barker AJ, et al. 4D flow magnetic resonance imaging in bicuspid aortic valve disease demonstrates altered distribution of aortic blood flow helicity. Magn Reson Med. 2014;71(4):1542–53. https://doi.org/10.1002/mrm.24802.

31. Hope MD, Hope TA, Crook SES, et al. 4D flow CMR in assessment of valve-related ascending aortic disease. JACC Cardiovasc Imaging. 2011;4(7):781–7. https://doi.org/10.1016/j.jcmg.2011.05.004.

32. Barker AJ, Lanning C, Shandas R. Quantification of hemodynamic wall shear stress in patients with bicuspid aortic valve using phase-contrast MRI. Ann Biomed Eng. 2010;38(3):788–800. https://doi.org/10.1007/s10439-009-9854-3.

33. Hope TA, Markl M, Wigström L, Alley MT, Miller DC, Herfkens RJ. Comparison of flow patterns in ascending aortic aneurysms and volunteers using four-dimensional magnetic resonance velocity mapping. J Magn Reson Imaging. 2007;26(6):1471–9. https://doi.org/10.1002/jmri.21082.

34. Dyverfeldt P, Bissell MM, Barker AJ, et al. 4D flow cardiovascular magnetic resonance consensus statement. J Cardiovasc Magn Reson. 2015;17(1):72. https://doi.org/10.1186/s12968-015-0174-5.

35. Cibis M, Potters WV, Gijsen FJ, et al. The effect of spatial and temporal resolution of cine phase contrast MRI on wall shear stress and oscillatory shear index assessment. PLoS One. 2016;11(9):1–15. https://doi.org/10.1371/journal.pone.0163316.

36. Markl M, Wallis W, Harloff A. Reproducibility of flow and wall shear stress analysis using flow-sensitive four-dimensional MRI. J Magn Reson Imaging. 2011;33(4):988–94. https://doi.org/10.1002/jmri.22519.

37. Sotelo J, Urbina J, Valverde I, et al. 3D quantification of wall shear stress and oscillatory shear index using a finite-element method in 3D CINE PC-MRI data of the thoracic aorta. IEEE Trans Med Imaging. 2016;48(10):1–1. https://doi.org/10.1109/TMI.2016.2517406.

38. Van Ooij P, Powell AL, Potters WV, Carr JC, Markl M, Barker AJ. Reproducibility and interobserver variability of systolic blood flow velocity and 3D wall shear stress derived from 4D flow MRI in the healthy aorta. J Magn Reson Imaging. 2016;43(1):236–48. https://doi.org/10.1002/jmri.24959.

11

Fully quantitative pixel-wise analysis of cardiovascular magnetic resonance perfusion improves discrimination of dark rim artifact from perfusion defects associated with epicardial coronary stenosis

Allison D. Ta[1,2], Li-Yueh Hsu[1], Hannah M. Conn[1], Susanne Winkler[1,3], Anders M. Greve[1], Sujata M. Shanbhag[1], Marcus Y. Chen[1], W. Patricia Bandettini[1] and Andrew E. Arai[1*]

Abstract

Background: Dark rim artifacts in first-pass cardiovascular magnetic resonance (CMR) perfusion images can mimic perfusion defects and affect diagnostic accuracy for coronary artery disease (CAD). We evaluated whether *quantitative* myocardial blood flow (MBF) can differentiate dark rim artifacts from true perfusion defects in CMR perfusion.

Methods: Regadenoson perfusion CMR was performed at 1.5 T in 76 patients. Significant CAD was defined by quantitative invasive coronary angiography (QCA) ≥ 50% diameter stenosis. Non-significant CAD (NonCAD) was defined as stenosis by QCA < 50% diameter stenosis or computed tomographic coronary angiography (CTA) < 30% in all major epicardial arteries. Dark rim artifacts had study specific and guideline-based definitions for comparison purposes. MBF was quantified at the pixel-level and sector-level.

Results: In a NonCAD subgroup with dark rim artifacts, stress MBF was lower in the subendocardial than midmyocardial and epicardial layers (2.17 ± 0.61 vs. 3.06 ± 0.75 vs. 3.24 ± 0.80 mL/min/g, both $p < 0.001$) and was also 30% lower than in remote regions (2.17 ± 0.61 vs. 2.83 ± 0.67 mL/min/g, $p < 0.001$). However, subendocardial stress MBF in dark rim artifacts was 37–56% higher than in true perfusion defects (2.17 ± 0.61 vs. 0.95 ± 0.43 mL/min/g, $p < 0.001$). Absolute stress MBF differentiated CAD from NonCAD with an accuracy ranging from 86 to 89% (all $p < 0.001$) using pixel-level analyses. Similar results were seen at a sector level.

Conclusion: Quantitative stress MBF is lower in dark rim artifacts than remote myocardium but significantly higher than in true perfusion defects. If confirmed in larger series, this approach may aid the interpretation of clinical stress perfusion exams.

Keywords: Myocardial perfusion, Dark-rim artifact, MRI, Coronary artery disease, Quantitative perfusion

* Correspondence: araia@nih.gov
[1]National Heart, Lung and Blood Institute, National Institutes of Health,
Department of Health and Human Services, Bldg 10, Rm B1D416, MSC 1061,
10 Center Drive, Bethesda, MD 20892-1061, USA
Full list of author information is available at the end of the article

Background

Stress tests remain an attractive approach for diagnosing coronary artery disease (CAD) [1]. Stress cardiovascular magnetic resonance (CMR) perfusion can detect CAD and additionally quantification improves the objectivity of interpretation [2].

A dark rim artifact that mimics a true defect is one important limitation in CMR perfusion. There are numerous causes of dark rim artifact including: Gibbs ringing [3], inadequate spatial resolution [4, 5], motion artifacts [6], non-uniformity across k-space [7], and partial volume errors. Higher heart rates can exacerbate cardiac motion creating larger dark rim artifacts [8]. To complicate matters, different artifacts from multiple causes can combine to exacerbate dark rim artifact.

Quantitative measurements of myocardial blood flow (MBF) might provide insight into differentiating dark rim artifacts from true perfusion defects. Our primary aim was to use fully quantitative analysis of perfusion CMR at the pixel-level to characterize dark rim artifacts, normal perfusion, and true perfusion defects. We also aimed to understand how well qualitative assessment of dark rim artifacts published by the Society for Cardiovascular Magnetic Resonance (SCMR) guidelines [9] differentiated CAD from those without CAD (NonCAD).

Methods

Patient population

The aim to characterize dark rim artifacts was a retrospective design we felt that could be addressed with the use of existing data. All CMR scans were prospectively acquired from under a research clinical trial (ClinicalTrials.gov Identifier: NCT00027170) but subjects were retrospectively selected for this analysis of dark rim artifacts. The clinical trial was approved by the institutional review board. All subjects gave written informed consent. Prospective exclusion criteria included contraindication to regadenoson, unstable angina within 48 h, hemodynamic instability, acute renal failure, estimated glomerular filtration rate < 30 ml/min/1.73m^2, claustrophobia, and certain metallic implants. Patients were referred to assess either a chest pain equivalent syndrome, had a prior equivocal nuclear stress test, or to assess the significance of a known coronary stenosis.

For this retrospective analysis of dark rim artifacts, studies were selected by finding the overlap between three clinical research databases summarizing stress perfusion CMR studies, Computed tomography (CT) coronary angiography studies, and invasive coronary angiography (CATH) exams (Fig. 1). Consecutive patients over a 1.3 year period (2010–2012) with a quantitative regadenoson perfusion CMR exam and correlative quantitative invasive coronary angiography (QCA) or CT coronary angiogram (CTA) within 90 days of CMR

were included in the retrospective analysis. Patients with coronary artery bypass, congenital heart disease, significant co-morbid conditions, or technical issues with the CMR acquisition were excluded. Patients with severe three-vessel CAD (QCA ≥ 70% stenosis in all three vessels) were also excluded by study design as we aimed to compare MBF in abnormal regions relative to the remote myocardium. NonCAD patients were excluded if they had a history of percutaneous coronary intervention or myocardial infarction.

Standard of reference

Significant CAD was defined by an intermediate stenosis (50–69% diameter) or severe stenosis (≥ 70% diameter) in any major coronary artery by QCA. Invasive QCA (Artis, Siemens AG, Berlin, Germany) was measured by a physician blinded to the clinical history and CMR perfusion results. NonCAD was defined by invasive QCA (< 50% diameter) or CTA stenosis (< 30% diameter). The attribution of vessel territories to each perfusion defect was performed unblinded after the QCA.

Vasodilator stress CMR perfusion

The CMR exam was performed on a 1.5 T scanner (Magnetom Avanto or Magnetom Espree, Siemens Healthineers, Erlangen, Germany) using a balanced steady state free procession (bSSFP) sequence with a 'dual sequence' technique to measure the arterial input function [10]. Three myocardial slice locations were imaged during every R-R interval over 60 heartbeats. Typical imaging parameters included: a three 90° sequel preparation pulse, 50° readout flip angle, 95 ms saturation recovery time, a 2.3 ms repetition time, a 1.22 ms echo time, a typical field of view of 360x270mm^2, an acquisition matrix of 128 × 96, an image matrix of 256 × 192 after interpolation, and 8 mm slice thickness. Parallel imaging was used with an acceleration factor of 2. Non-rigid motion correction was used to facilitate pixel-wise perfusion quantification.

Antianginal medications were held for the CMR scan and patients were instructed to avoid caffeine for 24 h. Stress perfusion imaging was performed 70 s after the 400 mcg bolus of regadenoson and rest imaging occurred 20 min later. Gadolinium-DTPA (Magnevist, Berlex Laboratories, Wayne, New Jersey, USA; 0.05 mmol/kg) was injected during the stress and rest first pass perfusion imaging at 5 ml/s.

Myocardial blood flow quantification and comparison

Quantitative pixel maps of perfusion were created as previously described [11] with a few refinements over those methods. The perfusion images had automated motion correction from the scanner. The user still needed to draw epicardial contours, endocardial contours, and select a most normal appearing myocardial region. The amount of labor involved was greatly reduced from prior methods.

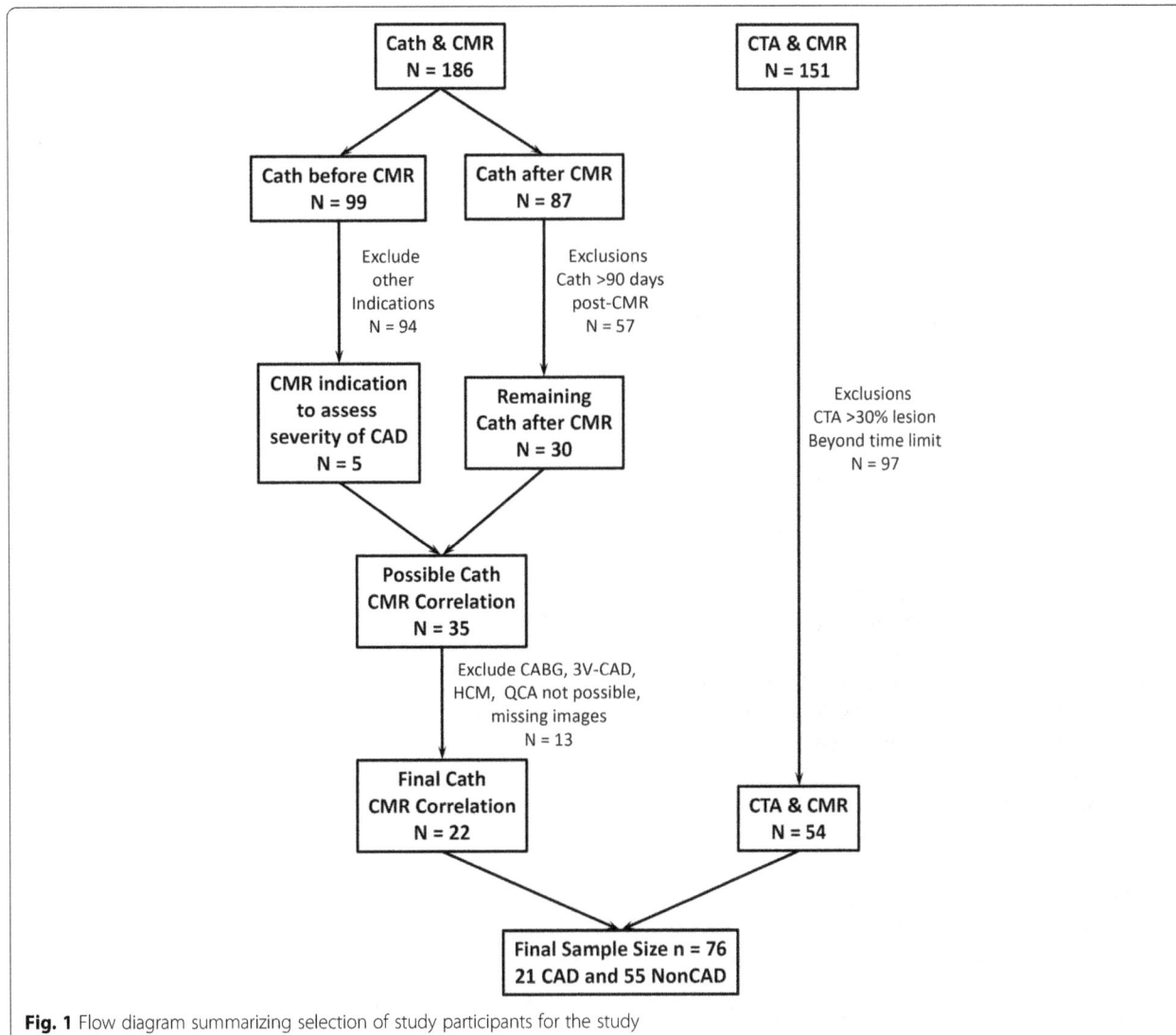

Fig. 1 Flow diagram summarizing selection of study participants for the study

The program used the same fundamental quantification steps but would process a circular field of view larger than the left ventricular (LV) myocardium. Results were displayed such that each myocardial pixel shows the estimated MBF value in units of mL/min/g.

Because the appearance of dark rim artifacts and true perfusion defects can be narrow, regional MBF were measured from the perfusion pixel maps by 3-layers: subendocardial, midmyocardial, and epicardial layers. Regions of interest in different layers were sized based on the extent of the dark rim artifact and perfusion defects. Sector level analysis was also performed by dividing the myocardium into 6 segments then dividing each segment into inner and outer subsectors.

Definitions of dark rim artifacts
Since this paper aimed to examine the characteristics of dark rim artifacts and whether they might explain some false positive perfusion defects, we defined a dark rim artifact as hypointense subendocardial regions on stress perfusion images in the NonCAD group. This definition is different from prior definitions, but benefits from the prior knowledge that this group of subjects cannot have true positive perfusion defects.

We also studied the diagnostic performance of dark rim artifact definitions as described in the SCMR Guidelines [9] which have three definitions of dark rim artifact: 1) An apparent perfusion defect seen in stress that lasts < 7 beats is considered a "dark rim artifact" while one that lasts ≥ 7 beats is called a "true positive perfusion defect," 2) An apparent perfusion defect seen at rest and at stress is a "dark rim artifact" while one at stress only is a "true positive defect," and 3) if myocardial signal intensity decreases below baseline prior to myocardial enhancement, the apparent defect is a dark rim artifact.

It is important to recognize this paper's specific focus in quantitative analysis goes beyond the SCMR guidelines [9]. We used the SCMR definition of a dark rim artifact only in qualitative diagnostic accuracy analyses of those specific criteria, while our quantitative MBF comparison was not restricted to those criteria.

Statistical analysis

For quantitative comparison of MBF measurements in dark rim artifact vs. true perfusion defects, the patients were divided into two distinct groups: CAD defined by QCA $\geq 50\%$ stenosis versus NonCAD subgroup with DRA.

All patients were analyzed using standard contingency tables, sensitivity, specificity, accuracy, positive predictive value, negative predictive value, and area under the curve. MedCalc (version 12.7.7.0, Mariakerke, Belgium) was used for statistical comparisons. Values were expressed as mean $\pm$ SD. The Kolmogorov-Smirnov test was used to test for Normal distribution. The Student's t-test was used for pairwise comparison of normally distributed data. The Wilcoxon and Mann-Whitney tests were applied to non-normally distributed data. The Fisher's Exact test was used to compare discrete variables. A Bonferroni correction was applied for multiple comparisons when necessary. Receiver operator characteristics curves were used to evaluate the discriminatory performance for prediction of CAD.

Results

Baseline characteristics of patient population

Patients ($N = 76$) averaged 55.9 ± 12.2 years of age and 55% (n = 41) were male (Table 1). Patient inclusion and exclusion is summarized in Fig. 1. On a per patient basis, 28% ($N = 21$) had significant QCA defined CAD and 18 of these 21 patients had at least one stenosis ≥ 70 by QCA (Table 2). A total of 84 coronary arteries were analyzed by QCA (left main, left anterior descending (LAD), circumflex (CX), and right coronary (RCA) arteries). There were 47 vessels with 0–49% stenosis, 13 vessels with intermediate stenosis (50–69%) and 24 vessels with severe stenosis ($\geq 70\%$). Within the NonCAD group, a subgroup of patients ($N = 45$) were identified as having dark rim artifact. Examples of normal, dark rim artifact, and true perfusion defects are shown in Figs. 2 and 3.

Stress myocardial blood flow in patients with CAD

Consistent with known subendocardial vulnerability to ischemia, there was a more severe decrease in stress MBF in the subendocardium compared with other layers in patients with CAD seen in both pixel and sector measurements (Figs. 4 and 5). In patients with either a $\geq 70\%$ QCA stenosis or a 50–69% QCA stenosis, stress MBF was lower downstream from the stenosis in all three layers of myocardium, but most severely affected in the

Table 1 Demographic summary stratified by coronary artery disease status

	NonCAD (N = 55)		CAD (N = 21)		p-value
Cardiovascular Risk Factors					
Age	53.0 ± 11.7		63.0 ± 10.1		**0.001**
Male	29	53%	15	71%	0.195
Hypertension	26	47%	14	67%	0.199
Hyperlipidemia	26	47%	18	86%	**0.004**
Diabetes	5	9%	5	24%	0.128
Smoking	21	38%	12	57%	0.196
Family history of CAD	14	25%	10	48%	0.097
Body mass index (kg/m²)	29.1 ± 6.6		28.3 ± 4.6		0.81
Past Medical History					
Prior PCI	0	0%	3	14%	**0.019**
CABG[a]	0	0%	0	0%	1.000
Prior cerebrovascular accident	0	0%	1	5%	0.276
Medications					
Aspirin or Anti-Platelet	29	53%	15	71%	0.25
Beta blocker	19	35%	11	52%	0.27
Calcium channel blocker	4	7%	1	5%	0.84
Nitrate	2	4%	1	5%	0.65
Diuretic	8	15%	2	19%	0.94
ACE inhibitor	13	24%	8	38%	0.35
ARB	4	7%	2	10%	0.97
Statin	22	40%	19	90%	**< 0.001**

Abbreviations: ACE angiotensin converting enzyme inhibitor, ARB angiotensin receptor blocker, BP blood pressure, CABG coronary artery bypass grafting, CAD coronary artery disease, LV left ventricular, LVEDV left ventricular end diastolic volume, LVESV left ventricular end systolic volume, LVEDMass left ventricular end diastolic mass, LGE late gadolinium enhancement, N/A not applicable, PCI percutaneous coronary intervention
p values that were significant (p<0.050 or lower) are in bold
[a]Patients with a prior history of coronary artery by-pass surgery and 3 vessel CAD were excluded from this study

subendocardium (Fig. 4, all comparisons either $p = 0.016$ or $p < 0.001$). The transmural gradient of lower perfusion toward the subendocardium was most prominent in patients with severe CAD ($\geq 70\%$ QCA stenosis), but also present in patients with intermediate CAD (50–69% QCA stenosis).

Quantitative analysis to characterize dark rim artifacts vs. perfusion defects associated with CAD

Pixel-wise analysis

In the NonCAD subgroup with dark rim artifacts, stress subendocardial MBF was lower in the dark rim artifact than in the remote myocardium (Fig. 4, $p < 0.001$).

Table 2 Summary of coronary artery disease status, hemodynamics, and CMR findings

	NonCAD (N = 55)	CAD (N = 21)		p-value
Extent of CAD by QCA				
Left main disease	N/A	0	0%	N/A
LAD disease	N/A	16	76%	N/A
CX disease	N/A	9	43%	N/A
RCA disease	N/A	12	57%	N/A
3-vessel CAD[a]	N/A	0[a]	0%[a]	N/A
2-vessel CAD	N/A	16	76%	N/A
1-vessel CAD	N/A	5	24%	N/A
Severity of stenosis				
0–49%	N/A	47	56%	N/A
50–69%	N/A	13	15%	N/A
≥ 70%	N/A	24	29%	N/A
Hemodynamics				
Baseline systolic BP (mmHg)	131.3 ± 14.7	137.0 ± 12.7		0.122
Baseline diastolic BP (mmHg)	79.5 ± 10.7	78.3 ± 13.3		0.875
Baseline heart rate (bpm)	67.1 ± 12.1	66.7 ± 10.7		0.891
Baseline rate pressure Product (bpm^{a}mmHg)	9148 ± 1784	8802 ± 1785		0.452
Stress systolic BP (mmHg)	128.8 ± 17.7	134.2 ± 16.7		0.224
Stress diastolic BP (mmHg)	74.5 ± 14.2	72.3 ± 14.5		0.548
Stress heart rate (bmp)	101.2 ± 14.0	94.7 ± 13.7		0.070
Stress rate pressure product (bmp^{a}mmHg)	12,709 ± 2472	13,053 ± 2743		0.617
CMR Findings				
LV ejection fraction (%)	64.1 ± 6.5	60.3 ± 6.5		**0.047**
LV stroke volume (ml)	100.4 ± 21.7	93.1 ± 25.0		0.213
LVEDV (ml)	159.2 ± 41.8	157.0 ± 45.1		0.841
LVESV (ml)	58.7 ± 25.5	63.9 ± 29.1		0.453
LVED Mass (g)	98.0 ± 28.8	107.7 ± 25.5		0.177
LGE evidence of infarction	0　　0%	8	38%	**< 0.001**

Abbreviations: BP blood pressure, *CX* circumflex coronary artery, *LGE* late gadolinium enhancement, *LV* left ventricular, *LVEDV* left ventricular end diastolic volume, *LVESV* left ventricular end systolic volume, *LVEDMass* left ventricular end diastolic mass, *LGE* late gadolinium enhancement, *N/A* not applicable
p values that were significant (*p*<0.050 or lower) are in bold
[a]Patients with a prior history of coronary artery by-pass surgery and 3 vessel *CAD* coronary artery disease were excluded from this study

However, stress MBF in the midmyocardium and epicardium were not significantly different in the dark rim artifact region versus remote myocardium.

Stress subendocardial MBF in dark rim artifact in the NonCAD subgroup was significantly higher than stress MBF downstream from either a ≥ 70% QCA stenosis or a 50–69% QCA stenosis (Fig. 4, $p < 0.001$). Thus, although dark rim artifacts visually look darker and had lower MBF measurements than remote regions, quantitative MBF in these regions differentiated dark rim artifacts from perfusion defects associated with CAD (Fig. 4).

Sector-wise analysis
Similar to the pixel-wise quantification, sector-wise MBF measurements were able to differentiate dark rim artifacts from intermediate and severe stenosis (Fig. 5). However, there was no statistically significant difference between dark rim artifacts and the remote regions within the NonCAD subgroup (Fig. 5). Since inner sectors extended halfway across the myocardium and were frequently larger in the circumferential direction than the dark rim artifacts, these 2-layers sector-level measurements included myocardium outside of the visually apparent dark rim artifacts. Thus the 3-layers of pixel-wise analyses were smaller in both transmural and circumferential extent than the two-layer sectors.

Implications for differentiating CAD from NonCAD
Using pixel-wise measurements, the group of patients with significant CAD on a per-territory basis could be differentiated from the NonCAD group by stress subendocardial MBF with an accuracy of 86% ($p < 0.0001$, Fig. 6). The sensitivity was 86% and the specificity was 85%. The stress MBF in the midmyocardium had an accuracy of 89% ($p < 0.0001$) with a sensitivity of 92% and specificity of 87%. The stress MBF in the epicardium had an accuracy of 86% ($p < 0.001$) with a sensitivity of 84% and specificity of 87%. Similar results were seen for sector-level results but with different optimal thresholds.

The optimal MBF threshold for distinguishing patients with CAD from NonCAD was 1.55 mL/min/g in the subendocardium, 2.13 mL/min/g in the midmyocardium, and 2.19 mL/min/g in the epicardium (Fig. 6). Higher thresholds apply to the sector-level analysis (Fig. 6).

Rest myocardial blood flow
While stress MBF clearly differentiated significant CAD from remote myocardium in all layers of myocardium, the rest perfusion metrics were not able to differentiate regional MBF differences in the distribution of coronary stenoses vs. remote myocardium ($p = NS$).

Performance of SCMR guideline advice for differentiating dark rim artifacts from true perfusion defects
Using the SCMR Guideline to define DRA persisting < 7 beats and "true perfusion defects" as ≥ 7 heartbeats had a sensitivity of 95%, but a specificity of only 18% for significant CAD. Thus, dark rim artifacts were *not* differentiated from true perfusion defects by the duration of dark region alone.

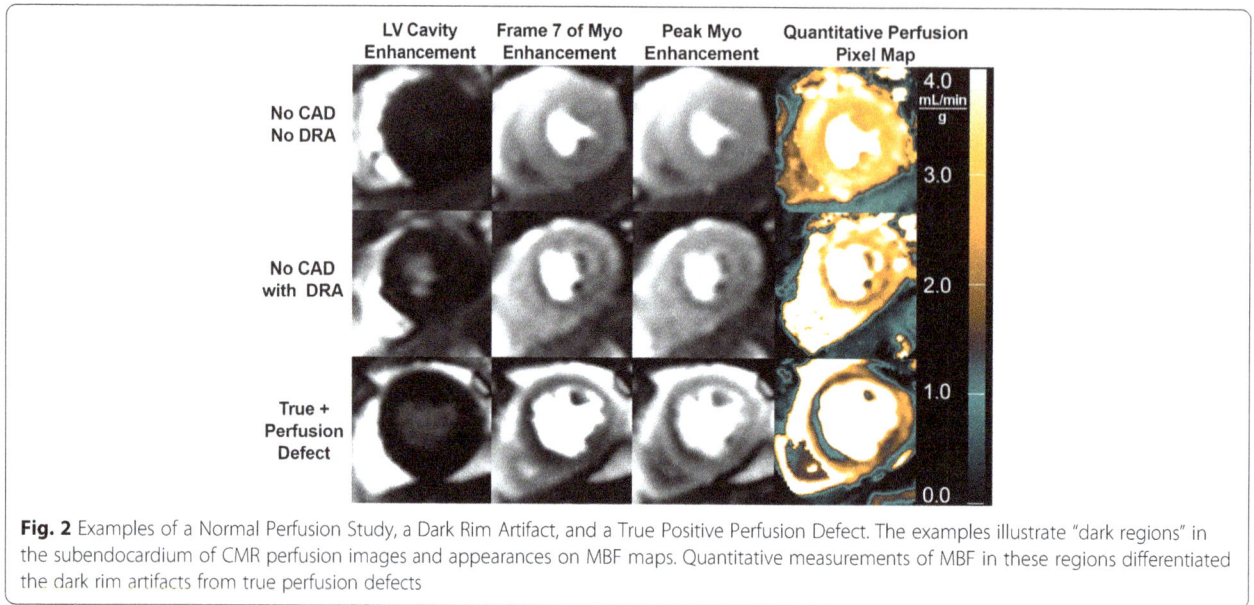

Fig. 2 Examples of a Normal Perfusion Study, a Dark Rim Artifact, and a True Positive Perfusion Defect. The examples illustrate "dark regions" in the subendocardium of CMR perfusion images and appearances on MBF maps. Quantitative measurements of MBF in these regions differentiated the dark rim artifacts from true perfusion defects

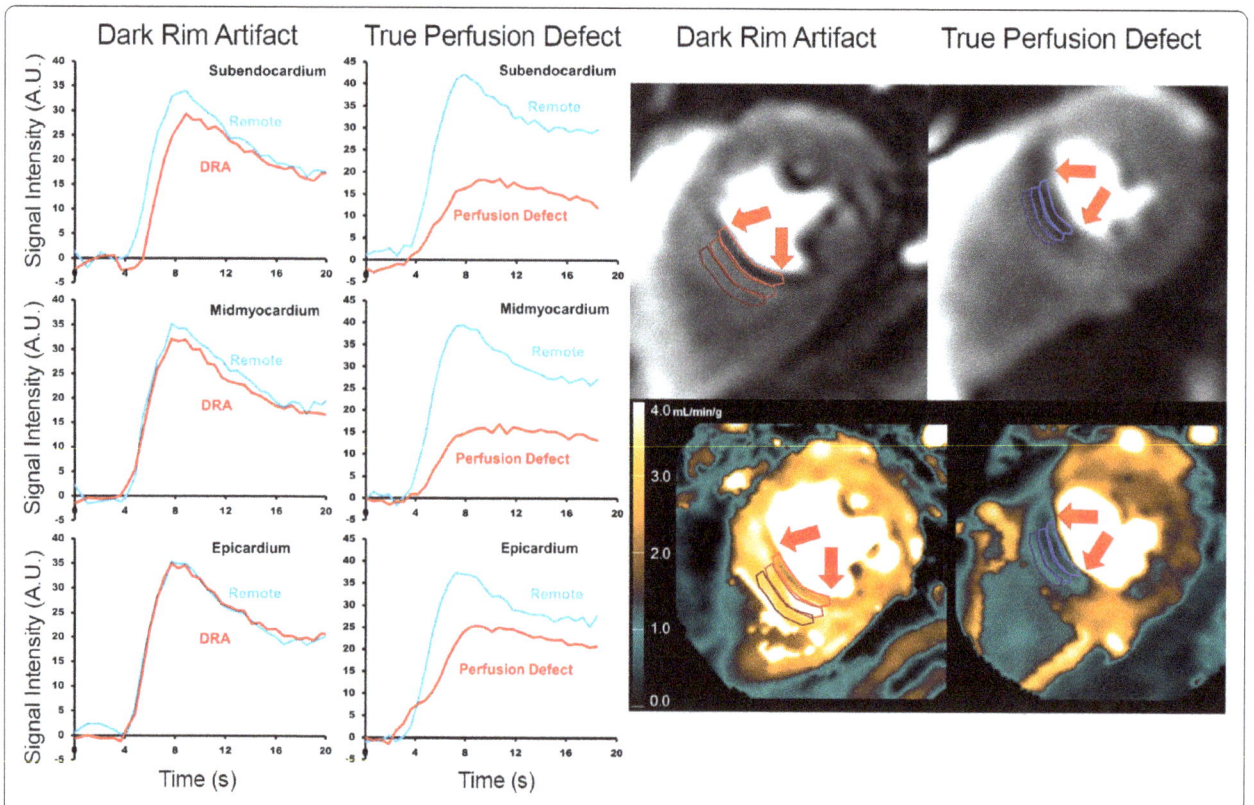

Fig. 3 Raw Stress Perfusion CMR images and Signal Intensity Curves in Dark Rim Artifacts and True Perfusion Defect. The dark rim artifacts in the septum (arrows) has three findings: (1) a decrease in the signal intensity curve prior to contrast arrival, (2) a delay in enhancement relative to the remote zone, and (3) a lower signal intensity throughout the upslope and peak of myocardial enhancement. However, the signal intensity curves in the midmyocardium and epicardium are not affected by the dark rim artifacts. In the true perfusion defect, the amplitude, upslope and persistence of the signal intensity abnormalities are all different than the remote region

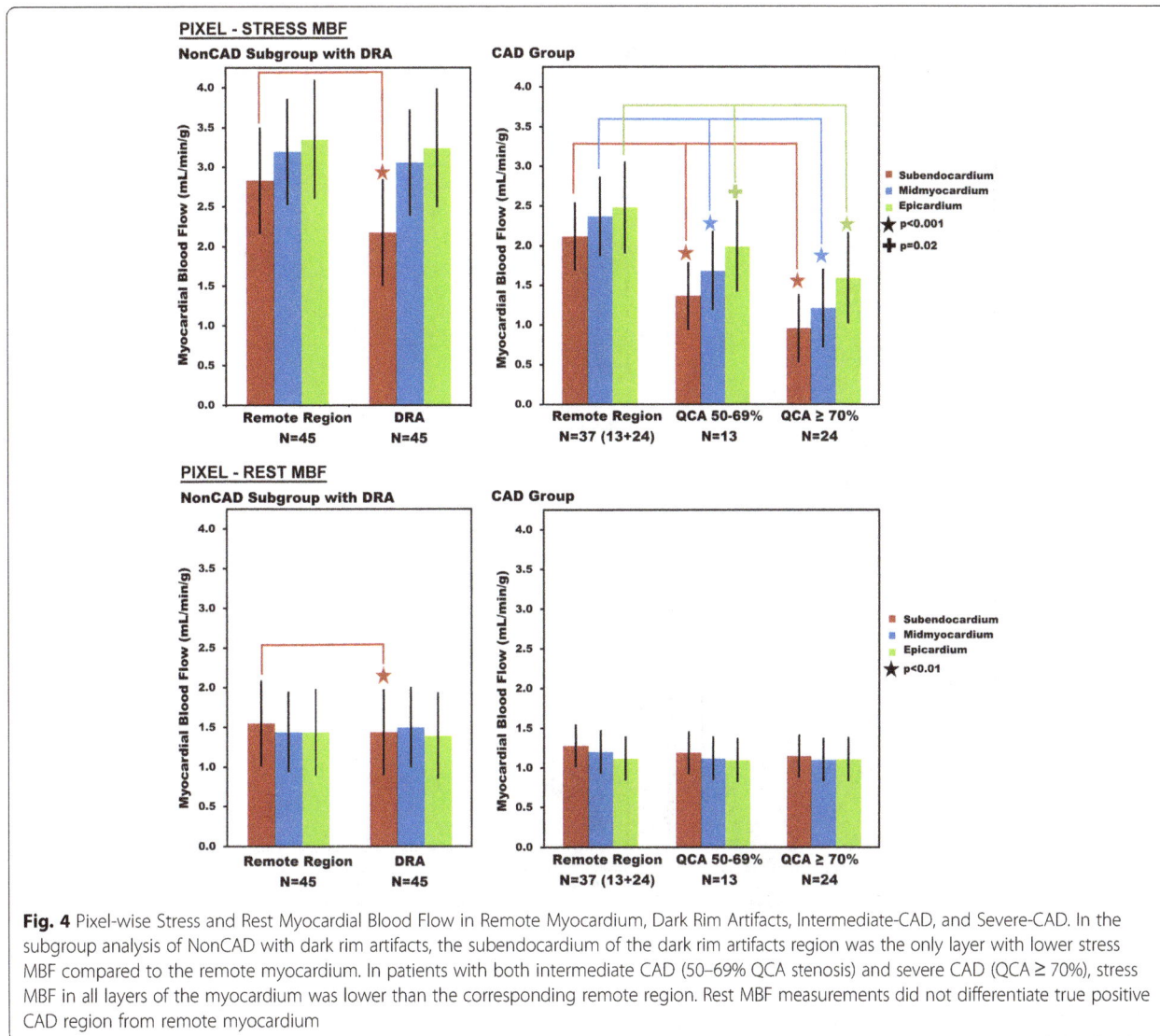

Fig. 4 Pixel-wise Stress and Rest Myocardial Blood Flow in Remote Myocardium, Dark Rim Artifacts, Intermediate-CAD, and Severe-CAD. In the subgroup analysis of NonCAD with dark rim artifacts, the subendocardium of the dark rim artifacts region was the only layer with lower stress MBF compared to the remote myocardium. In patients with both intermediate CAD (50–69% QCA stenosis) and severe CAD (QCA ≥ 70%), stress MBF in all layers of the myocardium was lower than the corresponding remote region. Rest MBF measurements did not differentiate true positive CAD region from remote myocardium

Combining an analysis of a dark region on the 7th frame of myocardial enhancement on both rest and stress perfusion images as a method of distinguishing a "perfusion defect" from a "dark rim artifact" improved the specificity to 75%, but decreased the sensitivity to 71%.

A decrease in signal intensity less than 2SD from the baseline prior to myocardial enhancement was found in only 6 of the 76 subjects. Using this measurement as an indicator of a dark rim artifact had poor diagnostic performance of a 90% sensitivity, but only a 7% specificity despite some excellent examples (Fig. 3).

Quality assurance metrics

Three observations support that the perfusion pixel-maps can differentiate about three layers across the myocardium:

1) For subjects with significant CAD during stress perfusion, myocardial wall thickness averaged (10.4 ± 2.24 mm) which was equivalent to 3.0 ± 0.6 non-interpolated pixels across the wall and twice as many interpolated pixels.

2) At rest, subendocardial MBF was greater than epicardial MBF within the remote myocardium of both NonCAD and CAD in pixel-level (Fig. 4, $p = 0.02$ and Fig. 4, $p = 0.002$ respectively) and sector-level ($p \leq 0.0001$ and $p = 0.003$ respectively, Fig. 5).

3) The difference between endocardial and epicardial MBF in patients with CAD was larger on the 3-layer pixel-wise comparison (Fig. 4) than the 2-layer sector-level analysis (Fig. 5). For the group of patients with a 50–69% QCA stenosis, endocardial MBF was only 12% lower than epicardial MBF on sector-level analysis, but 32% lower on pixel-level measurements. For a ≥ 70% stenosis, endocardial MBF was 12% lower than epicardial MBF on sector-level analysis but 40% lower on pixel-level measurements.

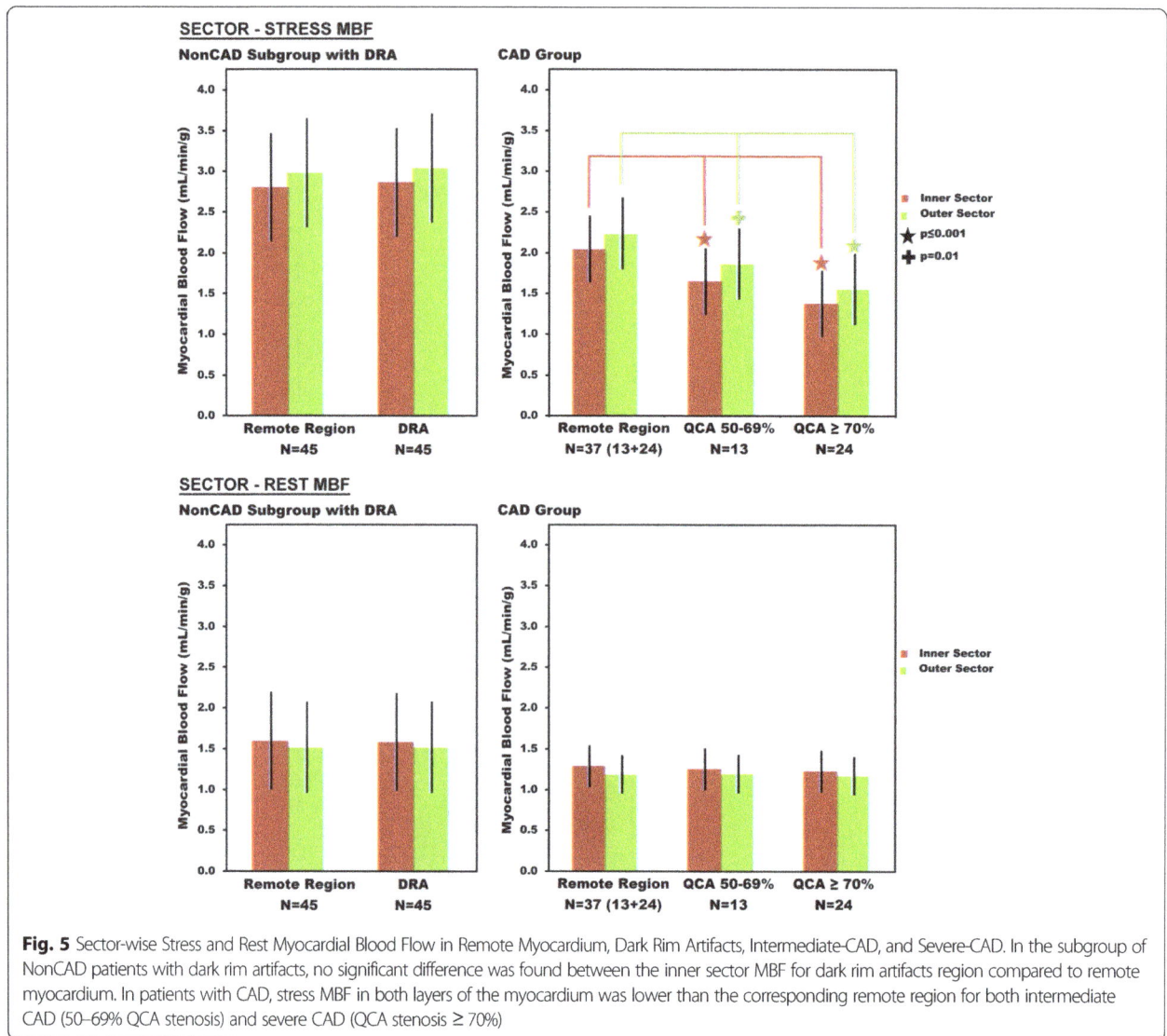

Fig. 5 Sector-wise Stress and Rest Myocardial Blood Flow in Remote Myocardium, Dark Rim Artifacts, Intermediate-CAD, and Severe-CAD. In the subgroup of NonCAD patients with dark rim artifacts, no significant difference was found between the inner sector MBF for dark rim artifacts region compared to remote myocardium. In patients with CAD, stress MBF in both layers of the myocardium was lower than the corresponding remote region for both intermediate CAD (50–69% QCA stenosis) and severe CAD (QCA stenosis ≥ 70%)

Discussion

This is the first perfusion CMR study that specifically measured MBF at the pixel-level in dark rim artifacts and compared them to the MBF measurements in true perfusion defects in a large series of patients. In our study, fully quantitative measurements of CMR stress MBF distinguished dark rim artifacts from true perfusion defects for both intermediate (50–69% QCA stenosis) and severe CAD (≥ 70% QCA stenosis). MBF measures in dark rim artifacts, despite being lower than remote myocardium, were quantitatively *less* severely decreased than true perfusion defects. From our perfusion pixel map analysis, dark rim artifacts typically did not extend into the midmyocardium or epicardium while true perfusion defects did. We found that measurable dark rim artifact frequently lasted longer than 7 heart beats after myocardial contrast arrival indicating that the SCMR recommended criterion for

differentiating a dark rim artifact from "true perfusion defects" associated with CAD is not sufficiently specific.

Dark rim artifacts could be one factor affecting the diagnostic accuracy of CMR perfusion trials. A dark rim artifact that mimics a subendocardial perfusion defect can lead to a false positive diagnosis of CAD. Conversely, minor perfusion defects may be underdiagnosed if they resemble a dark rim artifact. Thus, dark rim artifacts could adversely affect both specificity and sensitivity of stress CMR. From a recent meta-analysis, the diagnostic performance of CMR was comparable to single photon emission computed tomography (SPECT) and positron emission tomography (PET) [12]. However, 14 of 27 CMR stress perfusion studies had specificity < 80% and the multicenter MR-IMPACT II study had a sensitivity of 67% and specificity 61% [13]. On the other hand, the large CE-MARC study had higher sensitivity

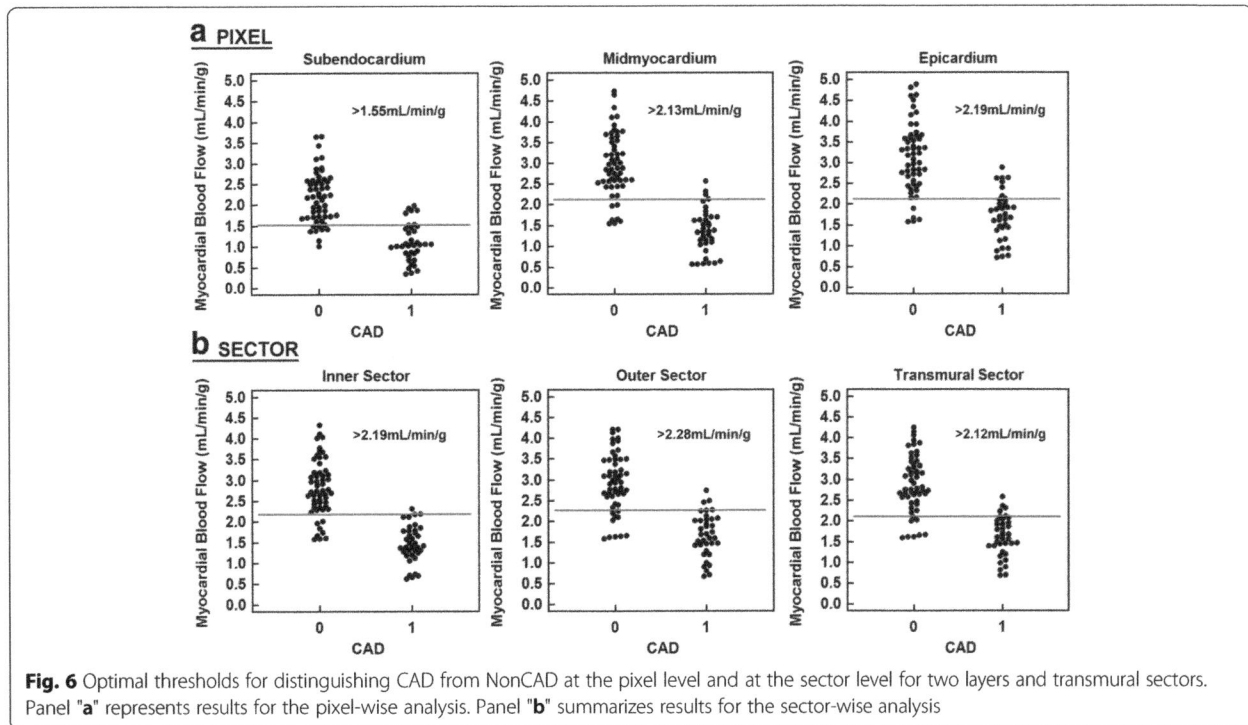

Fig. 6 Optimal thresholds for distinguishing CAD from NonCAD at the pixel level and at the sector level for two layers and transmural sectors. Panel "**a**" represents results for the pixel-wise analysis. Panel "**b**" summarizes results for the sector-wise analysis

(86.5%) and specificity (83.4%) [14]. Thus, expert readers can interpret stress perfusion studies with very good sensitivity and specificity and must have learned how to differentiate true perfusion defects from dark rim artifacts. For example, Greenwood et al. was able to reduce unnecessary invasive coronary angiography from 28.8% in the NICE Guideline Group to 7.5% in the CMR group. [15]

The prevalence of dark rim artifacts on CMR perfusion imaging has been reported to range from (55–100%) depending on the imaging technique and the method used to identify a dark rim artifacts [16, 17]. In our study, the NonCAD cohort had an 82% prevalence of hypointense subendocardial regions on stress perfusion images. While this prevalence was on the high end, a bSSFP sequence tends to cause more dark rim artifactsthan other CMR methods. The apparent severity of dark rim artifacts is also dependent on the contrast and brightness used to display gray scale perfusion images.

A number of acquisition improvements have been developed to reduce dark rim artifacts, including k-t SENSE accelerated parallel imaging [5], increased spatial resolution [7], non-Cartesian imaging [18, 19], and filtering [4]. Since dark rim artifacts have not been eliminated, alternative strategies are being explored.

Since eliminating dark rim artifacts has been difficult in CMR perfusion, there is a need for an objective, sensitive, and specific technique to differentiate true CAD from artifacts. Semi-quantitative MBF from CMR can perform comparably with other perfusion reference standards such

as SPECT and PET for diagnostic studies [14, 20, 21]. However, semi-quantitative methods tend to underestimate MBF which reduces the ability to differentiate normal from abnormal MBF [22].

In recent studies, quantitative CMR stress MBF outperformed qualitative and semi-quantitative methods [23]. Fully quantitative measurements more effectively described the extent of perfusion defects [24]. Quantification at the pixel level has been validated in canines by microspheres [11], in phantoms [25], and in humans by PET [26]. Pixel-wise quantification of MBF provides high resolution and may improve diagnostic accuracy.

Limitations

The limitations of this study include the lack of fractional flow reserve (FFR) as a comparison, the small single center design, and the lack of an independent validation dataset. The correlation between a vessel's physiologic significance and the percent stenosis measured by QCA is imperfect. However, QCA has been used commonly in studies evaluating the diagnostic performance of non-invasive stress testing. Fractional flow reserve wasn't available in most of the patients in this study. Use of CTA in the inclusion/exclusion criteria may be questioned but was justified by the high negative predictive value of the test. Use of CTA also helps reduce referral bias compared with studies that recruit patients scheduled for invasive coronary angiography and better represents the population undergoing stress tests.

The lack of an independent validation set mean these results should be confirmed in an independent dataset. Until such a study is performed, the thresholds depicted should be considered conceptually important (i.e. dark rim artifacts appear to have MBF between normal perfusion and perfusion defects associated with significant CAD). The absolute thresholds may not be applicable to other perfusion methods.

The bSSFP perfusion sequence has a higher contrast to noise ratio than other methods, but it may increase the appearance of dark rim artifacts causing more false positives. Further study is needed to address whether our findings are translatable to other methods used in CMR perfusion imaging.

Currently, there is no other technique to measure microvascular flow in dark rim artifact regions to evaluate whether dark rim artifacts represent a microvascular perfusion defect or an artifact. Invasive measurements of microvascular perfusion indices were not available in any patients in this study. Thus, some fraction of dark rim artifacts could represent real microvascular disease.

Conclusion

The ability to objectively differentiate between artifact and true perfusion defect potentially represents an important breakthrough for a common problem that affects confidence in interpretation of CMR perfusion. Larger prospective studies are needed to confirm our findings.

Abbreviations
BP: Blood pressure; bSSFP: Balanced steady state free precession; CAD: Coronary artery disease; CMR: Cardiovascular magnetic resonance; NonCAD: Patients *without* coronary artery disease; PCI: Percutaneous coronary intervention; PET: Positron emission tomography; QCA: Quantitative coronary angiography; RCA: Right coronary artery; SCMR: Society for Cardiovascular Magnetic Resonance; SPECT: Single photon emission computed tomography

Acknowledgements
We would like to thank the Sarnoff Cardiovascular Research Foundation for funding Allison Ta's research project. We would also like to thank Duke University Medical School for supporting Allison Ta.

Funding
This work was funded by the Division of Intramural Research, National Heart, Lung and Blood Institute, National Institutes of Health, Bethesda, MD, USA, HL006137–02, HL006137–03, and HL006137–04. Allison Ta was funded by the Sarnoff Cardiovascular Research Fellowship Program, Great Falls, Virginia, USA.

Authors' contributions
AT participated in design of project methods, carried out the quantification of data, analyzed results, and drafted manuscript. LH developed the quantification program, assisted with data analysis and drafting of manuscript. HC assisted with quantification of data and drafting of manuscript. SW performed quantitative coronary angiography. AG performed statistical analysis and drafting of manuscript. SS performed CMR data acquisition and interpretation. MC performed CTA data acquisition and interpretation. PB performed CMR data acquisition, interpretation, and drafting of manuscript. AA conceived project, participated in design and drafting of manuscript. All authors read and approved the final manuscript.

Competing interests
Dr. Arai has research agreements with Siemens (US Government Cooperative Research and Development Agreement HL-CR-05-004). No other conflicts of interest to disclose.

Author details
[1]National Heart, Lung and Blood Institute, National Institutes of Health, Department of Health and Human Services, Bldg 10, Rm B1D416, MSC 1061, 10 Center Drive, Bethesda, MD 20892-1061, USA. [2]Duke University School of Medicine, Durham, North Carolina, USA. [3]Medical University of Vienna, Vienna, Austria.

References
1. Douglas PS, Hoffmann U, Patel MR, Mark DB, Al-Khalidi HR, Cavanaugh B, et al. Outcomes of anatomical versus functional testing for coronary artery disease. N Engl J Med. 2015;372(14):1291–300.
2. Bratis K, Mahmoud I, Chiribiri A, Nagel E. Quantitative myocardial perfusion imaging by cardiovascular magnetic resonance and positron emission tomography. J Nucl Cardiol. 2013;20(5):860–70.
3. Ferreira P, Gatehouse P, Kellman P, Bucciarelli-Ducci C, Firmin D. Variability Of myocardial perfusion dark rim Gibbs artifacts due to sub-pixel shifts. J Cardiovasc Magn Reson. 2009;11(1):1–10.
4. Di Bella E, Parker D, Sinusas A. On the dark rim artifact in dynamic contrast-enhanced MRI myocardial perfusion studies. Magn Reson Med. 2005;54(5):1295–9.
5. Maredia N, Radjenovic A, Kozerke S, Larghat A, Greenwood JP, Plein S. Effect of improving spatial or temporal resolution on image quality and quantitative perfusion assessment with k-t SENSE acceleration in first-pass CMR myocardial perfusion imaging. Magn Reson Med. 2010;64(6):1616–24.
6. Storey P, Chen Q, Li W, Edelman RR, Prasad PV. Band artifacts due to bulk motion. Magn Reson Med. 2002;48(6):1028–36.
7. Kellman P, Arai AE. Imaging sequences for first pass perfusion-a review. J Cardiovasc Magn Reson. 2007;9(3):525–37.
8. Meloni A, Al-Saadi N, Torheim G, Hoebel N, Reynolds HG, De Marchi D, et al. Myocardial first-pass perfusion: influence of spatial resolution and heart rate on the dark rim artifact. Magn Reson Med. 2011;66(6):1731–8.
9. Schulz-Menger J, Bluemke DA, Bremerich J, Flamm SD, Fogel MA, Friedrich MG, et al. Standardized image interpretation and post processing in cardiovascular magnetic resonance: Society for Cardiovascular Magnetic Resonance (SCMR) Board of Trustees Task Force on standardized post processing. J Cardiovasc Magn Reson. 2013;15:35.
10. Gatehouse PD, Elkington AG, Ablitt NA, Yang GZ, Pennell DJ, Firmin DN. Accurate assessment of the arterial input function during high-dose myocardial perfusion cardiovascular magnetic resonance. J Magn Reson Imaging. 2004;20(1):39–45.
11. Hsu L-Y, Groves DW, Aletras AH, Kellman P, Arai AE. A quantitative pixel-wise measurement of myocardial blood flow by contrast-enhanced first-pass CMR perfusion ImagingMicrosphere validation in dogs and feasibility study in humans. J Am Coll Cardiol Img. 2012;5(2):154–66.
12. Jaarsma C, Leiner T, Bekkers SC, Crijns HJ, Wildberger JE, Nagel E, et al. Diagnostic performance of noninvasive myocardial perfusion imaging using single-photon emission computed tomography, cardiac magnetic resonance, and positron emission tomography imaging for the detection of obstructive coronary artery Disease. A meta-analysis. J Am Coll Cardiol. 2012;59(19):1719–28.
13. Schwitter J, Wacker CM, Wilke N, Al-Saadi N, Sauer E, Huettle K, et al. MR-IMPACT II: magnetic resonance imaging for myocardial perfusion assessment in coronary artery disease trial: perfusion-cardiac magnetic resonance vs. single-photon emission computed tomography for the detection of coronary artery disease: a comparative multicentre, multivendor trial. Eur Heart J. 2013;34(10):775–81.

14. Greenwood JP, Maredia N, Younger JF, Brown JM, Nixon J, Everett CC, et al. Cardiovascular magnetic resonance and single-photon emission computed tomography for diagnosis of coronary heart disease (CE-MARC): a prospective trial. Lancet. 2012;379(9814):453–60.

15. Greenwood JP, Ripley DP, Berry C, McCann GP, Plein S, Bucciarelli-Ducci C, et al. Effect of care guided by cardiovascular magnetic resonance, myocardial perfusion scintigraphy, or NICE guidelines on subsequent unnecessary angiography rates: the CE-MARC 2 randomized clinical trial. JAMA. 2016;316(10):1051–60.

16. Fenchel M, Helber U, Simonetti OP, Stauder NI, Kramer U, Nguyen CN, et al. Multislice first-pass myocardial perfusion imaging: comparison of saturation recovery (SR)-TrueFISP-two-dimensional (2D) and SR-TurboFLASH-2D pulse sequences. J Magn Reson Imaging. 2004;19(5):555–63.

17. Plein S, Ryf S, Schwitter J, Radjenovic A, Boesiger P, Kozerke S. Dynamic contrast-enhanced myocardial perfusion MRI accelerated with k-t sense. Magn Reson Med. 2007;58(4):777–85.

18. Salerno M, Taylor A, Yang Y, Kuruvilla S, Ragosta M, Meyer CH, et al. Adenosine stress cardiovascular magnetic resonance with variable-density spiral pulse sequences accurately detects coronary artery disease initial clinical evaluation. Circ Cardiovasc Imaging. 2014;7(4):639–46.

19. Sharif B, Dharmakumar R, LaBounty T, Arsanjani R, Shufelt C, Thomson L, et al. Towards elimination of the dark-rim artifact in first-pass myocardial perfusion MRI: removing Gibbs ringing effects using optimized radial imaging. Magn Reson Med. 2014;72(1):124–36.

20. Doyle M, Fuisz A, Kortright E, Biederman RW, Walsh EG, Martin ET, et al. The impact of myocardial flow reserve on the detection of coronary artery disease by perfusion imaging methods: an NHLBI WISE study: PERFUSION IMAGING. J Cardiovasc Magn Reson. 2003;5(3):475–85.

21. Ibrahim T, Nekolla SG, Schreiber K, Odaka K, Volz S, Mehilli J, et al. Assessment of coronary flow reserve: comparison between contrast-enhanced magnetic resonance imaging and positron emission tomography. J Am Coll Cardiol. 2002;39(5):864–70.

22. Hsu LY, Rhoads KL, Holly JE, Kellman P, Aletras AH, Arai AE. Quantitative myocardial perfusion analysis with a dual-bolus contrast-enhanced first-pass MRI technique in humans. J Magn Reson Imaging. 2006;23(3):315–22.

23. Mordini FE, Haddad T, Hsu L-Y, Kellman P, Lowrey TB, Aletras AH, et al. Diagnostic accuracy of stress perfusion CMR in comparison with quantitative coronary AngiographyFully quantitative, Semiquantitative, and qualitative assessment. J Am Coll Cardiol Img. 2014;7(1):14–22.

24. Patel AR, Antkowiak PF, Nandalur KR, West AM, Salerno M, Arora V, et al. Assessment of advanced coronary artery DiseaseAdvantages of quantitative cardiac magnetic resonance perfusion analysis. J Am Coll Cardiol. 2010;56(7):561–9.

25. Zarinabad N, Chiribiri A, Hautvast GL, Ishida M, Schuster A, Cvetkovic Z, et al. Voxel-wise quantification of myocardial perfusion by cardiac magnetic resonance. Feasibility and methods comparison. Magn Reson Med. 2012;68(6):1994–2004.

26. Miller CA, Naish JH, Ainslie MP, Tonge C, Tout D, Arumugam P, et al. Voxel-wise quantification of myocardial blood flow with cardiovascular magnetic resonance: effect of variations in methodology and validation with positron emission tomography. J Cardiovasc Magn Reson. 2014;16(1):11.

12

Diabetes mellitus and insulin resistance associate with left ventricular shape and torsion by cardiovascular magnetic resonance imaging in asymptomatic individuals from the multi-ethnic study of atherosclerosis

Kihei Yoneyama[1,5], Bharath A. Venkatesh[1], Colin O. Wu[2], Nathan Mewton[1], Ola Gjesdal[1], Satoru Kishi[1], Robyn L. McClelland[3], David A. Bluemke[4] and João A. C. Lima[1,6*]

Abstract

Background: Although diabetes mellitus (DM) and insulin resistance associate with adverse cardiac events, the associations of left ventricular (LV) remodeling and function with compromised glucose metabolism have not been fully evaluated in a general population. We used cardiovascular magnetic resonance (CMR) to evaluate how CMR indices are associated with DM or insulin resistance among participants before developing cardiac events.

Methods: We studied 1476 participants who were free of clinical cardiovascular disease and who underwent tagged CMR in the Multi-Ethnic Study of Atherosclerosis (MESA). LV shape and longitudinal myocardial shortening and torsion were assessed by CMR. A higher sphericity index represents a more spherical LV shape. Multivariable linear regression was used to evaluate the associations of DM or homeostasis model assessment-estimated insulin resistance (HOMA-IR) with CMR indices.

Results: In multiple linear regression, longitudinal shortening was lower in impaired fasting glucose than normal fasting glucose (NFG) (0.36% lower vs. NFG, $p < 0.05$); torsion was greater in treated DM (0.24 °/cm greater vs. NFG, $p < 0.05$) after full adjustments. Among participants without DM, greater log-HOMA-IR was correlated with greater LV mass (3.92 g/index, $p < 0.05$) and LV mass-to-volume ratio (0.05 /index, $p < 0.01$), and lower sphericity index (-1.26/index, $p < 0.01$). Greater log-HOMA IR was associated with lower longitudinal shortening (-0.26%/index, $p < 0.05$) and circumferential shortening (-0.30%/index, $p < 0.05$). Torsion was positively correlated with log-HOMA-IR until 1.5 of log-HOMA-IR (0.16 °/cm/index, $p = 0.030$).), and tended to fall once above 1.5 of log-HOMA-IR (-0.50 °/cm/index, $p = 0.203$). The sphericity index was associated negatively with LV mass-to-volume ratio (-0.02/%, $p < 0.001$) and torsion (-0.03°/cm/%, $p < 0.001$).

(Continued on next page)

* Correspondence: jlima@jhmi.edu
[1]Department of Cardiology, Johns Hopkins University, Baltimore, MD, USA
[6]Radiology and Epidemiology, Johns Hopkins University, Blalock 524D1,
Johns Hopkins Hospital, 600 North Wolfe Street, Baltimore, MD 21287, USA
Full list of author information is available at the end of the article

(Continued from previous page)
Conclusions: Glucose metabolism disorders are associated with LV concentric remodeling, less spherical shape, and reduced systolic myocardial shortening in the general population. Although torsion is higher in participants who are treated for DM and impaired insulin resistance, myocardial shortening was progressively decreased with higher HOMA-IR and torsion was increased only with less severe insulin resistance.

Keywords: Glucose tolerance, Heart failure, Metabolic disease, Obesity, Strain

Background
Type 2 diabetes mellitus (DM) is a group of metabolic diseases; insulin resistance is a condition characterized by the failure to respond appropriately to insulin. Chronic hyperglycemia may impair myocardial energy metabolism, induces cardiomyocyte systolic dysfunction and eventually cell death [1, 2]. Epidemiological studies have demonstrated that DM and insulin resistance are related to cardiovascular disease and heart failure [3–5].

Left ventricular (LV) structure, shape and myocardial shortening (myocardial strain) have been shown to have incremental predictive value for cardiovascular events beyond the traditional LV ejection fraction measures [6–10]. Although DM and insulin resistance associate with adverse cardiac events, the associations of LV remodeling and function with compromised glucose metabolism have not been fully evaluated in a general population. We hypothesized that DM or insulin resistance might associate with LV remodeling and systolic function before developing cardiac events.

The Multi-Ethnic Study of Atherosclerosis (MESA)—a prospective study sponsored by the National Heart Lung and Blood Institute (NHLBI) of the National Institutes of Health—is a large cohort study of ethnically diverse individuals free of cardiovascular disease at baseline, and was primarily designed to study the progression of subclinical cardiovascular disease [11]. MESA is the largest cardiovascular magnetic resonance (CMR) tagging study to allow unique investigation of cardiac mechanics at the population level. To test the hypothesis, we used MESA CMR tagging examination to evaluate how CMR indices are associated with DM or insulin resistance among participants free of clinical cardiovascular disease.

Methods
Participants
MESA evaluated the mechanisms that underlie the development and progression of subclinical cardiovascular diseases among asymptomatic individuals. Details of the MESA study design have been previously described [11]. In brief, between July 2000 and August 2002, 6814 men and women—who identified themselves as Caucasian, African American, Hispanic, or Chinese and were 45–

84 years of age and free of clinically apparent cardiovascular disease—were recruited. CMR was performed in 5004 participants as part of the baseline examination. In an ancillary study, 1773 consecutive participants underwent tagged CMR studies at enrollment in six centers: Wake Forest University, Columbia University, Johns Hopkins University, the University of Minnesota, Northwestern University, and the University of California. Of these, torsion data were available for 1478 participants as previously described [12]; of those, two cases were excluded because of lack of clinical information. A total of 1476 participants were thus enrolled in the study. None of those were known type 1 DM. All participants gave informed consent, and the study protocol was approved by the institutional review board at each site.

Cine CMR data analysis
LV end-systolic volume and end-diastolic volume (LVEDV), LV mass, and LV ejection fraction were obtained (Additional file 1) [6, 13]. LV mass-to-volume ratio was calculated as LV mass divided by LVEDV. LV length at end-diastole was calculated as the average distance from the epicardial apex to the mitral valve insertion as measured from the 2 and 4 chamber views. The LV sphericity index at end-diastole was calculated as the percentage of the LVEDV relative to the volume of a calculated sphere with the LV length [14]. A higher index represents a more spherical shape of the ventricle and a lower reduced spericity. LV longitudinal shortening (long-axis fractional shortening) was calculated as (LV length at diastole – LV length at systole)/LV length at diastole*100 (%) [15]. A higher value represents an increased shortening of the ventricle.

Tagged CMR was performed using a segmented k-space electrocardiogram (ECG)-gated fast low angle shot pulse sequence (Additional file 1). Circumferential shortening was represented by the absolute peak strain. Positive numbers of shortening represent more contraction. Torsion (°/cm) was calculated by dividing the peak systolic twist by the inter-slice distance. CMR indices are dysplayed in Additional file 1.

Risk factor measures
Risk factors measures are provided in Additional file 1. Body mass index (BMI) was calculated as weight over

height squared. Untreated DM was defined as fasting glucose ≥126 mg/dl without any use of hypoglycemic medication or insulin. Treated DM was defined as use of hypoglycemic medication or insulin. Impaired fasting glucose (IFG) was defined as fasting glucose levels between 100 mg/dl and 125 mg/dl. All other participants were defined as having normal fasting glucose (NFG). Serum insulin was determined by a radioimmunoassay method using the Linco Human Insulin-Specific RIA kit (MilliporeSigma, Burlington, Massachusetts, USA.). Homeostasis model assessment-estimated insulin resistance (HOMA-IR) was calculated as insulin (mU/

l) × (glucose [mg/dl] × 0.055)/22.5 [16, 17]. Participants with DM were excluded from the HOMA-IR calculation.

Statistical analysis

Summary statistics were presented using median (interquartile range; 25 to 75%) for continuous variables, and percent for categorical variables. The chi-square test was used for comparison of categorical variables. Wilcoxon's rank-sum test was used to test the differences to compare each DM fasting glucose state. Multivariable linear regression models were used to compare CMR indices by DM fasting glucose criteria. We also used

Table 1 Baseline demographic characteristics according to DM state ($n = 1476$)

Variable	DM state*			
	NFG ($n = 1004$)	IFG ($n = 262$)	Untreated DM ($n = 47$)	Treated DM ($n = 163$)
Age, year	65 (56 to 72)	67 (61 to 72)†	66 (58 to 72)	68 (64 to 75)†
Male sex, %§	509 (50.7)	158 (60.3)	35 (74.5)	90 (55.2)
Ethnic, n (%)§				
Caucasian	336 (33)	65 (25)	12 (26)	24 (15)
Black	124 (12)	51 (19)	7 (15)	26 (16)
Hispanic	271 (27)	66 (25)	16 (34)	56 (34)
Chinese	273 (27)	80 (31)	12 (26)	57 (35)
Smoking status, n (%)				
Never	513 (51)	142 (54)	22 (47)	88 (54)
Former	376 (38)	87 (33)	20 (43)	54 (33)
Current	109 (11)	32 (12)	5 (11)	20 (12)
Alcohol status, n (%)§				
Never	195 (20)	47 (18)	8 (17)	44 (27)
Former	240 (24)	61 (23)	9 (20)	56 (35)
Current	558 (56)	152 (58)	29 (63)	61 (38)
Body mass index, kg/m²	27 (24 to 30)	29 (26 to 32)†	28 (25 to 32)	29 (26 to 32)†
Systolic BP, mmHg	124 (111 to 139)	131 (118 to 145)†	125 (115 to 145)	132 (120 to 146)†
Diastolic BP, mmHg	72 (65 to 78)	74 (67 to 82)†	73 (68 to 85)	70 (64 to 77)‡
Resting heart rate, bpm	60 (55 to 67)	64 (58 to 71)†	66 (60 to 71)†	66 (58 to 73)†
Hypertension, n (%)§	417 (42)	145 (55)	23 (49)	120 (74)
Current smoker, n (%)	109 (11)	32 (12)	5 (11)	20 (12)
Total-cholesterol, mg/dl	193 (172 to 215)	195 (170 to 220)	200 (170 to 218)	184 (161 to 205)
HDL-cholesterol, mg/dl	50 (42 to 60)	45 (38 to 53)†	42 (33 to 54)†	44 (38 to 54)†
Triglyceride, mg/dl	104 (74 to 150)	125 (86 to 186)†	128 (79 to 233)	128 (83 to 202)†
Lipid-lowering medication, n (%)§	160 (16)	53 (20)	12 (26)	53 (33)
Anti-hypertensive medication, n (%)§	337 (34)	128 (49)	16 (35)	122 (75)
eGFR, mL/min	76 (66 to 87)	76 (64 to 88)	83 (66 to 97)	77 (63 to 91)
Walking, MET-min/week	945 (360 to 1920)	788 (315 to 1770)	1245 (315 to 1995)	2243 (735 to 3750)

Values are median (interquartile range). BP, blood pressure; DM, diabetes mellitus; eGFR, estimated glomerular filtration rate
HDL, high-density lipoprotein; IFG, impaired fasting glucose; NFG, normal fasting glucose
*DM was defined as fasting glucose ≥126 mg/dl or use of hypoglycemic medication or insulin; IFG was defined as fasting glucose levels between 100 mg/dl and 125 mg/dl; all other participants were defined as having NFG
†p < 0.0125 vs. NFG in in Wilcoxon test, ‡p < 0.0125 vs. untreated DM in Wilcoxon test. §p < 0.05 in chi-square

Table 2 Association of CMR LV indices by DM state ($n = 1476$)

Dependent variables (LV indices)	Multivariable liner regression; coefficients			
	IFG (vs. NFG)	Untreated DM (vs. NFG)	Treated DM (vs. NFG)	R^2
End-diastolic volume, ml	−1.86 (1.81)	2.89 (3.82)	0.17 (2.26)	0.41
Mass, g	1.64 (2.00)	5.01 (4.22)	4.42 (2.50)*	0.55
Mass-to-volume	0.04 (0.02)†	0.01 (0.04)	0.04 (0.02)*	0.19
Sphericity index, %	−0.44 (0.43)	0.94 (0.90)	−0.27 (0.54)	0.10
Ejection fraction, %	−0.33 (0.51)	−1.27 (1.08)	0.76 (0.64)	0.19
Longitudinal shortening, %	−0.36 (0.17)†	−0.63 (0.37)*	−0.17 (0.22)	0.17
Circumferential shortening, %	−0.03 (0.18)	−0.43 (0.39)	−0.17 (0.23)	0.15
Torsion, °/cm	0.13 (0.08)	−0.25 (0.18)	0.24 (0.11)†	0.18

Coefficients (standard errors) represents the difference in depend variables compared to NFG as a reference in DM fasting glucose criteria. Model include age, gender, race, height, obesity (BMI ≥ 30 kg/m²), smoking status (non, former, and current), heart rate, systolic blood pressure, total cholesterol, use of medication for hypertension and dyslipidemia, estimated glomerular filtration rate, walking in METs per week, and alcoholic status (non-drinker, former, or current)

Abbreviations and definition of DM state as in Table 1

* $p < 0.1$, †$p < 0.05$

multivariable linear regression to evaluate the associations of HOMA-IR with CMR indices. Potential covariates included age, gender, race, height, obesity (BMI ≥ 30 kg/m²), smoking status (never, former, or current), heart rate, systolic blood pressure, total cholesterol, use of medication for hypertension and dyslipidemia, estimated glomerular filtration rate, walking in METs per week, and alcoholic status (non-drinker, former, or current). Significant nonlinearity was present between the torsion and HOMA-IR with a knot at 1.5 of log-HOMA-IR. Therefore, we used a linear spline model to estimate the relationship as a piecewise linear function with adjustments for the same covariates, as described above. Standardized values were defined by dividing the differences between the observed values and the sample means by the corresponding standard deviations. Statistical

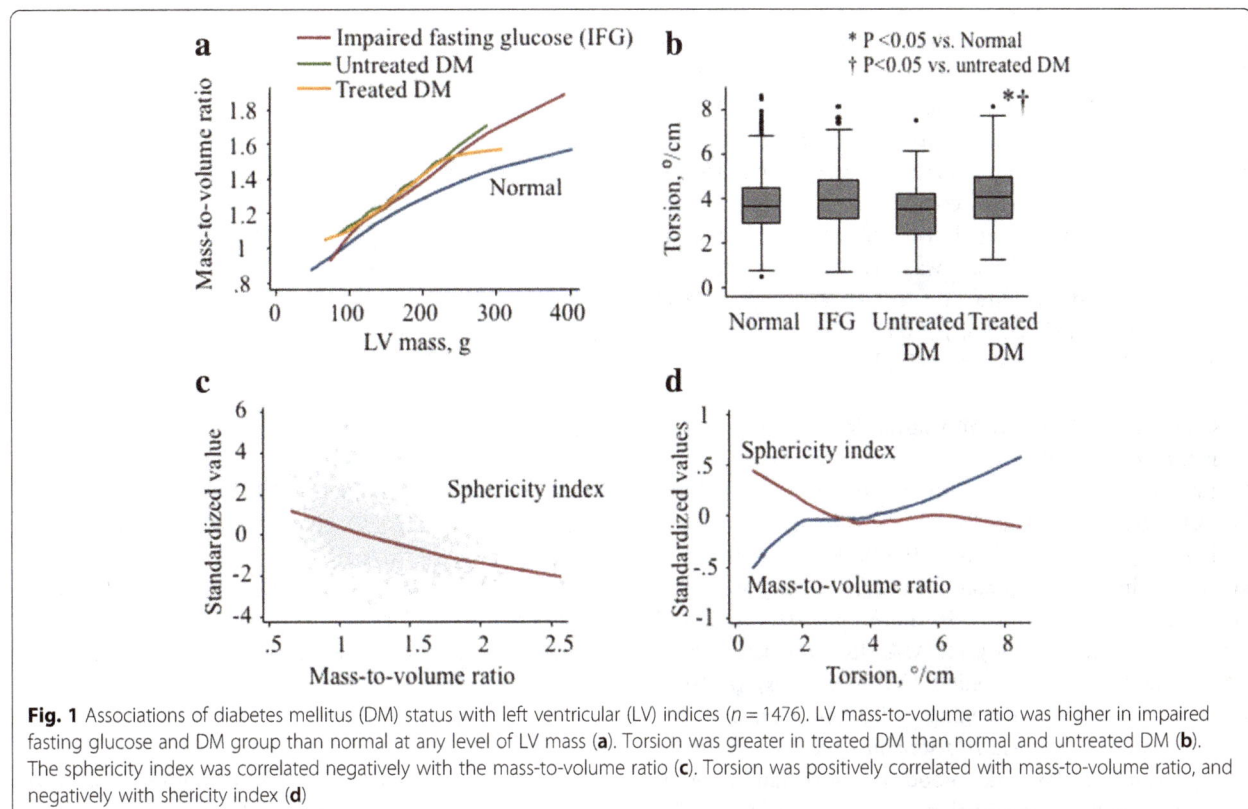

Fig. 1 Associations of diabetes mellitus (DM) status with left ventricular (LV) indices ($n = 1476$). LV mass-to-volume ratio was higher in impaired fasting glucose and DM group than normal at any level of LV mass (**a**). Torsion was greater in treated DM than normal and untreated DM (**b**). The sphericity index was correlated negatively with the mass-to-volume ratio (**c**). Torsion was positively correlated with mass-to-volume ratio, and negatively with shericity index (**d**)

analyses were performed using the Stata statistical software package (Version 14, College Station, Texas, USA). A two-sided p-value < 0.05 was considered statistically significant.

Results

Of the total 1476 participants population, 210 (14%) had DM and 262 (18%) had IFG.

Baseline characteristics according to DM fasting glucose criteria are shown in Table 1. Age and systolic blood pressure were higher in the IFG group and in the Treated DM group than in the NFG group. Diastolic blood pressure was greater in the IFG group and lower in the treated DM group than in the NFG group. Hypertension was common in treated DM (NFG; 42%, IFG; 55%, untreated DM; 49%, treated DM; 74%, $p < 0.05$). Use of lipid-lowering medication was common in treated DM (NFG; 16%, IFG; 20%, untreated DM; 26%, treated DM; 33%, $p < 0.05$).

Differences in LV structure and function in DM fasting glucose criteria compared to NFG

The median LV ejection fraction was 70% interquartile range (64, 74%) in the whole study population, and did not differ among DM fasting glucose criteria. Compared to NFG, treated DM tended to have greater LV mass (4.4 g greater vs. NFG, $p = 0.077$) and mass-to-volume ratio (0.04 greater vs. NFG, $p < 0.05$) with a lower longitudinal shortening (0.36% lower vs. NFG, p < 0.05) after adjustments for all prespecified confounders (Table 2). But torsion was greater in treated DM (0.24°/cm greater vs. NFG, $p < 0.05$) than NFG after full adjustments (Fig. 1). Circumferential shortening did not differ in DM status compared to NFG. The association of LV shape with concentric remodeling and torsion are shown in Fig. 1. In multiple linear regression, the sphericity index was associated negatively with LV mass-to-volume ratio ($- 0.02$/%, $p < 0.001$) and torsion ($- 0.03$°/cm/%, $p < 0.001$) after full adjustments (models included as in Table 2).

LV structure and function with serum fasting glucose, insulin, and HOMA-IR

Multivariable linear regression models in Table 3 indicate that greater log-transformed HOMA-IR was associated with greater LV mass (3.9 g/index, $p < 0.05$) and mass-to-volume ratio (0.05 /index, $p < 0.01$), and with lower sphericity index ($- 1.26$/index, p < 0.01) after full adjustments. Greater log-HOMA IR associated with lower longitudinal shortening ($- 0.26$%/index, p < 0.05) and circumferential shortening ($- 0.30$%/index, p < 0.05) after adjustments. These relationships were confounded by hypertension (systolic blood pressure, and use of anti-hypertensive medication) and obesity. The

Table 3 Association of LV remodeling and function by HOMA-IR among participants without diabetes mellitus ($n = 1266$)*

Dependent variables (LV indices)	Multivariable liner regression coefficients	
	Log-HOMA-IR	R^2
End-diastolic volume, ml		
Model 1	2.66 (1.40)	0.36
Model 2	−2.53 (1.48)	0.41
Mass, g		
Model 1	11.58 (1.58)‡	0.49
Model 2	3.92 (1.61)†	0.56
Mass-to-volume		
Model 1	0.07 (0.01)‡	0.18
Model 2	0.05 (0.01)‡	0.20
Sphericity index, %		
Model 1	−1.06 (0.33)‡	0.11
Model 2	−1.26 (0.35)‡	0.11
Ejection fraction, %		
Model 1	0.15 (0.38)	0.18
Model 2	0.25 (0.41)	0.18
Longitudinal shortening, %		
Model 1	−0.26 (0.13)†	0.16
Model 2	−0.22 (0.14)	0.17
Circumferential shortening, %		
Model 1	−0.30 (0.14)†	0.13
Model 2	−0.08 (0.15)	0.14
Torsion, °/cm		
Model 1	0.13 (0.06)†	0.16
Model 2	0.11 (0.07)	0.17

Coefficients (standard error) represents the change in dependent variables corresponds to 1 unit increase in independent variables. Model 1 included age, gender, race, height, smoking status(never, former, or current), heart rate, hypertension, total cholesterol, use of medication for dyslipidemia, estimated glomerular filtration rate, walking in METs per week, and alcohol status (non-drinker, former, or current). Model 2 included systolic blood pressure, anti-hypertensive medication use, and obesity (BMI ≥ 30 kg/m²) in addition to Model 1
Homeostasis model assessment-estimated insulin resistance (HOMA-IR) was calculated as insulin (mU/l) × (glucose [mg/dl] × 0.055)/22.5. [16, 17]
*Participants with diabetes mellitus were excluded because participants with DM were excluded from the HOMA-IR calculation
†p < 0.05, ‡p < 0.01

association between torsion and HOMA-IR was nonlinear (Fig. 2 and Table 4). Torsion was correlated positively with log-HOMA-IR until 1.5 of log-HOMA-IR (0.16 °/cm/index, $p = 0.030$), and tended to fall once above 1.5 of log-HOMA-IR ($- 0.50$ °/cm/index, $p = 0.203$) after full adjustments (models included as in Table 2).

Discussion

DM and insulin resistance are two of the most powerful risk factors for cardiovascular disease; however, the

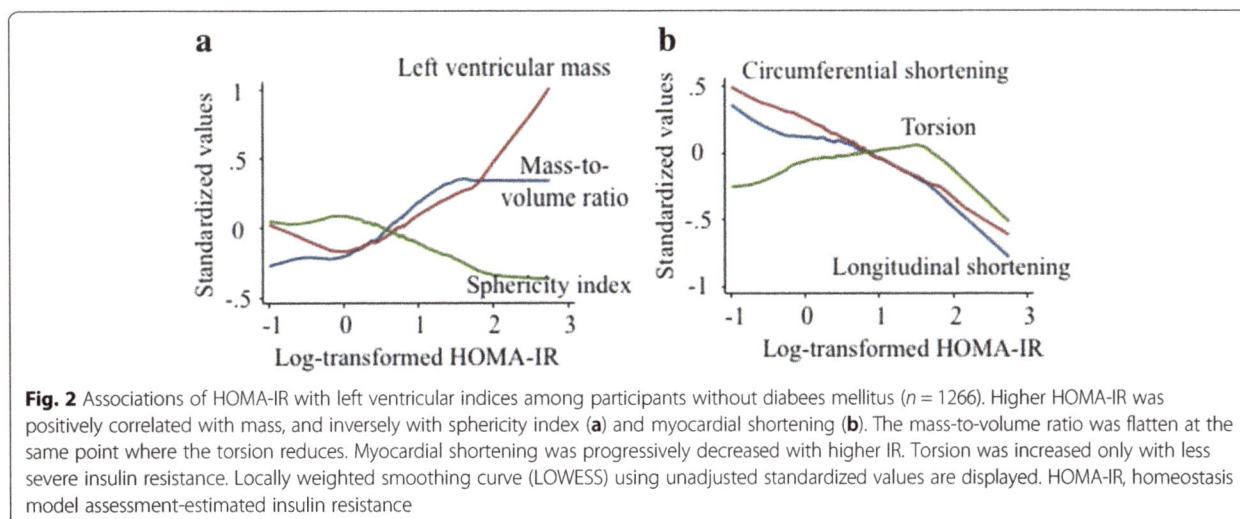

Fig. 2 Associations of HOMA-IR with left ventricular indices among participants without diabees mellitus ($n = 1266$). Higher HOMA-IR was positively correlated with mass, and inversely with sphericity index (**a**) and myocardial shortening (**b**). The mass-to-volume ratio was flatten at the same point where the torsion reduces. Myocardial shortening was progressively decreased with higher IR. Torsion was increased only with less severe insulin resistance. Locally weighted smoothing curve (LOWESS) using unadjusted standardized values are displayed. HOMA-IR, homeostasis model assessment-estimated insulin resistance

mechanisms of adaptation that alter the cardiovascular system in subjects with glucose metabolism disorders remain largely unknown. In MESA participants without known heart disease or clinical evidence of coronary artery disease at inclusion, we found the following: (1) participants with treated DM had greater LV concentric remodeling and greater torsion compared to participants with normal fasting glucose (NFG); (2) insulin resistance (non-DM) was related to a more conical LV shape and concentric remodeling with impaired systolic longitudinal myocardial shortening, but torsion was higher in advance with insulin resistance and was mirrored in a somewhat parallel manner with higher LV mass-to-volume ratio and conical shape. These observations suggest that DM or impaired insulin resistance are associated with adverse LV concentric remodeling, conical LV shape, and impaired systolic function. Increased torsion may be a key compensation mechanism to maintain global systolic function despite the alteration of myocardial shortening and structure due to compromised glucose metabolism in the general population (Fig. 3).

In the present study, subjects with treated DM had a more concentric LV than those with NFG subjects. In the Strong Heart Study, DM patients had increased LV mass and wall thickness by conventional echocardiography than normal glucose tolerance [18]. According to data from the Diabetes Control and Complication Trial/Epidemiology of Diabetes Intervention and Complications (DCC/EDIC) study, the mean Hemoglobin A1c levels are correlated positively with increased concentric remodeling defined by CMR among type 1 DM patients [19]. Our results are consistent with observations of previous large studies. We also found that higher HOMA-IR, a pre-diabetic status, was associated with concentric remodeling. The following studies also support our results: (a) in the Framingham Heart Study, LV mass and wall thickness by echocardiography were positively associated with an increase in HOMA-IR despite the relations being attenuated by BMI [20]; (b) in the Strong Heart Study, echocardiography indices demonstrated that insulin glucose tolerance was associated with higher LV mass and relative wall thickness [21]; (c) in the Coronary Artery Risk Development in Young Adults (CARDIA) study, high insulin resistance was associated with worse relative wall thickness [22]; (d) in a recent report from our study, central obesity and HOMA-IR were also associated with concentric remodeling [23].

Table 4 Association of left ventricular torsion with HOMA-IR ($n = 1266$)*

Depend variable	Multivariable spline liner regression		R^2
	Log HOMA-IR < 1.5 mg/dl	Log HOMA-IR > 1.5 mg/dl	
Torsion, °/cm			
Model 1	0.16 (0.07)†	−0.51 (.40)	0.15
Model 2	0.16 (0.08)†	−0.50 (0.40)	0.17

Coefficients (standard error) represents the change in torsion corresponds to 1 unite increase in log-HOMA-IR

Model1 included age, gender, race and height

Model 2 included age, gender, race, height, obesity (BMI ≥ 30 kg/m2), smoking status (non, former, and current), heart rate, systolic blood pressure, total cholesterol, use of medication for hypertension and dyslipidemia, estimated glomerular filtration rate, walking in METs per week, and alcoholic status (non-drinker, former, or current) as in Table 3

*Participants with diabetes mellitus were excluded as in Table 3

† $P < 0.05$

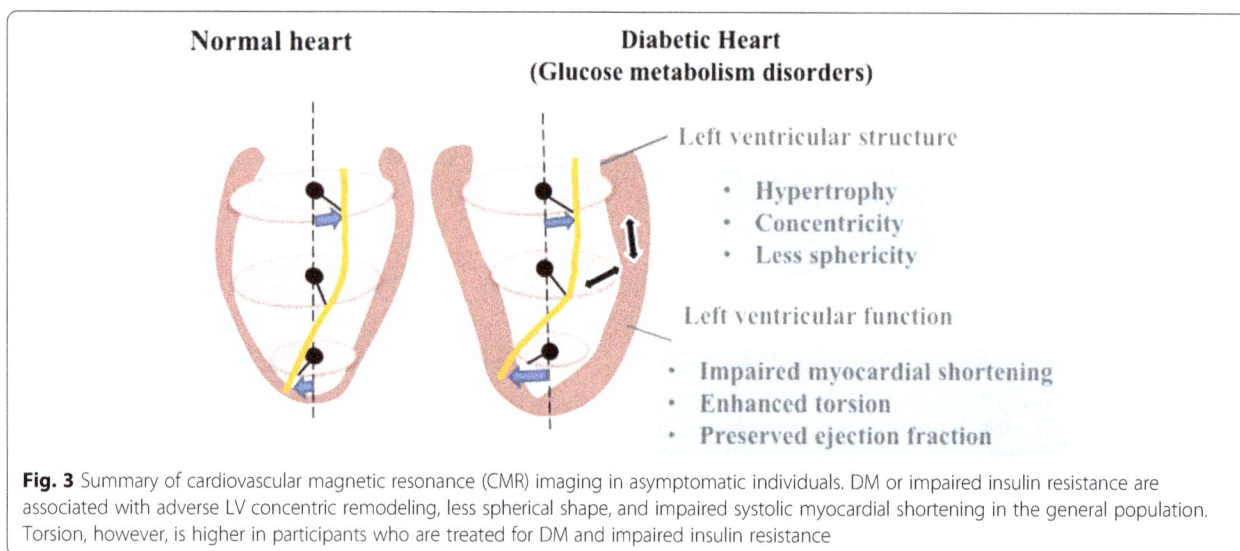

Fig. 3 Summary of cardiovascular magnetic resonance (CMR) imaging in asymptomatic individuals. DM or impaired insulin resistance are associated with adverse LV concentric remodeling, less spherical shape, and impaired systolic myocardial shortening in the general population. Torsion, however, is higher in participants who are treated for DM and impaired insulin resistance

Although the effect of LV sphericity shape has been described in LV severe systolic dysfunction [24] or in women's hearts [12], we found that higher HOMA-IR was related to lower LV sphericity (reduced sphericity). Since the more conical the LV becomes, the more the relative wall thickness increases, there might be a link between LV conical shape and torsion with respect to the lever-arm theory. In this theory, a greater radius difference between the endocardium and the epicardium would result in increased torsion (Fig. 4). Another mechanism of enhanced torsion in DM could be altered myocardial perfusion by subclinical coronary artery atherosclerosis or by coronary microvascular disease [25]. It has been reported that the apical rotation angle

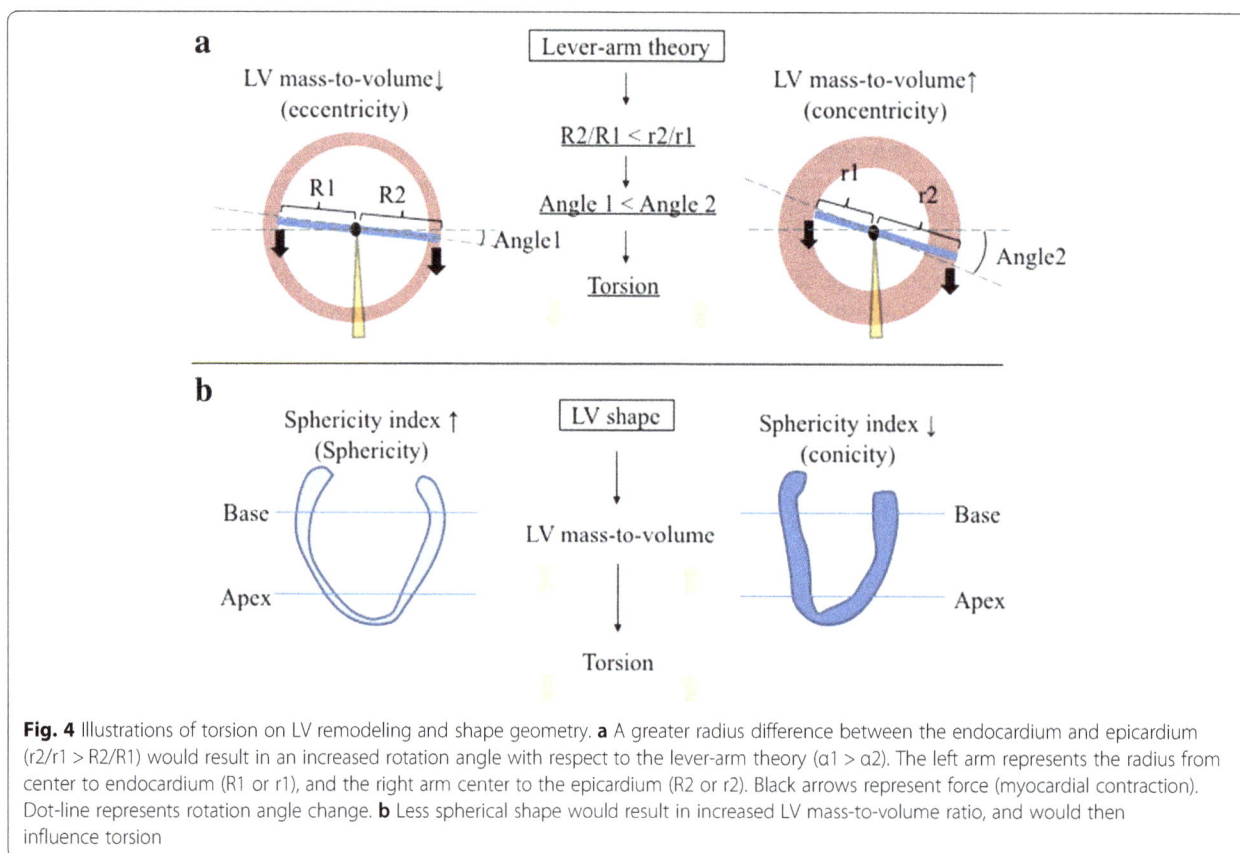

Fig. 4 Illustrations of torsion on LV remodeling and shape geometry. **a** A greater radius difference between the endocardium and epicardium (r2/r1 > R2/R1) would result in an increased rotation angle with respect to the lever-arm theory (α1 > α2). The left arm represents the radius from center to endocardium (R1 or r1), and the right arm center to the epicardium (R2 or r2). Black arrows represent force (myocardial contraction). Dot-line represents rotation angle change. **b** Less spherical shape would result in increased LV mass-to-volume ratio, and would then influence torsion

is internally increased by coronary occlusion in an early phase of myocardial ischemia [26], but the angle might be decreased by long-standing coronary occlusion. Shivu et al. [27] reported that enhanced torsion was associated with lower myocardial perfusion reserve assessed by adenosine stress CMR among type 1 DM patients. Since the structure of the endocardium and epicardium are oriented in different directions, reduced subendocardial function may alter the balance between the opposing rotational forces and thus result in increased torsion [28].

In the present study, torsion was not enhanced in the untreated DM group. It has been noticed in a clinical practice that the direct pathway from DM to dilated cardiac failure (increased LV sphericity and eccentricity change) can occur without a myocardial infarction [29]. Chronic exposure to disturbances of glucose metabolism in DM might negatively affect LV mechanics through myocardial fibrosis and microvascular disease [29, 30]. The spherical and eccentricity change in LV wall could attenuate enhanced torsion.

In our data, longitudinal and circumferential shortening were impaired with insulin resistance despite the relations being confounded by obesity and hypertension. In the Strong Heart Study, DM had lower fractional shortening by echocardiography than normal glucose tolerance [18]. Others have reported alterations in longitudinal and circumferential shortening by cine DENSE and 3D tag analysis in type 2 DM with small sample sizes [31, 32]. Their results agree to the current study, in that circumferential and longitudinal shortening were reduced but torsion increased, with increased mass to volume ratio. High glucose level induces an increased oxidative stress that facilitates cardiomyocyte damage and hypertrophy, and interstitial fibrosis [2]. This is in accordance with our results that reduced longitudinal and circumferential shortening are associated with increased HOMA-IR. In contrast, the data from the Framingham study of fractional shortening by M-mode did not correlate with HOMA-IR [20]. Type-1 DM with normoalbuminuria have longitudinal shortening similar to healthy control subjects [33]. Other studies have found that type-1 DM with mean hemoglobin A1c of 6.8%, had no difference in longitudinal and circumferential shortening, but torsion was increased [34]. The relatively preserved myocardial shortening in DM or insulin resistance may be partly compensated for by increased torsion. Indeed, torsion reflects the circumferential-longitudinal (CL) shear direction of the LV; therefore, the increase in torsion compensates the decrease in longitudinal and circumferential contractility.

LV torsion and myocardial strain are a principle for quantification of LV function which is also feasible with speckle-tracking echocardiography. Global LV torsion may be used to identify subclinical systolic dysfunction in patients with DM in addition to myocardial shortening. Although LV torsion has yet not been included in clinical practice guidelines, it is likely to become a useful application when evaluating patients with heart failure symptoms. Therefore, future studies should investigate if LV torsion may be useful marker of the predicting heart failure.

Our study has several limitations. First, because of the cross-sectional design, we cannot establish causal relations between glucose metabolism disorders and LV indices; however, MESA is the largest CMR tagging study to evaluate these associations so far, allowing unique investigation of cardiac mechanics at the population level. Second, the small number of untreated DM participants affects the power to detect differences in LV indices compared to NFG. This might be a factor explaining why torsion was not increased in the untreated DM group.

Although some investigators have also expressed torsion as the representing the shear deformation angle, wich torsion normalized by twist angle and LV radius [35], we did not assess the torsional shear angle.

Conclusions

Glucose metabolism disorders are associated with LV concentric remodeling, less spherical shape, and reduced systolic myocardial shortening in the general population. Although torsion is higher in participants who are treated for DM and impaired insulin resistance, torsion was increased only with less severe insulin resistance. Increased torsion may be a key compensation mechanism to maintain global systolic function despite impaired myocardial shortening, and be explained by the changes in LV concentric remodeling with less spherical shape due to compromised glucose metabolism.

Abbreviations
BMI: Body mass index; CMR: Cardiovascular magnetic resonance; DM: Diabetes mellitus; ECG: Electrocardiogram; HOMA-IR: Homeostasis model assessment-estimated insulin resistance; IFG: Impaired fasting glucose; LV: Left ventricle/left ventricular; LVEDV: Left ventricluar end-diastolic volume; NFG: Normal fasting glucose; MESA: Multi-Ethnic Study of Atherosclerosis

Acknowledgements
The authors thank the other investigators, staff, and participants of the MESA study for their valuable contributions. A full list of participating MESA investigators and institutions can be found at http://www.mesa-nhlbi.org.

Funding
This research was supported by contracts N01-HC-95159 through N01-HC-95160, N01-HC-95161, N01-HC-95162, N01-HC-95163, N01-HC-95164, N01-HC-95165, N01-HC-95166, N01-HC-95167, N01-HC-95168, and N01-HC-95169 from the National Heart, Lung, and Blood Institute and by grants UL1-TR-000040 and UL1-TR-001079 from NCRR.

Declarations
The views expressed in this manuscript are those of the authors and do not necessarily represent the views of the National Heart, Lung, and Blood Institute; the National Institutes of Health; or the U.S. Department of Health and Human Services.

Authors' contributions
KY, BAV, NM, OG, SK, and JACL all made all made substantial contributions to conception and design of the study. KY, NM, and OG analyzed and interpreted the data. KY, BAV, NM, and OG drafted the manuscript. COW, RLM, DAB, and JACL edited the manuscript. All authors revised the manuscript critically for important intellectual content. All authors read and approved the final manuscript

Competing interests
The authors declare that they have no competing interests.

Author details
[1]Department of Cardiology, Johns Hopkins University, Baltimore, MD, USA. [2]Offices of Biostatistics Research, National Heart, Lung, and Blood Institute, Bethesda, MD, USA. [3]Department of Biostatistics, University of Washington, Seattle, WA, USA. [4]National Institute of Biomedical Imaging and Bioengineering, National Institutes of Health Clinical Center, Bethesda, MD, USA. [5]St. Marianna University School of Medicine, Kawasaki, Japan. [6]Radiology and Epidemiology, Johns Hopkins University, Blalock 524D1, Johns Hopkins Hospital, 600 North Wolfe Street, Baltimore, MD 21287, USA.

References
1. Ren J, Davidoff AJ. Diabetes rapidly induces contractile dysfunctions in isolated ventricular myocytes. Am J Phys. 1997;272:H148–58.
2. Mortuza R, Chakrabarti S. Glucose-induced cell signaling in the pathogenesis of diabetic cardiomyopathy. Heart Fail Rev. 2014;19:75–86.
3. Kannel WB, McGee DL. Diabetes and cardiovascular disease. The Framingham study. JAMA. 1979;241:2035–8.
4. Chahal H, Bluemke DA, Wu CO, et al. Heart failure risk prediction in the multi-ethnic study of atherosclerosis. Heart. 2015;101:58–64.
5. Ingelsson E, Sundstrom J, Arnlov J, et al. Insulin resistance and risk of congestive heart failure. JAMA. 2005;294:334–41.
6. Bluemke DA, Kronmal RA, Lima JA, et al. The relationship of left ventricular mass and geometry to incident cardiovascular events: the MESA (multi-ethnic study of atherosclerosis) study. J Am Coll Cardiol. 2008;52:2148–55.
7. McMurray JJ, Adamopoulos S, Anker SD, et al. ESC Guidelines for the diagnosis and treatment of acute and chronic heart failure 2012: The Task Force for the Diagnosis and Treatment of Acute and Chronic Heart Failure 2012 of the European Society of Cardiology. Developed in collaboration with the Heart Failure Association (HFA) of the ESC. Eur Heart J. 2012;33: 1787–847.
8. Choi EY, Rosen BD, Fernandes VR, et al. Prognostic value of myocardial circumferential strain for incident heart failure and cardiovascular events in asymptomatic individuals: the multi-ethnic study of atherosclerosis. Eur Heart J. 2013;34:2354–61.
9. Yoneyama K, Venkatesh BA, Bluemke DA, et al. Cardiovascular magnetic resonance in an adult human population: serial observations from the multi-ethnic study of atherosclerosis. J Cardiovasc Magn Reson. 2017;19:52.
10. Ambale-Venkatesh B, Yoneyama K, Sharma RK, et al. Left ventricular shape predicts different types of cardiovascular events in the general population. Heart. 2017;103:499–507.
11. Bild DE, Bluemke DA, Burke GL, et al. Multi-ethnic study of atherosclerosis: objectives and design. Am J Epidemiol. 2002;156:871–81.
12. Yoneyama K, Gjesdal O, Choi EY, et al. Age, sex, and hypertension-related remodeling influences left ventricular torsion assessed by tagged cardiac magnetic resonance in asymptomatic individuals: the multi-ethnic study of atherosclerosis. Circulation. 2012;126:2481–90.
13. Natori S, Lai S, Finn JP, et al. Cardiovascular function in multi-ethnic study of atherosclerosis: normal values by age, sex, and ethnicity. AJR Am J Roentgenol. 2006;186:S357–65.

14. Lamas GA, Vaughan DE, Parisi AF, et al. Effects of left ventricular shape and captopril therapy on exercise capacity after anterior wall acute myocardial infarction. Am J Cardiol. 1989;63:1167–73.
15. Gjesdal O, Yoneyama K, Mewton N, et al. Reduced long axis strain is associated with heart failure and cardiovascular events in the multi-ethnic study of atherosclerosis. J Magn Reson Imaging. 2016;44:178–85.
16. Matthews DR, Hosker JP, Rudenski AS, et al. Homeostasis model assessment: insulin resistance and beta-cell function from fasting plasma glucose and insulin concentrations in man. Diabetologia. 1985;28:412–9.
17. Bertoni AG, Wong ND, Shea S, et al. Insulin resistance, metabolic syndrome, and subclinical atherosclerosis: the multi-ethnic study of atherosclerosis (MESA). Diabetes Care. 2007;30:2951–6.
18. Devereux RB, Roman MJ, Paranicas M, et al. Impact of diabetes on cardiac structure and function: the strong heart study. Circulation. 2000;101:2271–6.
19. Turkbey EB, Backlund JY, Genuth S, et al. Myocardial structure, function, and scar in patients with type 1 diabetes mellitus. Circulation. 2011;124:1737–46.
20. Rutter MK, Parise H, Benjamin EJ, et al. Impact of glucose intolerance and insulin resistance on cardiac structure and function: sex-related differences in the Framingham heart study. Circulation. 2003;107:448–54.
21. Ilercil A, Devereux RB, Roman MJ, et al. Relationship of impaired glucose tolerance to left ventricular structure and function: the strong heart study. Am Heart J. 2001;141:992–8.
22. Kishi S, Gidding SS, Reis JP, et al. Association of Insulin Resistance and Glycemic Metabolic Abnormalities with LV structure and function in middle age: The CARDIA Study. JACC Cardiovasc Imaging. 2017;10:105–14.
23. Shah RV, Abbasi SA, Heydari B, et al. Insulin resistance, subclinical left ventricular remodeling, and the obesity paradox: MESA (multi-ethnic study of atherosclerosis). J Am Coll Cardiol. 2013;61:1698–706.
24. Hung J, Papakostas L, Tahta SA, et al. Mechanism of recurrent ischemic mitral regurgitation after annuloplasty: continued LV remodeling as a moving target. Circulation. 2004;110:II85–90.
25. Budoff MJ, Raggi P, Beller GA, et al. Noninvasive cardiovascular risk assessment of the asymptomatic diabetic patient: The Imaging Council of the American College of Cardiology. JACC Cardiovasc Imaging. 2016;9:176–92.
26. Kroeker CA, Tyberg JV, Beyar R. Effects of ischemia on left ventricular apex rotation. An experimental study in anesthetized dogs. Circulation. 1995;92: 3539–48.
27. Shivu GN, Abozguia K, Phan TT, et al. Increased left ventricular torsion in uncomplicated type 1 diabetic patients: the role of coronary microvascular function. Diabetes Care. 2009;32:1710–2.
28. Claus P, Omar AM, Pedrizzetti G, et al. Tissue tracking Technology for Assessing Cardiac Mechanics: principles, normal values, and Clinical Applications. JACC Cardiovasc Imaging. 2015;8:1444–60.
29. Coughlin SS, Pearle DL, Baughman KL, et al. Diabetes mellitus and risk of idiopathic dilated cardiomyopathy. The Washington, DC dilated cardiomyopathy study. Ann Epidemiol. 1994;4:67–74.
30. Ohkubo Y, Kishikawa H, Araki E, et al. Intensive insulin therapy prevents the progression of diabetic microvascular complications in Japanese patients with non-insulin-dependent diabetes mellitus: a randomized prospective 6-year study. Diabetes Res Clin Pract. 1995;28:103–17.
31. Ernande L, Thibault H, Bergerot C, et al. Systolic myocardial dysfunction in patients with type 2 diabetes mellitus: identification at MR imaging with cine displacement encoding with stimulated echoes. Radiology. 2012;265: 402–9.
32. Fonseca CG, Dissanayake AM, Doughty RN, et al. Three-dimensional assessment of left ventricular systolic strain in patients with type 2 diabetes mellitus, diastolic dysfunction, and normal ejection fraction. Am J Cardiol. 2004;94:1391–5.
33. Jensen MT, Sogaard P, Andersen HU, et al. Global longitudinal strain is not impaired in type 1 diabetes patients without albuminuria: the thousand & 1 study. JACC Cardiovasc Imaging. 2015;8:400–10.
34. Chung J, Abraszewski P, Yu X, et al. Paradoxical increase in ventricular torsion and systolic torsion rate in type I diabetic patients under tight glycemic control. J Am Coll Cardiol. 2006;47:384–90.
35. Young AA, Cowan BR. Evaluation of left ventricular torsion by cardiovascular magnetic resonance. J Cardiovasc Magn Reson. 2012;14:49.

13

3D whole-brain vessel wall cardiovascular magnetic resonance imaging: a study on the reliability in the quantification of intracranial vessel dimensions

Na Zhang[1,2,3], Fan Zhang[2], Zixin Deng[2,4], Qi Yang[2], Marcio A. Diniz[5], Shlee S. Song[6], Konrad H. Schlick[6], M. Marcel Maya[7], Nestor Gonzalez[8], Debiao Li[2,4,9], Hairong Zheng[1,3], Xin Liu[1,3*] and Zhaoyang Fan[2,9*]

Abstract

Background: One of the potentially important applications of three-dimensional (3D) intracranial vessel wall (IVW) cardiovascular magnetic resonance (CMR) is to monitor disease progression and regression via quantitative measurement of IVW morphology during medical management or drug development. However, a prerequisite for this application is to validate that IVW morphologic measurements based on the modality are reliable. In this study we performed comprehensive reliability analysis for the recently proposed whole-brain IVW CMR technique.

Methods: Thirty-four healthy subjects and 10 patients with known intracranial atherosclerotic disease underwent repeat whole-brain IVW CMR scans. In 19 of the 34 subjects, two-dimensional (2D) turbo spin-echo (TSE) scan was performed to serve as a reference for the assessment of vessel dimensions. Lumen and wall volume, normalized wall index, mean and maximum wall thickness were measured in both 3D and 2D IVW CMR images. Scan-rescan, intra-observer, and inter-observer reproducibility of 3D IVW CMR in the quantification of IVW or plaque dimensions were respectively assessed in volunteers and patients as well as for different healthy subjectsub-groups (i.e. < 50 and ≥ 50 years). The agreement in vessel wall and lumen measurements between the 3D technique and the 2D TSE method was also investigated. In addition, the sample size required for future longitudinal clinical studies was calculated.

Results: The intra-class correlation coefficient (ICC) and Bland-Altman plots indicated excellent reproducibility and inter-method agreement for all morphologic measurements (All ICCs > 0.75). In addition, all ICCs of patients were equal to or higher than that of healthy subjects except maximum wall thickness. In volunteers, all ICCs of the age group of ≥50 years were equal to or higher than that of the age group of < 50 years. Normalized wall index and mean and maximum wall thickness were significantly larger in the age group of ≥50 years. To detect 5% - 20% difference between placebo and treatment groups, normalized wall index requires the smallest sample size while lumen volume requires the highest sample size.

Conclusions: Whole-brain 3D IVW CMR is a reliable imaging method for the quantification of intracranial vessel dimensions and could potentially be useful for monitoring plaque progression and regression.

Keywords: Intracranial vessel wall morphology, Vessel wall imaging, Whole-brain, Reliability, Magnetic resonance imaging, Intracranial atherosclerotic disease

* Correspondence: xin.liu@siat.ac.cn; fanzhaoyang@gmail.com
[1]Paul C. Lauterbur Research Center for Biomedical Imaging, Shenzhen Institutes of Advanced Technology, Chinese Academy of Sciences, 1068 Xueyuan Ave., Shenzhen University Town, Shenzhen 518055, China
[2]Biomedical Imaging Research Institute, Department of Biomedical Sciences, Cedars-Sinai Medical Center, 8700 Beverly Blvd., PACT 400, Los Angeles, CA 90048, USA
Full list of author information is available at the end of the article

Background

Intracranial atherosclerotic disease (ICAD) is one of the major causes for cerebrovascular events such as stroke and transient ischemic attack [1, 2]. Luminography imaging, routinely used in the diagnostic workup of ICAD, is restricted to the detection of luminal stenosis, which is, however, not a specific marker for confirming and risk-stratifying atherosclerotic plaques [3]. In contrast, high-resolution black-blood cardiovascular magnetic resonance (CMR) can directly visualize the intracranial vessel wall (IVW) and has demonstrated the potential to characterize plaque features that are intimately associated with clinical events [4–8].

Three-dimensional (3D) turbo spin-echo (TSE) with variable refocusing flip angles, as a black-blood CMR technique, has recently gained growing interest among the IVW imaging research community [9–15]. Compared with a conventionally used two-dimensional (2D) TSE method, the 3D approach provides larger spatial coverage, higher spatial resolution and signal-to-noise ratio (SNR), and the flexibility in image visualization, which are all desirable for visualizing small, tortuous, and deep-seated intracranial arteries. Continued technical improvements are being introduced to the technique, primarily in signal suppression of the cerebrospinal fluid (CSF) [16–19] and arterial blood [17], spatial coverage [16, 18], and scan efficiency [20]. Notably, a whole-brain IVW CMR imaging method was recently developed by incorporating non-selective excitation and a trailing magnetization flip-down module with a commercially available 3D TSE sequence - Sampling Perfection with Application-optimized Contrast using different flip angle Evolutions (SPACE) [18]. Remarkable CSF signal attenuation and enhanced image SNR and T1 contrast weighting make the technique well suited for evaluating vessel wall morphology and revealing plaque features with a characteristic hyper-intense appearance such as intra-plaque hemorrhage and post-contrast wall enhancement. With additional optimization at 3 Tesla, a 3D scan with a whole-brain spatial coverage and isotropic 0.5-mm spatial resolution can be completed within 7–8 min [20]. Such improved imaging efficiency further strengthens its applicability for clinical settings.

One of the potentially important applications of 3D IVW CMR is to monitor ICAD progression and regression via quantitative measurement of vessel wall morphology during medical management or drug development. Demonstrated in extracranial vascular beds, several plaque morphologic measures derived by high-resolution black-blood CMR, such as mean wall thickness, plaque burden, and wall remodeling ratio, may serve as imaging surrogates for therapeutic responses [21–24]. A key prerequisite for 3D IVW CMR to become an imaging tool for longitudinal ICAD assessment is the reliability of the technique in vessel wall and lumen dimension quantification. However, there is a paucity of data reported on the aspect [9, 25].

The purpose of this study was to perform comprehensive reliability analysis for 3D IVW CMR, particularly the recently proposed whole-brain IVW CMR imaging technique [20]. Scan-rescan, intra-observer, and inter-observer reproducibility in the quantification of intracranial vessel dimensions were respectively assessed for healthy subjects and patients with ICAD as well as for different sub-groups (i.e. age < 50 and ≥ 50 years). The agreement in vessel wall and lumen measurements between the 3D technique and the conventionally used 2D TSE method was also investigated in a subgroup of the subjects. In addition, the sample size required for future longitudinal clinical studies was calculated. The findings from this study are expected to indicate the performance of the method in general populations and to provide insights into planning future studies on clinical patients.

Methods

Study population

The prospective study was approved by the local institutional review board. Thirty-four healthy subjects (24 males; 14 aged 31–49 years and 20 aged 50–66 years) without known cerebrovascular diseases and 10 patients (7 males; 42–69 years, mean 51.2 years) with known ICAD were recruited. Written informed consent was obtained from all subjects.

Imaging protocol

All CMR examinations were performed on a 3-Tesla whole-body system (MAGNETOM Verio, Siemens Healthineers, Erlangen, Germany) with a 32-channel head coil. Subjects were scanned in a supine position with a foam padding to minimize head movement. Two repeated 3D IVW CMR scans were performed with an off-table break for healthy subjects and 7 to 11-day intervals for patients [18, 20]. When any of the two scans exhibited motion-related image blurring at the discretion of the CMR technologist, reacquisition was attempted only once to simulate real clinical settings. Relevant imaging parameters were as follows: sagittal imaging orientation, repetition time (TR) /echo time (TE) = 900/ 15 ms, receiver bandwidth = 488 Hz/pixel, field of view = 170 × 170 × (110–127) mm^3, matrix size = 320 × 320 × (208–240) with 7.7–6.7% partition oversampling, spatial resolution = 0.53 × 0.53 × 0.53 mm^3 (without zero-filled interpolation), turbo factor = 52, echo train duration = 271 ms, 6/8 partial Fourier in the partition-encoding direction, parallel imaging (GRAPPA) acceleration rate = 2 in the phase-encoding direction, scan time = 7 min 10 s – 8 min 10 s depending on the head size.

In 19 out of the 34 healthy subjects, T1-weighted 2D TSE was also performed during the rescan session to provide an CMR imaging reference for assessing the inter-method agreement. Due to its relatively poor scan efficiency, the acquisition was prescribed only for three arterial segments that often present with ICAD in patients, including the distal basilar artery (BA), distal internal carotid artery (ICA) supraclinoid segment (C4), and proximal middle cerebral artery (MCA) M1 segment. Immediately after the 3D IVW CMR rescan, 3D images were reconstructed into three contiguous 2-mm-thick cross-sections at each of the three segments by an experienced CMR technologist using the multiplanar reconstruction (MPR) functionality available on the imaging console. A 2D TSE image was then acquired for each of these cross-sections with following imaging parameters: TR/TE = 800/12 ms, receiver bandwidth = 411 Hz/pixel, field of view = 170×170 mm^3, matrix size = 320×320, spatial resolution = 0.53×0.53 mm^2, slice thickness = 2 mm, turbo factor = 9, signal averages = 4, scan time per slice = 1 min 37 s.

Image analysis

All images were transferred to a workstation (Syngo MultiModality Workplace, Siemens Healthineers). The scan and rescan 3D IVW CMR image sets were first co-registered using an image fusion functionality to account for head repositioning. At the same locations on both image sets, 5 following vessel segments were analyzed for each healthy subject: the distal BA, the distal vertebral artery (VA; V4), the distal ICA C4, the proximal MCA M1, and the proximal anterior cerebral artery (ACA) A1. Three contiguous cross-sections of 2-mm thickness were generated via MPR for each segment. For each patient, 3 contiguous cross-sections of 2-mm thickness centered at the thickest location of the most stenotic plaque were also generated via MPR.

All these reconstructed cross-sectional images and corresponding 2D TSE images underwent vessel wall and lumen dimension quantification using commercial software (VesselMass, Leiden University Medical Center, Leiden, the Netherlands). Each image was magnified 4–6 times with bilinear interpolation. Lumen and outer wall boundaries were traced manually along the interfaces between the lumen and wall and between the wall and surrounding tissue respectively, generating two contours (Fig. 1). When part of a boundary was invisible, the contour was completed to maintain the continuity of the vessel's curvature [9]. The entire vessel wall region encased by the two contours were automatically divided into ten evenly spaced segments. The software generated the following measurements: the average and maximum wall thickness (i.e. the mean and maximum value of the ten distances between contours), the lumen area (i.e. the area inside the luminal contour), and the wall area (i.e. subtracting the inner contour area from the outer contour area). Additionally, normalized wall index was calculated as the ratio of the wall area to the outer contour

area. Contouring and determination of the above wall and lumen dimensions for any 3 consecutive slices required a processing time of approximately 2.5 min per scan. For each vessel segment or plaque, the measured normalized wall index and mean/maximum wall thickness were, respectively, averaged over the three slices; lumen volume and wall volume were obtained by summing the area measurements of the three slices and multiplying by 2 mm.

Two readers (with 6-year and more than 10-year experience in vascular CMR imaging, respectively) independently performed above vessel wall and lumen measurements on the images from the first 3D IVW CMR scan. After two weeks, one of the readers performed a second-round measurement on the same data, and the other performed measurement on the images from the second scan followed by measurement another 2 weeks later for the 2D TSE scan when available.

Statistical analysis

All statistical analyses were performed using SPSS (version 19.0, International Business Machines, Armonk, New York, USA) and R (version 3.4.1). Intra-class correlation coefficient (ICC) was obtained from a two-way random model with two raters for inter-rater reproducibility and a two-way mixed model with two raters for intra-rater and scan-rescan reproducibility. Confidence intervals for the overall ICC were calculated by bootstrap taking in account the correlation between segments in the same patient. An ICC value of less than 0.4 was considered poor agreement, a value of 0.4–0.75 was considered good agreement, and a value of 0.75 or greater was considered excellent agreement [26]. Bland-Altman analysis was also used to determine the scan-rescan, intra-, and inter-observer reproducibility of 3D IVW CMR as well as inter-method agreement between 3D IVW CMR and 2D TSE in quantifying vessel dimensions for volunteers.

In addition, the healthy cohort was further categorized by age into two groups, i.e. < 50 years and ≥50 years. All above reproducibility were determined for each group. Morphologic measurements averaged over the two readers were used to determine the differences between the two groups based on independent t-test. A two-tailed P value of 0.05 or less was considered to indicate a significant difference.

Based on the scan-rescan data analysis, the sample size required for each of dimension measurements to compare placebo and treatment group in a clinical trial with 80% of power at 5% significance level was calculated using a t-test with equal variances. It was assumed that the mean of the placebo group would be equal to the mean from the healthy subjects in our study and that the mean of the treatment group would be 5, 10, 15, and

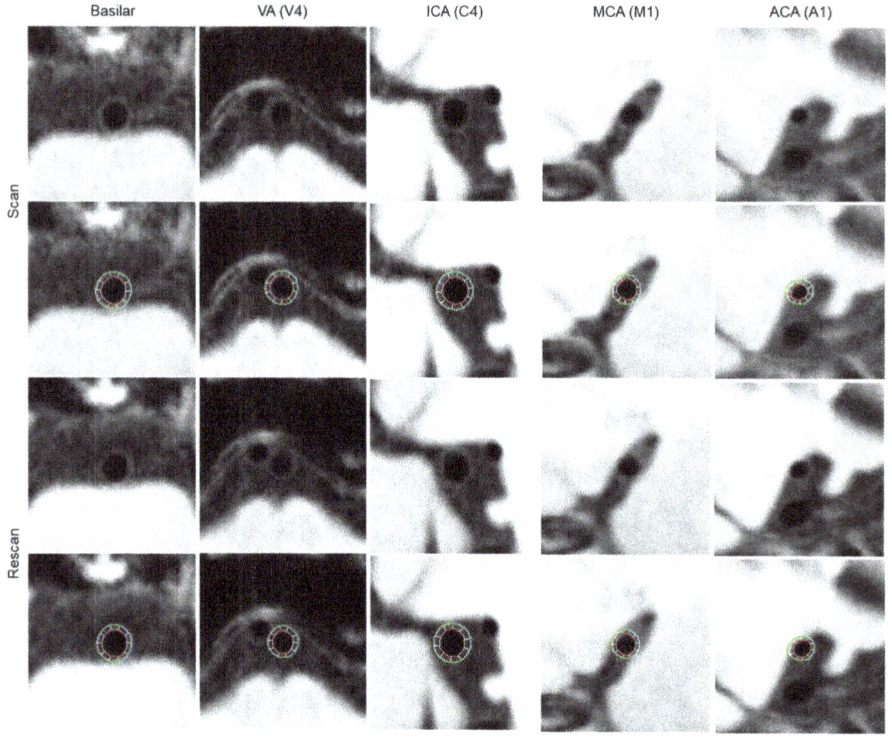

Fig. 1 Representative images of scan and rescan analysis of lumen and outer wall boundaries for the five designated arterial segments: the distal basilar artery, the distal vertebral artery (VA (V4)), the distal internal carotid artery (ICA) supraclinoid segment (C4), the middle cerebral artery (MCA) M1 segment, and anterior cerebral artery (ACA) A1 segments, from a 55-year-old male healthy subject

20% different. The standard deviations for placebo and treatment groups were assumed to be equal and given by the subject variance estimated from a linear mixed model with subject as fixed effect and scan as random effect.

Results

Motion-related vessel wall blurring was observed by the CMR technologist in either of the two 3D IVW CMR scans in 6 healthy subjects and 2 patients. Reacquisitions in these subjects were performed and yielded acceptable image quality in all but 2 healthy subjects (51 and 49 years) and 1 patient (61 years) who were excluded from image analysis. Hence, a total of 160 paired arterial segments from 32 healthy subjects (13: age < 50 years and 19: age ≥ 50 years) and 9 plaques (5 on MCA, 2 on BA, and 2 on VA) were available for reproducibility analysis; a total of 54 paired arterial segments from 18 healthy subjects were available for inter-method agreement analysis.

Measurement reproducibility

3D IVW CMR provided visually consistent delineation of the vessel wall (Fig. 2) and plaques (Fig. 3) in both scans. In some plaques, high signal-intensity features were observed (Fig. 3 case A). For healthy subjects, morphologic measurements and corresponding ICC values,

when combining all assessed segments, are summarized in Table 1 (Segment-based results are summarized in Additional file 1: Table S1). Each of the assessed morphologic indices had all ICCs greater than 0.75, indicating excellent reproducibility. More specifically, for the intra-observer reproducibility, all ICCs were equal to or greater than 0.93. For the scan-rescan and inter-observer reproducibility, all ICCs except for that for the inter-observer reproducibility on normalized wall index were equal to or greater than 0.83. For patients, vessel wall and lumen measurements at the most stenotic plaque and corresponding ICC values are summarized in Table 2. All ICCs except for that for the inter-observer reproducibility on maximum wall thickness (ICC = 0.87) were equal to or greater than 0.91, indicating excellent reproducibility.

The Bland-Altman plots for all arterial segments of healthy subjects are shown in Fig. 4 for lumen volume, normalized wall index, and mean wall thickness, respectively. Random error scattering patterns and independence of the difference on the mean value were observed.

All ICCs of the healthy subgroup age ≥ 50 years were equal to or higher than that of the < 50 years subgroups, but in most cases, were lower than that of patients (Fig. 5). As shown in Table 3, there were no significant difference in lumen or wall volume between

3D whole-brain vessel wall cardiovascular magnetic resonance imaging: a study on the reliability...

133

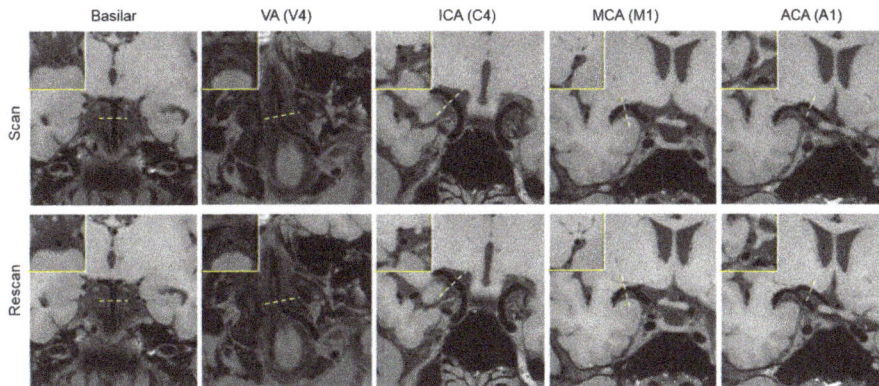

Fig. 2 Representative 3D intracranial vessel wall MR images acquired in two scans from a 55-year-old male healthy subjects and reformatted cross-sections (upper left in the yellow box) for each designated arterial segment in the location indicated by the dashed lines. Both scans provide exquisite vessel wall depiction for the five designated arterial segments: the distal basilar artery, distal vertebral artery (VA (V4)), the distal internal carotid artery (ICA) supraclinoid segment (C4), the middle cerebral artery (MCA) M1 segment right after the trifurcation, and the anterior cerebral artery (ACA) A1 segments

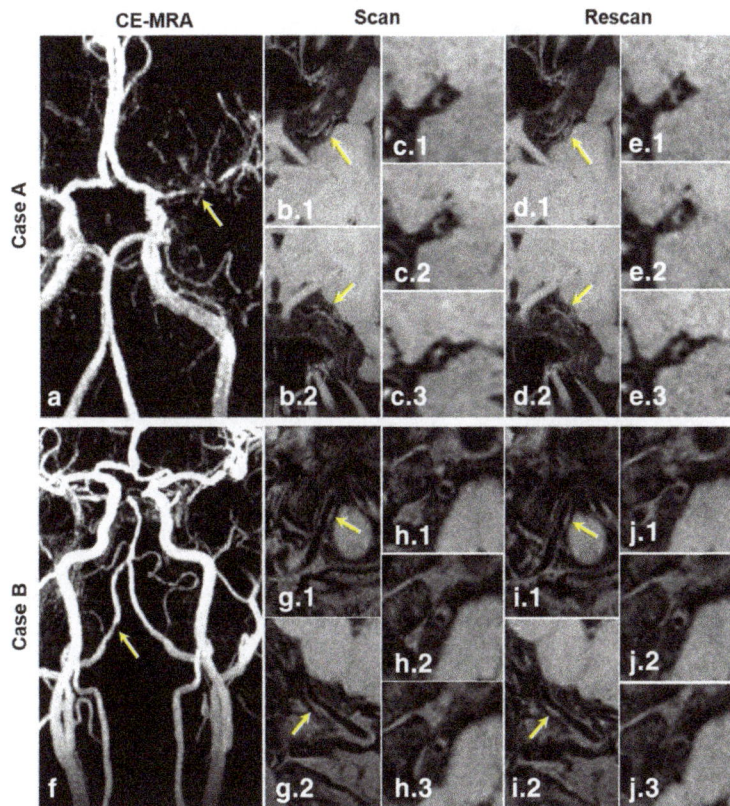

Fig. 3 Two representative clinical cases imaged with 3D intracranial vessel wall (IVW) CMR. Contrast-enhanced MRA demonstrates a severe stenosis at the left middle cerebral artery (MCA) M1 segment (arrow in **a**) in a 42-year-old male patient and a moderate stenosis at the right vertebral artery (VA) (arrow in **f**) in a 48-year-old female patient. Reconstructed long-axis images from 3D whole-brain IVW scan and rescan reveal wall thickening at both stenoses (arrows in **b** and **d**, **g** and **i**). Reconstructed short-axis (cross-section) images for the MCA plaque (**c** and **e**) and VA plaque (**h** and **j**) demonstrate the eccentric wall thickening. Note that the delineation quality of these plaques from scan and rescan are visually comparable

Table 1 Vessel wall and lumen measurements averaged over all assessed segments and corresponding ICC values of inter-scan, intra-observer, and inter-observer reproducibilities of 3D intracranial vessel wall MR in healthy subjects

		inter-scan (n = 160)		Intra-observer (n = 160)		Inter-observer (n = 160)	
	1st scan, 1st observer, 1st measurement (mean ± SD)	2nd scan, 1st observer (mean ± SD)	ICC (95% CI)	1st scan, 1st observer, 2nd measurement (mean ± SD)	ICC (95% CI)	1st scan, 2nd observer (mean ± SD)	ICC (95% CI)
Lumen volume (mm³)	42.0 ± 16.4	42.9 ± 16.8	0.99 (0.98–0.99)	43.3 ± 16.6	0.99 (0.98–0.99)	40.4 ± 17.4	0.98 (0.97–0.99)
Wall volume (mm³)	49.7 ± 15.8	49.5 ± 16.6	0.98 (0.98–0.99)	50.1 ± 15.4	0.99 (0.98–0.99)	45.7 ± 17.2	0.93 (0.80–0.96)
Normalized wall index	0.55 ± 0.04	0.54 ± 0.05	0.87 (0.80–0.91)	0.54 ± 0.04	0.93 (0.89–0.95)	0.53 ± 0.06	0.76 (0.63–0.83)
Mean wall thickness (mm)	0.71 ± 0.11	0.70 ± 0.13	0.95 (0.93–0.96)	0.71 ± 0.11	0.96 (0.95–0.97)	0.67 ± 0.14	0.83 (0.67–0.89)
Maximum wall thickness (mm)	0.86 ± 0.12	0.85 ± 0.15	0.93 (0.90–0.95)	0.86 ± 0.13	0.95 (0.93–0.96)	0.85 ± 0.18	0.84 (0.78–0.88)

SD standard deviation, *ICC* intra-class correlation coefficient, *CI* confidence intervals

the two age groups. However, normalized wall index and mean and maximum wall thickness were significantly larger in the age group of ≥50 years ($P ≤ 0.05$).

Inter-method agreement

Figure 6 shows representative 3D IVW images and reformatted vessel wall cross-sections as well as slice thickness- and location-matched 2D TSE images for three arterial segments. The two acquisition methods provided visually comparable vessel wall delineation. When all three segments were evaluated together, all paired morphologic measurements exhibited an excellent agreement as indicated by an ICC with 95% CI of 0.98 (0.95–0.99), 0.96 (0.84–0.98), 0.96 (0.92–0.97), 0.92 (0.82–0.96), and 0.88 (0.32–0.96) for lumen volume, wall volume, normalized wall index, mean wall thickness, and maximum wall thickness, respectively. Segment-based morphologic measurements and corresponding ICC values for 3D and 2D IVW CMR are summarized in Additional file 1: Table S2. The differences between 3D and 2D IVW

CMR and the mean values with limits of agreement for all segments are illustrated in Bland-Altman plots (Fig. 7). The mean differences between 3D and 2D IVW CMR were 2.4 mm³ for lumen volume, 3.0 mm³ for vessel wall volume, 0.002 for normalized wall index, 0.02 mm for mean wall thickness, and 0.04 mm for maximum wall thickness. Bland-Altman analysis demonstrated good agreement with small bias between the two techniques.

Sample size

Table 4 shows sample size required to compare placebo and treatment group for all measures means considering MCA segment with 80% of power at 5% significance level using a t-test for two independent samples with equal variance. The sample sizes required for the measures in other segments are also presented in Additional file 1: Table S3. Normalized wall index requires the smallest sample size while lumen volume requires the highest sample size to compare two groups. The large-sized segments (ICA, VA,

Table 2 Vessel wall and lumen measurements at the most stenotic plaques and corresponding ICC values of inter-scan, intra-observer, and inter-observer reproducibilities of 3D intracranial vessel wall MR in patients

		Inter-scan (n = 9)		Intra-observer (n = 9)		Inter-observer (n = 9)	
	1st scan, 1st observer, 1st measurement (mean ± SD)	2nd scan, 1st observer (mean ± SD)	ICC (95% CI)	1st scan, 1st observer, 2nd measurement (mean ± SD)	ICC (95% CI)	1st scan, 2nd observer (mean ± SD)	ICC (95% CI)
Lumen volume (mm³)	25.1 ± 18.2	26.57 ± 21.33	0.99 (0.94–0.99)	25.7 ± 17.6	0.99 (0.99–0.99)	23.7 ± 18.0	0.99 (0.96–0.99)
Wall volume (mm³)	54.2 ± 32.6	55.36 ± 31.82	0.99 (0.97–0.99)	54.5 ± 29.4	0.99 (0.96–0.99)	50.2± 26.3	0.98 (0.90–0.99)
Normalized wall index	0.69 ± 0.08	0.69 ± 0.10	0.93 (0.66–0.98)	0.69 ± 0.09	0.98 (0.89–0.99)	0.69 ± 0.10	0.92 (0.65–0.98)
Mean wall thickness (mm)	0.90 ± 0.29	0.92 ± 0.28	0.97 (0.89–0.99)	0.91 ± 0.25	0.97 (0.89–0.99)	0.88 ± 0.25	0.97 (0.86–0.99)
Maximum wall thickness (mm)	1.35 ± 0.37	1.39 ± 0.31	0.91 (0.59–0.98)	1.44 ± 0.37	0.94 (0.76–0.99)	1.25 ± 0.29	0.87 (0.49–0.97)

SD standard deviation, *ICC* intra-class correlation coefficient, *CI* confidence intervals

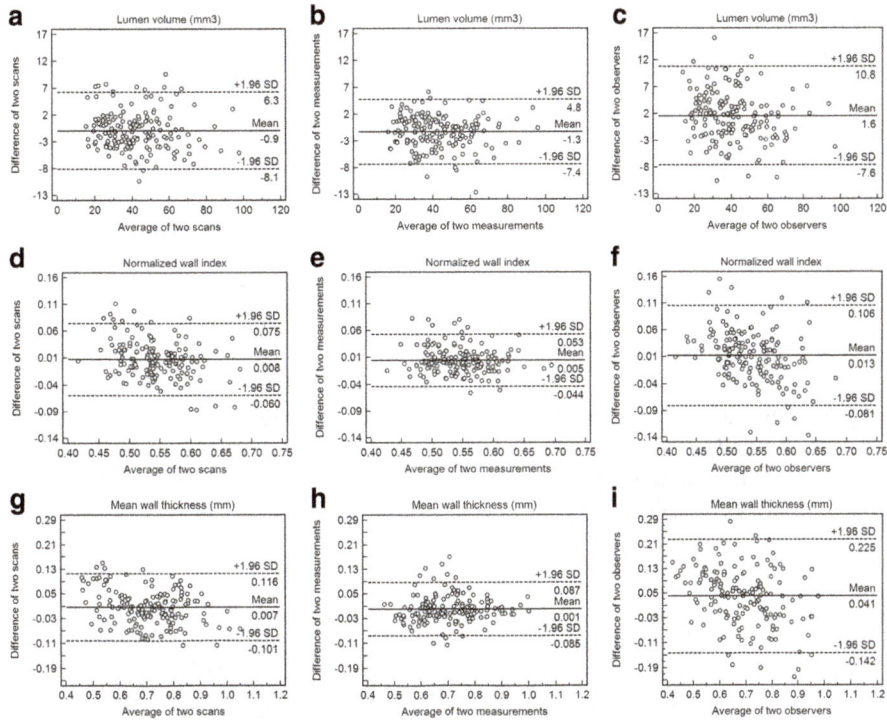

Fig. 4 Bland-Altman plots for lumen volume (**a** inter-scan, **b** intra-observer, **c** inter-observer), normalized wall index (**d** inter-scan, **e** intra-observer, **f** inter-observer), and mean wall thickness (**g** inter-scan, **h** intra-observer, **i** inter-observer). The solid lines represent the mean difference, and the dashed lines indicate the 95% limits of agreement. SD = standard deviation

and BA) requires the smaller sample size than small-sized segments (MCA and ACA).

Discussion

A non-invasive imaging method for reliably quantifying longitudinal morphologic changes in ICAD is potentially useful in medical management or drug development. High-resolution black-blood 2D CMR, traditionally used for ICAD imaging, has been shown to be a morphology-probing tool with good intra- and inter-observer agreement [27] as well as low scan-rescan variability [28]. With aforementioned technical advantages that are more relevant to vessel wall morphologic assessments, 3D IVW CMR has increasingly been advocated as a non-invasive imaging modality for ICAD research [9–15]. However, its applicability in longitudinal imaging evaluations has yet to

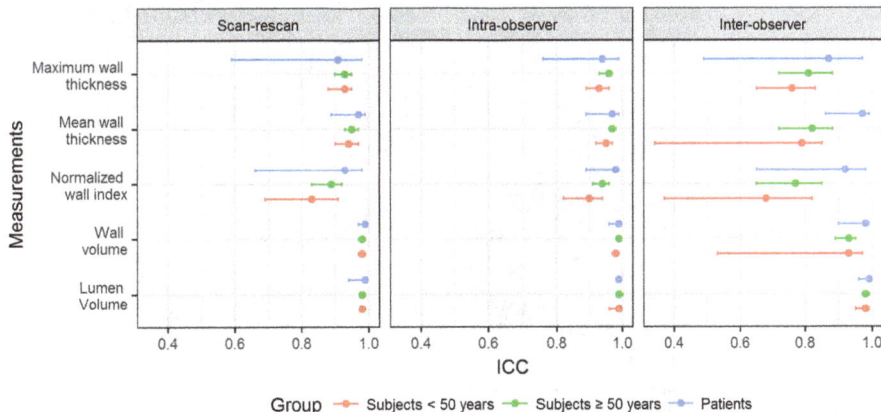

Fig. 5 The comparison of ICCs (95% CI) for all vessel wall and lumen measurements among patients and different age groups of healthy subjects. ICC = intra-class correlation coefficient; CI = confidence interval

Table 3 The comparison for the vessel wall and lumen measurements averaged over two observers between different age subgroups. Data are presented as means ± standard deviations

Age group	Lumen volume (mm³)	Wall volume (mm³)	Normalized wall index[a]	Mean wall thickness (mm)[a]	Maximum wall thickness (mm)[a]
≥50 years	41.2 ± 16.7	50.5 ± 16.0	0.55 ± 0.06	0.69 ± 0.14	0.88 ± 0.18
< 50 years	47.7 ± 16.1	48.9 ± 15.5	0.51 ± 0.04	0.63 ± 0.14	0.80 ± 0.17
P value	0.23	0.61	< 0.001	0.05	0.03

[a]denotes statistical significance

be established. Thus, the present study sought to conduct a comprehensive investigation on its reliability in the quantification of intracranial vessel dimensions.

Scan-rescan reproducibility is a paramount requirement for an imaging modality to be used for serial examinations. Our results showed excellent scan-rescan reproducibility in measuring the dimensions of major intracranial arterial segments for healthy subjects and plaques for patients with all ICCs ≥0.87 and 0.91, respectively. A previous study on using 2D IVW CMR for evaluating MCA lumen and plaque area/volume showed better ICCs (0.97 or higher) [28]. This is likely because the 3D technique is more susceptible to any errors caused by, for example, image registration, reformation, and vessel wall contouring, particularly in healthy subjects where the vessel wall is thinner. A more recent

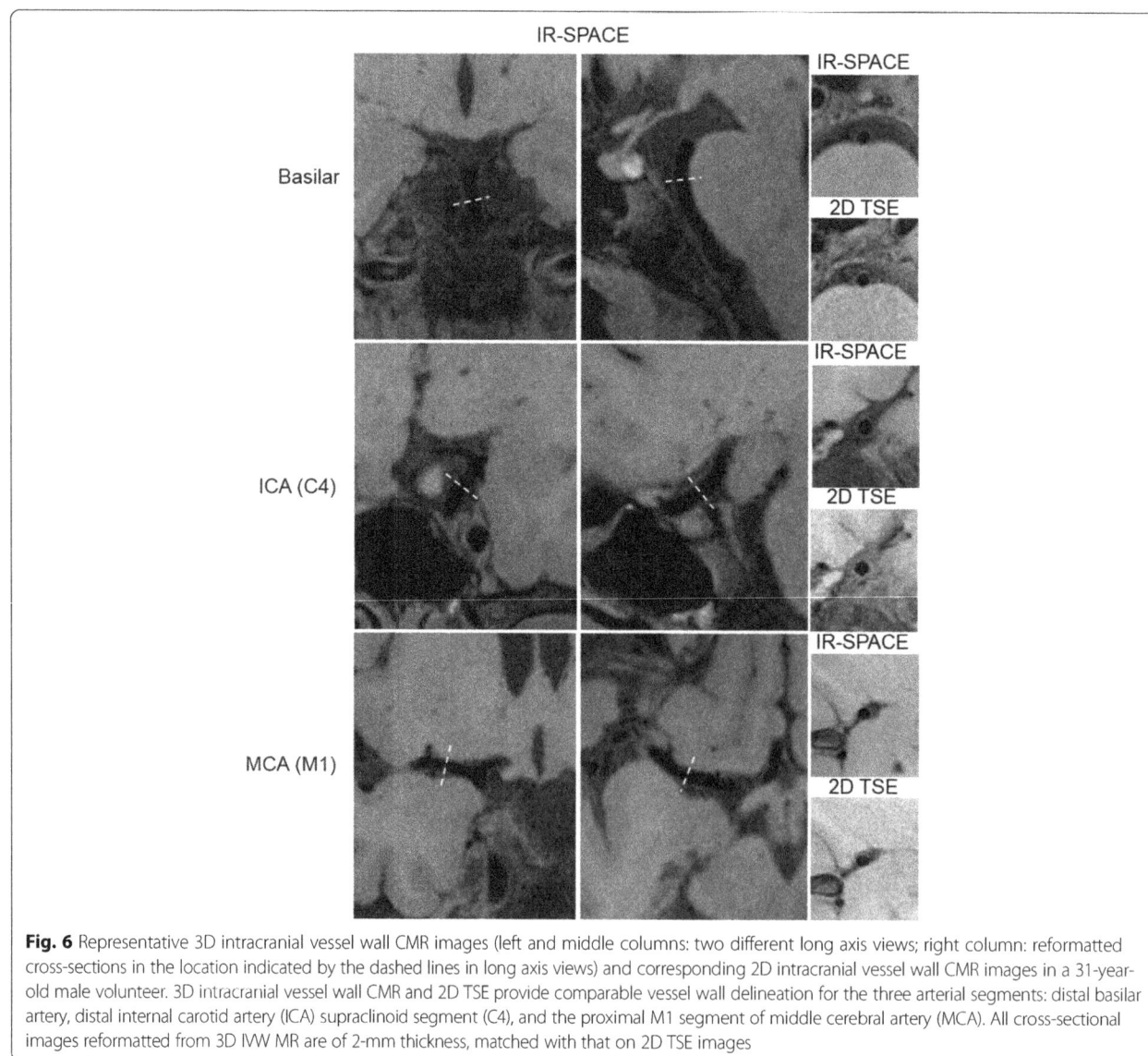

Fig. 6 Representative 3D intracranial vessel wall CMR images (left and middle columns: two different long axis views; right column: reformatted cross-sections in the location indicated by the dashed lines in long axis views) and corresponding 2D intracranial vessel wall CMR images in a 31-year-old male volunteer. 3D intracranial vessel wall CMR and 2D TSE provide comparable vessel wall delineation for the three arterial segments: distal basilar artery, distal internal carotid artery (ICA) supraclinoid segment (C4), and the proximal M1 segment of middle cerebral artery (MCA). All cross-sectional images reformatted from 3D IVW MR are of 2-mm thickness, matched with that on 2D TSE images

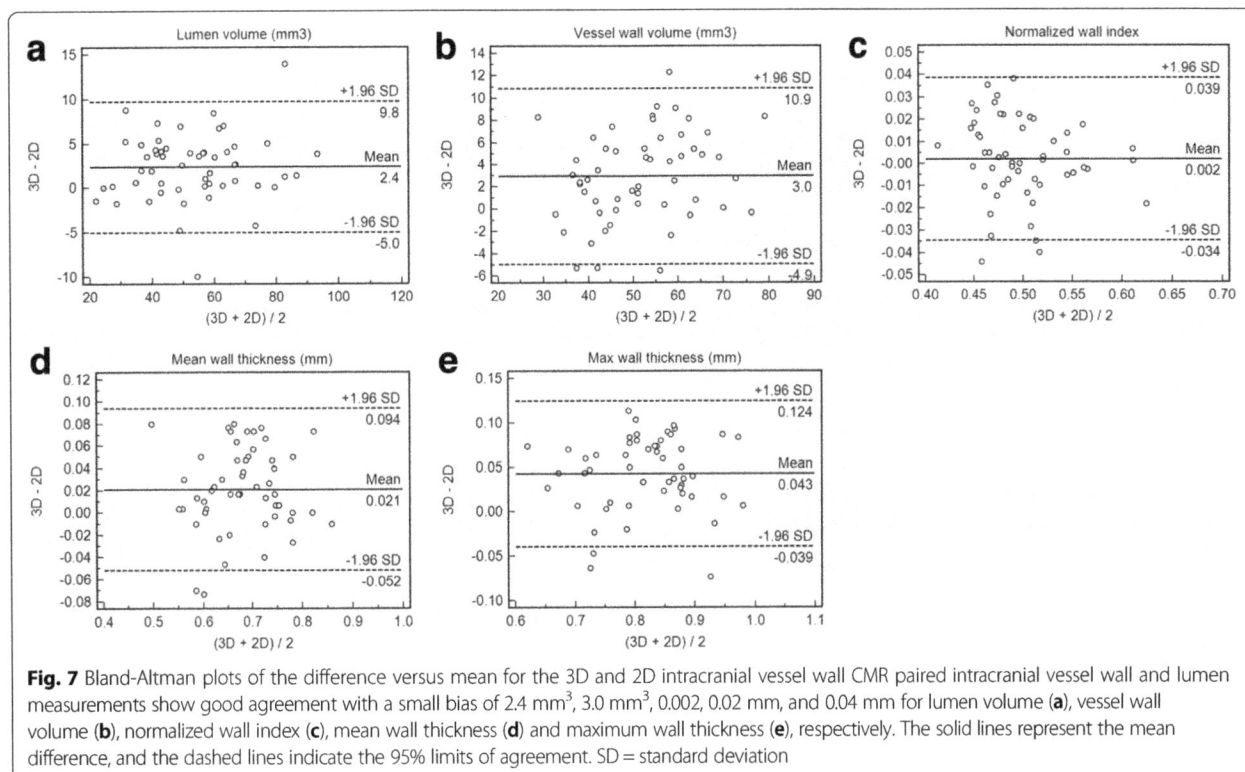

Fig. 7 Bland-Altman plots of the difference versus mean for the 3D and 2D intracranial vessel wall CMR paired intracranial vessel wall and lumen measurements show good agreement with a small bias of 2.4 mm³, 3.0 mm³, 0.002, 0.02 mm, and 0.04 mm for lumen volume (**a**), vessel wall volume (**b**), normalized wall index (**c**), mean wall thickness (**d**) and maximum wall thickness (**e**), respectively. The solid lines represent the mean difference, and the dashed lines indicate the 95% limits of agreement. SD = standard deviation

population-based study has reported considerably lower reproducibility in wall volume, normalized wall index, and mean wall thickness for a 3D IVW CMR sequence [25]. One of major possible reasons for the better performance of the whole-brain IVW CMR sequence in our study is that two repeat scans were in the same imaging session in healthy volunteers or days apart in patients.. Clearly this same-session investigation strategy for healthy subjects only reveals the scan-rescan repeatability instead of the true longitudinal repeatability of a technique, but has commonly been used in many previous studies [26, 28, 29]. Nevertheless, our findings suggest the possibility for reliable serial examination of IVW using the 3D whole-brain IVW CMR technique as previous carotid studies did [26, 29, 30].

Table 4 Sample Sizes per Group for differences of 5%, 10%, 15%, and 20% from placebo group mean estimated in the middle cerebral artery segment based on the inter-scan analysis

	Placebo group (mean ± SD)	Sample size			
		5%	10%	15%	20%
Lumen volume (mm³)	38.9 ± 8.9	329	83	38	22
Wall volume (mm³)	41.1 ± 7.6	215	55	25	15
Normalized wall index	0.52 ± 0.05	60	16	8	5
Mean wall thickness (mm)	0.63 ± 0.08	103	27	13	8
Maximum wall thickness (mm)	0.77 ± 0.1	107	28	13	8

SD standard deviation

Our study also revealed excellent intra- and inter-observer reproducibility in quantifying intracranial vessel dimensions. In general, all ICCs were better than those reported by the recent population-based study whereby a slab-selective 3D IVW CMR sequence was used [25]. Our evaluations were focused on a recently developed whole-brain vessel wall CMR imaging method because of its several technical advantages over other existing slab-selective 3D IVW imaging techniques [18]. A noteworthy feature is its more superior delineation of the outer vessel wall boundary due to an improved signal suppression in surrounding CSF [18]. Additionally, relatively short echo time due to the use of a non-selective excitation radio-frequency pulse may contribute to better overall image SNR. Hence, quantification of vessel area, wall area, and wall thickness would potentially be more accurate.

As part of reliability analysis, the present study investigated the inter-method agreement between 3D IVW CMR and conventionally used 2D TSE. The lumen and vessel wall volume and normalized wall index measured from 3D IVW CMR showed excellent accordance with those measured from conventional 2D TSE (ICC > 0.96) despite potential registration errors. This corroborates the findings reported in the previous study [9]. The ICCs of mean and maximum wall thickness, particularly the latter, were slightly lower, which could be explained by the fact that these measurements are more prone to outliers [26]. Nevertheless, they generally showed excellent agreement between the two techniques. While the accuracy of the 3D technique is questionable due to the lack of histology validation, our finding suggests that this technique is at least comparable to the 2D technique and can be utilized as a more time-efficient ICAD imaging method. Given the much higher and isotropic spatial resolution and flexibility in image reformation with 3D imaging, the geometry of small lesions from the tortuous intracranial arteries would, in theory, be quantified more accurately.

In general, relatively large-sized segments exhibited higher reproducibility and smaller sample size required than small-sized segments, and the age group of ≥50 years demonstrated equal or higher reproducibility than the younger group. Additionally, the patient group demonstrated an even better reproducibility than the age group of ≥50. This is perhaps explained by the thicker vessel wall in large-sized segments and in older subjects or patients that is favorable for morphologic quantification. Our results did show that normalized wall index and mean and maximum wall thickness were significantly larger in the age group of ≥50 years versus the younger group and in the patient group versus the healthy group. The limit in spatial resolution and associated errors in image registration and contouring are thought of as major factors influencing the measurement consistency. It is noteworthy that in clinical patients who have ICAD lesions or dramatically thickened vessel wall, such an effect might be alleviated. Additionally, 0. 5 mm spatial resolution provided by the whole-brain IVW CMR technique is currently the best choice given the trade-off between imaging time and diagnostic quality as recommended [31].

With such high reproducibility of vessel dimension measurements, whole-brain IVW CMR imaging can potentially be translated into research and clinical applications for monitoring disease progression and therapeutic response. More importantly, higher inter-scan reproducibility promises fewer participants for therapeutic trial enrollment and reduced cost. Sample sizes for MCA segment presented are higher than Zhang et al. [28] because they based their calculations on the standard deviation between scans while we used standard deviations resulting from the total variance decreased by the variance between scans as Mihai et al. [32].

There are limitations with this work. First, we focused reliability analyses on healthy subjects and only 9 patients were included. Despite relatively large vessel wall dimension in ICAD patients which favors morphologic measurement, reproducibility could be compromised by, for example, reduced image quality due to motion. Reproducibility studies based on healthy subjects have commonly been investigated in the field of vessel wall

CMR imaging [9, 26, 29, 33]. The results from this type of study may provide indication of the technical performance in general populations as well as insights into planning future studies on clinical patients. Second, the 3D technique is still susceptible to motion artifacts which occurred in 6 out of 34 healthy subjects and in 1 out of 10 patients. Four of the 6 healthy subjects were still eligible for analysis as reacquisition was of acceptable image quality. Hence, our conclusion holds valid when only considering cases with acceptable diagnostic quality. Further improvement in motion resistance is clearly necessary to foster the technique's clinical reliability. Third, the scan and rescan were performed on the same CMR scanner with the same CMR technologist. Thus, we could not estimate any variation caused by imaging scanners or between MR technologists.

Conclusion
In conclusion, whole-brain 3D IVW CMR is a reliable CMR imaging method for the quantification of intracranial vessel dimensions and could potentially be useful for monitoring plaque progression and regression.

Abbreviations
2D: Two-dimensional; 3D: Three-dimensional; A1: Proximal ACA; ACA: Anterior cerebral artery; BA: Basilar artery; C4: Distal ICA supraclinoid segment; CMR: Cardiovascular magnetic resonance; CSF: Cerebrospinal fluid; ICA: Internal carotid artery; ICAD: Intracranial atherosclerotic disease; ICC: Intra-class correlation coefficient; IR: Inversion-recovery; IVW: Intracranial vessel wall; M1: Proximal middle cerebral artery; MCA: Middle cerebral artery; MPR: Multiplanar reconstruction; SNR: Signal-to-noise ratio; SPACE: Sampling Perfection with Application-optimized Contrast using different flip angle Evolutions; TE: Echo time; TR: Repetition time; TSE: Turbo spin-echo; V4: Distal vertebral artery; VA: vertebral artery

Acknowledgements
The authors thank Laura G. Smith and Gill Edward for their help in conducting the imaging experiments.

Funding
This work was supported in part by American Heart Association (15SDG25710441), National Institutes of Health (NHLBI 2R01HL096119), National Natural Science Foundation of China (81301216 and 81327801), National Key R&D Program of China (2016YFC0100100), Key Laboratory for Magnetic Resonance and Multimodality Imaging of Guangdong Province (2014B030301013), Shenzhen Science and Technology Program (JCYJ20170413161350892).

Authors' contributions
NZ performed data acquisition, analysis, and interpretation and drafted the manuscript. FZ, ZD, and QY made substantial contribution to data acquisition and analysis. MD was in charge of statistical analysis and interpretation of data. SS, KS, MM, and NG have made a substantial contribution to the study design and data interpretation and helped revise the manuscript critically for important intellectual content. DL and HZ have made substantial contributions to conception and design of the study. ZF and XL conceived of the study design and provided supervision of the whole project and critical review of the manuscript. All authors read and approved the final manuscript.

Competing interests

The authors declare that they have no competing interests.

Author details

[1]Paul C. Lauterbur Research Center for Biomedical Imaging, Shenzhen Institutes of Advanced Technology, Chinese Academy of Sciences, 1068 Xueyuan Ave., Shenzhen University Town, Shenzhen 518055, China. [2]Biomedical Imaging Research Institute, Department of Biomedical Sciences, Cedars-Sinai Medical Center, 8700 Beverly Blvd., PACT 400, Los Angeles, CA 90048, USA. [3]Shenzhen College of Advanced Technology, University of Chinese Academy of Sciences, Shenzhen, China. [4]Department of Bioengineering, University of California, Los Angeles, CA, USA. [5]Biostatistics and Bioinformatics Research Center, Cedars-Sinai Medical Center, Los Angeles, CA, USA. [6]Department of Neurology, Cedars-Sinai Medical Center, Los Angeles, CA, USA. [7]Department of Radiology, Cedars-Sinai Medical Center, Los Angeles, CA, USA. [8]Department of Neurosurgery, Cedars-Sinai Medical Center, Los Angeles, CA, USA. [9]Department of Medicine, University of California, Los Angeles, CA, USA.

References

1. Go AS, Mozaffarian D, Roger VL, Benjamin EJ, Berry JD, Blaha MJ, Dai S, Ford ES, Fox CS, Franco S, et al. Heart disease and stroke statistics–2014 update: a report from the American Heart Association. Circulation. 2014;129(3):e28-e292.
2. Wong LK. Global burden of intracranial atherosclerosis. Int J Stroke. 2006; 1(3):158–9.
3. Alexander MD, Yuan C, Rutman A, Tirschwell DL, Palagallo G, Gandhi D, Sekhar LN, Mossa-Basha M. High-resolution intracranial vessel wall imaging: imaging beyond the lumen. J Neurol Neurosurg Psychiatry. 2016;87(6):589–97.
4. Chung GH, Kwak HS, Hwang SB, Jin GY. High resolution MR imaging in patients with symptomatic middle cerebral artery stenosis. Eur J Radiol. 2012;81(12):4069–74.
5. Niizuma K, Shimizu H, Takada S, Tominaga T. Middle cerebral artery plaque imaging using 3-tesla high-resolution MRI. J Clin Neurosci. 2008;15(10): 1137–41.
6. Xu WH, Li ML, Gao S, Ni J, Zhou LX, Yao M, Peng B, Feng F, Jin ZY, Cui LY. In vivo high-resolution MR imaging of symptomatic and asymptomatic middle cerebral artery atherosclerotic stenosis. Atherosclerosis. 2010;212(2):507–11.
7. Skarpathiotakis M, Mandell DM, Swartz RH, Tomlinson G, Mikulis DJ. Intracranial atherosclerotic plaque enhancement in patients with ischemic stroke. AJNR Am J Neuroradiol. 2013;34(2):299–304.
8. Klein IF, Lavallee PC, Mazighi M, Schouman-Claeys E, Labreuche J, Amarenco P. Basilar artery atherosclerotic plaques in paramedian and lacunar pontine infarctions: a high-resolution MRI study. Stroke. 2010;41(7):1405–9.
9. Qiao Y, Steinman DA, Qin Q, Etesami M, Schar M, Astor BC, Wasserman BA. Intracranial arterial wall imaging using three-dimensional high isotropic resolution black blood MRI at 3.0 tesla. J Magn Reson Imaging. 2011;34(1): 22–30.
10. Qiao Y, Zeiler SR, Mirbagheri S, Leigh R, Urrutia V, Wityk R, Wasserman BA. Intracranial plaque enhancement in patients with cerebrovascular events on high-spatial-resolution MR images. Radiology. 2014;271(2):534–42.
11. Ryoo S, Cha J, Kim SJ, Choi JW, Ki CS, Kim KH, Jeon P, Kim JS, Hong SC, Bang OY. High-resolution magnetic resonance wall imaging findings of Moyamoya disease. Stroke. 2014;45(8):2457–60.
12. Natori T, Sasaki M, Miyoshi M, Ohba H, Katsura N, Yamaguchi M, Narumi S, Kabasawa H, Kudo K, Ito K, et al. Evaluating middle cerebral artery atherosclerotic lesions in acute ischemic stroke using magnetic resonance T1-weighted 3-dimensional vessel wall imaging. J Stroke Cerebrovasc Dis. 2014;23(4):706–11.
13. Sakurai K, Miura T, Sagisaka T, Hattori M, Matsukawa N, Mase M, Kasai H, Arai N, Kawai T, Shimohira M, et al. Evaluation of luminal and vessel wall abnormalities in subacute and other stages of intracranial vertebrobasilar artery dissections using the volume isotropic turbo-spin-echo acquisition (VISTA) sequence: a preliminary study. J Neuroradiol. 2013;40(1):19–28.
14. van der Kolk AG, Zwanenburg JJ, Brundel M, Biessels GJ, Visser F, Luijten PR, Hendrikse J. Intracranial vessel wall imaging at 7.0-T MRI. Stroke. 2011;42(9): 2478–84.
15. Dieleman N, Yang W, Abrigo JM, Chu WC, van der Kolk AG, Siero JC, Wong KS, Hendrikse J, Chen XY. Magnetic resonance imaging of plaque morphology,

16. burden, and distribution in patients with symptomatic middle cerebral artery stenosis. Stroke. 2016;47(7):1797–802.
16. van der Kolk AG, Hendrikse J, Brundel M, Biessels GJ, Smit EJ, Visser F, Luijten PR, Zwanenburg JJ. Multi-sequence whole-brain intracranial vessel wall imaging at 7.0 tesla. Eur Radiol. 2013;23(11):2996–3004.
17. Wang J, Helle M, Zhou Z, Bornert P, Hatsukami TS, Yuan C. Joint blood and cerebrospinal fluid suppression for intracranial vessel wall MRI. Magn Reson Med. 2016;75(2):831–8.
18. Fan Z, Yang Q, Deng Z, Li Y, Bi X, Song S, Li D. Whole-brain intracranial vessel wall imaging at 3 tesla using cerebrospinal fluid-attenuated T1-weighted 3D turbo spin echo. Magn Reson Med. 2017;77(3):1142–50.
19. Yang H, Zhang X, Qin Q, Liu L, Wasserman BA, Qiao Y. Improved cerebrospinal fluid suppression for intracranial vessel wall MRI. J Magn Reson Imaging. 2016; 44(3):665–72.
20. Yang Q, Deng Z, Bi X, Song SS, Schlick KH, Gonzalez NR, Li D, Fan Z. Whole-brain vessel wall MRI: a parameter tune-up solution to improve the scan efficiency of three-dimensional variable flip-angle turbo spin-echo. J Magn Reson Imaging. 2017;46(3):751–7.
21. Zhao XQ, Dong L, Hatsukami T, Phan BA, Chu B, Moore A, Lane T, Neradilek MB, Polissar N, Monick D, et al. MR imaging of carotid plaque composition during lipid-lowering therapy a prospective assessment of effect and time course. JACC Cardiovasc Imaging. 2011;4(9):977–86.
22. Underhill HR, Yuan C, Zhao XQ, Kraiss LW, Parker DL, Saam T, Chu B, Takaya N, Liu F, Polissar NL, et al. Effect of rosuvastatin therapy on carotid plaque morphology and composition in moderately hypercholesterolemic patients: a high-resolution magnetic resonance imaging trial. Am Heart J. 2008; 155(3):584. e581–588
23. Corti R, Fuster V, Fayad ZA, Worthley SG, Helft G, Chaplin WF, Muntwyler J, Viles-Gonzalez JF, Weinberger J, Smith DA, et al. Effects of aggressive versus conventional lipid-lowering therapy by simvastatin on human atherosclerotic lesions: a prospective, randomized, double-blind trial with high-resolution magnetic resonance imaging. J Am Coll Cardiol. 2005;46(1):106–12.
24. Fernandes JL, Serrano CV Jr, Blotta MH, Coelho OR, Nicolau JC, Avila LF, Rochitte CE, Parga Filho JR. Regression of coronary artery outward remodeling in patients with non-ST-segment acute coronary syndromes: a longitudinal study using noninvasive magnetic resonance imaging. Am Heart J. 2006;152(6):1123–32.
25. Qiao Y, Guallar E, Suri FK, Liu L, Zhang Y, Anwar Z, Mirbagheri S, Xie YJ, Nezami N, Intrapiromkul J, et al. MR imaging measures of intracranial atherosclerosis in a population-based study. Radiology. 2016;280(3):860–8.
26. Kroner ES, Westenberg JJ, van der Geest RJ, Brouwer NJ, Doornbos J, Kooi ME, van der Wall EE, Lamb HJ, Siebelink HJ. High field carotid vessel wall imaging: a study on reproducibility. Eur J Radiol. 2013;82(4):680–5.
27. Yang WQ, Huang B, Liu XT, Liu HJ, Li PJ, Zhu WZ. Reproducibility of high-resolution MRI for the middle cerebral artery plaque at 3T. Eur J Radiol. 2014;83(1):e49–55.
28. Zhang X, Zhu C, Peng W, Tian B, Chen L, Teng Z, Lu J, Sadat U, Saloner D, Liu Q. Scan-rescan reproducibility of high resolution magnetic resonance imaging of atherosclerotic plaque in the middle cerebral artery. PLoS One. 2015;10(8):e0134913.
29. Alizadeh Dehnavi R, Doornbos J, Tamsma JT, Stuber M, Putter H, van der Geest RJ, Lamb HJ, de Roos A. Assessment of the carotid artery by MRI at 3T: a study on reproducibility. J Magn Reson Imaging. 2007;25(5):1035–43.
30. Li F, Yarnykh VL, Hatsukami TS, Chu B, Balu N, Wang J, Underhill HR, Zhao X, Smith R, Yuan C. Scan-rescan reproducibility of carotid atherosclerotic plaque morphology and tissue composition measurements using multicontrast MRI at 3T. J Magn Reson Imaging. 2010;31(1):168–76.
31. Mandell DM, Mossa-Basha M, Qiao Y, Hess CP, Hui F, Matouk C, Johnson MH, Daemen MJ, Vossough A, Edjlali M, et al. Intracranial Vessel Wall MRI: principles and expert consensus recommendations of the American Society of Neuroradiology. AJNR Am J Neuroradiol. 2017;38(2):218–29.
32. Mihai G, Varghese J, Lu B, Zhu H, Simonetti OP, Rajagopalan S. Reproducibility of thoracic and abdominal aortic wall measurements with three-dimensional, variable flip angle (SPACE) MRI. J magn reson Imaging. 2015;41(1):202–12.
33. Eikendal AL, Blomberg BA, Haaring C, Saam T, van der Geest RJ, Visser F, Bots ML, den Ruijter HM, Hoefer IE, Leiner T. 3D black blood VISTA vessel wall cardiovascular magnetic resonance of the thoracic aorta wall in young, healthy adults: reproducibility and implications for efficacy trial sample sizes: a cross-sectional study. J cardiovasc Magn Reson. 2016;18:20.

14

Evaluation of skeletal muscle microvascular perfusion of lower extremities by cardiovascular magnetic resonance arterial spin labeling, blood oxygenation level-dependent, and intravoxel incoherent motion techniques

Shiteng Suo[1†], Lan Zhang[2†], Hui Tang[1], Qihong Ni[2], Suqin Li[1], Haimin Mao[1], Xiangyu Liu[1], Shengyun He[1], Jianxun Qu[3], Qing Lu[1*] and Jianrong Xu[1*]

Abstract

Background: Noninvasive cardiovascular magnetic resonance (CMR) techniques including arterial spin labeling (ASL), blood oxygenation level-dependent (BOLD), and intravoxel incoherent motion (IVIM), are capable of measuring tissue perfusion-related parameters. We sought to evaluate and compare these three CMR techniques in characterizing skeletal muscle perfusion in lower extremities and to investigate their abilities to diagnose and assess the severity of peripheral arterial disease (PAD).

Methods: Fifteen healthy young subjects, 14 patients with PAD, and 10 age-matched healthy old subjects underwent ASL, BOLD, and IVIM CMR perfusion imaging. Healthy young and healthy old participants were subjected to a cuff-induced ischemia experiment with pressures of 20 mmHg and 40 mmHg above systolic pressure during imaging. Perfusion-related metrics, including blood flow, T2* relaxation time, perfusion fraction f, diffusion coefficient D, and pseudodiffusion coefficient D^*, were measured in the anterior, lateral, soleus, and gastrocnemius muscle groups. Friedman, Mann-Whitney, Wilcoxon signed rank, and Spearman rank correlation tests were used for statistical analysis.

Results: In cases of significant differences determined by the Friedman test ($P < 0.05$), blood flow, T2*, and D values gradually decreased, while f values showed a tendency to increase in healthy subjects under cuff compression. No significant correlations were found among the ASL, BOLD, and IVIM parameters (all $P > 0.05$). Blood flow and T2* values showed significant positive correlations with transcutaneous oxygen pressure measurements ($\rho = 0.465$ and 0. 522, respectively; both $P \leq 0.001$), while f values showed a significant negative correlation in healthy young subjects ($\rho = -0.351$; $P = 0.018$). T2* was independent of age in every muscle group. T2* values were significantly decreased in PAD patients compared with healthy old subjects and severe PAD patients compared with mild-to-moderate PAD patients (all $P < 0.0125$). Significant correlations were found between T2* and ankle–brachial index values in all muscle groups in PAD patients ($\rho = 0.644–0.837$; all $P < 0.0125$). Other imaging parameters failed to show benefits towards the diagnosis and disease severity evaluation of PAD.

(Continued on next page)

* Correspondence: drluqingsjtu@163.com; xujianrong_renji@163.com
†Equal contributors
[1]Department of Radiology, Renji Hospital, School of Medicine, Shanghai Jiao Tong University, No. 160, Pujian Rd, Shanghai 200127, China
Full list of author information is available at the end of the article

(Continued from previous page)

Conclusions: ASL, BOLD, and IVIM provide complementary information regarding tissue perfusion. Compared with ASL and IVIM, BOLD may be a more reliable technique for assessing PAD in the resting state and could thus be applied together with angiography in clinical studies as a tool to comprehensively assess microvascular and macrovascular properties in PAD patients.

Keywords: Cardiovascular magnetic resonance, Perfusion, Oxygenation, Blood flow, Diffusion-weighted imaging

Background

Peripheral arterial disease (PAD) is a highly prevalent and severe atherosclerotic condition characterized by progressive peripheral arterial development of lower extremeity stenosis/occlusions [1]. Patients affected with PAD suffer from reduced quality of life, and more importantly, increased risk of cardiovascular and cerebrovascular events [2]. Therefore, a noninvasive and objective method is desirable for diagnostic, prognostic, and therapeutic purposes, such as early detection of physiological function changes, clinical risk stratification for predicting myocardial infarction or stroke, and intervention planning for symptomatic patients.

Noninvasive testing of flow-limiting stenosis typically includes measurement of the ankle–brachial index (ABI), the ratio of ankle systolic blood pressure to arm systolic pressure [3]. PAD is considered to be present when the ABI is ≤0.90 and severe when the ABI is ≤0.50 [3]. However, ABI has low sensitivity for PAD diagnosis and may not be necessarily associated with symptom relief after interventions [4, 5]. Transcutaneous oxygen pressure (TcPO2) measurement is an additional method used to indirectly assess the degree of ischemia in ischemic skeletal muscle by measuring tissue oxygenation [6]. The use of TcPO2 measurement is limited because it is confined to the skin and thus does not accurately reflect muscle perfusion [7].

Medical imaging has emerged as an important tool in the diagnosis and management of PAD. Imaging modalities, including computer tomography (CT) angiography, cardiovascular magnetic resonance (CMR) angiography, and digital subtraction angiography, are commonly used to assess abnormal blood vessels and blood flow to the lower extremities. These techniques fail to provide information regarding skeletal muscle microvascular perfusion in the affected extremity [8]. However, as PAD extends beyond the large-vessels, blood flow impairment leads to microvascular dysfunction. Precise assessment of skeletal muscle perfusion would facilitate the comprehensive evaluation of PAD and could be combined with conventional angiography to reveal both functional and anatomical characteristics.

Several CMR techniques can noninvasively measure microvascular perfusion using endogenous tracers, including arterial spin labeling (ASL), blood oxygenation level-dependent (BOLD), and intravoxel incoherent motion (IVIM). ASL magnetically tags arterial blood using radiofrequency pulses, and the perfusion contrast is given by the signal difference between the tagged image and the non-tagged control image obtained without net magnetization perturbation in arterial blood [9]. BOLD uses the paramagnetic effect of deoxygenated hemoglobin as an intrinsic contrast agent, which decreases the $T2^*$ relaxation signal [10]. IVIM is a variant of conventional diffusion-weighted imaging by separating the effect of blood flow in the randomly oriented capillary network from that of thermally driven water molecular diffusion [11]. ASL, BOLD, and IVIM have been successfully applied to measure skeletal muscle perfusion in previous studies [12–14]. Since perfusion-related metrics derived from these different CMR techniques are based on completely distinct mechanisms, they may depict different aspects of muscle perfusion properties. ASL is more related to the function of blood delivery to target tissues, BOLD is related to tissue oxygenation, and IVIM is related to pseudodiffusion within capillary beds. We hypothesize that multi-parametric CMR techniques, including ASL, BOLD, and IVIM, could provide complementary information regarding perfusion in skeletal muscles and would represent various alteration patterns in the presence of perfusion deficits.

Hence, this study aimed to 1) test the feasibility of using ASL, BOLD, and IVIM to measure perfusion changes in the lower extremities of healthy subjects under different external compression statuses; 2) validate the associations between ASL-, BOLD-, and IVIM-derived parameters and TcPO2 measurements; 3) evaluate the effects of age on imaging parameter measurements of ASL, BOLD, and IVIM in healthy subjects at rest; 4) use ASL, BOLD, and IVIM to compare perfusion in affected and contralateral (asymptomatic) lower extremities in PAD patients at rest; 5) compare the capabilities of resting-state ASL, BOLD, and IVIM in detecting perfusion differences between PAD patients and age-matched healthy subjects and between mild-to-moderate and severe PAD patients; and 6) investigate the associations between ASL-, BOLD-, and IVIM-derived parameters and ABI in PAD patients.

Methods

The local institutional review board approved the prospective study, and written consent was obtained from all subjects prior to participation. Technical support for imaging sequence optimization was provided by a GE Healthcare employee (JQ). Authors not associated with GE Healthcare had full control of the data and information submitted for publication.

Subjects

Between February 2016 and October 2017, three groups of subjects were enrolled: 1) healthy young subjects ($n = 15$); 2) PAD patients ($n = 14$); and 3) age-matched healthy old subjects ($n = 10$). None of the healthy subjects showed clinical evidence of PAD, cardiac insufficiency, hypoxic pulmonary diseases, or lower extremity venous disorders. Each of these subjects had a normal peripheral pulse status and an ABI > 0.90, and they were all non-smokers. The healthy old group was age-matched to the PAD group to eliminate the confounding effect of age on CMR perfusion parameter measurements. Patients with PAD were recruited from the department of vascular surgery with symptoms of intermittent claudication, rest pain, or critical limb ischemia and an ABI ≤ 0.90. The PAD group was then stratified into two disease severity subgroups based on ABI: 1) the mild-to-moderate group corresponded to an ABI of 0.51 to 0.90 ($n = 7$); and 2) the severe group corresponded to an ABI ≤ 0.50 (n = 7). Details for each group are listed in Table 1.

Imaging protocol

In preparation for the scans, all subjects were asked to refrain from alcohol, caffeine, and vigorous exercise 12 h before imaging. The healthy young and healthy old subjects were subjected to a cuff-induced arterial occlusion experiment during the CMR imaging scans to test the sensitivities of ASL, BOLD, and IVIM to pressure variations. Ischemia via arterial occlusion was induced in the lower extremity by a sphygmomanometer cuff tied around the middle of one thigh. The contralateral lower extremity without intervention was imaged simultaneously as the control side. ASL, BOLD, and IVIM were conducted four times in the following order: baseline (Pre), cuff compression with a pressure of 20 mmHg above systolic pressure

(Cuff-20), cuff compression with a pressure of 40 mmHg above systolic pressure (Cuff-40), and recovery period (Post). Two different cuff pressures were used to verify whether different air pressures could modulate the perfusion signal intensity and thus provoke different degrees of ischemia. The pressure of 40 mmHg above systolic pressure was chosen in accordance with the previously reported range of 30–50 mmHg above systolic pressure, which is recommended for provoking complete and reproducible ischemia [15]. During the Cuff-20 and Cuff-40 sessions, the cuff was kept inflated until all scans were completed (6 min 20 s). The last three sessions were performed at 30-min intervals to avoid the interference from the preceding session (Fig. 1). To test the interscan reproducibility, 5 healthy subjects were subjected to a second scan within 1 week. Patients with PAD received baseline examinations only at rest. All subjects were asked to lie still in the supine position for approximately 15 min before the onset of CMR imaging to ensure that their legs were at heart height [16], and remain still during the entire examination.

All the CMR measurements were carried out on a 3-T CMR system (HDxt, General Electric Healthcare, Waukesha, Wisconsin, USA) with an eight-channel cardiac coil. The subjects were investigated in the supine position. Prior to acquisition of the CMR perfusion images, axial three-dimensional (3D) spoiled gradient-recalled echo T1-weighted images (repetition time ms/echo time ms 4.1/1.5; flip angle = 12°; matrix, 320 × 320; FOV, 32 × 32 mm²; slice thickness = 5 mm; number of slices = 12) were acquired for use as anatomical landmarks. A FOV of 32 × 32 mm² could cover both legs without leaving anything outside, thus prohibiting wrapping artifacts [17]. Pseudocontinuous ASL was performed using an interleaved 3D stack of spiral fast spin-echo sequence with background suppression. Each spiral arm included 512 sampling points in k-space and a total of 6 spiral arms were acquired. Background suppression was achieved via 5 inversion pulses placed 0, 1465, 2100, 2600, and 2880 ms after the labeling start point to suppress a broad range of T1 values [18]. Other ASL parameters were as follows:

Table 1 Demographics

Subjects	Number	Sex (M/F)	Age	ABI	Hypertension	Diabetes mellitus
Healthy Young	15	7/8	24 (20–28)	All ABI > 1	0	0
Healthy Old	10	6/4	60 (50–67)	1.09 (0.96–1.22)	1	0
PAD	14	9/5	65 (55–79)	0.52 (0.00–0.90)	10	8
Mild-to-moderate	7	4/3	59 (55–66)	0.65 (0.55–0.90)	5	5
Severe	7	5/2	69 (57–79)	0.35 (0.00–0.48)	5	3

Data are medians with ranges in parentheses or n
ABI ankle-brachial index, *PAD* peripheral arterial disease

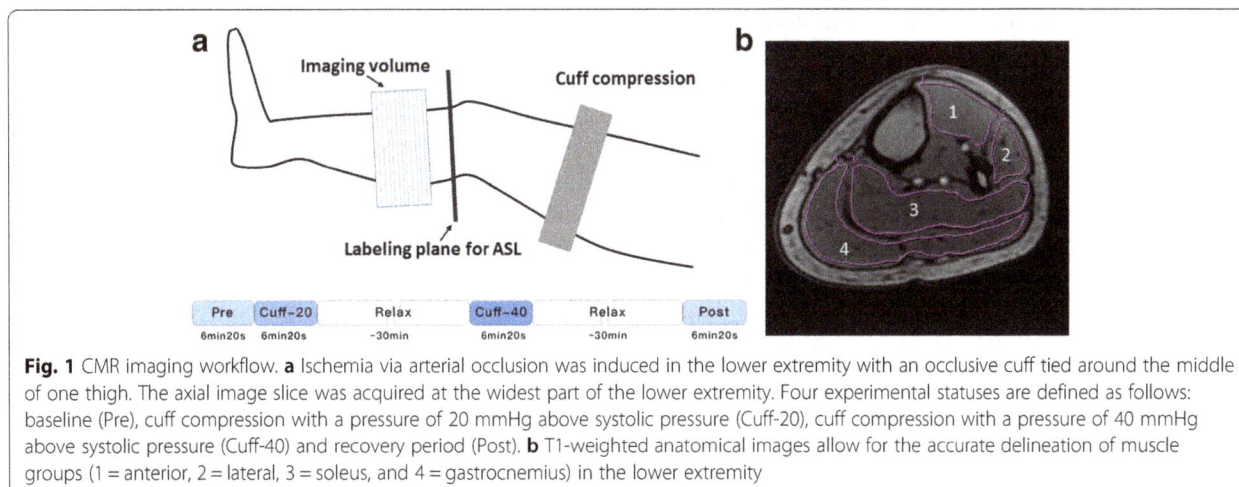

Fig. 1 CMR imaging workflow. **a** Ischemia via arterial occlusion was induced in the lower extremity with an occlusive cuff tied around the middle of one thigh. The axial image slice was acquired at the widest part of the lower extremity. Four experimental statuses are defined as follows: baseline (Pre), cuff compression with a pressure of 20 mmHg above systolic pressure (Cuff-20), cuff compression with a pressure of 40 mmHg above systolic pressure (Cuff-40) and recovery period (Post). **b** T1-weighted anatomical images allow for the accurate delineation of muscle groups (1 = anterior, 2 = lateral, 3 = soleus, and 4 = gastrocnemius) in the lower extremity

repetition time ms/echo time ms = 4316/9.4; bandwidth = 62.5 kHz; FOV = 32 × 32 mm^2; slice thickness = 5 mm; number of slices = 12; number of averages = 2; post-labeling delay time = 1525 ms. A post-labeling delay time of 1525 ms before imaging was used to allow the blood to perfuse all muscle groups, which was similar to that used in a previous study [19]. BOLD was performed using a multi-echo gradient-recalled echo sequence implementing the following parameters: repetition time ms/echo times ms 875/ (2.5, 6.7, 10.9, 15.1, 19.3, 23.5, 27.7, 31.9, 36.1, 40.3, 44.5, 48.7, 52.9, 57.1, 61.3, and 65.5); matrix = 256 × 128; FOV = 32 × 32 mm^2; slice thickness/gap = 5/ 0 mm; number of slices = 12. IVIM imaging was performed using a single shot spin-echo echo-planar imaging sequence at 9 b-values (0, 20, 50, 100, 150, 200, 300, 500, and 800 s/mm^2) in three orthogonal gradient directions, with the following parameters: repetition time ms/echo time ms = 2800/70; matrix = 192 × 192; FOV = 32 × 32 mm^2; slice thickness/gap = 5/ 0 mm; number of slices = 12; number of averages = 3; parallel imaging factor = two. A standard monopolar Stejskal-Tanner diffusion encoding scheme was applied with diffusion gradient pulse duration of 16 ms. The acquisition times for ASL, BOLD, and IVIM were 2 min 18 s, 1 min 59 s, and 2 min 3 s, respectively. All imaging was performed in the axial plane at the level of the middle calf.

Image analysis

ASL, BOLD, and IVIM data were post-processed on a pixel-by-pixel basis on a workstation (Advantage Workstation 4.5; General Electric Healthcare) to obtain corresponding parametric maps of blood flow, T2* relaxation time, perfusion fraction f, diffusion coefficient D, and pseudodiffusion coefficient D^*.

Pseudocontinuous ASL perfusion was calculated using a one-compartment model for blood after subtracting the tagged images from the nontagged control images. Blood flow was quantified using the following equation:

$$BF = \frac{\lambda \cdot (SI_{control} - SI_{label}) \cdot e^{\frac{PLD}{T_{1,blood}}}}{2 \cdot \alpha \cdot T_{1,blood} \cdot SI_{PD} \cdot \left(1 - e^{-\frac{\tau}{T_{1,blood}}}\right)},$$

where PLD is the post-labeling delay (1525 ms), λ is the tissue partition coefficient (0.9 ml/g) [19], $T_{1,\,blood}$ is the longitudinal relaxation time of blood (1600 ms) [19], α is the labeling efficiency (0.80 × 0.75) (label pseudocontinuous ASL × background suppression) [18], τ is the labeling duration (1450 ms), SI_{PD} is the proton density reference without labeling or background saturation, and $SI_{control}$ and SI_{label} are the control and tagged signals, respectively. The arterial transit time was ignored in the quantification.

T2* relaxation time was calculated from the multi-echo T2* gradient-recalled echo data using the least-square fit of monoexponential decay [20], according to the following equation: $S(TE) = S_{TE0} \cdot \exp(-TE/T2^*)$, where TE is the gradient echo time and S(TE) and S_{TE0} are the measured signal intensities for TE ≠ 0 and TE = 0, respectively.

The multi-b-value diffusion-weighted images were analyzed using the IVIM model according to the following equation: $S(b) = S_{b0} \cdot [f \cdot \exp(-bD^*) + (1-f) \cdot \exp(-bD)]$, where $S(b)$ is the measured signal intensity obtained with a nonzero b-value and S_{b0} is the measured signal intensity for $b = 0$. With this equation, perfusion fraction f together with diffusion coefficient D and pseudodiffusion coefficient D^* were calculated using a nonlinear biexponential fit based on the Levenberg-Marquardt technique [21].

For BOLD and IVIM analysis, goodness of fit was assessed using $R^2 = 1 - ESS/TSS$, where ESS is the sum of squared errors between the data points and the fitting curve and *TSS* is the sum of squared differences between the data points and the mean value of all data points. Additional computations were performed to assess the signal-to-noise ratios (SNRs) of the images obtained with TE of 65.5 ms for BOLD and *b*-value of 800 s/mm^2 for IVIM. Noisy images were excluded from curve fitting.

Regions of interest (ROIs) were manually drawn on T1-weighted images around the 4 muscle groups (anterior, lateral, soleus, and gastrocnemius) at the largest cross-sectional area of the calf on both the experimental and control sides (Fig. 1). Attention was given to exclude areas influenced by bones and large vessels, and the inter-osseous muscle was not investigated because it contains a relatively large number of vessels [22]. ROIs were then copied and pasted into the corresponding functional perfusion maps. Average values within ROIs were recorded. Independent analysis of perfusion maps (from 7 randomly selected healthy subjects) by 2 radiologists blinded to the clinical outcomes was conducted to evaluate the interreader reproducibility. In addition, the repeat scans of 5 healthy subjects were analyzed by the same blinded radiologist to test the interscan reproducibility. Normalized values were obtained by dividing each imaging parameter value obtained under the experimental statuses (Cuff-20/Cuff-40/Post) by the baseline measurement (Pre).

TcPO2 measurements

TcPO2 measurements were acquired in all healthy young subjects the day after the CMR examinations using a TcPO2 monitoring system (Periflux System 5000; Perimed, Jarfalla, Sweden) in an air-conditioned room maintained at 22 °C. The cuff-induced ischemia paradigm followed the same process as that described for the CMR experiments. One author (LZ, 12 years of experience in TcPO2 measurement) placed the electrode at the same spot at which the CMR measurements were taken (i.e., the medial upper third of the calf adjacent to the gastrocnemius muscle at the maximal calf diameter) [7].

Statistical analysis

Statistical analyses were performed using SPSS version 20 (International Business Machines, Armonk, New York, USA), OriginPro 2016 (OriginLab Corp., Northampton, Massachusetts, USA), and Prism 5 (GraphPad Software Inc., La Jolla, California, USA). *P*-values less than 0.05 were considered to indicate statistical significance.

All data were expressed as the median (range) owing to non-normal data distributions. To assess interreader and interscan reproducibility, the intraclass correlation coefficient (ICC) was calculated. ICC values less than 0.40 indicated poor reproducibility, those ranging from 0.40 to

0.75 indicated fair to good reproducibility, and those higher than 0.75 indicated excellent reproducibility.

To determine whether differences existed in each imaging parameter value under different statuses (Pre/Cuff-20/Cuff-40/Post) in the experimental and control lower extremities, the Friedman test was used. In cases of statistical significance, further pairwise comparisons with the Dunn test were performed. The Wilcoxon signed rank test was used to compare imaging parameter measurements between left and right lower extremities in all healthy subjects under different statuses. The non-parametric Spearman rank correlation test was performed to assess correlations between imaging parameters derived from different methods, as well as between imaging parameters in gastrocnemius and TcPO2 measurements. Strength of correlation based on the Spearman rank correlation coefficient (ρ) was interpreted as follows: 0.00 to 0.20, very weak to negligible correlation; 0.21 to 0.40, weak correlation; 0.41 to 0.70, moderate correlation; 0.71 to 0.90, strong correlation; and 0.91 to 1.00, very strong correlation [23]. The effects of age on the baseline imaging parameter measurements were investigated by comparing the values between the healthy young and healthy old groups with the Mann-Whitney *U* test. The Wilcoxon signed rank test was used for comparisons of imaging parameter measurements between the left and right lower extremities in PAD patients. Then, imaging parameters were compared between PAD patients and healthy old subjects, as well as between mild-to-moderate and severe PAD patients using the Mann-Whitney *U* test. Finally, correlations between imaging parameters and ABI in PAD patients were assessed using the Spearman rank correlation test. Bonferroni correction for multiple comparisons for the number of muscle groups was applied when necessary.

The sample size of patients included in this study was estimated using one-sided calculations with α of 0.05 and a power of 80% to detect an absolute T2* decrease of 4 ms (compared with normal) with a standard deviation of 2 ms based on the results of previous studies [24, 25]. Assuming a 20% dropout rate, it was determined that 10 participants were required.

Results

All subjects successfully completed the CMR examinations (Table 1). Cuff compression of the thigh was well tolerated. Quantitative image analysis was conducted for each participant. Representative source images and parametric maps are illustrated in Additional file 1: Figure S1. The median R^2 values for BOLD and IVIM fittings were 0.90 (range, 0.80–0.98) and 0.98 (range, 0.92–1.00), respectively. The median SNR values on the

TE = 65.5 ms and $b = 800$ s/mm^2 images were 19.2 (range, 14.4–23.5) and 17.2 (range, 14.2–32.0), respectively. The overall interreader reproducibility was fair to excellent, with ICC values of 0.83 for blood flow, 0.93 for T2*, 0.77 for f, 0.92 for D, and 0.64 for D^*. The overall interscan reproducibility was fair to excellent, with ICC values of 0.73 for blood flow, 0.85 for T2*, 0.67 for f, 0.84 for D, and 0.55 for D^*.

Functional imaging parameter variation under the cuff compression paradigm

Changes in quantitative imaging parameters under the cuff compression paradigm in the healthy young and healthy old groups are illustrated in Figs. 2 and 3 for the experimental lower extremity and in Additional file 2: Figure S2 and Additional file 3: Figure S3 for the control side.

In the healthy young group on the experimental side, only blood flow and T2* values showed significant differences among the 4 statuses in all muscle groups (all $P < 0.01$ for blood flow, and all $P < 0.001$ for T2*). f and D values showed significant differences in the lateral, soleus, and gastrocnemius muscle groups, and D^* values were significantly different in the soleus and gastrocnemius muscle groups (all $P <$ 0.05). Under the Cuff-20/Cuff-40 compression statuses, T2* values were significantly lower than the baseline measurements in all muscle groups (all $P <$ 0.05), and blood flow, f, D, and D^* values showed marked differences in only some muscle groups. No significant differences for any parameter in either muscle group were observed between the Post and Pre statuses (all $P > 0.05$) (Fig. 2).

In the healthy old group on the experimental side, only T2*, f, and D values showed significant differences among the 4 statuses in all muscle groups (all $P < 0.001$ for T2*, and all $P < 0.01$ for f and D). D^* values showed significant differences in the soleus and gastrocnemius muscle groups (both $P < 0.01$). Blood flow values did not significantly differ in any muscle group (all $P > 0.05$). Under the Cuff-20/Cuff-40 compression statuses, significant differences were found for T2* values compared with those at baseline in all muscle groups except for the anterior muscle group under the 20-mmHg status (all $P < 0.05$). Furthermore, f, D, and D^* values were significantly different in several muscle groups under these statuses (all $P < 0.05$). Additionally, no significant differences between Pre and Post measurements were observed for any of the parameters (all $P > 0.05$) (Fig. 3).

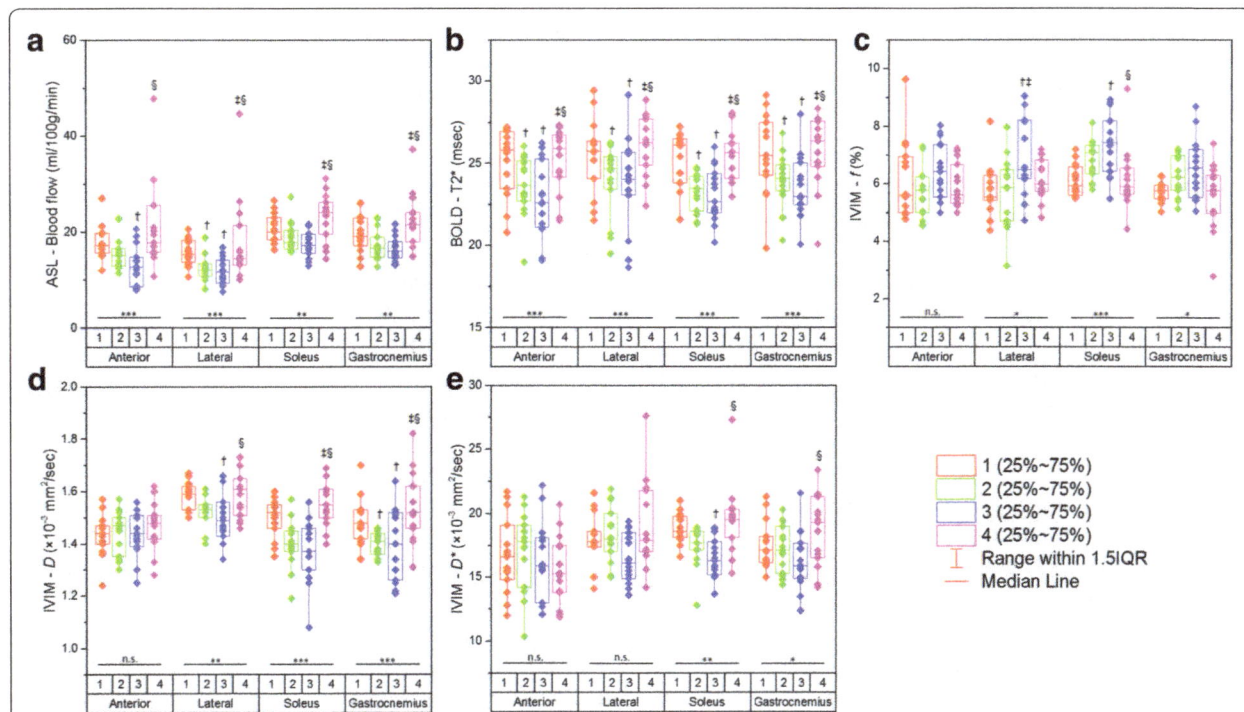

Fig. 2 Graphs presenting serial measurements of imaging parameters from ASL (**a**), BOLD (**b**), and IVIM (**c, d, e**) for the anterior, lateral, soleus, and gastrocnemius muscle groups in healthy young subjects. Comparisons among all four statuses (1 = baseline; 2 = 20-mmHg cuff compression; 3 = 40-mmHg cuff compression; 4 = recovery) for every muscle group were performed using the Friedman test (n.s. = not significant; * = $P < 0.05$; ** = $P <$ 0.01; *** = $P < 0.001$). Further pairwise comparisons were made with the Dunn test († = $P < 0.05$ compared with baseline; ‡ = $P < 0.05$ compared with 20-mmHg cuff compression; § = $P < 0.05$ compared with 40-mmHg cuff compression)

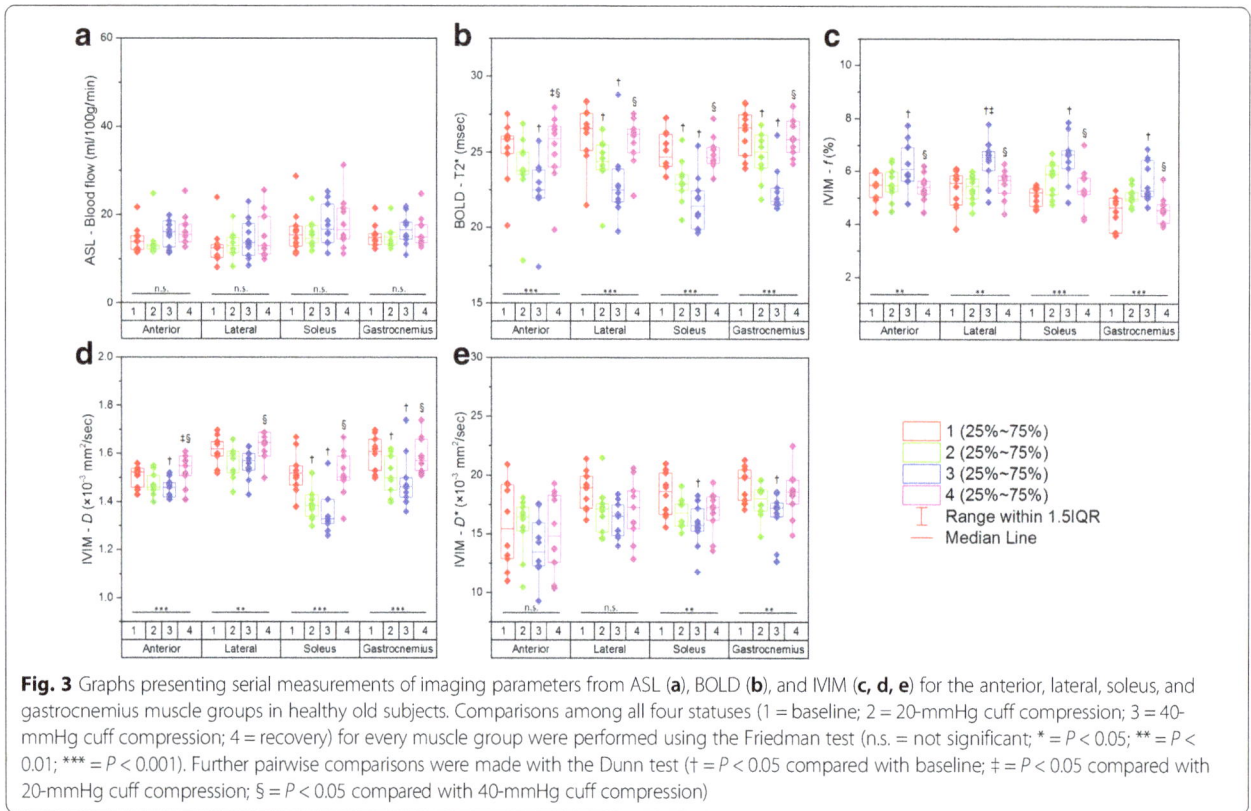

Fig. 3 Graphs presenting serial measurements of imaging parameters from ASL (**a**), BOLD (**b**), and IVIM (**c, d, e**) for the anterior, lateral, soleus, and gastrocnemius muscle groups in healthy old subjects. Comparisons among all four statuses (1 = baseline; 2 = 20-mmHg cuff compression; 3 = 40-mmHg cuff compression; 4 = recovery) for every muscle group were performed using the Friedman test (n.s. = not significant; * = $P < 0.05$; ** = $P < 0.01$; *** = $P < 0.001$). Further pairwise comparisons were made with the Dunn test († = $P < 0.05$ compared with baseline; ‡ = $P < 0.05$ compared with 20-mmHg cuff compression; § = $P < 0.05$ compared with 40-mmHg cuff compression)

In both the healthy young and healthy old groups on the experimental side, in the cases of significant differences, blood flow, T2*, and D values gradually decreased under the Cuff-20 and Cuff-40 compression statuses, while f values showed a tendency to increase. During the recovery period, all parameters nearly returned to normal (Figs. 2 and 3).

In both the healthy young and healthy old groups on the control side, among all parameters, only T2* values in some muscle groups showed significant differences among the 4 statuses ($P < 0.05$) (Additional file 2: Figure S2 and Additional file 3: Figure S3).

Comparison of imaging parameters between the experimental and control sides

Results of Wilcoxon signed rank test comparing functional imaging parameters between the experimental and control sides under different statuses are illustrated in Table 2. No significant differences in any parameter were observed between the left and right lower extremities in healthy subjects at rest (all $P > 0.0125$). Most muscle groups exhibited significant differences in perfusion-related parameter values especially when the cuff compression pressure was increased to 40 mmHg above systolic pressure.

Correlation between functional imaging parameters derived from ASL, BOLD, and IVIM

No significant correlations between functional imaging parameters derived from the different methods were observed (all $P > 0.05$) (Additional file 4: Table S1).

Correlation between functional imaging parameters and TcPO2 measurements

The normalized CMR imaging parameters blood flow, T2*, and f were all correlated with normalized TcPO2 measurements (Fig. 4). Blood flow and T2* showed significant moderate correlations with TcPO2 measurements ($\rho = 0.465$ ($P = 0.001$) and $\rho = 0.522$ ($P < 0.001$), respectively). A significant negative correlation was observed between f and TcPO2 measurements ($P = 0.018$), although the correlation was weak ($\rho = -0.351$). No significant correlation was found for D ($P = 0.054$) or D^* values ($P = 0.340$).

Effects of age on resting-state functional imaging parameter measurements in healthy subjects

Within the muscle groups studied, blood flow for all muscle groups, f for the soleus and gastrocnemius groups, and D and D^* for the gastrocnemius group demonstrated significant differences between the healthy young and healthy old groups at rest (all $P < 0.0125$).

Table 2 Comparison of functional perfusion parameters between experimental and control sides under different statuses in healthy subjects

Parameter	Test	P-value			
		Anterior	Lateral	Soleus	Gastrocnemius
ASL-Blood flow	Pre	0.040	0.779	0.657	0.819
	Cuff-20	0.619	0.104	0.074	**0.011**
	Cuff-40	0.545	0.026	**0.006**	**0.004**
	Post	0.020	0.339	0.026	0.088
BOLD-T2*	Pre	0.093	0.135	0.040	0.710
	Cuff-20	0.946	0.030	**< 0.001**	**0.007**
	Cuff-40	**0.009**	**0.001**	**< 0.001**	**< 0.001**
	Post	0.023	0.051	**0.007**	0.015
IVIM-f	Pre	0.036	0.104	0.853	0.767
	Cuff-20	0.231	0.333	0.018	0.059
	Cuff-40	**0.003**	0.023	**< 0.001**	**0.001**
	Post	0.363	0.786	0.757	0.216
IVIM-D	Pre	0.909	0.057	0.840	0.449
	Cuff-20	0.543	0.440	**0.002**	**0.005**
	Cuff-40	0.483	0.495	**< 0.001**	**0.002**
	Post	0.078	**0.001**	**0.007**	**0.004**
IVIM-D*	Pre	0.648	0.407	0.872	0.553
	Cuff-20	0.590	0.313	**0.011**	0.027
	Cuff-40	0.427	**0.003**	**0.001**	**0.002**
	Post	0.174	0.338	0.607	0.288

Data are P-values derived from the Wilcoxon signed rank test. After Bonferroni correction, $P < 0.0125$ denotes statistical significance. The statistically significant values are presented in bold

Only T2* was found to be independent of age in every muscle group (all $P > 0.0125$) (Table 3).

Comparison of resting-state functional imaging parameters between the affected and contralateral sides in PAD patients

In PAD patients, T2* was markedly reduced on the affected side compared with that on the contralateral side; significance was reached in the anterior muscle group ($P = 0.005$), and no significance was reached in the lateral, soleus, or gastrocnemius muscle groups (all $P > 0.0125$) (Additional file 5: Table S2).

Using ASL, BOLD, and IVIM to measure perfusion in PAD patients

Results of Mann-Whitney U tests comparing functional perfusion parameters between PAD patients and age-matched healthy subjects and between mild-to-moderate and severe PAD patients at rest are illustrated in Table 4. Among all parameters, T2* showed the best performance for the discrimination, with significantly reduced values observed in PAD patients compared with age-matched

healthy old subjects and severe PAD patients compared with mild-to-moderate patients in all muscle groups (all $P < 0.0125$). No significant differences in other parameters in any muscle group were observed except D^* values between PAD patients and healthy old subjects in the lateral muscle group.

Spearman rank correlation analysis showed that in PAD patients, T2* was significantly correlated with ABI in the anterior ($\rho = 0.837$; $P < 0.001$), lateral ($\rho = 0.820$; $P < 0.001$), soleus ($\rho = 0.785$; $P = 0.001$), and gastrocnemius ($\rho = 0.644$; $P = 0.012$) muscle groups (Fig. 5), whereas no significant correlation was observed for the other parameters (all $P > 0.05$).

Discussion

Noninvasive monitoring of skeletal muscle perfusion in the lower extremities is critical for PAD patient management as perfusion can provide insight into microvascular function and endothelial integrity [5]. Advanced CMR techniques, including ASL, BOLD, and IVIM, have been utilized in the assessment of skeletal muscle perfusion [12–14]; however, to our knowledge, few studies have been performed to directly compare these techniques in the same subject cohort [5, 26]. Furthermore, there is limited literature on comparisons of these CMR parameters with routinely used parameters in clinical practice such as TcPO2 and ABI [5, 7, 13]. The results of our study suggested that 1) ASL, BOLD, and IVIM could respond to cuff-induced ischemia in healthy subjects—that is, when the difference reached a significant level, ASL-derived blood flow values, BOLD-derived T2* values, and IVIM-derived D values tended to decrease with increasing external pressure while IVIM-derived f values tended to increase under cuff compression; 2) blood flow, T2*, and f values were all correlated with TcPO2 measurements; 3) ASL of all muscle groups and IVIM of the gastrocnemius group were influenced by age; only BOLD was independent of age in every muscle group; 4) BOLD could detect perfusion differences between the affected and contralateral lower extremities in PAD patients; 5) BOLD could separate PAD patients from healthy old subjects and PAD patients with different severities; and 6) BOLD-derived T2* was correlated with ABI in PAD patients.

Similar to the results in published literature [19, 27], baseline blood flow in skeletal muscle as measured by ASL in the lower extremity was mostly near or less than 20 ml/100 g/min in our study. For BOLD CMR, we observed a baseline mean T2* value of approximately 25 ms in healthy subjects, which lies within the previously reported range of 22–27 ms [13, 25, 28, 29]. IVIM imaging of skeletal muscle in the lower extremity has rarely been studied. In other parts of the body, IVIM-derived f, D, and D^* values were reported to be 3%,

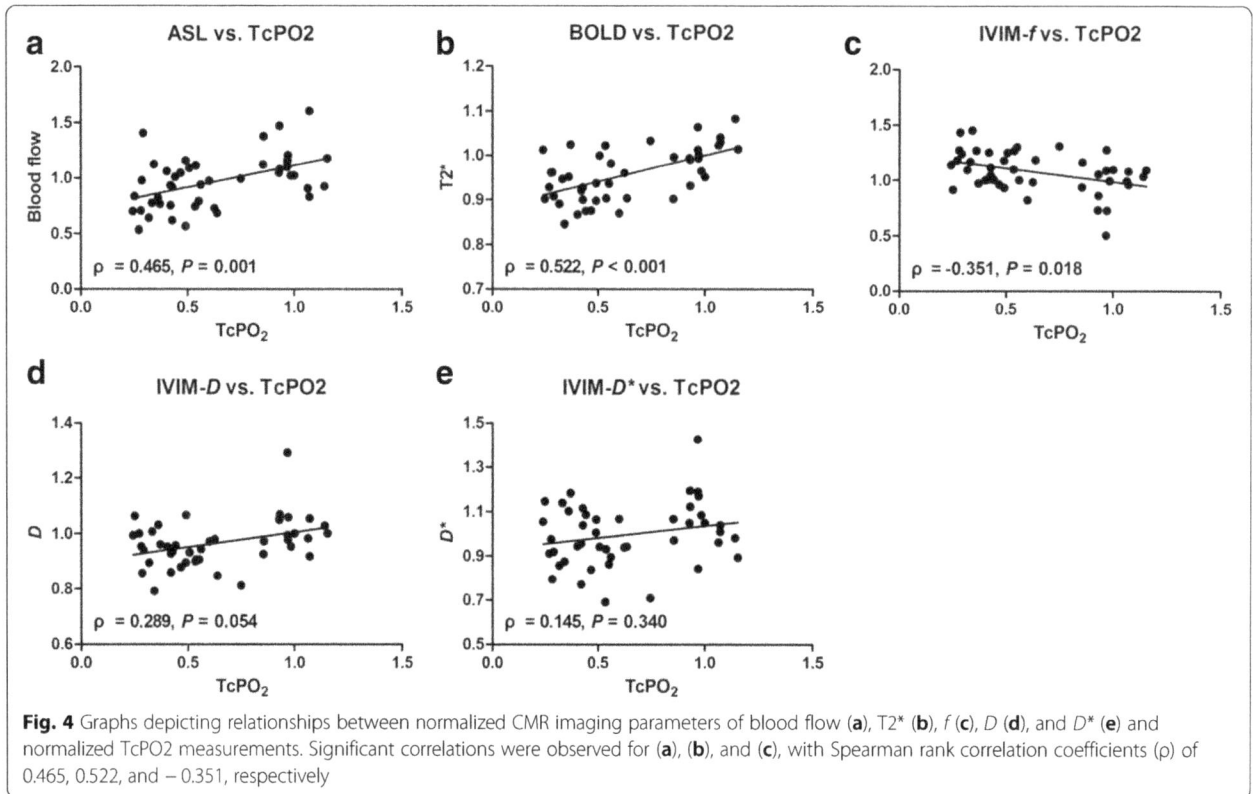

Fig. 4 Graphs depicting relationships between normalized CMR imaging parameters of blood flow (**a**), T2* (**b**), f (**c**), D (**d**), and D^* (**e**) and normalized TcPO2 measurements. Significant correlations were observed for (**a**), (**b**), and (**c**), with Spearman rank correlation coefficients (ρ) of 0.465, 0.522, and − 0.351, respectively

1.45×10^{-3} mm^2/s, and 28.5×10^{-3} mm^2/s, respectively, in the forearm muscle at rest by Filli et al. [14], and 6.6%, 1.45×10^{-3} mm^2/s, and 11.7×10^{-3} mm^2/s, respectively, in the shoulder muscle by Nguyen et al. [30]. These findings are consistent with our observations (e.g., 5.9%, 1.52×10^{-3} mm^2/s, and 18.6×10^{-3} mm^2/s, respectively, in the soleus muscle in healthy young subjects).

Under cuff compression conditions, negative ASL and BOLD contrasts in healthy young subjects developed due to ischemic insult, which agreed with previous

Table 3 Comparison of functional imaging parameters between healthy young and healthy old subjects

Parameter	P-value			
	Anterior	Lateral	Soleus	Gastrocnemius
ASL-Blood flow	**0.005**	**0.007**	**0.004**	**0.003**
BOLD-T2*	0.978	0.367	0.531	0.567
IVIM-f	0.216	0.285	**< 0.001**	**< 0.001**
IVIM-D	0.014	0.160	0.807	**0.012**
IVIM-D^*	0.567	0.338	0.683	**0.011**

Data are P-values derived from the Mann-Whitney U test. After Bonferroni correction, $P < 0.0125$ denotes statistical significance. The statistically significant values are presented in bold
ASL arterial spin labeling, *BOLD* blood oxygenation level-dependent, *IVIM* intravoxel incoherent motion

studies [7, 12, 13, 25, 31]. ASL is capable of measuring blood flow through muscle tissue microvasculature given that ASL and radiolabeled microsphere measurements in rat leg muscle have shown good correlation for perfusion [32]. Cuff compression interrupted both arterial inflow and venous outflow simultaneously, thus provoking reduced blood flow obtained by ASL. Although the exact source of the BOLD signal in skeletal muscle is not yet fully understood, it is generally accepted that the signal is primarily associated with capillary and blood oxygenation state [7]. Lebon et al. also found that the T2* signal in muscle rapidly decreased during ischemia and attributed this change to early hemoglobin desaturation [33]. This finding is logical given that the BOLD signal changed almost synchronously with hemoglobin desaturation but preceded myoglobin desaturation [33], as the dissociation constant of hemoglobin is more than 10 times higher than that of myoglobin. IVIM-derived D values also showed a decreasing trend under cuff-induced ischemic conditions. Local ischemia leads to decreased diffusivity of water molecules within muscles, and this decreased D was mostly likely attributed to this physical effect. Conversely, the perfusion fraction f derived from IVIM showed a tendency to increase in the case of arterial occlusion. Given that f reflects the signal fraction of capillary blood flow in entire water molecule diffusion pool within each voxel [11], it can be hypothesized that

Table 4 Associations of the presence and severity of PAD with functional imaging parameters

Parameter		AHO vs. PAD			Mild-to-moderate vs. Severe PAD		
		AHO	PAD	P-value	Mild-to-moderate	Severe	P-value
ASL-Blood flow (ml/100 g/min)	Anterior	14.0 (11.6–21.8)	15.2 (8.1–34.2)	0.666	16.3 (9.9–23.7)	14.5 (8.1–34.2)	0.318
	Lateral	12.6 (8.3–24.0)	12.9 (8.2–34.0)	0.886	13.7 (8.2–19.7)	12.0 (9.2–34.0)	0.805
	Soleus	15.5 (11.3–28.8)	14.7 (12.0–40.1)	0.796	16.5 (12.0–26.7)	14.2 (12.3–40.1)	0.456
	Gastrocnemius	14.9 (12.4–21.6)	14.5 (10.5–25.5)	0.625	14.4 (11.0–19.0)	14.8 (10.5–25.5)	0.805
BOLD-T2* (ms)	Anterior	25.9 (20.2–27.5)	21.9 (13.4–26.8)	**0.002**	22.3 (21.7–26.8)	19.4 (13.4–23.5)	**0.011**
	Lateral	26.6 (21.5–28.3)	21.8 (11.5–28.7)	**0.011**	25.2 (19.9–28.7)	16.6 (11.5–22.9)	**0.004**
	Soleus	24.7 (23.4–27.3)	22.5 (14.8–26.6)	**0.007**	24.3 (22.1–26.6)	17.4 (14.8–22.8)	**0.001**
	Gastrocnemius	26.7 (23.9–28.3)	22.5 (13.5–26.1)	**0.001**	24.7 (20.2–26.1)	19.3 (13.5–24.8)	**0.011**
IVIM-f (%)	Anterior	5.5 (4.5–6.0)	5.7 (4.5–12.0)	0.235	5.7 (4.5–12.0)	6.6 (5.2–7.7)	0.383
	Lateral	5.6 (3.8–6.1)	5.6 (4.4–14.5)	0.371	4.8 (4.4–14.5)	5.7 (5.1–8.8)	0.535
	Soleus	5.2 (4.6–5.5)	5.2 (3.7–14.2)	0.472	4.9 (3.7–14.2)	5.4 (5.0–6.7)	0.456
	Gastrocnemius	4.7 (3.6–5.3)	5.6 (3.7–7.7)	0.016	5.8 (3.7–7.7)	5.4 (4.3–5.8)	0.209
IVIM-D ($\times 10^{-3}$ mm^2/s)	Anterior	1.53 (1.43–1.56)	1.48 (1.24–2.02)	0.122	1.54 (1.24–2.02)	1.38 (1.33–1.52)	0.053
	Lateral	1.62 (1.52–1.70)	1.51 (0.97–1.72)	0.186	1.65 (0.97–1.72)	1.48 (1.18–1.55)	0.165
	Soleus	1.52 (1.38–1.67)	1.44 (1.28–1.99)	0.235	1.47 (1.42–1.99)	1.32 (1.28–1.58)	0.038
	Gastrocnemius	1.61 (1.50–1.70)	1.51 (1.33–1.88)	0.371	1.61 (1.45–1.88)	1.40 (1.33–1.74)	0.073
IVIM-D* ($\times 10^{-3}$ mm^2/s)	Anterior	15.5 (11.0–20.9)	17.2 (11.0–20.5)	0.437	17.4 (11.0–20.5)	17.0 (14.9–19.9)	0.620
	Lateral	19.0 (16.2–21.4)	14.8 (9.1–18.1)	**0.001**	14.2 (9.1–17.7)	17.3 (10.6–18.1)	0.318
	Soleus	18.7 (15.6–21.0)	17.2 (9.4–27.5)	0.235	17.1 (9.4–21.8)	17.3 (14.4–27.5)	0.902
	Gastrocnemius	19.8 (17.1–21.3)	17.3 (12.5–21.9)	0.391	17.6 (12.5–21.8)	16.4 (14.3–21.9)	0.902

Data are medians with ranges in parentheses. After Bonferroni correction, $P < 0.0125$ denotes statistical significance. The statistically significant values are presented in bold

AHO age-matched healthy old subjects, PAD peripheral arterial disease, ASL arterial spin labeling, BOLD blood oxygenation level-dependent, IVIM intravoxel incoherent motion

obstruction of venous reflux is probably responsible for the altered f values. In addition, it has been suggested that decrease in venous oxygen saturation may release relaxing factors than can cause microvascular dilation [34], which may also increase the f value. In healthy old subjects, changing trends for the imaging parameters were similar to those observed in the healthy young group except for ASL. ASL is limited by the intrinsic low SNR in skeletal muscle, wherein the ASL signal represents only 0.5%–1% of the raw image intensity [8]. This notion may account for the lack of statistical significance of ASL measurements, especially given that the healthy old sample number was small ($n = 10$).

Interestingly, we also observed aberrant T2* signal changes on the control sides of healthy subjects during the cuff compression experiment on the other lower extremity, in accordance with the findings of a previous study [35]. Yeung et al. suggested that this might be because of the high sensitivity of BOLD CMR imaging to local magnetic field disturbances caused by magnetic susceptibility effects, which may be induced by oxygen in the air at high pressure during cuff inflation [35].

Ledermann et al. reported that BOLD CMR imaging correlated with TcPO2 measurements in healthy volunteers during muscle ischemia [7], which was consistent with our results. However, the correlation observed by Ledermann et al. was stronger (correlation coefficient, 0.96) than that in our study (correlation coefficient, 0.522), primarily because Ledermann et al. averaged signal intensities across all volunteers for statistics, not for individuals. In addition, ASL-derived blood flow and IVIM-derived f values were also found to correlate with TcPO2 measurements in our study, with correlation coefficients of 0.465 and − 0.351, respectively. The correlation between BOLD-derived T2* and TcPO2 measurements was stronger than those between the other parameters, which may be attributed to the fact that both BOLD CMR imaging and TcPO2 examination are directly associated with the oxygenation state at the microvascular level.

Age effects on parameter measurements varied among the different sequences and muscles. In our study, no significant differences between the healthy young and healthy old groups were observed for the baseline T2* value, indicating that age did not appear to affect BOLD

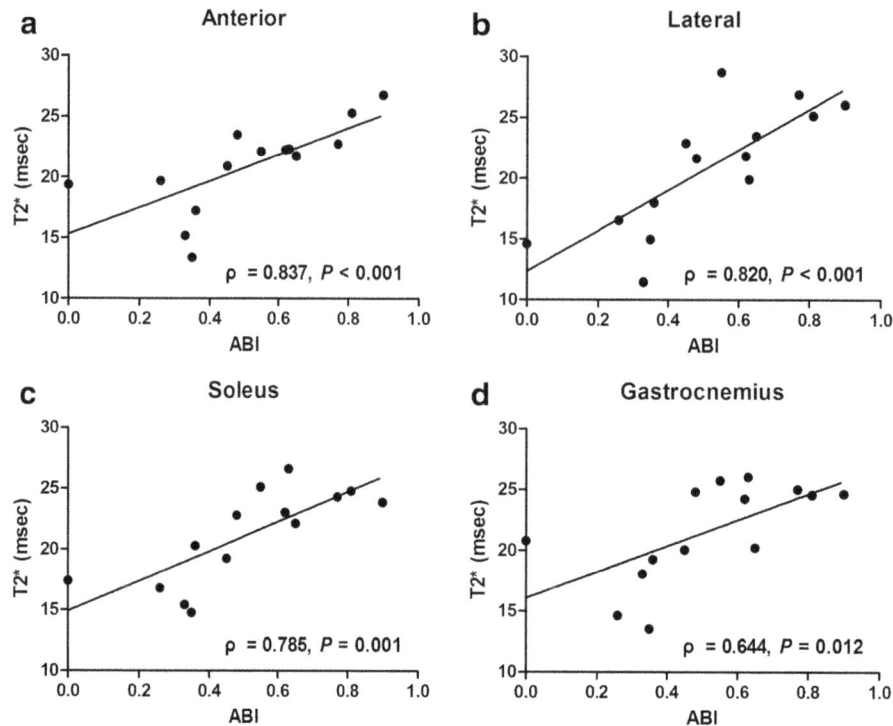

Fig. 5 Graphs depicting relationships between T2* in the anterior (**a**), lateral (**b**), soleus (**c**), and gastrocnemius (**d**) muscle groups and ABI in PAD patients. Significant correlations were observed for all muscle groups, with Spearman rank correlation coefficients (ρ) of 0.837, 0.820, 0.785, and 0.644, respectively

in healthy subjects at rest. This finding was in accordance with other observations [28]. In contrast, ASL and IVIM were more easily influenced by the age factor especially in the gastrocnemius muscle group. The gastrocnemius is a fast-twitch type muscle, whereas the soleus belongs to the slow-twitch type. Degenerative processes of muscle fibers have been demonstrated to differ with fiber type, and the fast-twitch muscle is more prone to aging and fatigue [36, 37].

The ABI is a measure providing objective data for diagnosing PAD. When applying these imaging techniques on PAD patients, we found that BOLD was capable of detecting perfusion deficits at rest better than ASL and IVIM. Lower T2* values were related to the presence of PAD and more disease severity stratified by ABI. As discussed earlier, BOLD effect is generally assumed to reflect blood oxygenation state influenced by the ratio of oxygenated to deoxygenated hemoglobin, which is determined by the balance between oxygen supply and consumption [15]. In PAD, arterial blood flow in the lower extremities is limited, leading to reduced oxygenated hemoglobin. Moreover, the impaired vascular function causes a longer contact time between blood and myocytes, leading to more efficient deoxygenation of hemoglobin [15]. These two effects both contribute to a reduced T2* value. In a previous study by Englund et

al., BOLD-derived metrics under the ischemia-reperfusion paradigm were also found to be correlated with ABI, suggestive of disease severity-dependent impairment of vascular response in PAD patients [5]. Our results suggest that even at rest, vascular function at the tissue level could be indicative of disease progression. However, unlike CMR imaging, ABI cannot be obtained from all patients especially in patients with critical limb ischemia.

In the cuff-induced arterial occlusion experiment on healthy subjects, varying degrees of ischemia were factitiously induced by different pressures above the systolic pressure, and CMR imaging techniques were able to detect these changes. However, in healthy old subjects and PAD patients with differing degrees of ischemia, only BOLD was effective for this discrimination at rest. One possible explanation for this finding could be that the degree of ischemic insult in PAD patients was less severe than that induced by cuff occlusion. Additionally, collateral arteries developed in skeletal muscles in PAD patients would compensate for the perfusion deficit. BOLD is more sensitive to these less dramatic changes, which may be ASL- or IVIM-insensitive.

Numerous previous studies have used ASL or BOLD to monitor dynamic perfusion changes in skeletal muscles at rest and during ischemia and hyperemia, which allows the measurement of key parameters, such as peak hyperemic value (PHV) and time-to-peak (TTP). In our study, we did not measure continuous temporal changes of ASL, BOLD, and IVIM in our subjects mainly because it was not technically feasible to perform these three sequences sequentially at a high temporal resolution. Nevertheless, our protocol can be regarded as a simplified approach to the dynamic scanning method; a similar approach was also used in a previous study [38]. Although PHV and TTP proved useful for the assessment of PAD in most published studies, conflicting results also exist [13]. In addition, the reproducibility of the data is another concern. Versluis et al. investigated the reproducibility of BOLD-derived PHV and TTP values in healthy subjects and PAD patients [39]. The reproducibility was unsatisfying with a coefficient of variation up to 26.7% and an ICC value as low as 0.59 [39]. Moreover, due to massive pain or risk of worsening the clinical condition caused by cuff compression, patients with critical limb ischemia, ulceration, necrosis, or gangrene should be considered with caution or even excluded from the study [40]. Compared with the cuff compression paradigm, the resting-state imaging scheme is simple to perform, less time-consuming, and more acceptable to PAD patients [24]. In our study, we wanted to investigate and were most concerned with whether the baseline measurements of these techniques had value in assessing PAD.

The present study has several limitations. First, the number of study subjects was relatively small. Second, no gold standard for blood flow, oxygenation, or microvascular perfusion in skeletal muscle could be established in our subjects. For example, mixed venous oxygen saturation measurements would be informative regarding the confirmation of BOLD results. Nevertheless, our results revealed significant relationships with TcPO2 measurements, which are commonly used in clinical routines. However, the use of TcPO2 measurement is limited since it is confined to the skin microvasculature and thus fails to directly analyze the skeletal muscle [7]. Therefore, once further validated, noninvasive CMR techniques might be used to gain direct information regarding skeletal muscle perfusion in lower extremities. Third, the cuff compression paradigm was used in the study instead of exercise. Exercise is more physiologically and clinically relevant. A previous study showed that muscle perfusion at peak exercise was correlated with 6-min walk distance in lower extremities [41]. Compared with exercise, cuff compression has improved test-retest reproducibility [42] and less motion artifacts [40]. Moreover, cuff compression allow the assessment of muscles which respond less to commonly used ankle flexion exercise [42]. Lopez et al. suggested the use of cuff compression in a more general study

population and the use of exercise in specific PAD therapies in claudicants based on its physiologic and clinical relevance [42]. Fourth, skeletal muscle energetics were not investigated in the current study. [31]P CMR spectroscopy is a useful tool to noninvasively probe skeletal muscle energetics, including adenosine triphosphate and creatine phosphate metabolism [43], which would help to better understand the perfusion results in our study. Further studies are warranted. Finally, CMR angiography was not performed in the current study.

Conclusions
In conclusion, the present study shows that multiparametric CMR techniques including ASL, BOLD, and IVIM provide useful and complementary information regarding tissue perfusion in the lower extremities of healthy subjects. Perfusion-related metrics derived from these techniques correlate with TcPO2 measurements. In PAD patients, BOLD is a more reliable imaging technique for the detection and stratification of alterations in microvascular function at rest compared with ASL and IVIM.

Abbreviations
3D: Three dimensional; ABI: Ankle-brachial index; ASL: Arterial spin labeling; BOLD: Blood oxygenation level-dependent; CMR: Cardiovascular magnetic resonance; CT: Computer tomography; ESS: Sum of squared errors; FOV: Field of view; ICC: Intraclass correlation coefficient; IVIM: Intravoxel incoherent motion; PAD: Peripheral arterial disease; PHV: Peak hyperemic value; PLD: Post-labeling delay; ROI: Region of interest; SNR: Signal-to-noise ratio; TcPO2: Transcutaneous oxygen pressure; TE: Echo time; TSS: Sum of squared differences; TTP: Time-to-peak

Acknowledgements
Not applicable

Funding
This work was supported by National Natural Science Foundation of China (grants 81501458, 81271638, and 81571630) and the Shanghai Pujiang Program (grant 15PJ1405200).

Authors' contributions
SS, LZ, QL and JX contributed to the conception and study design. HT, SH and SL performed the CMR examinations and acquired CMR data. QN, HM and XL performed the TcPO2 examinations and ABI tests. JQ contributed to the CMR sequence and image postprocessing development. SS and QL analyzed and interpreted the CMR data and performed statistical analysis. SS and LZ drafted the manuscript. All authors participated in revising the manuscript and read and approved the final manuscript.

Competing interests
The authors declare that they have no competing interests.

Author details
[1]Department of Radiology, Renji Hospital, School of Medicine, Shanghai Jiao Tong University, No. 160, Pujian Rd, Shanghai 200127, China. [2]Department of Vascular Surgery, Renji Hospital, School of Medicine, Shanghai Jiao Tong University, Shanghai, China. [3]GE Healthcare China, Shanghai, China.

References

1. Hirsch AT, Criqui MH, Treat-Jacobson D, Regensteiner JG, Creager MA, Olin JW, et al. Peripheral arterial disease detection, awareness, and treatment in primary care. JAMA. 2001;286:1317–24.
2. Criqui MH, Langer RD, Fronek A, Feigelson HS, Klauber MR, McCann TJ, et al. Mortality over a period of 10 years in patients with peripheral arterial disease. New Engl J Med. 1992;326:381–6.
3. Kullo IJ, Rooke TW. Peripheral artery disease. N Engl J Med. 2016;374:861–71.
4. Stein R, Hriljac I, Halperin JL, Gustavson SM, Teodorescu V, Olin JW. Limitation of the resting ankle-brachial index in symptomatic patients with peripheral arterial disease. Vasc Med. 2006;11:29–33.
5. Englund EK, Langham MC, Ratcliffe SJ, Fanning MJ, Wehrli FW, Mohler ER, et al. Multiparametric assessment of vascular function in peripheral artery disease dynamic measurement of skeletal muscle perfusion, blood-oxygen-level dependent signal, and venous oxygen saturation. Circ Cardiovasc Imaging. 2015;8:e002673.
6. Bunt T, Holloway GA. TcPO2 as an accurate predictor of therapy in limb salvage. Ann Vasc Surg. 1996;10:224–7.
7. Ledermann HP, Heidecker H-G, Schulte A-C, Thalhammer C, Aschwanden M, Jaeger KA, et al. Calf muscles imaged at BOLD MR: correlation with TcPo2 and Flowmetry measurements during ischemia and reactive hyperemia—initial experience. Radiology. 2006;241:477–84.
8. Bajwa A, Wesolowski R, Patel A, Saha P, Ludwinski F, Smith A, et al. Assessment of tissue perfusion in the lower limb current methods and techniques under development. Circ Cardiovasc Imaging. 2014;7:836–43.
9. Detre JA, Leigh JS, Williams DS, Koretsky AP. Perfusion imaging. Magn Reson Med. 1992;23:37–45.
10. Ogawa S, Lee T-M, Kay AR, Tank DW. Brain magnetic resonance imaging with contrast dependent on blood oxygenation. Proc Natl Acad Sci U S A. 1990;87:9868–72.
11. Le Bihan D, Breton E, Lallemand D, Aubin M, Vignaud J, Laval-Jeantet M. Separation of diffusion and perfusion in intravoxel incoherent motion MR imaging. Radiology. 1988;168:497–505.
12. Wu W-C, Mohler E, Ratcliffe SJ, Wehrli FW, Detre JA, Floyd TF. Skeletal muscle microvascular flow in progressive peripheral artery disease: assessment with continuous arterial spin-labeling perfusion magnetic resonance imaging. J Am Coll Cardiol. 2009;53:2372–7.
13. Bajwa A, Wesolowski R, Patel A, Saha P, Ludwinski F, Ikram M, et al. Blood oxygenation level-dependent CMR-derived measures in critical limb ischemia and changes with revascularization. J Am Coll Cardiol. 2016;67:420–31.
14. Filli L, Boss A, Wurnig MC, Kenkel D, Andreisek G, Guggenberger R. Dynamic intravoxel incoherent motion imaging of skeletal muscle at rest and after exercise. NMR Biomed. 2015;28:240–6.
15. Jacobi B, Bongartz G, Partovi S, Schulte AC, Aschwanden M, Lumsden AB, et al. Skeletal muscle BOLD MRI: from underlying physiological concepts to its usefulness in clinical conditions. J Magn Reson Imaging. 2012;35:1253–65.
16. Duteil S, Wary C, Raynaud JS, Lebon V, Lesage D, Leroy-Willig A, et al. Influence of vascular filling and perfusion on BOLD contrast during reactive hyperemia in human skeletal muscle. Magn Reson Med. 2006;55:450–4.
17. Loughran T, Higgins DM, McCallum M, Coombs A, Straub V, Hollingsworth KG. Improving highly accelerated fat fraction measurements for clinical trials in muscular dystrophy: origin and quantitative effect of R2* changes. Radiology. 2015;275:570–8.
18. Mutsaerts HJ, Steketee RM, Heijtel DF, Kuijer JP, van Osch MJ, Majoie CB, et al. Inter-vendor reproducibility of pseudo-continuous arterial spin labeling at 3 tesla. PLoS One. 2014;9:e104108.
19. Grozinger G, Pohmann R, Schick F, Grosse U, Syha R, Brechtel K, et al. Perfusion measurements of the calf in patients with peripheral arterial occlusive disease before and after percutaneous transluminal angioplasty using MR arterial spin labeling. J Magn Reson Imaging. 2014;40:980–7.
20. Ledermann H-P, Schulte A-C, Heidecker H-G, Aschwanden M, Jäger KA, Scheffler K, et al. Blood oxygenation level–dependent magnetic resonance imaging of the skeletal muscle in patients with peripheral arterial occlusive disease. Circulation. 2006;113:2929–35.
21. Cao M, Suo S, Han X, Jin K, Sun Y, Wang Y, et al. Application of a simplified method for estimating perfusion derived from diffusion-weighted MR imaging in glioma grading. Front Aging Neurosci. 2018;9:432.
22. Schulte AC, Aschwanden M, Bilecen D. Calf muscles at blood oxygen level-dependent MR imaging: aging effects at postocclusive reactive hyperemia. Radiology. 2008;247:482–9.
23. Heye S, Maleux G, Oyen RH, Claes K, Kuypers DR. Occupational radiation

24. dose: percutaneous interventional procedures on hemodialysis arteriovenous fistulas and grafts. Radiology. 2012;264:278–84.
24. Zuo CS, Sung YH, Simonson DC, Habecker E, Wang J, Haws C, et al. Reduced T2* values in soleus muscle of patients with type 2 diabetes mellitus. PLoS One. 2012;7:e49337.
25. Englund EK, Langham MC, Li C, Rodgers ZB, Floyd TF, Mohler ER, et al. Combined measurement of perfusion, venous oxygen saturation, and skeletal muscle T2* during reactive hyperemia in the leg. J Cardiovasc Magn Reson. 2013;15:70.
26. Andreisek G, White LM, Sussman MS, Langer DL, Patel C, Su JW, et al. T2*-weighted and arterial spin labeling MRI of calf muscles in healthy volunteers and patients with chronic exertional compartment syndrome: preliminary experience. AJR Am J Roentgenol. 2009;193:W327–33.
27. Wu WC, Wang J, Detre JA, Ratcliffe SJ, Floyd TF. Transit delay and flow quantification in muscle with continuous arterial spin labeling perfusion-MRI. J Magn Reson Imaging. 2008;28:445–52.
28. Kos S, Klarhofer M, Aschwanden M, Scheffler K, Jacob AL, Bilecen D. Simultaneous dynamic blood oxygen level-dependent magnetic resonance imaging of foot and calf muscles: aging effects at ischemia and postocclusive hyperemia in healthy volunteers. Investig Radiol. 2009;44:741–7.
29. Partovi S, Schulte AC, Jacobi B, Klarhofer M, Lumsden AB, Loebe M, et al. Blood oxygenation level-dependent (BOLD) MRI of human skeletal muscle at 1.5 and 3 T. J Magn Reson Imaging. 2012;35:1227–32.
30. Nguyen A, Ledoux JB, Omoumi P, Becce F, Forget J, Federau C. Application of intravoxel incoherent motion perfusion imaging to shoulder muscles after a lift-off test of varying duration. NMR Biomed. 2016;29:66–73.
31. Yu G, Floyd TF, Durduran T, Zhou C, Wang J, Detre JA, et al. Validation of diffuse correlation spectroscopy for muscle blood flow with concurrent arterial spin labeled perfusion MRI. Opt Express. 2007;15:1064–75.
32. Pohmann R, Künnecke B, Fingerle J, Kienlin MV. Fast perfusion measurements in rat skeletal muscle at rest and during exercise with single-voxel FAIR (flow-sensitive alternating inversion recovery). Magn Reson Med. 2006;55:108–15.
33. Lebon V, Brillault-Salvat C, Bloch G, Leroy-Willig A, Carlier PG. Evidence of muscle BOLD effect revealed by simultaneous interleaved gradient-echo NMRI and myoglobin NMRS during leg ischemia. Magn Reson Med. 1998;40:551–8.
34. Clifford PS, Hellsten Y. Vasodilatory mechanisms in contracting skeletal muscle. J Appl Physiol. 2004;97:393–403.
35. Yeung DK, Griffith JF, Li AF, Ma HT, Yuan J. Air pressure-induced susceptibility changes in vascular reactivity studies using BOLD MRI. J Magn Reson Imaging. 2013;38:976–80.
36. Ishihara A, Naitoh H, Katsuta S. Effects of ageing on the total number of muscle fibers and motoneurons of the tibialis anterior and soleus muscles in the rat. Brain Res. 1987;435:355–8.
37. Noseworthy MD, Bulte DP, Alfonsi J. BOLD magnetic resonance imaging of skeletal muscle. Semin Musculoskelet Radiol. 2003;7:307–15.
38. Wang C, Zhang R, Zhang X, Wang H, Zhao K, Jin L, et al. Noninvasive measurement of lower extremity muscle oxygen extraction fraction under cuff compression paradigm. J Magn Reson Imaging. 2016;43:1148–58.
39. Versluis B, Backes WH, van Eupen MG, Jaspers K, Nelemans PJ, Rouwet EV, et al. Magnetic resonance imaging in peripheral arterial disease: reproducibility of the assessment of morphological and functional vascular status. Investig Radiol. 2011;46:11–24.
40. Partovi S, Karimi S, Jacobi B, Schulte AC, Aschwanden M, Zipp L, et al. Clinical implications of skeletal muscle blood-oxygenation-level-dependent (BOLD) MRI. MAGMA. 2012;25:251–61.
41. Anderson JD, Epstein FH, Meyer CH, Hagspiel KD, Wang H, Berr SS, et al. Multifactorial determinants of functional capacity in peripheral arterial disease: uncoupling of calf muscle perfusion and metabolism. J Am Coll Cardiol. 2009;54:628–35.
42. Lopez D, Pollak AW, Meyer CH, Epstein FH, Zhao L, Pesch AJ, et al. Arterial spin labeling perfusion cardiovascular magnetic resonance of the calf in peripheral arterial disease: cuff occlusion hyperemia vs exercise. J Cardiovasc Magn Reson. 2015;17:23.
43. Weiss K, Schar M, Panjrath GS, Zhang Y, Sharma K, Bottomley PA, et al. Fatigability, exercise intolerance, and abnormal skeletal muscle energetics in heart failure. Circ Heart Fail. 2017;10:e004129.

15

Cardiovascular magnetic resonance black-blood thrombus imaging for the diagnosis of acute deep vein thrombosis at 1.5 Tesla

Hanwei Chen[1,2†], Xueping He[1,2†], Guoxi Xie[3,4*] (ID), Jianke Liang[1], Yufeng Ye[1], Wei Deng[1], Zhuonan He[1], Dexiang Liu[1], Debiao Li[5], Xin Liu[6] and Zhaoyang Fan[5]

Abstract

Background: The aim was to investigate the feasibility of a cardiovascular magnetic resonance (CMR) black-blood thrombus imaging (BBTI) technique, based on delay alternating with nutation for tailored excitation black-blood preparation and a variable flip angle turbo-spin-echo readout, for the diagnosis of acute deep vein thrombosis (DVT) at 1.5 T.

Methods: BBTI was conducted in 15 healthy subjects and 30 acute DVT patients. Contrast-enhanced CMR venography (CE-CMRV) was conducted for comparison and only performed in the patients. Apparent contrast-to-noise ratios between the thrombus and the muscle/lumen were calculated to determine whether BBTI could provide an adequate thrombus signal for diagnosis. Two blinded readers assessed the randomized BBTI images from all participants and made independent decisions on the presence or absence of thrombus at the segment level. Images obtained by CE-CMRV were also randomized and assessed by the two readers. Using the consensus CE-CMRV as a reference, the sensitivity, specificity, positive and negative predictive values, and accuracy of BBTI, as well as its diagnostic agreement with CE-CMRV, were calculated. Additionally, diagnostic confidence and interobserver diagnostic agreement were evaluated.

Results: The thrombi in the acute phase exhibited iso- or hyperintense signals on the BBTI images. All the healthy subjects were correctly identified from the participants based on the segment level. The diagnostic confidence of BBTI was comparable to that of CE-CMRV (3.69 ± 0.52 vs. 3.70 ± 0.47). High overall sensitivity (95.2%), SP (98.6%), positive predictive value (96.0%), negative predictive value (98.3%), and accuracy (97.7%), as well as excellent diagnostic and interobserver agreements, were achieved using BBTI.

Conclusion: BBTI is a reliable, contrast-free technique for the diagnosis of acute DVT at 1.5 T.

Keywords: Magnetic resonance imaging, Deep vein thrombosis, Venous thrombosis, Venography

Background

Deep vein thrombosis (DVT) is a common clinical disease that can lead to severe complications such as pulmonary embolism, post-thrombotic syndrome, venous ulcer, and chronic pulmonary artery hypertension [1–3]. Early detection of newly formed thrombus is important for timely thrombolytic therapy and minimizing the occurrence of life-threating pulmonary embolism [4–6].

Several medical imaging techniques have been developed for diagnosing DVT in recent decades. X-ray contrast venography has traditionally been the gold standard [7]; however, the need for iodinated contrast agent and radiation exposure, as well as the technique's invasive nature, have led to its rare use in purely diagnostic settings [8]. Ultrasonography is currently a first-line technique used for the diagnosis in patients with clinically suspected DVT because of operation convenience, low cost, and high diagnostic sensitivity (94%) and specificity (98%) [9].

However, the disadvantages of ultrasound include operator dependence, limited visualization in the pelvis station, and an inability to differentiate the phases of thrombus [8, 10, 11] Cardiovascular magnetic resonance

* Correspondence: guoxixie@163.com
†Hanwei Chen and Xueping He contributed equally to this work.
3The Sixth Affiliated Hospital, Guangzhou Medical University, Xinzao, Panyu District, Qingyuan 511518, Guangdong, China
4Department of Biomedical Engineering of Basic Medical School, Guangzhou Medical University, Guangzhou 511436, Guangdong, China
Full list of author information is available at the end of the article

(CMR) imaging may serve as an alternative or complementary imaging tool to ultrasoiund [8, 12]. Previous studies have demonstrated that contrast-enhanced CMR venography (CE-CMRV) is reliable for assessing deep and superficial venous systems and has a high sensitivity (92%) and specificity (94.8%) for detecting DVT [13–15]. However, this technique may be contraindicated in patients with an allergy to gadolinium, and in pregnancy or severe renal dysfunction.

Other CMRV techniques that do not need contrast agent can also be used for the diagnosis of DVT. These techniques include time-of-flight, phase contrast, and balanced steady-state free precession (bSSFP), which all allow the indirect identification of thrombus because the stationary tissue shows a signal void within the venous lumen [16–18]. However, these techniques cannot directly visualize the thrombus signal, which is important for clinical decision-making in DVT treatment [19].

In 1997, Moody et al. introduced a contrast-free CMR technique called MR direct thrombus imaging (MRDTI) for the diagnosis of DVT [20]. The technique utilizes the short-T1 methemoglobin within the thrombus at certain phases (primarily acute and subacute) to generate a bright thrombus signal on T1-weighted images, thus allowing DVT to be readily identified [6]. However, owing to the low concentration in methemoglobin, hyperacute or chronic thrombi appear relatively dark on MRDTI, and their visualization can be confounded by the surrounding venous blood, potentially leading to an inaccurate estimation of DVT distribution. This necessitates a combination of the technique with MR venography when characterizing DVT progression [21].

Recently, three-dimensional (3D) T1-weighted black-blood CMR techniques have been developed for the diagnosis of DVT without the use of a contrast agent [22, 23]. The principle underlying the techniques is that venous blood flow signal is suppressed to allow the intra-luminal thrombus to be visualized within the venous lumen. The technique proposed by Treil et al. relies on the inherent black-blood effect of the 3D variable-flip-angle turbo spin-echo sequence, which may be inadequate for suppressing the signal from extremely slow venous blood flow [22]. An improved technique called black-blood thrombus imaging (BBTI) combines the same 3D turbo spin echo readout with an additional black-suppressing preparation, i.e., delay alternating with nutation for tailored excitation (DANTE), to achieve better DVT visualization [23]. A preliminary study demonstrated that BBTI can detect non-acute DVT at 3 Tesla (T) with high sensitivity (90.4%) and specificity (99.0%), using CE-CMRV as a reference.

The performance of BBTI for detecting acute (particularly hyperacute) DVT at a lower but more commonly used field strength (i.e., 1.5 T) remains unknown. A thrombus in the hyperacute phase is rich in deoxyhemoglobin rather than methemoglobin and can therefore have short T2

relaxation values [24, 25]. This may lead to lower signal intensity in acute DVT and reduced contrast between DVT and the surrounding venous blood and vessel wall. Lower signal-to-noise ratio (SNR) at 1.5 T may further impair the visualization of DVT. The purpose of this prospective study was to assess the image quality and diagnostic performance of BBTI at 1.5 T in patients with acute DVT, using CE-CMRV as the reference standard.

Methods
Subjects
Fifteen healthy subjects (38.1 ± 14.2 years, 7 women) with no history of peripheral vascular disease, and 30 acute DVT patients (54.1 ± 17.0 years, 22 women) were studied. The patients were consecutively enrolled from a local hospital from September 2015 to May 2017 (Table 1) and were all inpatients at the time of participation. One of the patients was first diagnosed with DVT 9 years ago and had a symptomatic recurrent ipsilateral DVT for 10 days. All the others were experiencing symptoms for the first time. The duration of symptoms was 7.3 ± 4.0 days (range, 2–14 days), and therefore all cases were deemed acute, according to the duration from symptom onset to CMR scan, as follows: acute phase (≤ 14 days), subacute phase (15–28 days), subacute-to-chronic phase (29–180 days), and chronic phase (> 180 days) [23, 26]. The initial diagnosis of DVT was made using the D-dimer test and ultrasound performed by experienced sonographers as part of routine standard of care. The ultrasound test only targeted the leg(s) with DVT symptoms, and the duration between

Table 1 Patient characteristics

Characteristics	
Age, mean ± SD (range), (years)	54.1 ± 17.0 (27–84)
Sex	8 male, 22 female
Body mass index	23.7 ± 1.4 (20.3–27.0)
Symptom duration, mean ± SD (range), (days)	7.3 ± 4.0 (2–14)
Symptom duration ≤7 days, n (%)	16 (53.3%)
Symptoms:	
Leg pain, n (%)	27 (90.0%)
Swollen leg, n (%)	30 (100%)
Local warmth, n (%)	24 (80.0%)
Recurrence (%), n (%)	1 (3.3%)
Pulmonary embolism, n (%)	4 (13.3%)
Recent trauma (< 1 month), n (%)	1 (3.3%)
Recent surgery (< 1 month), n (%)	6 (20.0%)
Previous venous thromboembolism, (pulmonary embolism or DVT), n (%)	1 (3.3%)

Note: *SD* standard deviation, *DVT* deep vein thrombosis

the ultrasound test and CMR scan was less than 24 h. The exclusion criteria were known contraindications to CMR (e.g., claustrophobia, pregnancy, gadolinium allergy or renal failure). This prospective study was approved by the institutional review board, and written informed consent was obtained from all the subjects.

CMR imaging

CMR imaging was performed on a 1.5 T scanner (MAGNE-TOM Avanto, Siemens Helathineers, Erlangen, Germany). BBTI was performed on both patients and healthy subjects. To scan the entire lower limb, each of the subjects was placed in the supine position (feet first) and underwent 3-station scanning using a 6-channel body coil and an 8-channel peripheral vascular coil, as well as integrated spine coils. The coverage of the first station was from the lower inferior vena cava to the proximal femoral vein, the second station from the femoral vein and deep femoral vein to the proximal popliteal vein, and the third station from the popliteal vein to the distal calf vein. The scan time of each station was 3–5 min. To evaluate the accuracy of BBTI for the diagnosis of DVT, CE-CMRV using a 3D gradient echo fast low-angle shot (FLASH) pulse sequence for data acquisition served as the reference standard and was only performed in the patients. Following a mask measurement, the FLASH sequence was initiated when contrast agent (gadopentetate dimeglumine [Magnevist; Bayer Pharmaceuticals, Leverkusen, Germany]) arrived at the iliac artery, as detected using the Care Bolus technique (Siemens Healthineers). A fixed dose of 30 mL (469 mg/mL) of contrast agent was administered intravenously at a speed of 3.0 mL/second in the median cubital vein using a remote-controlled injection system (Medrad Spectris, Indianola, Pennsylvania, USA). The contrast injection was followed by a 20 mL saline flush injected at the same rate. The scan was continuously repeated three times to capture a well-enhanced time frame. The scan parameters are presented in Table 2.

Image analysis

All the images were loaded onto a workstation (Leonardo, Siemens Healthineers) for post-processing and qualitative and quantitative evaluations by two readers (Y. Y. and W. D) with over 10 years' of CMR experience.

Qualitative image analysis at the vessel segment level was performed on both healthy subjects and DVT patients. The venous system of each lower limb was divided into the inferior vena cava (IVC), common, internal and external iliac veins, common femoral vein, femoral vein, deep femoral vein, popliteal vein, tibiofibular trunk vein, anterior and posterior tibial veins, fibular vein, and the great and small saphenous veins on both sides. If vessel collateralization was identified, the collateral segments were also assessed. Collateralization is defined as the growth of new veins that serve the same vascular bed as

Table 2 Imaging parameters of black blood thrombus imaging (BBTI) and contrast-enhanced cardiovascular magnetic resonance venography (CE-CMRV)

	BBTI	CE-CMRV
Repetition time (ms)	650	4.37
Echo time (ms)	11	1.41
Turbo factor	40	NA
Fat suppression	yes	no
Flip angle (degree)	T1 variable	25
FOV read (mm)	352	500
Number of partitions	208–256	112
Voxel size (mm^3)	$1.4 \times 1.4 \times 1.4$	$1.5 \times 1.1 \times 1.2$
Interpolated voxel size (mm^3)	$0.7 \times 0.7 \times 0.7$	$0.75 \times 0.55 \times 0.6$
Bandwidth (Hz/pixel)	698	250
DANTE pulse train length	125	NA
DANTE flip angle	15	NA

Note: *FOV* field-of-view, *DANTE* delay alternating with nutation for tailored excitation, *NA* non applicable

the original veins, which cannot themselves adequately supply the vascular bed. As collateral segments are usually too small or complex to be correctly identified, only the clots that blocked the collateral segments that were dilated large enough to be identified on both the BBTI and CE-CMRV images were considered for analysis.

All the images obtained from the healthy subjects and patients were mixed and randomized in preparation for reading on a per-segment vessel basis by two independent readers for the absence or presence of thrombus, without knowledge of each subject's information or the ultrasound test results. A time interval of 2 weeks was required for image review of BBTI and CE-CMRV to avoid memory bias. The image quality and diagnostic confidence of each observed venous segment in all the subjects were assessed on a 4-point scale (1: poor; 4: excellent) [22, 23]. If two readers disagreed with each other regarding the presence or absence of DVT on standard CE-MRV, the readers reached a consensus after checking all the available information, including the ultrasound results.

To illustrate that the thrombus in the acute phase had adequate signal intensity (SI) on the BBTI images for diagnosis, the apparent SNR of the thrombus, muscle, and the dark venous lumen were calculated as the mean SI divided by the noise (σ_n), and the apparent contrast-to-noise ratio (CNR) between the thrombus and the muscle ([$SI_{thrombus} - SI_{muscle}$]/$\sigma_n$) and between the thrombus and the venous lumen ([$SI_{thrombus} - SI_{lumen}$]/$\sigma_n$) were also calculated. The noise was the standard deviation of the SI determined in four artefact-free background regions to minimize bias due to the inhomogeneous signal. SI was measured as the mean signal intensity within a manually drawn region of interest (ROI). Notably, the ROIs of the thrombus and dark lumen were determined in consensus by the two readers. If visually different SI of the thrombi (i.e., iso- or hyper-intense signal relative to the muscle) were observed in the same patient, the SI was measured separately for the SNR and CNR calculations.

The feasibility of using BBTI for thrombus volume measurement and understanding thrombus progression in the acute phase was explored. Specifically, thrombi in each patient were segmented in a semiautomatic fashion using VesselMass (Vessel Mass, Leiden University Medical Center, Leiden,,The Netherlands), and iso–/hyperintense thrombi were measured separately for each patient. The percentage of the iso-intense thrombus in the total thrombus volume was calculated and reported for each patient.

Statistics

The image quality and diagnostic confidence scores of both healthy subjects and DVT patients were presented as the mean ± standard deviation (SD). Interobserver agreement using the kappa statistic was performed for the healthy subjects and patients in all the venous segments for the presence or absence of thrombus, image quality, and diagnostic confidence of BBTI.

The sensitivity, specificity, positive and negative predictive values, and accuracy of BBTI in the diagnosis of DVT patients were calculated using a standard 4×4 contingency table, with the consensus CE-CMRV as a reference. A paired sample Student's t test was used to compare the continuous variables, and the data were presented as the mean ± SD. Interobserver agreement and agreement between BBTI and the consensus CE-CMRV were tested using Cohen's κ test. Agreement was rated as fair (kappa value κ = 0.21–0.40), moderate (κ = 0.41–0.6), substantial (κ = 0.61–0.80), or excellent (κ > 0.80) [27]. Of note, $p < 0.05$ indicated statistical significance. Linear regression was used to demonstrate the trends of the thrombus signal variation along with the duration of symptom onset increase. The Statistical Package for the Social Sciences (SPSS 17.0, International Business Machines, Armonk, New York, USA) software was used for the statistical analysis.

Results

All participants successfully completed the CMR examinations, and no adverse events occurred. The thrombi within the black-blood venous lumen appeared iso- and/or hyper-intense relative to the muscle signal intensity on the BBTI images. Both large thrombi (Figs. 1 and 2) and small thrombi (Fig. 3) were correctly visualized by BBTI. Their location and size were visually matched with those detected using CE-CMRV. According to the apparent SNR and CNR analysis, both the iso- and hyperintense thrombi had

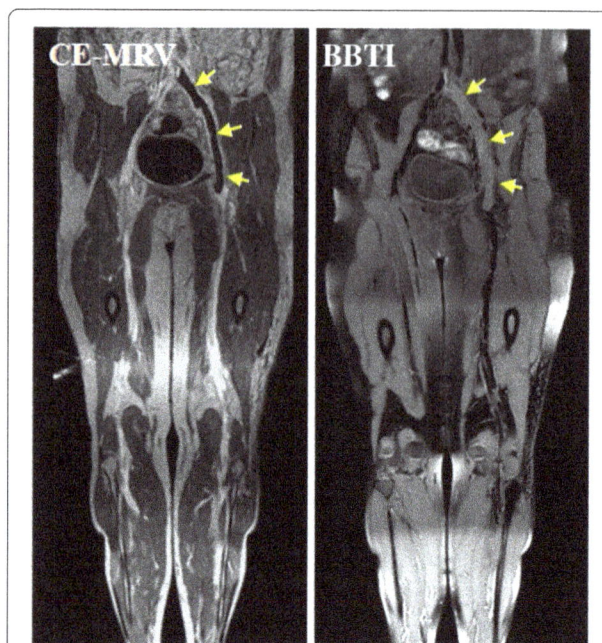

Fig. 1 Representative images obtained by contrast-enhanced cardiovascular magnetic resonance (CE-CMRV) and black blood thrombus imaging (BBTI) from a 55-year-old woman with deep venous thrombosis (DVT) symptom onset at 5 days. The thrombus detected by BBTI showed iso-intense signals within the black-blood venous lumen. The locations and sizes of the thrombi between BBTI and CE-CMRV matched (yellow arrows)

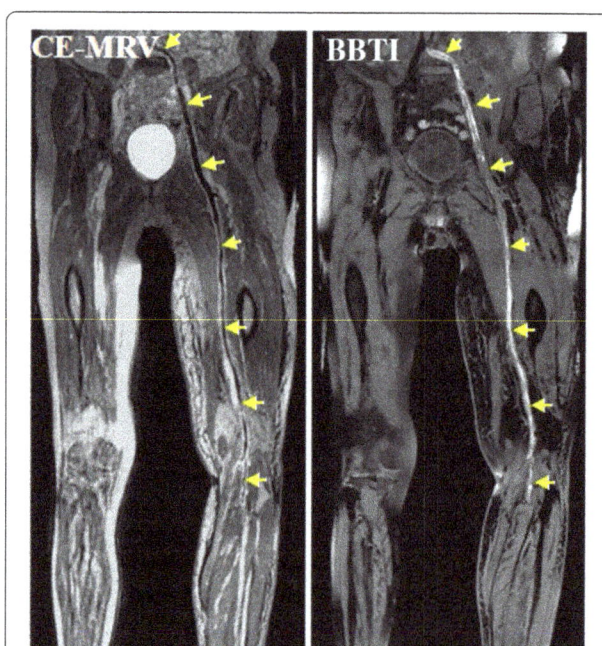

Fig. 2 Representative images obtained by CE-CMRV and BBTI from a 68-year-old woman with DVT symptom onset at 8 days. The thrombus detected by BBTI showed iso- and hyperintense signals within the black-blood venous lumen. The locations and sizes of the thrombi between BBTI and CE-CMRV matched (yellow arrows)

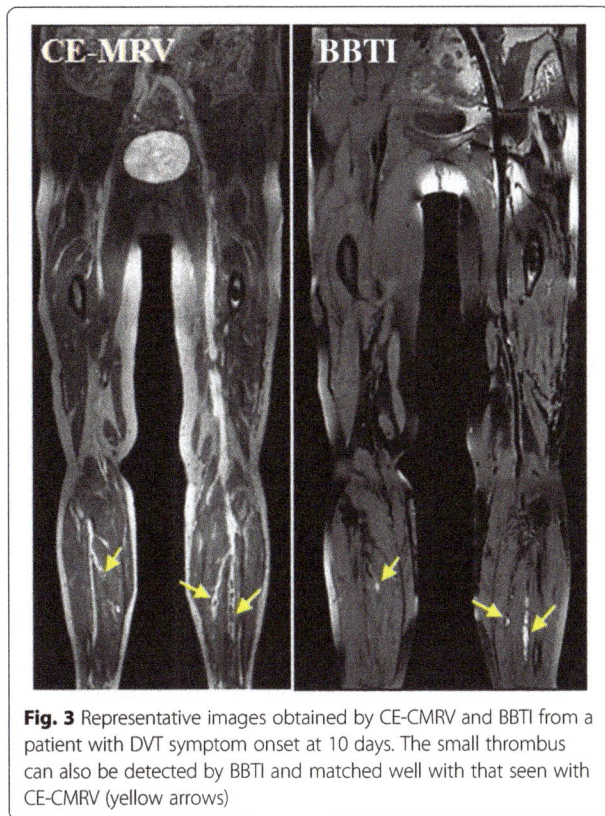

Fig. 3 Representative images obtained by CE-CMRV and BBTI from a patient with DVT symptom onset at 10 days. The small thrombus can also be detected by BBTI and matched well with that seen with CE-CMRV (yellow arrows)

adequate signal intensities for diagnosis (Fig. 4). According to the linear regression analysis, the thrombus signal intensity has the tendency to become higher as the duration of symptom onset increases (Figs. 5 and 6).

The image quality (3.62 ± 0.50 vs. 3.62 ± 0.59) and diagnostic confidence (3.68 ± 0.48 vs. 3.67 ± 0.56) of BBTI were good or excellent for the healthy subjects and patients. No part of any venous segment from the

healthy subjects was misidentified as being positive by either reader. In other words, all the healthy subjects were correctly identified from among the participants by both readers, using only the BBTI images. The interobserver agreements of BBTI were excellent in all the venous segments of the healthy subjects and patients regarding the presence or absence of thrombus, image quality, and diagnostic confidence (Table 3).

In total, 870 venous segments from thirty patients were observed by both BBTI and CE-CMRV. Eight of these (i.e., one popliteal vein, 2 anterior tibial veins, 1 posterior tibial veins, 3 fibular veins, and 1 small saphenous vein) demonstrated poor diagnostic confidence (i.e., score < 2) on the BBTI images and three (i.e., one popliteal vein, 1 posterior tibial vein, and 1 fibular vein) were seen on the CE-CMRV images. Thus, these eight segments were excluded, and the other 862 segments were used for statistical analysis. BBTI provided a comparable diagnostic confidence score for patients compared with CE-CMRV (average over the two readers: 3.69 ± 0.52 vs. 3.70 ± 0.47, $p = 0.23$). All the patients were confirmed to have thrombi on both the BBTI and CE-CMRV images. According to the consensus reading of CE-CMRV, thrombi were identified in 227 of 862 venous segments (26.3%) (Table 4). No free-floating thrombus was detected by either BBTI or CE-CMRV. The underlying reason may be related to the limits of spatial resolution and the lack of dynamic information provided by BBTI and CE-CMRV. The locations of the thrombi in the 227 venous segments included 65 abdominopelvic venous segments (28.6%), 92 femoral-popliteal venous segments (40.5%), 43 calf venous segments (18.9%), 9 superficial venous segments (4.0%), and 18 collateral branch venous segments (7.9%). Both CE-CMRV and BBTI showed above-knee DVT in 8 patients, calf DVT associated with

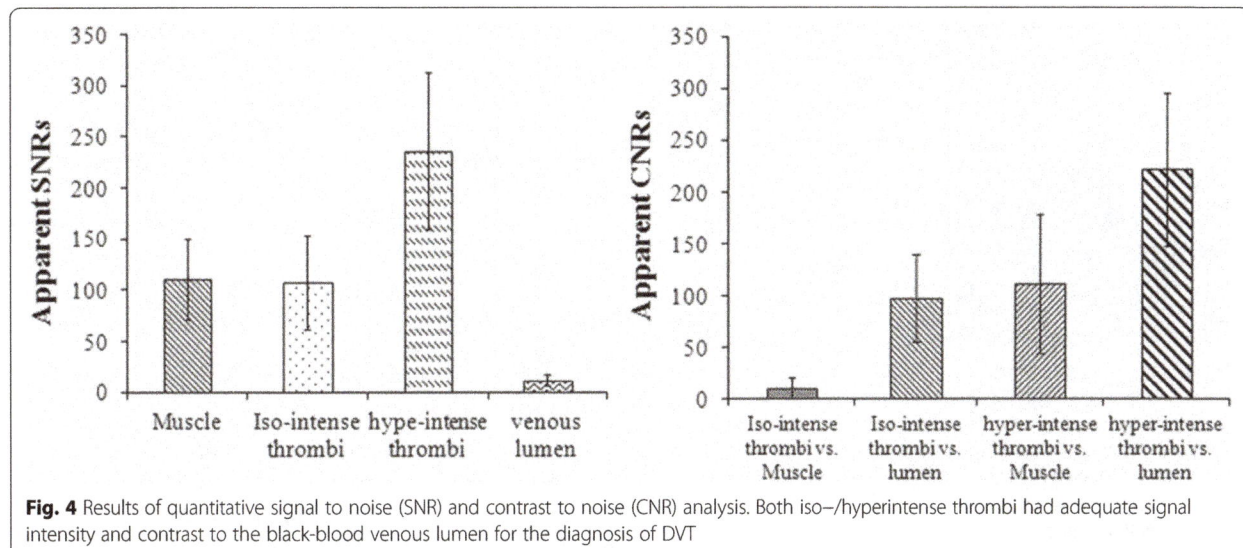

Fig. 4 Results of quantitative signal to noise (SNR) and contrast to noise (CNR) analysis. Both iso–/hyperintense thrombi had adequate signal intensity and contrast to the black-blood venous lumen for the diagnosis of DVT

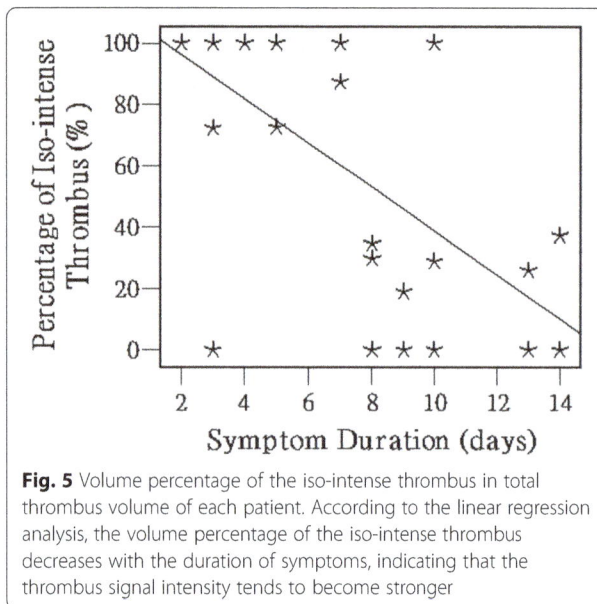

Fig. 5 Volume percentage of the iso-intense thrombus in total thrombus volume of each patient. According to the linear regression analysis, the volume percentage of the iso-intense thrombus decreases with the duration of symptoms, indicating that the thrombus signal intensity tends to become stronger

above-knee DVT in 22 patients, and 8 of the 30 patients had IVC thrombosis. Using the consensus CE-CMRV diagnosis as the reference standard, the overall sensitivity (95.2%), SP (98.6%), positive predictive value (96.0%), negative predictive value (98.3%), and accuracy (97.7%) were obtained by BBTI (Table 5). In addition, BBTI had a higher sensitivity (97.4 vs.

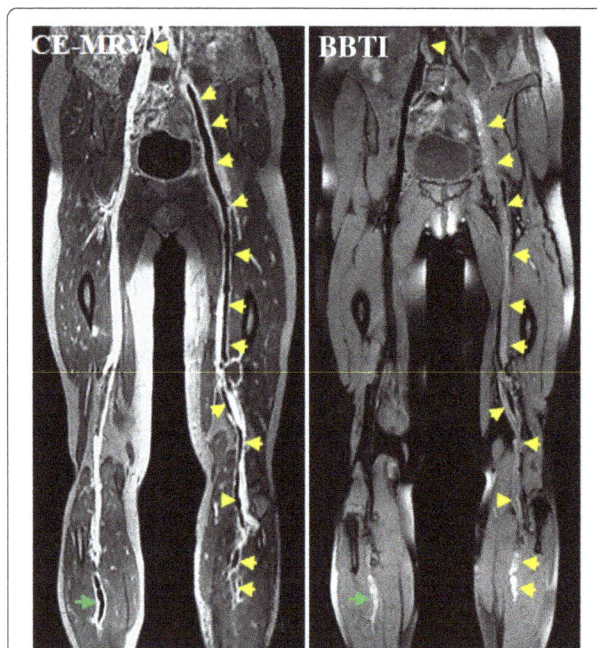

Fig. 6 Example images obtained in 50-year-old woman with DVT symptom onset at 3 days. The thrombus (green arrows) was detected by BBTI at the asymptomatic right leg, which was missed by the initial ultrasound and confirmed by CE-CMRV. Most parts of the thrombi (yellow arrows) appeared as isointense signals on the BBTI images. The locations and sizes of the thrombi between BBTI and CE-CMRV matched

81.4%), specificity (99.3 vs. 99.0%), and accuracy (98.7 vs. 95.7%) for the diagnosis of DVT above the knee compared to that below the knee. Notably, thrombus was also identified in the asymptomatic legs of three patients using BBTI; this was not identified by the initial ultrasound test and confirmed by CE-CMRV (Fig. 6).

Excellent agreement was noted between BBTI and CE-CMRV regarding the presence or absence of thrombus (reader 1, $\kappa = 0.94$, $p < 0.001$; and reader 2, $\kappa = 0.92$, $p < 0.001$).

Discussion

In this prospective study, BBTI demonstrated a high sensitivity, specificity, and accuracy for the diagnosis of acute DVT at 1.5 T, without the use of a CMR contrast agent. Additionally, excellent diagnostic confidence scores and agreement with CE-CMRV on the diagnosis of DVT were achieved by BBTI. These findings were consistent with those of a previous study at 3 T [23] Thus, BBTI has the capacity to diagnose acute DVT at 1.5 T.

BBTI has some remarkable technical advantages for the diagnosis of DVT. If the venous blood flow signals are effectively suppressed while the thrombus has adequate signal intensity, the thrombus can be directly identified within the venous lumen. BBTI not only exploits the inherent black-blood effect of the SPACE readout but also the DANTE black-blood preparation for a more robust signal suppression of venous blood flow [28, 29]. Additionally, the SPACE readout used in BBTI is a variant of a spin echo sequence for 3D imaging that has an intrinsically high SNR and rapid data acquisition, which allows for the BBTI scan within a reasonable scan duration (i.e., less than 15 min for the entire lower limbs) and provides adequate thrombus signals for detection, even if the scan is performed at 1.5 T. Moreover, SPACE was configured as a T1-weighted readout. Because the image weighting of a DANTE sequence is dominated by the readout (not the DANTE preparation), [30, 31] BBTI is a T1-weighted technique that has advantages for the diagnosis of DVT. Thus, the diagnostic confidence score of BBTI is comparable to that of CE-CMRV, and an overall high sensitivity, specificity, negative/positive predictive value and accuracy can be obtained by BBTI at 1.5 T for the diagnosis of acute DVT.

BBTI may have a specific role in several scenarios for the diagnosis of DVT. First, unlike ultrasound, which often exclusively scans the symptomatic leg(s) with the goal of time efficiency, [32, 33] BBTI with a 3-station scan can cover both lower limbs. This feature is important for the diagnosis of asymptomatic DVT. In this study, DVT was detected in the asymptomatic contralateral legs of three patients, lesions that were not identified in the initial ultrasound test. Second, BBTI may be useful for the identification of thrombus in the pelvis, which is challenging for ultrasound [34]. In this study, a

Table 3 Results of interobserver agreement between the two readers for diagnosis of DVT, image quality, and diagnostic confidence of BBTI

Vessel segments	Diagnosis of DVT Interobserver agreement ((κ / p))	Image Quality Interobserver agreement ((κ / p))	Diagnostic Confidence Interobserver agreement ((κ / p))
Abdominopelvic veins	1.00 / < 0.001	0.78 / < 0.001	0.61 / < 0.001
Femoral-popliteal veins	0.95 / < 0.001	0.69 / < 0.001	0.65 / < 0.001
Calf veins	0.87 / < 0.001	0.73 / < 0.001	0.75 / < 0.001
Superficial veins	0.88 / < 0.001	0.79 / < 0.001	0.77 / < 0.001
Collateral branch veins	0.91 / < 0.001	0.95 / < 0.001	0.83 / < 0.001
Overall	0.94 / < 0.001	0.82 / < 0.001	0.80 / < 0.001

Note: DVT deep vein thrombosis, BBTI black-blood magnetic resonance thrombus imaging

high sensitivity (98.5%) and specificity (100%) in the abdominopelvic segments without the use of a gadolinium based contrast agent were achieved using BBTI. Third, unlike the time-of flight, phase contrast, and bSSFP techniques, which indirectly identify the thrombus through blood filling defects, BBTI allows the direct visualization of the thrombus and measurement of thrombus signal intensity. This is beneficial for DVT treatment decision-making and could be complimentary to time of flight, phase contrast, and bSSFP imaging. Lastly, BBTI is more suited than ultrasound for the differentiation of acutely formed thrombus

compared with chronic thrombus. The recurrence rate of DVT remains high (20–40%) [21, 35]. It is necessary to identify newly formed thrombus during monitoring of the progression of DVT and guide therapy for avoiding further complications such as pulmonary embolism [36]. As a noninvasive, contrast-free and time-efficient technique, BBTI could be suitable for this evaluation.

Signal variation of the thrombus in the acute phase was observed on the BBTI images. The thrombus signal change has the tendency to increase with the duration of symptom onset. This signal variation may result from variation in the

Table 4 Results of BBTI and CE-CMRV examinations in 862 vessel segments

Vessel segments	BBTI(Reader1/Reader2) Thrombus present	Thrombus absent	Consensus of CE-CMRV Thrombus present	Thrombus absent
Abdominopelvic veins				
Inferior vena cava	8/8	22/22	8	22
Common iliac vein	18/18	42/42	18	42
Internal iliac vein	16/16	44/44	18	42
External iliac vein	21/21	39/39	21	39
Femoral-popliteal veins				
Common femoral vein	23/24	37/36	24	36
Femoral vein	27/27	33/33	27	33
Deep femoral vein	17/15	43/45	16	44
Popliteal vein	27/25	32/34	25	34
Calf veins				
Tibiofibular trunk vein	14/17	46/43	16	44
Anterior tibial vein	1/2	57/56	3	55
Posterior tibial vein	11/11	48/48	11	48
Fibular vein	11/8	46/49	13	44
Superficial veins				
Great saphenous vein	9/8	51/52	9	51
Small saphenous vein	0/1	59/58	0	59
Collateral branch veins	22/21	38/39	18	42
Total	225/222	637/640	227	635

Note: BBTI black-blood magnetic resonance thrombus imaging, CE-CMRV contrast-enhanced cardiovascular magnetic resonance venography

Table 5 Qualitative and statistical analysis results of BBTI for the diagnosis of DVT using consensus CE-CMRV as the reference standard

Vessel segments	Sensitivity (%) Reader1 /Reader 2	Specificity (%) Reader1 /Reader 2	Positive predictive value (%) Reader1 /Reader 2	Negative predictive value (%) Reader1 /Reader 2	Accuracy (%) Reader1 /Reader 2
Abdominopelvic veins	98.5 / 98.5	100 / 100	100 / 100	99.3 / 99.3	99.5 / 99.5
Femoral-popliteal veins	98.9 / 96.7	98.0 / 98.6	96.8 / 97.8	99.3 / 98.0	98.3 / 97.9
Calf veins	81.4 / 79.1	99.0 / 97.9	94.6 / 89.5	95.9 / 95.4	95.7 / 94.4
The superficial veins	100 / 88.9	100 / 99.1	100 / 88.9	100 / 99.1	100 / 98.3
Collateral branch veins	100 / 94.4	90.5 / 90.5	81.8 / 81.0	100 / 97.4	93.3 / 91.7
Overall	95.2 / 93.0	98.6 / 98.3	96.0 / 95.0	98.3 / 97.5	97.7 / 96.9

Note: *BBTI* black-blood magnetic resonance thrombus imaging, *CE-CMRV* contrast-enhanced cardiovascular magnetic resonance venography

concentration of methemoglobin in the thrombus. Previous studies have demonstrated that T1-weighted contrast is superior in the detection of thrombus because there is a linear relationship between the concentration of methemoglobin and T1 shortening of the venous thrombus [19, 37]. The higher the concentration of methemoglobin, the shorter the T1 relaxation time of the thrombus and thus, the brighter the thrombus signals on the T1-weighted image. BBTI may serve as a useful imaging tool for understanding thrombus progression because BBTI is a T1-weighed imaging technique and has the capacity for excellent separation between DVT and the surrounding venous lumen. This should be evaluated in a systematic study with a larger patient cohort.

BBTI provides a higher sensitivity above the knee than below the knee in acute DVT patients. Only two thrombi presenting as isointense in the internal iliac vein went unrecognized by either reader. However, a reassessment of the misinterpreted venous segments above the knee showed consistent results with CE-CMRV. Interpretation of the thrombus below the knee is more difficult. This may be caused by the small and complex anatomy of the calf vessel, the insufficient spatial resolution provided by BBTI, and the thrombus appearing as isointense relative to the adjacent muscle signals. Improving the spatial resolution is possible but would prolong the scan time and reduce the image SNR. Nevertheless, the interobserver agreement was excellent, and the findings in this study were consistent with current CMR techniques and ultrasound [18, 32, 38, 39].

It should be noted that some residual blood signals remain apparent on the BBTI images because there is little or no blood flow. This is not a problem unique to the BBTI technique, but is a common problem when the contrast is based on blood flow suppression or enhancement, such as with the widely used technique of ultrasound. Nevertheless, the thrombus and residual blood can be differentiated by an experienced radiologist. This is because DVT is often characterized by obstruction/ dilatation of the involved veins and the clot is heterogeneous. Thus, the thrombus appeared as a signal with isolated and/or inhomogeneity intensity within the black venous lumen. In contrast, the residual blood often appeared as an iso- and homogeneous intense signal at the tortuous popliteal vein and the small calf vein.

There were several limitations to this work. First, the leg fat on the BBTI images was not suppressed well due to B0/B1 field inhomogeneity. However, the thrombus was within the venous lumen and the BBTI images could be reformatted with arbitrary orientation. Both the qualitative and quantitative analysis results demonstrated that fat suppression was not a significant issue in the identification of the thrombus. Second, conventional x-ray venography was not available for comparison as the reference standard. That for our study was established by consensus with CE-CMRV and, if necessary, with the assistance of ultrasound. This is because conventional x-ray venography is rarely used as a purely diagnostic modality in clinical settings. CE-CMRV has been shown in multiple studies to have an extremely high sensitivity and specificity compared with contrast venography [12, 14, 34]. Third, gadopentetate dimeglumine was used as the contrast agent because it is a globally recognized agent with a history of wide use, and it possesses the most comprehensive safety database. However, gadobenate dimeglumine could be considered for as a contrast agent in future studies because it can achieve the same contrast effect at a lower dose. Fourth, the current data only focused on acute DVT patients. Further evaluation of the diagnostic performance for thrombus at different phases should be performed on a larger group of DVT patients in future studies.

Conclusions

BBTI exhibits excellent diagnostic performance on acute DVT at 1.5 T. BBTI is a promising technique that can be used for the diagnosis in clinical practice of acute DVT without the use of a contrast agent.

Abbreviations

3D: Three-dimensional; BBTI: Black-blood thrombus imaging; bSSFP: Balanced steady state free precession; CE-CMRV: Contrast-enhanced cardiovascular magnetic resonance venography; CMR: Cardiovascular magnetic Resonance; CNR: Contrast-to-noise ratio; DANTE: Delay alternating with nutation for tailored excitation; DVT: Deep vein thrombosis; FLASH: Fast low-angle shot; IVC: Inferior vena cava; MRDTI: Magnetic resonance direct thrombus imaging; PTS: Post-thrombotic syndrome; ROI: Region-of-interest; SD: Standard deviation; SI: Signal intensity; SNR: Signal-to-noise ratio; SPACE: three-dimensional variable flip angle turbo-spin-echo; T: Tesla

Funding
This work was supported in part by the National Science Foundation of China (81571669, 81729003), the Natural Science Foundation of Shenzhen (JCYJ20160331185933583, JCYJ20160531174850658), and the Natural Science Foundation of Guangdong (2017A050501026, 2014A030313691).

Authors' contributions
HC, XH, and GX designed the experiments, performed the data collection, and drafted the manuscript. ZH and JL were responsible for data collection. YY and WD conducted image analysis. DL was responsible for the statistical analysis. DL, XL, and ZF contributed to the writing and editing of the manuscript. ZF provided BBTI sequence support. All the authors gave final approval of the version to be published.

Competing interests
The authors declare that they have no competing interests.

Author details
[1]Department of Radiology, Guangzhou Panyu Central Hospital, Guangzhou 511400, Guangdong, China. [2]Medical Imaging Institute of Panyu, Guangzhou 511400, Guangdong, China. [3]The Sixth Affiliated Hospital, Guangzhou Medical University, Xinzao, Panyu District, Qingyuan 511518, Guangdong, China. [4]Department of Biomedical Engineering of Basic Medical School, Guangzhou Medical University, Guangzhou 511436, Guangdong, China. [5]Biomedical Imaging Research Institute, Cedars-Sinai Medical Center, Los Angeles, CA 90048, USA. [6]Lauterbur Research Center for Biomedical Imaging, Shenzhen Institutes of Advanced Technology, Chinese Academy of Sciences, Shenzhen 518055, Guangdong, China.

References
1. Heit JA, Silverstein MD, Mohr DN, Petterson TM, O'Fallon WM, Melton LJ. Predictors of survival after deep vein thrombosis and pulmonary embolism: a population-based, cohort study. Arch Intern Med. 1999;159:445–53.
2. Heit JA. The epidemiology of venous thromboembolism in the community. Arterioscler Thromb Vasc Biol. 2008;28:370–2.
3. Beckman MG, Hooper WC, Critchley SE, Ortel TL. Venous thromboembolism: a public health concern. Am J Prev Med. 2010;38:S495–501.
4. Zhang X, Ren Q, Jiang X, Sun J, Gong J, Tang B, et al. A prospective randomized trial of catheter-directed thrombolysis with additional balloon dilatation for iliofemoral deep venous thrombosis: a single-center experience. Cardiovasc Intervent Radiol. 2014;37:958–68.
5. Janssen MC, Wollersheim H, Schultze-Kool LJ, Thien T. Local and systemic thrombolytic therapy for acute deep venous thrombosis. Neth J Med. 2005;63:81–90.
6. Tan M, Mol GC, van Rooden CJ, Klok FA, Westerbeek RE, del Sol AI, et al. Magnetic resonance direct thrombus imaging differentiates acute recurrent ipsilateral deep vein thrombosis from residual thrombosis. Blood. 2014;124: 623–7.
7. Carpenter JP, Holland GA, Baum RA, Owen RS, Carpenter JT, Cope C. Magnetic resonance venography for the detection of deep venous

thrombosis: comparison with contrast venography and duplex Doppler ultrasonography. J Vasc Surg. 1993;18:734–41.
8. Tan M, van Rooden CJ, Westerbeek RE, Huisman MV. Diagnostic management of clinically suspected acute deep vein thrombosis. Br J Haematol. 2009;146:347–60.
9. Goodacre S, Sampson F, Thomas S, van Beek E, Sutton A. Systematic review and meta-analysis of the diagnostic accuracy of ultrasonography for deep vein thrombosis. BMC Med Imaging. 2005;5:6.
10. Righini M. Is it worth diagnosing and treating distal deep vein thrombosis? No. J Thromb Haemost. 2007;5:55–9.
11. El Kheir D, Büller H. One-time comprehensive ultrasonography to diagnose deep venous thrombosis: is that the solution? Ann Intern Med. 2004;140:1052–3.
12. Huisman MV, Klok FA. Diagnostic management of acute deep vein thrombosis and pulmonary embolism. J Thromb Haemost. 2013;11:412–22.
13. Huang SY, Kim CY, Miller MJ, Gupta RT, Lessne ML, Horvath JJ, et al. Abdominopelvic and lower extremity deep venous thrombosis: evaluation with contrast-enhanced MR venography with a blood-pool agent. AJR Am J Roentgenol. 2013;201:208–14.
14. Ruehm S, Zimny K, Debatin J. Direct contrast-enhanced 3D MR venography. Eur Radiol. 2001;11:102–12.
15. Sampson FC, Goodacre SW, Thomas SM, van Beek EJ. The accuracy of MRI in diagnosis of suspected deep vein thrombosis: systematic review and meta-analysis. Eur Radiol. 2007;17:175–81.
16. Orbell JH, Smith A, Burnand KG, Waltham M. Imaging of deep vein thrombosis. Br J Surg. 2008;95:137–46.
17. Li W, Salanitri J, Tutton S, Dunkle EE, Schneider JR, Caprini JA, et al. Lower extremity deep venous thrombosis: evaluation with ferumoxytol-enhanced MR imaging and dual-contrast mechanism–preliminary experience. Radiology. 2007;242:873–81.
18. Cantwell CP, Cradock A, Bruzzi J, Fitzpatrick P, Eustace S, Murray JG. MR Venography with true fast imaging with steady-state precession for suspected Lowerlimb deep vein thrombosis. J Vasc Interv Radiol. 2006;17:1763–70.
19. Saha P, Andia ME, Modarai B, Blume U, Humphries J, Patel AS, et al. Magnetic resonance T1 relaxation time of venous thrombus is determined by iron processing and predicts susceptibility to lysis. Circulation. 2013;128:729–36.
20. Moody AR. Direct imaging of deep-vein thrombosis with magnetic resonance imaging. Lancet. 1997;350:1073.
21. Mendichovszky IA, Priest AN, Bowden DJ, Hunter S, Joubert I, Hilborne S, et al. Combined MR direct thrombus imaging and non-contrast magnetic resonance venography reveal the evolution of deep vein thrombosis: a feasibility study. Eur Radiol. 2017;27:2326–32.
22. Treitl KM, Treitl M, Kooijman-Kurfuerst H, Kammer NN, Coppenrath E, Suderland E, et al. Three-dimensional black-blood T1-weighted turbo spin-echo techniques for the diagnosis of deep vein thrombosis in comparison with contrast-enhanced magnetic resonance imaging: a pilot study. Investig Radiol. 2015;50:401–8.
23. Xie GX, Chen HW, He XP, Liang JK, Deng W, He ZN, et al. Black-blood thrombus imaging (BTI): a contrast-free cardiovascular magnetic resonance approach for the diagnosis of non-acute deep vein thrombosis. J Cardiovasc Magn Reson. 2017;19:4.
24. Kimura K, Iguchi Y, Shibazaki K, Watanabe M, Iwanaga T, Aoki J. M1 susceptibility vessel sign on T2* as a strong predictor for no early recanalization after IV-t-PA in acute ischemic stroke. Stroke. 2009;40:3130–2.
25. Bradley WG Jr. MR appearance of hemorrhage in the brain. Radiology. 1993; 189:15–26.
26. Vedantham S, Grassi CJ, Ferral H, Patel NH, Thorpe PE, Antonacci VP, et al. Reporting standards for endovascular treatment of lower extremity deep vein thrombosis. J Vasc Interv Radiol. 2009;20:S391–408.
27. Landis JR, Koch GG. The measurement of observer agreement for categorical data. Biometrics. 1977;33:159–74.
28. Xie Y, Yang Q, Xie G, Pang J, Fan Z, Li D. Improved black-blood imaging using DANTE-SPACE for simultaneous carotid and intracranial vessel wall evaluation. Magn Reson Med. 2016;75:2286–94.
29. Wang J, Helle M, Zhou Z, Bornert P, Hatsukami TS, Yuan C. Joint blood and cerebrospinal fluid suppression for intracranial vessel wall MRI. Magn Reson Med. 2016;75:831–8.
30. Li L, Chai JT, Biasiolli L, Robson MD, Choudhury RP, Handa AI, et al. Black-blood multicontrast imaging of carotid arteries with DANTE-prepared 2D and 3D MR imaging. Radiology. 2014;273:560–9.

31. Li L, Miller KL, Jezzard P. DANTE-prepared pulse trains: a novel approach to motion-sensitized and motion-suppressed quantitative magnetic resonance imaging. Magn Reson Med. 2012;68:1423–38.

32. Fraser DG, Moody AR, Morgan PS, Martel AL, Davidson I. Diagnosis of lower-limb deep venous thrombosis: a prospective blinded study of magnetic resonance direct thrombus imaging. Ann Intern Med. 2002;136:89–98.

33. Hulle TVD, Dronkers CEA, Huisman MV, Klok FA. Current standings in diagnostic management of acute venous thromboembolism: still rough around the edges. Blood Rev. 2016;30:21–6.

34. Aschauer M, Deutschmann HA, Stollberger R, Hausegger KA, Obernosterer A, Schöllnast H, et al. Value of a blood pool contrast agent in MR venography of the lower extremities and pelvis: preliminary results in 12 patients. Magn Reson Med. 2003;50:993–1002.

35. Goldhaber SZ, Bounameaux H. Pulmonary embolism and deep vein thrombosis. Lancet. 2012;379:1835–46.

36. Bates SM, Jaeschke R, Stevens SM, Goodacre S, Wells PS, Stevenson MD, et al. Diagnosis of DVT: antithrombotic therapy and prevention of thrombosis, 9th ed: American College of Chest Physicians evidence-based clinical practice guidelines. Chest. 2012;141:e351S–418S.

37. Blume U, Orbell J, Waltham M, Smith A, Razavi R, Schaeffter T. 3D T 1-mapping for the characterization of deep vein thrombosis. MAGMA. 2009;22:375–83.

38. Evans AJ, Sostman HD, Witty LA, Paulson EK, Spritzer CE, Hertzberg BS, et al. Detection of deep venous thrombosis: prospective comparison of MR imaging and sonography. J Magn Reson Imaging. 1996;6:44–51.

39. Larsson E-M, Sundén P, Olsson C-G, Debatin Jr, Duerinckx AJ, Baum R, et al. MR venography using an intravascular contrast agent: results from a multicenter phase 2 study of dosage. AJR Am J Roentgenol. 2003;180:227–32.

16

Noninvasive hematocrit assessment for cardiovascular magnetic resonance extracellular volume quantification using a point-of-care device and synthetic derivation

Sean Robison[1], Gauri Rani Karur[1], Rachel M. Wald[1,2], Paaladinesh Thavendiranathan[1,2], Andrew M. Crean[1,2] and Kate Hanneman[1*]

Abstract

Background: Calculation of cardiovascular magnetic resonance (CMR) extracellular volume (ECV) requires input of hematocrit, which may not be readily available. The purpose of this study was to evaluate the diagnostic accuracy of ECV calculated using various noninvasive measures of hematocrit compared to ECV calculated with input of laboratory hematocrit as the reference standard.

Methods: One hundred twenty three subjects (47.7 ± 14.1 years; 42% male) were prospectively recruited for CMR T1 mapping between August 2016 and April 2017. Laboratory hematocrit was assessed by venipuncture. Noninvasive hematocrit was assessed with a point-of-care (POC) device (Pronto-7® Pulse CO-Oximeter®, Masimo Personal Health, Irvine, California, USA) and by synthetic derivation based on the relationship with blood pool T1 values. Left ventricular ECV was calculated with input of laboratory hematocrit (Lab-ECV), POC hematocrit (POC-ECV), and synthetic hematocrit (synthetic-ECV), respectively. Statistical analysis included Wilcoxon signed-rank test, Bland-Altman analysis, receiver-operating curve analysis and intra-class correlation (ICC).

Results: There was no significant difference between Lab-ECV and POC-ECV ($27.1 \pm 4.7\%$ vs. $27.3 \pm 4.8\%$, $p = 0.106$), with minimal bias and modest precision (bias $- 0.18\%$, 95%CI [$- 2.85$, 2.49]). There was no significant difference between Lab-ECV and synthetic-ECV ($26.7 \pm 4.4\%$ vs. $26.5 \pm 4.3\%$, $p = 0.084$) in subjects imaged at 1.5 T, although bias was slightly higher and limits of agreement were wider (bias 0.23%, 95%CI [$- 2.82$, 3.27]). For discrimination of abnormal Lab-ECV $\geq 30\%$, POC-ECV had good diagnostic performance (sensitivity 85%, specificity 96%, accuracy 94%, and AUC 0.902) and synthetic-ECV had moderate diagnostic performance (sensitivity 71%, specificity 98%, accuracy 93%, and AUC 0.849). POC-ECV had excellent test-retest (ICC 0.994, 95%CI[0.987, 0.997]) and inter-observer agreement (ICC 0.974, 95%CI[0.929, 0.991]).

Conclusions: Myocardial ECV can be accurately and reproducibly calculated with input of hematocrit measured using a noninvasive POC device, potentially overcoming an important barrier to implementation of ECV. Further evaluation of synthetic ECV is required prior to clinical implementation.

Keywords: Cardiovascular magnetic resonance (CMR), T1 mapping, Extracellular volume (ECV), Noninvasive hemoglobin monitoring, Hematocrit

* Correspondence: kate.hanneman@uhn.ca
[1]Department of Medical Imaging, Toronto General Hospital, University Health Network, University of Toronto, 585 University Ave, 1PMB-298, Toronto, ON M5G 2N2, Canada
Full list of author information is available at the end of the article

Background

Myocardial extracellular volume (ECV) fraction derived from cardiovascular magnetic resonance (CMR) T1 mapping has been validated based on histology [1–3], with demonstrated prognostic significance in several conditions [4–6]. Calculation of ECV requires accurate and timely assessment of hematocrit, to correct for the blood contrast volume of distribution [7]. Traditional laboratory determination of hematocrit via venipuncture in the setting of ECV evaluation is costly, mildly uncomfortable for the patient, and often inconvenient. Therefore, rapid noninvasive determination of hematocrit would be beneficial in the setting of ECV analysis.

Noninvasive point-of-care (POC) devices have recently become commercially available, providing immediate hemoglobin and hematocrit results without the need for blood sampling by venipuncture or finger prick [8–10]. Additionally, synthetic derivation of hematocrit has recently been described based on the relationship between hematocrit and non-contrast blood pool T1 values [11]. However, there are important limitations to synthetic analysis, as each specific acquisition scheme requires derivation and validation [12]. A recent study suggests that synthetic ECV may result in miscategorization of individual patients [13].

The purpose of this study was to evaluate the diagnostic accuracy of CMR ECV calculated using noninvasive measures of hematocrit (determined with a POC device and synthetic derivation) compared to ECV calculated with input of laboratory hematocrit as the reference standard. We hypothesized that there would be no significant difference in myocardial ECV calculated using noninvasive measures of hematocrit as compared with ECV derived from laboratory hematocrit.

Methods

Study population

Institutional research ethics board approval was obtained for this prospective study. Between August 2016 and April 2017, 149 subjects undergoing clinical or research CMR were prospectively recruited for T1 mapping with calculation of ECV. Written informed consent was obtained from all study subjects. Exclusion criteria included incomplete or aborted CMR ($n = 4$), subject refusal of intravenous contrast administration ($n = 2$), substantial artifact precluding image analysis ($n = 4$), and failure of POC device analysis (due to the presence of gel nail polish, marked hand tremor, and/or inadequate signal) ($n = 16$). The final cohort of 123 subjects included both patients and healthy subjects (47.7 ± 14.1 years; 42% male). Clinical and demographic information were extracted from the electronic patient record.

CMR technique

CMR was performed at 1.5 T ($n = 74$, Magnetom Avanto, Siemens Healthineers, Erlangen, Germany) or 3 T ($n = 34$, Magnetom Skyra, Siemens Healthineers; and $n = 15$ Biograph mMR, Siemens Healthineers). Retrospectively gated balanced steady-state free precession (bSSFP) cine images were obtained for assessment of left ventricular (LV) size and function by a stack of short-axis slices with coverage from cardiac base to the apex with 8-mm thickness and 2-mm inter-slice gap. T1 mapping was performed using a bSSFP readout modified Look-Locker inversion recovery (MOLLI) acquisition scheme with three short-axis slices (8 mm slice thickness) acquired at basal, mid and apical locations, pre-contrast and 12–15 min after administration of 0.15 mmol/kg body weight of gadobuterol (Gadovist; Bayer Healthcare, Berlin, Germany) [14]. Multi-plane late gadolinium enhanced (LGE) imaging was performed approximately 15 min following contrast administration employing a 2D inversion recovery gradient-recalled echo sequence (slice thickness 8 mm and 2 mm inter-slice gap).

CMR analysis

All studies were analyzed by a fellowship trained radiologist (SR, with 3 years CMR experience) blinded to all identifying clinical and imaging data. Evaluation of LV volumes and function was performed using commercially available software (QMASS MRI, Medis Medical Imaging Systems, Leiden, The Netherlands).

After inline, non-rigid motion correction of individual T1 mapping images, an inline T1 map was generated using standard 3-parameter fitting. Analysis was performed off-line using commercially available software (cvi42; Circle Cardiovascular Imaging, Calgary, Alberta, Canada). Regions of interest were drawn manually in the LV blood pool on pre- and post-contrast T1 maps with care taken to avoid the myocardium and papillary muscles. Myocardial T1 values were calculated by contouring epicardial and endocardial borders at basal, mid and apical slices, with care taken to avoid blood pool and epicardial fat, Fig. 1. Myocardial segments with LGE were not excluded from T1 analysis. Blood pool and myocardial T1 values were averaged across the three slices.

Hematocrit assessment

A small blood sample (< 30 mL) was collected by venipuncture within 24 h of CMR for the purpose of central hospital laboratory determination of hemoglobin and hematocrit (Lab-Hct). The time between laboratory blood sampling and CMR start time was recorded. Samples were analyzed by a hematology analyzer (CELL-DYN, Sapphire, Abbott Core Laboratory, Abbott Park,

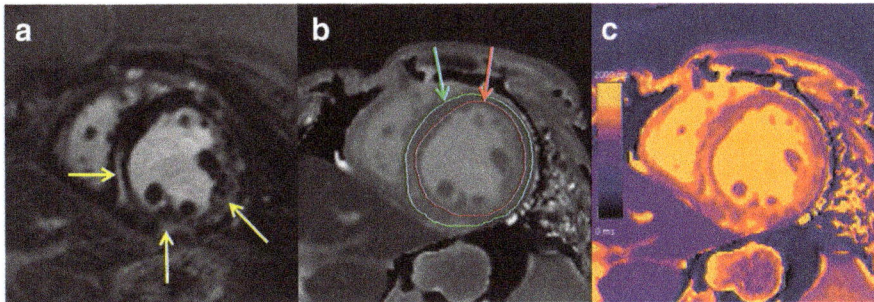

Fig. 1 Example short axis late gadolinium enhanced (LGE) image (**a**), non-contrast T1 map with contours (**b**), and color non-contrast T1 map (**c**) in a 30-year-old female with cardiac sarcoidosis. Yellow arrows indicate the presence of LGE. Endocardial (red arrow) and epicardial (green arrow) contours are shown

Illinois, USA), with reported bias and standard deviation of − 0.07 ± 1.17 g/dL [15]. Laboratory hemoglobin and hematocrit results were recorded blinded to clinical information and the results of POC and synthetic derivation analysis. Anemia was defined as a laboratory hemoglobin level < 122 g/L for females, < 132 g/L for males ≥60 years of age, and < 137 g/L for males < 60 years of age [16].

POC analysis was performed within 1 h of CMR using a Pronto-7° Pulse CO-Oximeter (Masimo Personal Health, Irvine, California, USA), by an experienced observer (SR) blinded to all identifying information and the results of laboratory analysis and synthetic derivation. The POC probe was applied to the fingertip of the ring or middle finger according to the manufacturer's guidelines. If the first attempt was unsuccessful with no result displayed, up to four additional attempts at POC analysis were performed. The total number of POC analysis attempts was recorded for each subject. The displayed hemoglobin value was recorded with subsequent derivation of hematocrit (POC-Hct) using a conversion of 0.3, according to previously published guidelines [17]. In a subset of subjects (n = 32), the total time for POC device analysis was determined, timed from turning the device on to recording the displayed hemoglobin value.

In the subgroup of subjects scanned at 1.5 T, synthetic hematocrit (synthetic-Hct) was calculated from the relationship between hematocrit and non-contrast blood pool T1 values as described previously, using a published linear regression formula for MOLLI acquisition schemes at 1.5 T [11]:

$$\text{Synthetic–Hct} = (866.0 * [1/\text{T1}_{\text{blood}}]) - 0.1232$$

Synthetic hematocrit was calculated by an experienced observer (SR) who was blinded to clinical information and the results of POC and laboratory analysis.

Synthetic-hematocrit was not evaluated in subjects imaged at 3 T due to lack of previously published formulas using the same CMR scanner that was used in this study. We did not fit a linear regression equation to our data given the relatively small number of subjects imaged at each field strength and acquisition scheme.

ECV derivation

Myocardial ECV was calculated based on pre- and post-contrast myocardial and blood pool T1 values and hematocrit, as proposed by Arheden et al. [18]. ECV was calculated with input of Lab-Hct (Lab-ECV), POC-Hct (POC-ECV), and synthetic-Hct (synthetic-ECV), respectively. The same myocardial and blood pool T1 values were used in each ECV calculation.

Test-retest and inter-observer agreement

To evaluate test-retest variability of POC measures, three POC analyses were performed in immediate succession in a subset of subjects (n = 42) without removal of the probe. In these subjects, the first result obtained was used in the general analysis.

To assess inter-observer agreement of POC measures, a second POC analysis was performed in a subset of subjects (n = 16) by a second experienced CMR fellowship trained reader (GK) independent from the first analysis, blinded to all identifying clinical data and the first set of measurements.

Comparison of POC devices

Evaluation of hematocrit using a second POC device (Pronto° Pulse CO-Oximeter, Masimo Personal Health) was performed in a group of 10 subjects. These 10 subjects also underwent parallel assessment using the Pronto-7° POC device and central hospital laboratory determination. Myocardial ECV was calculated in this group with input of hematocrit from the Pronto° device, Pronto-7° device, and laboratory determination.

Statistical analysis

Statistical analysis was performed using STATA v14.1 (Stata Corporation, College Station, Texas, USA). The sample size was calculated to detect a difference in ECV measurements between techniques of 1% with a standard deviation of ECV measurements of 3% using a paired t-test [19]. To detect this difference with a power of 95% and alpha error of 0.05, a total of 119 subjects were needed. All continuous data were first tested for normal distribution using the Shapiro-Wilk test. Continuous variables are described using mean and standard deviation or median and interquartile range (IQR), and categorical variables using numbers and percentage. Comparisons between values were made by paired t-test for continuous values with normal distribution and Wilcoxon signed-rank test for continuous values with non-normal distribution. Correlations between continuous variables were assessed with Pearson or Spearman correlation coefficient, as appropriate. Bias and precision were evaluated using Bland-Altman analysis. Test-retest and inter-observer agreement were assessed via the intra-class correlation coefficient (ICC) with two-way random effects model. Sensitivity analysis was performed, restricting the analysis to subjects in different subgroups including those with anemia, different field strengths (1.5 T and 3 T), gender (males and females) and clinical status (healthy subjects and patients). Diagnostic test performance of POC-ECV and synthetic-ECV in comparison to Lab-ECV as the reference standard was assessed using a Lab-ECV cut-off value of ≥30% as abnormal, including sensitivity, specificity, accuracy and area under the receiver operating curve (ROC) [20, 21]. A two-tailed p-value of < 0.05 was considered statistically significant.

Results

Baseline characteristics and clinical details are summarized in Table 1. CMR findings are summarized in Table 2.

Hematocrit assessment and ECV derivation

Hemoglobin, hematocrit and ECV values are detailed in Table 2. The median interval between blood sampling and CMR was 1.3 h (IQR 1.0–2.8 h). Mean laboratory hemoglobin and Lab-Hct values were 134.1 ± 17.0 g/L (range 79-169 g/L) and 0.399 ± 0.048 (range 0.239–0.509), respectively. The mean ratio of Lab-Hct to laboratory hemoglobin was 0.30 ± 0.01. A minority of subjects met criteria for anemia ($n = 31$, 25%). Mean Lab-ECV was 27.1 ± 4.7% (range 19.4–44.9%).

POC analysis was successfully performed in 63% ($n = 77$) of subjects on the first attempt, in 70% ($n = 86$) within two attempts, and in 91% ($n = 112$) within three attempts. The mean duration for POC analysis was 82 ± 9 s (range 70–105 s). Mean POC-Hct was 0.395 ± 0.044 with no

Table 1 Baseline Characteristics

Characteristic	Subjects ($n = 123$)
Age (years)	47.7 ± 14.1
Male	52 (42%)
BSA (m2)	1.9 ± 0.3
Heart rate (bpm)	69 ± 12
Indication for CMR	
Chemotoxicity	34 (28%)
Hypertrophic cardiomyopathy	24 (20%)
Anderson-Fabry disease	11 (9%)
Myocarditis/pericarditis	10 (8%)
Sarcoid	8 (7%)
Cardiomyopathy, cause unspecified	17 (14%)
Healthy subjects	19 (15%)
Field Strength	
1.5 T	74 (60%)
3 T	49 (40%)

Data are mean ± standard deviation or number of patients with percentage in parentheses
BPM beats per minute, *BSA* body surface area, *CMR* cardiovascular magnetic resonance

Table 2 Hemoglobin, Hematocrit and CMR Results

Measurement	Subjects ($n = 123$)
CMR Values	
LVEDV (mL)	152 (IQR 126–184)
Indexed LVEDV (mL/m^2)	80 (IQR 71–96)
LVESV (mL)	64 (IQR 50–80)
Indexed LVESV (mL/m^2)	34 (IQR 27–43)
LVSV (mL)	82 (IQR 69–103)
LVEF (%)	58 (IQR 52–64)
Laboratory Values	
Laboratory hemoglobin (g/L)	134.1 ± 17.0
Laboratory hematocrit	0.399 ± 0.048
Laboratory ECV (%)	27.1 ± 4.7
POC Values	
POC hemoglobin (g/L)	131.6 ± 14.7
POC hematocrit	0.395 ± 0.044
POC ECV (%)	27.3 ± 4.8
Synthetic Values	
Synthetic hematocrit	0.398 ± 0.031
Synthetic ECV (%)	26.5 ± 4.3
Elevated Laboratory ECV (≥30%)	31 (25%)
Anemia	31 (25%)

Data are mean ± standard deviation, median and interquartile range (IQR), or number of patients with percentage in parentheses
CMR cardiovascular magnetic resonance, *ECV* extracellular volume, *LVEDV* left ventricular end diastolic volume, *LVEF* left ventricular ejection fraction, *LVESV* left ventricular end systolic volume, *LVSV* left ventricular stroke volume, *POC* point-of-care

significant difference between POC-Hct and Lab-Hct ($p = 0.149$). Mean POC-ECV was $27.3 \pm 4.8\%$ with no significant difference between POC-ECV and Lab-ECV ($p = 0.106$). There was good correlation between laboratory and POC measures of hematocrit ($r = 0.81$, $p < 0.001$) and excellent correlation between laboratory and POC measures of ECV ($r = 0.94$, $p < 0.001$), Fig. 2a. On Bland-Altman analysis, there was minimal bias for POC-ECV in comparison to Lab-ECV with modest precision (bias = $- 0.18\%$, 95%CI [$- 2.85$, 2.49], confidence limit 5.34%), Fig. 3a.

Synthetic-Hct was derived from blood pool T1 values in all subjects imaged at 1.5 T ($n = 74$). There was no statistically significant difference between Lab-Hct and synthetic-Hct (0.392 ± 0.042 vs. 0.398 ± 0.031, $p = 0.074$) or Lab-ECV and synthetic-ECV ($26.7 \pm 4.4\%$ vs. $26.5 \pm 4.3\%$, $p = 0.084$) in the subgroup imaged at 1.5 T. There was moderate correlation between laboratory and synthetic measures of hematocrit ($r = 0.60$, $p < 0.001$) and excellent correlation between laboratory and synthetic measures of ECV ($r = 0.92$, p < 0.001), Fig. 2b. On Bland-Altman analysis, there was slightly larger bias for synthetic-ECV in comparison to Lab-ECV and slightly wider limits of agreement (bias = 0.23%, 95%CI [$- 2.82$, 3.27], confidence limit 6.09%), Fig. 3b.

Sensitivity analysis

There was no statistically significant difference between POC-ECV and Lab-ECV when analysis was restricted to different subgroups, including subjects imaged at 1.5 T ($n = 74$, $p = 0.410$), imaged at 3 T ($n = 49$, $p = 0.120$), females ($n = 71$, $p = 0.458$), males ($n = 52$, $p = 0.087$), healthy subjects ($n = 19$, $p = 0.376$), and patients ($n = 104$, $p = 0.164$). However, there was a significant difference between POC-ECV and Lab-ECV when analysis was restricted to subjects with anemia ($n = 31$, $p = 0.009$).

There was no significant difference between synthetic-ECV and Lab-ECV when analysis was restricted to males ($n = 22$, $p = 0.249$) and healthy subjects ($n = 12$, $p = 0.182$). However, there were significant differences between synthetic-ECV and Lab-ECV when analysis was restricted to females ($n = 52$, $p = 0.008$), patients ($n = 62$, $p = 0.018$), and subjects with anemia ($n = 22$, $p = 0.001$), suggesting that synthetic-ECV may be less robust compared to POC-ECV.

Diagnostic performance

ROC curves were used to evaluate the diagnostic performance of POC-ECV and synthetic-ECV in comparison to Lab-ECV as the reference standard using a cut-off of Lab-ECV $\geq 30\%$ as abnormal. POC-ECV had good diagnostic test performance for discriminating Lab-ECV $\geq 30\%$ (sensitivity 85%, specificity 96%, accuracy 94%, and area under the curve (AUC) 0.902, 95%CI[0.829, 0.976]). Synthetic-ECV had moderate diagnostic test performance (sensitivity 71%, specificity 98%, accuracy 93%, and AUC 0.849, 95%CI[0.725, 0.973]). There was no significant difference in AUC between the two noninvasive measures when analysis was restricted to studies performed at 1.5 T ($p = 0.629$).

Test-retest and inter-observer agreement

Excellent test-retest (ICC 0.951, 95%CI[0.905, 0.977]) and inter-observer agreement (ICC 0.900, 95%CI[0.719, 0.965]) were demonstrated for POC-Hct. Excellent test-retest (ICC 0.994, 95%CI[0.987, 0.997]) and inter-observer agreement (ICC 0.974, 95%CI[0.929, 0.991]) were demonstrated for POC-ECV.

Comparison of POC devices

In the group of subjects who underwent parallel hematocrit assessment with two POC devices and

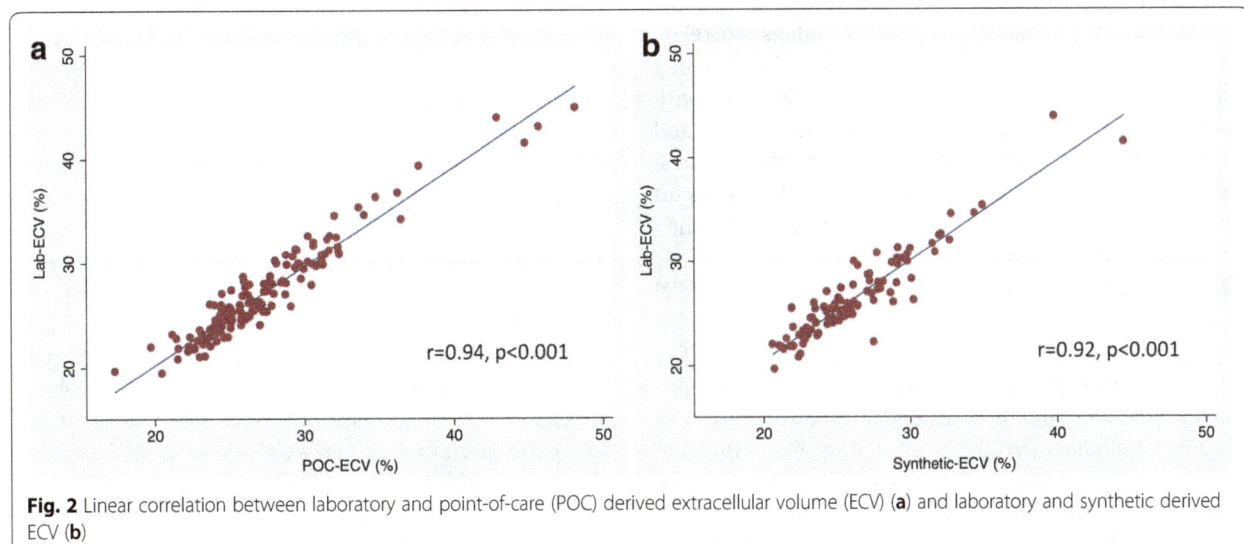

Fig. 2 Linear correlation between laboratory and point-of-care (POC) derived extracellular volume (ECV) (**a**) and laboratory and synthetic derived ECV (**b**)

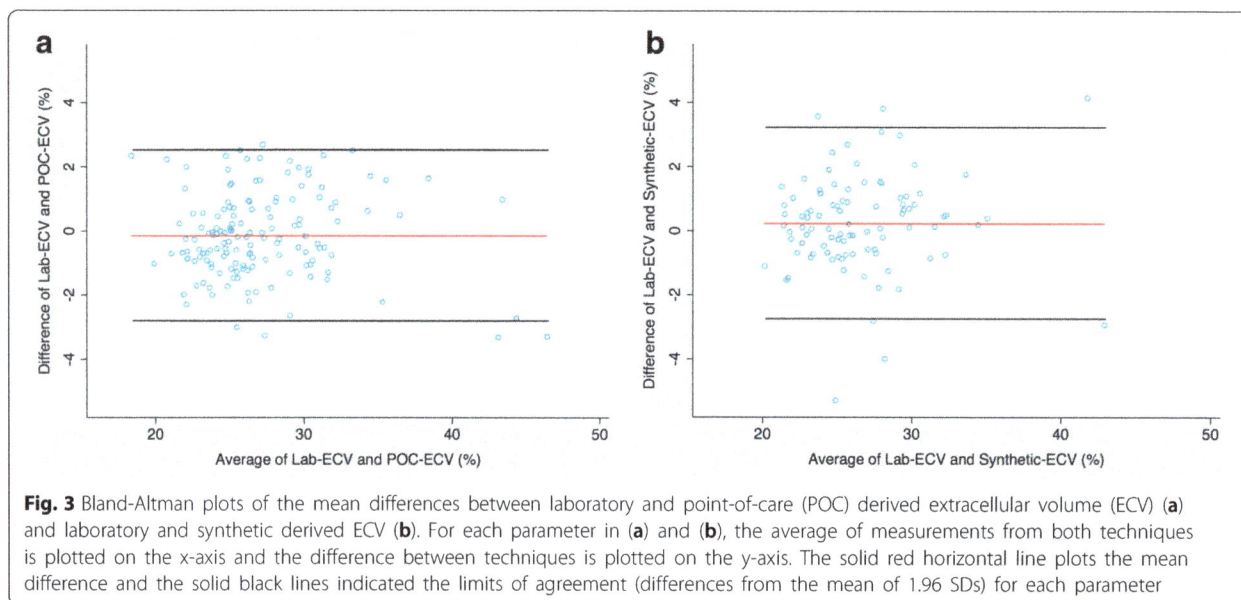

Fig. 3 Bland-Altman plots of the mean differences between laboratory and point-of-care (POC) derived extracellular volume (ECV) (**a**) and laboratory and synthetic derived ECV (**b**). For each parameter in (**a**) and (**b**), the average of measurements from both techniques is plotted on the x-axis and the difference between techniques is plotted on the y-axis. The solid red horizontal line plots the mean difference and the solid black lines indicated the limits of agreement (differences from the mean of 1.96 SDs) for each parameter

laboratory determination, there was no significant difference in hematocrit assessed using the Pronto* device (0.408 ± 0.045) compared to the Pronto-7* device (0.392 ± 0.045, $p = 0.135$) and compared to Lab-Hct (0.405 ± 0.044, $p = 0.830$). Similarly, there was no significant difference in ECV derived using hematocrit from the Pronto* POC device (24.3 ± 3.0%) compared to ECV derived using hematocrit from the Pronto-7* POC device (25.0 ± 2.9%, $p = 0.124$) and compared to ECV derived from Lab-Hct (24.3 ± 2.2%, $p = 0.959$).

Discussion

The results of this prospective study demonstrate that accurate and reproducible CMR ECV values can be calculated with input of hematocrit measured using a noninvasive POC device, potentially eliminating the need for blood collection by venipuncture for the purpose of ECV analysis. POC-ECV values correlate strongly with conventionally calculated ECV using laboratory hematocrit as the reference standard, with good diagnostic test performance, minimal bias and good agreement with Lab-ECV in both genders. Synthetic-ECV has slightly larger bias, wider limits of agreement and is less robust on sensitivity analyses when compared to POC-ECV.

There is growing interest in quantifying myocardial ECV as a marker of diffuse interstitial myocardial changes including fibrosis [22]. Myocardial ECV correlates with histologic measures of diffuse myocardial fibrosis [23, 24], and is independently associated with adverse outcomes including mortality [4]. However, clinical implementation of myocardial ECV may be limited by the requirement for timely hematocrit assessment [25]. Hematocrit is conventionally assessed by a

peripheral blood sample obtained by venipuncture which is often inconvenient and uncomfortable for the patient. Several methods of noninvasive hematocrit evaluation have recently become commercially available which could be implemented to streamline CMR ECV evaluation.

Noninvasive POC devices provide rapid on the spot measures of hemoglobin without the need for blood sampling [15, 26]. Most noninvasive POC devices rely on a spectrophotometer finger probe sensor to analyze light absorption characteristics of different hemoglobin species [27]. Prior studies utilizing earlier POC devices reported conflicting results [28, 29]. However, comparison of earlier results to current POC device performance is limited given ongoing software and hardware revisions [30]. More recent generations of POC devices (including the device used in this study), have been evaluated in subjects in a variety of clinical settings [9, 31, 32] and in healthy volunteers [33, 34], with good correlation between POC hemoglobin and laboratory reference measures. A recent large meta-analysis evaluating the accuracy and precision of current POC devices against central laboratory hemoglobin measurements reported a pooled random-effects mean difference of POC minus central laboratory hemoglobin values of 0.10 ± 1.37 g/dL (limits of agreement – 2.59 to 2.80 g/dL) [15]. Similarly, the results of our study demonstrate a small mean difference between POC-ECV and Lab-ECV of – 0.18% with relatively narrow limits of agreement (– 2.85 to 2.49%). Notably, previous publications have not evaluated the diagnostic performance of POC derived ECV values, which is an important strength of the current study.

We evaluated POC device performance in the calculation of myocardial ECV in a relatively diverse cohort of subjects, and therefore results are applicable in a relatively broad range of clinical and research settings. POC analysis was quick, with most measurements acquired with a single analysis attempt. This noninvasive measure of hematocrit was easily incorporated into the CMR workflow and can be implemented in myocardial ECV calculation with the following caveats. POC analysis was not possible in a small subset of subjects, including subjects with applied gel nail polish, marked hand tremor and poor peripheral perfusion, which are recognized limitations of POC device analysis [28, 35]. Additionally, in the subset of subjects with anemia, there was a significant difference between laboratory and POC ECV values. This may be explained by the fact that low hemoglobin levels have been shown to impair perfusion analysis [36]. Given this finding, POC derived hematocrit is not recommended for CMR ECV calculation in subjects with anemia. This finding can be further explored in future studies that include a larger number of subjects with anemia.

A few recent studies have reported synthetic derivation of hematocrit and ECV based on the linear relationship between hematocrit and non-contrast R1 of blood [11, 13]. Automated inline derivation of synthetic hematocrit with subsequent calculation of myocardial ECV could potentially improve workflow, eliminating the need to acquire an invasive hematocrit value at the time of CMR. Treibel et al. demonstrated moderate correlation between synthetic and laboratory hematocrit ($r^2 = 0.51$–0.45, $p < 0.001$) and strong correlation between synthetic and laboratory derived ECV ($r^2 = 0.97$, $p < 0.001$) [11]. Our study similarly demonstrates excellent correlation between synthetic and laboratory ECV, although the mean difference between synthetic-ECV and Lab-ECV was slightly greater and the limits of agreement were slightly wider when compared to POC-ECV. A recent study investigating synthetic ECV in a pediatric population reported 41 (25%) false negatives and 4 (2%) false positives for mid-septal synthetic ECV using a published model and cut-off value of 28.5% [13]. The authors conclude that use of synthetic hematocrit for the calculation of ECV results in miscategorization of individual patients. Similarly, the results of the current study demonstrate that synthetic-ECV values are less robust on sensitivity analysis compared to POC-ECV, with significant differences between laboratory and synthetic ECV values when restricted to females, patients and those with anemia. Synthetic hematocrit and ECV values are affected by factors that affect non-contrast blood pool T1 values, such as changes in oxygen and iron concentration and body temperature [37–40]. There are also important practical limitations to synthetic analysis, as formulas to calculate synthetic hematocrit should be derived at each institution in a large sample of patients

imaged on each individual scanner and with each specific acquisition scheme to which the results will be applied [12]. We conclude that synthetic-ECV is less robust compared to POC-ECV, and requires further evaluation prior to clinical implementation.

Our study has a number of limitations. First, the non-invasive POC device used in this study became commercially unavailable after this study was completed. However, multiple other non-invasive hemoglobin monitoring devices are currently available, including Pronto˙ Pulse CO-Oximeter˙ (Masimo Personal Health), Radical-7˙ Pulse CO-Oximeter˙ (Masimo Personal Health), NBM-200 (OrSense, Petah-Tikva, Israel) and Haemospect˙ (MRB Optical Systems GmbH & Co. KG, Wuppertal, Germany). Several prior studies have compared hemoglobin results from the Pronto-7˙ device used in this study and NBM-200 device, with similar accuracy and bias reported between devices [26, 41–43]. A recent meta-analysis evaluating the accuracy of non-invasive hemoglobin monitoring devices reported that pooled mean differences and standard deviations were similar among three devices included in the analysis (Radical-7˙, Pronto-7˙, and NBM-200 devices) [15]. We demonstrate no significant difference in hematocrit or ECV assessed using the Pronto˙ Pulse CO-Oximeter˙ compared to the Pronto-7˙ Pulse CO-Oximeter˙ and to laboratory values. These results suggest that currently available non-invasive hemoglobin monitoring devices will most likely lead to similar findings as reported in this study. Second, diurnal and monthly within-subject fluctuations in hematocrit are a recognized phenomenon, estimated at 3% [44, 45], with additional variations in hematocrit values linked to season, age, hydration and physical activity [46–49]. Our study used a single laboratory hematocrit measure within 24 h of CMR as the reference standard. It is possible that slight fluctuations in hematocrit between the time of CMR, POC device acquisition and peripheral blood sampling for laboratory analysis could have influenced the results. The median interval between laboratory hematocrit analysis and CMR was only 1.3 h and therefore the impact of potential variations in hematocrit between analysis methods is likely minimal. Third, non-invasive hemoglobin measurements may vary between POC devices and settings. However, a recent meta-analysis has demonstrated good agreement in hemoglobin between various POC devices [15]. The presence of an arrhythmia, including atrial fibrillation, was not recorded at the time of CMR. Therefore, the accuracy of POC devices in the setting of an arrhythmia has not been evaluated. Finally, the sample size was modest and all data were acquired at a single institution. Further multi-center studies including a larger number of patients with anemia should be performed to validate these results.

Conclusions

CMR ECV calculated with input of hematocrit measured using a noninvasive POC device is accurate and reproducible compared to conventionally calculated ECV using laboratory hematocrit, potentially overcoming an important barrier to clinical implementation of ECV measurements. Further evaluation of synthetic ECV is required prior to clinical implementation.

Abbreviations

AUC: Area under the curve; bSSFP: Balanced steady-state free precession; CMR: Cardiovascular magnetic resonance; ECV: Extracellular volume; Hct: Hematocrit; ICC: Intra-class correlation coefficient; IQR: Interquartile range; Lab-ECV: Laboratory extracellular volume; Lab-Hct: Laboratory hematocrit; LGE: Late gadolinium enhancement; LV: Left ventricle/left ventricular; MOLLI: MOdified Look-Locker Inversion; POC: Point-of-care; POC-ECV: Point-of-care extracellular volume; POC-Hct: Point-of-care hematocrit; ROC: Receiver operating curve; Synthetic-ECV: Synthetic extracellular volume; Synthetic-Hct: Synthetic hematocrit

Acknowledgements

Rosanna Chan, Research MRI Technologist.

Funding

KH: Radiological Society of North America Research Scholar Grant (RSCH1608) - salary support for corresponding author.
KH: Academic Innovation Fund (AIF) grant from the Joint Department of Medical Imaging, University of Toronto – support for design of the study and data collection, data analysis, and POC device acquisition.
RW: Canadian Institutes of Health Research Operating Grant (MOP 119353) - salary support.
PT: Canadian Institutes of Health Research New Investigator Award (FRN 147814) – support for data collection and analysis.

Authors' contributions

SR and KH were responsible for conception and design of the study. SR and GK contributed to subject recruitment and data acquisition. SR and KH analyzed and interpreted the data. SR, KH and PT contributed to statistical analysis. All authors made substantial contributions to analysis and interpretation of data. SR and KH drafted the manuscript. All authors critically revised and reviewed the manuscript. All authors read and approved the final manuscript and agree to be accountable for all aspects of the work.

Competing interests

The authors declare that they have no competing interests.

Author details

[1]Department of Medical Imaging, Toronto General Hospital, University Health Network, University of Toronto, 585 University Ave, 1PMB-298, Toronto, ON M5G 2N2, Canada. [2]Division of Cardiology, Department of Medicine, Peter Munk Cardiac Center, Toronto General Hospital, University of Toronto, Toronto, Canada.

References

1. de Meester de Ravenstein C, Bouzin C, Lazam S, Boulif J, Amzulescu M, Melchior J, Pasquet A, Vancraeynest D, Pouleur A-C, Vanoverschelde J-LJ, Gerber BL. Histological validation of measurement of diffuse interstitial myocardial fibrosis by myocardial extravascular volume fraction from modified look-locker imaging (MOLLI) T1 mapping at 3 T. J Cardiovasc Magn Reson. 2015;17:48.
2. Flett AS, Hayward MP, Ashworth MT, Hansen MS, Taylor AM, Elliott PM, McGregor C, Moon JC. Equilibrium contrast cardiovascular magnetic resonance for the measurement of diffuse myocardial fibrosis: preliminary validation in humans. Circulation. 2010;122:138–44.
3. Diao K-Y, Yang Z-G, Xu H-Y, Liu X, Zhang Q, Shi K, Jiang L, Xie L-J, Wen L-Y, Guo Y-K. Histologic validation of myocardial fibrosis measured by T1 mapping: a systematic review and meta-analysis. J Cardiovasc Magn Reson. 2016;18:1407.
4. Wong TC, Piehler K, Meier CG, Testa SM, Klock AM, Aneizi AA, Shakesprere J, Kellman P, Shroff SG, Schwartzman DS, Mulukutla SR, Simon MA, Schelbert EB. Association between extracellular matrix expansion quantified by cardiovascular magnetic resonance and short-term mortality. Circulation. 2012;126:1206–16.
5. Wong TC, Piehler KM, Kang IA, Kadakkal A, Kellman P, Schwartzman DS, Mulukutla SR, Simon MA, Shroff SG, Kuller LH, Schelbert EB. Myocardial extracellular volume fraction quantified by cardiovascular magnetic resonance is increased in diabetes and associated with mortality and incident heart failure admission. Eur Heart J. 2014;35:657–64.
6. Ambale-Venkatesh B, Lima JA, Cardiac MRI. A central prognostic tool in myocardial fibrosis. Nat Rev Cardiol. 2014;12:18–29.
7. Jellis CL, Kwon DH. Myocardial T1 mapping: modalities and clinical applications. Cardiovasc Diagn Ther. 2014;4:126–37.
8. Berkow L, Rotolo S, Mirski E. Continuous noninvasive hemoglobin monitoring during complex spine surgery. Anesth Analg. 2011;113:1396–402.
9. Joseph B, Pandit V, Aziz H, Kulvatunyou N, Zangbar B, Tang A, O' keeffe T, Jehangir Q, Snyder K, Rhee P. Transforming hemoglobin measurement in trauma patients: noninvasive spot check hemoglobin. J Am Coll Surg. 2015; 220:93–8.
10. Frasca D, Dahyot-Fizelier C, Catherine K, Levrat Q, Debaene B, Mimoz O. Accuracy of a continuous noninvasive hemoglobin monitor in intensive care unit patients. Crit Care Med. 2011;39:2277–82.
11. Treibel TA, Fontana M, Maestrini V, Castelletti S, Rosmini S, Simpson J, Nasis A, Bhuva AN, Bulluck H, Abdel-Gadir A, White SK, Manisty C, Spottiswoode BS, Wong TC, Piechnik SK, Kellman P, Robson MD, Schelbert EB, Moon JC. Automatic measurement of the myocardial interstitium: synthetic extracellular volume quantification without hematocrit sampling. J Am Coll Cardiol Img. 2016;9:54–63.
12. Bluemke DA, Kawel-Boehm N. Can a MR imaging scanner accurately measure hematocrit to determine ECV fraction? J Am Coll Cardiol Img. 2016;9:64–6.
13. Raucci FJ, Parra DA, Christensen JT, Hernandez LE, Markham LW, Xu M, Slaughter JC, Soslow JH. Synthetic hematocrit derived from the longitudinal relaxation of blood can lead to clinically significant errors in measurement of extracellular volume fraction in pediatric and young adult patients. J Cardiovasc Magn Reson. 2017;19:58.
14. Messroghli DR, Greiser A, Fröhlich M, Dietz R, Schulz-Menger J. Optimization and validation of a fully-integrated pulse sequence for modified look-locker inversion-recovery (MOLLI) T1 mapping of the heart. J Magn Reson Imaging. 2007;26:1081–6.
15. Kim S-H, Lilot M, Murphy LS-L, Sidhu KS, Yu Z, Rinehart J, Cannesson M. Accuracy of continuous noninvasive hemoglobin monitoring. Anesth Analg. 2014;119:332–46.
16. Beutler E, Waalen J. The definition of anemia: what is the lower limit of normal of the blood hemoglobin concentration? Blood. 2006;107:1747–50.
17. Anaemias N. Report of a WHO scientific group. World health organ tech. Ser. 1968;405:5–37.
18. Arheden H, Saeed M, Higgins CB, Gao DW, Bremerich J, Wyttenbach R, Dae MW, Wendland MF. Measurement of the distribution volume of gadopentetate dimeglumine at echo-planar MR imaging to quantify myocardial infarction: comparison with 99mTc-DTPA autoradiography in rats. Radiology. 1999;211:698–708.

19. Neilan TG, Coelho-Filho OR, Shah RV, Abbasi SA, Heydari B, Watanabe E, Chen Y, Mandry D, Pierre-Mongeon F, Blankstein R, Kwong RY, Jerosch-Herold M. Myocardial extracellular volume fraction from T1 measurements in healthy volunteers and mice. J Am Coll Cardiol Img. 2013;6:672–83.

20. Liu S, Han J, Nacif MS, Jones J, Kawel N. Diffuse myocardial fibrosis evaluation using cardiac magnetic resonance T1 mapping: sample size considerations for clinical trials. J Cardiovasc Magn. 2012;14:90.

21. Kellman P, Wilson JR, Xue H, Bandettini WP, Shanbhag SM, Druey KM, Ugander M, Arai AE. Extracellular volume fraction mapping in the myocardium, part 2: initial clinical experience. J Cardiovasc Magn Reson. 2012;14:64.

22. Taylor AJ, Salerno M, Dharmakumar R, Jerosch-Herold M. T1 mapping: basic techniques and clinical applications. J Am Coll Cardiol Img. 2016;9:67–81.

23. Miller CA, Naish JH, Bishop P, Coutts G, Clark D, Zhao S, Ray SG, Yonan N, Williams SG, Flett AS, Moon JC, Greiser A, Parker GJM, Schmitt M. Comprehensive validation of cardiovascular magnetic resonance techniques for the assessment of myocardial extracellular volume. Circ Cardiovasc Imaging. 2013;6:373–83.

24. Siepen FAD, Buss SJ, Messroghli D, Andre F, Lossnitzer D, Seitz S, Keller M, Schnabel PA, Giannitsis E, Korosoglou G, Katus HA, Steen H. T1 mapping in dilated cardiomyopathy with cardiac magnetic resonance: quantification of diffuse myocardial fibrosis and comparison with endomyocardial biopsy. Eur Heart J Cardiovasc Imaging. 2015;16:210–6.

25. Moon JC, Messroghli DR, Kellman P, Piechnik SK, Robson MD, Ugander M, Gatehouse PD, Arai AE, Friedrich MG, Neubauer S, Schulz-Menger J, Schelbert EB. Society for Cardiovascular Magnetic Resonance Imaging, cardiovascular magnetic resonance working Group of the European Society of cardiology. Myocardial T1 mapping and extracellular volume quantification: a Society for Cardiovascular Magnetic Resonance (SCMR) and CMR working Group of the European Society of cardiology consensus statement. J Cardiovasc Magn Reson. 2013;15:92.

26. Gayat E, Aulagnier J, Matthieu E, Boisson M, Fischler M. Non-invasive measurement of hemoglobin: assessment of two different point-of-care technologies. PLoS One. 2012;7:e30065.

27. McMurdy JW, Jay GD, Suner S, Crawford G. Noninvasive optical, electrical, and acoustic methods of total hemoglobin determination. Clin Chem. 2008; 54:264–72.

28. Miller RD, Ward TA, Shiboski SC, Cohen NHA. Comparison of three methods of hemoglobin monitoring in patients undergoing spine surgery. Anesth Analg. 2011;112:858–63.

29. Riess ML, Pagel PS. Noninvasively measured hemoglobin concentration reflects arterial hemoglobin concentration before but not after cardiopulmonary bypass in patients undergoing coronary artery or valve surgery. J Cardiothorac Vasc Anesth. 2016;30:1167–71.

30. Hiscock R. Systematic review and meta-analysis of method comparison studies of Masimo pulse co-oximeters (Radical-7™ or Pronto-7™) and HemoCue® absorption spectrometers (B-hemoglobin or 201+) with laboratory haemoglobin estimation. Anaesth Intensive Care. 2015;43:3.

31. DeBarros M, Shawhan R, Bingham J, Sokol K, Izenberg S, Martin M. Assessing serum hemoglobin levels without venipuncture: accuracy and reliability of Pronto-7 noninvasive spot-check device. Amer J Surg. 2015;209:848–55.

32. Erdogan Kayhan G, Colak YZ, Sanli M, Ucar M, Toprak H. Accuracy of non-invasive hemoglobin monitoring by pulse co-oximeter during liver transplantation. Minerva Anestesiol. 2017;83(5):485–92.

33. Shah N, Osea EA, Martinez GJ. Accuracy of noninvasive hemoglobin and invasive point-of-care hemoglobin testing compared with a laboratory analyzer. Int J Lab Hematol. 2013;36:56–61.

34. Vyas KJ, Danz D, Gilman RH, Wise RA, León-Velarde F, Miranda JJ, Checkley W. Noninvasive assessment of excessive Erythrocytosis as a screening method for Chronic Mountain sickness at high altitude. High Alt Med Biol. 2015;16:162–8.

35. Yamaura K, Nanishi N, Higashi M, Hoka S. Effects of thermoregulatory vasoconstriction on pulse hemoglobin measurements using a co-oximeter in patients undergoing surgery. J Clin Anesth. 2014;26:643–7.

36. Khalafallah AA, Chilvers CR, Thomas M, Chilvers CM, Sexton M, Vialle M, Robertson IK. Usefulness of non-invasive spectrophotometric haemoglobin estimation for detecting low haemoglobin levels when compared with a standard laboratory assay for preoperative assessment. Br J Anaesth. 2015; 114:669–76.

37. Barth M, Moser E. Proton NMR Relaxation times of human blood samples at 1.5 T and implications for functional MRI. Cell Mol Biol (Noisy-le-grand). 1997;43:783–91.

38. Tadamura E, Hatabu H, Li W, Prasad PV, Edelman RR. Effect of oxygen inhalation on relaxation times in various tissues. J Magn Reson Imaging. 1997;7:220–5.

39. Yilmaz A, Bucciolini M, Longo G, Franciolini F, Ciraolo L, Renzi R. Determination of dependence of spin-lattice relaxation rate in serum upon concentration of added iron by magnetic resonance imaging. Clin Phys Physiol Meas. 1990;11:343–9.

40. Silvennoinen MJ, Kettunen MI, Kauppinen RA. Effects of hematocrit and oxygen saturation level on blood spin-lattice relaxation. Magn Reson Med. 2003;49:568–71.

41. Belardinelli A, Benni M, Tazzari PL, Pagliaro P. Noninvasive methods for haemoglobin screening in prospective blood donors. Vox Sang 16 ed. 2013; 105:116–20.

42. Ardin S, Störmer M, Radojska S, Oustianskaia L, Hahn M, Gathof BS. Comparison of three noninvasive methods for hemoglobin screening of blood donors. Transfusion. 2014;55:379–87.

43. Pajares-Herraiz AL, Rodriguez-Gambarte JD, Eguia-Lopez B, Fernandez-Maqueda CT. Coello de Portugal C, Flores-Sanz MDV. A comparative study of three non-invasive Systems for Measurement of hemoglobin with HemoCue system having coulter LH750 as reference value. Hematol Transfus Int J MedCrave Online. 2015;1:1–10.

44. Jones AR, Twedt D, Swaim W, Gottfried E. Diurnal change of blood count analytes in normal subjects. Am J Clin Pathol. 1996;106:723–7.

45. Pocock SJ, Ashby D, Shaper AG, Walker M, Broughton PM. Diurnal variations in serum biochemical and haematological measurements. J Clin Pathol. 1989;42:172–9.

46. Wennesland R, Brown E, Hopper J, Hodges JL, Guttentag OE, Scott KG, Tucker IN, Bradley B. Red cell, plasma and blood volume in healthy men measured by radiochromium (Cr51) cell tagging and hematocrit: influence of age, somatotype and habits of physical activity on the variance after regression of volumes to height and weight combined. J Clin Invest. 1959; 38:1065–77.

47. Schumacher YO, Grathwohl D, Barturen JM, Wollenweber M, Heinrich L, Schmid A, Huber G, Haemoglobin KJ. Haematocrit and red blood cell indices in elite cyclists. Are the control values for blood testing valid? Int J Sports Med. 2000;21:380–5.

48. Thirup P. Haematocrit: within-subject and seasonal variation. Sports Med. 2003;33:231–43.

49. Schmidt W, Biermann B, Winchenbach P, Lison S, Böning D. How valid is the determination of hematocrit values to detect blood manipulations? Int J Sports Med. 2000;21:133–8.

17

Myocardial tissue characterization and strain analysis in healthy pregnant women using cardiovascular magnetic resonance native T1 mapping and feature tracking technique

Masafumi Nii[1*], Masaki Ishida[2], Kaoru Dohi[3], Hiroaki Tanaka[1], Eiji Kondo[1], Masaaki Ito[3], Hajime Sakuma[2] and Tomoaki Ikeda[1]

Abstract

Background: Peripartum cardiomyopathy is a life-threatening condition that occurs during the peripartum period in previously healthy women. Cardiovascular magnetic resonance (CMR) T1 mapping permits sensitive detection of tissue edema and fibrosis, and it may be useful in identifying altered myocardial tissue characteristics in peripartum cardiomyopathy. However, left ventricular (LV) volumes and mass increase considerably even in normal pregnancy, and it is not known whether altered tissue characteristics can be found in normal pregnancy. The aim of this study was to investigate whether the LV remodeling observed in normal pregnancy is associated with altered tissue characteristics determined by CMR.

Methods: Twelve normal pregnant women and 15 non pregnant women underwent cine CMR and myocardial T1 measurement at 1.5 T. Pregnant women were scanned three times, in the 2nd and 3rd trimesters of pregnancy and at 1 month postpartum. LV volumes, LV mass (LVM), and global longitudinal strain (GLS) were analyzed by cine CMR. Native myocardial T1 was determined using modified Look-Locker inversion recovery (MOLLI) images.

Results: LV end-diastolic volume (EDV) was significantly greater in the 3rd trimester (126 ± 22 mL) than in non-pregnant women (108 ± 14 mL, $p < 0.05$). LVM was significantly greater in the 3rd trimester (88.7 ± 11.8 g) than at 1 month postpartum (70.0 ± 9.8 g, $p < 0.05$) and in non-pregnant women (66.3 ± 13.9 g, $p < 0.05$). Myocardial native T1 among the 2nd and 3rd trimesters, 1 month postpartum, and non-pregnant women were similar (1133 ± 55 ms, 1138 ± 86 ms, 1105 ± 45 ms, and 1129 ± 52 ms, respectively, $p = 0.59$) as were GLS ($- 19.5 \pm 1.8$, $- 19.7\% \pm 2.2$, $- 19.0\% \pm 2.0\%$, and $- 19.3\% \pm 1.9\%$, respectively, $p = 0.66$).

Conclusions: LV remodeling during normal pregnancy is associated with myocardial hypertrophy, but not with edema or diffuse fibrosis of the myocardium or LV contractile dysfunction. These results observed in normal pregnancy will serve as an important basis for identifying myocardial abnormalities in patients with peripartum cardiomyopathy and other pregnancy-related myocardial diseases.

Keywords: Cardiovascular magnetic resonance, Cardiac function, Native myocardial T1 mapping, Pregnancy, Myocyte mass, Peripartum cardiomyopathy

* Correspondence: doaldosleeping@yahoo.co.jp
[1]Department of Obstetrics and Gynecology, Mie University Hospital, 2-174 Edobashi, Tsu, Mie 514-8507, Japan
Full list of author information is available at the end of the article

Background

Peripartum cardiomyopathy (PPCM) is a life-threatening condition that occurs during the peripartum period in previously healthy women [1, 2]. In Western countries, 0.02–0.03% of pregnant women develop PPCM [1, 2]. The precise mechanism that leads to PPCM remains uncertain [3]. Moreover, the early recognition of cardiomyopathy remains elusive, and it often only becomes apparent when the woman is symptomatic and already has well-established disease. Early diagnosis by non-invasive imaging techniques would have considerable value because it would permit early interventions to prevent disease progression.

Cardiovascular magnetic resonance (CMR) can be used during the second or third trimester of pregnancy for both the mother and fetus because no adverse effects of CMR during those periods for both mother and fetus have been reported in the literature [4–6]. CMR can provide a non-invasive assessment of cardiac structure, function, and tissue characteristics without the limitations imposed by variations in ventricular geometry or exposure to ionizing radiation. Cine CMR is a highly accurate and reproducible technique in the determination of cardiac volume and mass [7]. While late gadolinium enhancement (LGE) CMR is an effective and reproducible method of assessing focal myocardial fibrosis [8] and acute myocardial damage [9], LGE CMR requires administration of gadolinium contrast medium.

Native T1 mapping is a novel technique allowing quantitative assessment of diffuse myocardial tissue properties without use of gadolinium-based contrast medium [10]. Native T1 is influenced by the presence of edema, diffuse fibrosis, and protein deposition in the myocardium, showing increases in values [11]. Recognition of myocardial edema in acute myocarditis or Takotsubo cardiomyopathy by native T1 mapping was shown to be superior to that by T2-weighted sequences and LGE [12]. A prolonged native T1 in dilated cardiomyopathy patients correlates closely with histological fibrosis [13]. Native myocardial T1 values are increased in patients with various types of myocardial diseases, including dilated cardiomyopathy, hypertrophic cardiomyopathy, and aortic stenosis etc., reflecting the degree of diffuse myocardial fibrosis [14].

The prevalence of LGE in PPCM, which represents focal replacement fibrosis, varies substantially, ranging from 5 to 71% in the literature [15–19]. Thus, the utility of LGE CMR in clinical practice remains controversial. Native T1 mapping might be useful in the detection of PPCM in the early disease stage, since native T1 is a quantitative measure that can detect the subtle changes of diffuse myocardial fibrosis or edema.

Circulating blood volume increases by approximately 40% in normal pregnancy [20]. The increased blood volume in normal pregnancy leads to morphological and functional changes in the heart, such as increased left ventricular (LV) mass (LVM), [21–23] increased LV and atrial (LA) volumes, [21, 22] and reduced LV diastolic function [23]. Thus, in response to the major physiologic alterations in the maternal cardiovascular system throughout pregnancy, reversible morphological alterations, known as cardiac remodeling, are provoked in the maternal heart, ensuring a normotensive course of pregnancy [4, 7, 24]. The drastic changes in heart morphology and function in normal pregnancy may be associated with alterations of myocardial tissue characteristics. Therefore, CMR, especially T1 mapping, might have great potential in the management of PPCM and other pregnancy-related myocardial diseases. However, it is essential to understand the reference values of CMR parameters, including native T1, in normal pregnancy to identify myocardial abnormalities in patients with PPCM and other pregnancy-related myocardial diseases.

Consequently, the aim of this study was to investigate whether the LV remodeling observed in normal pregnancy is associated with altered tissue characteristics determined by CMR.

Methods

This prospective study was conducted in accordance with the principles of the Declaration of Helsinki and with the approval of the Institutional Review Board (2858, February 5, 2014). All women gave their written, informed consent prior to participation in this study.

Participants

Fourteen healthy pregnant women were prospectively recruited from between June 2015 and August 2016. Eligible subjects were between the age of 20 and 39 years at their last normal menstrual period, carrying a healthy singleton pregnancy. Exclusion criteria included any history of hypertension, diabetes mellitus, smoking, thyroid disease, known cardiac disease, any pregnancy-related complications including preeclampsia, hypertensive disorders of pregnancy, gestational diabetes, and the presence of a pacemaker or general contraindications to CMR. Of the 14 pregnant women, two were subsequently excluded because of hypertensive disorders of pregnancy. All 12 remaining women (33 ± 4 years) had a normal delivery between September 2015 and November 2016. This population was compared with 15 age-matched healthy non-pregnant women (31 ± 3 years). All 12 pregnant women underwent CMR three times, in the 2nd and 3rd trimesters of pregnancy and at 1 month postpartum, with a simultaneous 5.0 mL blood sample drawn to determine concentrations of hemoglobin (Hb) and brain type natriuretic peptide (BNP). Fifteen non-pregnant women also underwent CMR and provided a 5.0 mL blood sample immediately after the CMR examination and served as control women.

CMR image acquisition

CMR studies were performed on a 1.5 T CMR scanner (Achieva 1.5 T, Philips Healthcare, Best, The Netherlands) using a body coil for signal reception. No sedative medications or contrast agents were used, and all participants were imaged in the half left lateral decubitus position to minimize aortocaval compression. The CMR study protocol included cine CMR and native T1 mapping using a modified Look-Locker inversion recovery (MOLLI) sequence. Cine MR images were acquired with a retrospective electrocardiographic gating and a segmented steady-state-free precession sequence during brief periods of breath-holding at a shallow expiration in the following planes: LV 2-chamber and 4-chamber views and short-axis planes covering the entire LV and right ventricle (RV) (repetition time [TR] 2.9 ms; echo time [TE] 1.44 ms; flip angle [FA] 55°; field of view [FOV] 350×350 mm^2; acquisition matrix 176×176; reconstruction matrix 256×256; slice thickness 10 mm). All cine images were acquired with 20 phases per cardiac cycle. The short-axis plane was defined as the perpendicular plane to the horizontal and vertical long-axis views. Single-slice native T1 mapping was performed using a 17-heartbeat steady-state-free procession MOLLI sequence on the short-axis imaging plane at the level of the mid LV (TR, 2.3 ms; TE, 0.83 ms; FA, 35°; FOV, 300×327 mm^2; acquisition matrix, 176×140; reconstruction matrix, 288×288; slice thickness, 10 mm) [25].

CMR image analysis

CMR image analyses were carried out by an expert observer who had 15 years of CMR experience (M.I.) using CMR analysis software, cvi42 (Circle Cardiovascular Imaging Inc., Calgary, Canada). LV volume and function were analyzed based on the short-axis cine stack (Fig. 1). The endocardial and epicardial borders of the LV wall were manually traced on cine CMR images in end-diastolic and end-systolic phases. LVM was calculated as the volume of the LV myocardium multiplied by the specific gravity of the myocardium (1.05 g/ml) [26]. Mean LV wall thickness was measured in the end-diastolic phase on the short-axis view. The papillary muscles and trabeculations were not included in the myocardial mass calculation. Then, RV volume and function were analyzed based on the short-axis cine stack. LV and RV measurements were indexed to body surface area (BSA). Strain analysis was performed by a feature-tracking algorithm [11]. The endocardial and epicardial borders of LV and RV myocardium were manually traced in the end-diastolic phase of a 4-chamber view cine CMR image. Then, the software automatically propagated the endocardial and epicardial contours and tracked the motion of the in-plane tissue voxels through the entire cardiac cycle. Consequently, peak longitudinal strain values were recorded at global levels for the LV and RV. Native T1 measurement was performed pixel-wise. After correcting for respiratory motion of the images by non-rigid image registration, T1 maps were generated by fitting pixels to the equation $s(t) = a\text{-}b \exp.(-t/T1^*)$, and $T1 = (b/a\text{-}1) T1^*$, where a and b are constants, t is time, and $s(t)$ is signal intensity at time t [27]. The resulting pixel-wise native T1 maps were stored in

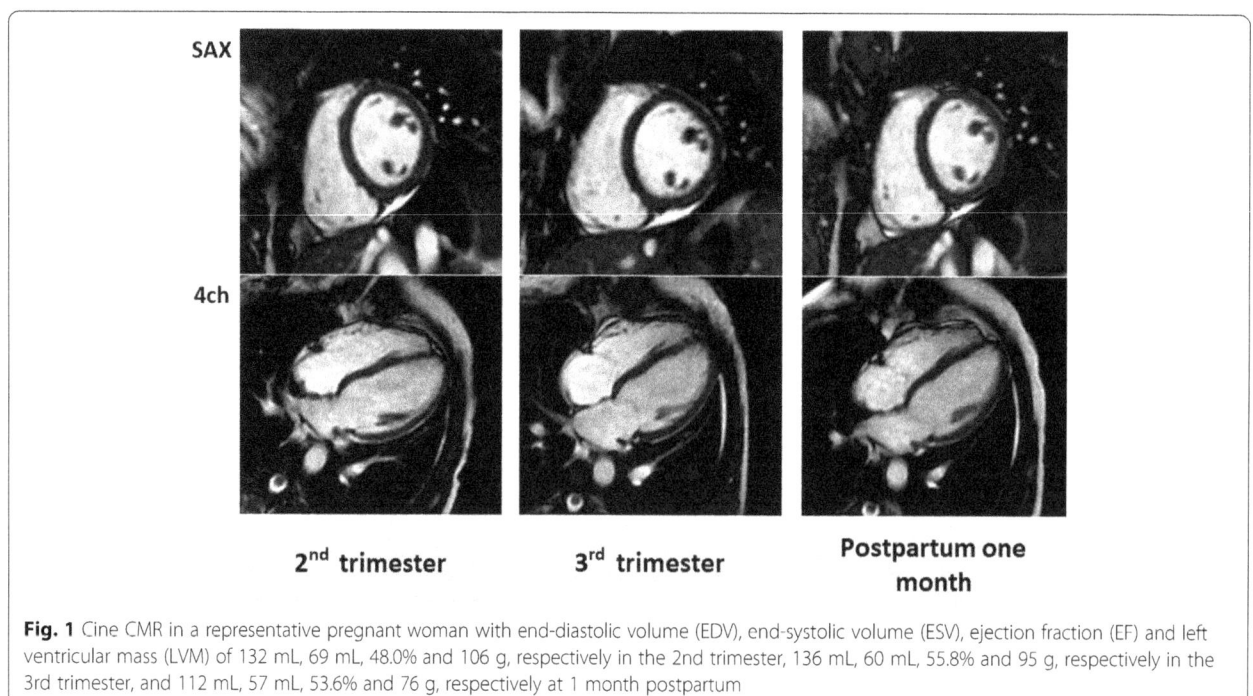

Fig. 1 Cine CMR in a representative pregnant woman with end-diastolic volume (EDV), end-systolic volume (ESV), ejection fraction (EF) and left ventricular mass (LVM) of 132 mL, 69 mL, 48.0% and 106 g, respectively in the 2nd trimester, 136 mL, 60 mL, 55.8% and 95 g, respectively in the 3rd trimester, and 112 mL, 57 mL, 53.6% and 76 g, respectively at 1 month postpartum

DICOM format, and native T1 values were averaged for all pixels (Fig. 2).

Statistical methods

The statistical analyses were performed using SPSS Statistics 20.0 (International Business Machiens, Armonk, New York, USA). Data were normally distributed (Kolmogorov-Smirnov test), and all data are therefore presented as means ± standard deviation (SD). Changes in variables within a group were compared using the paired t-test with the post hoc Tukey-Kramer method. Analysis of variance (ANOVA) was used for comparisons of multiple groups. Pearson's product-moment correlation coefficient was used to measure linear correlations between two variables. In all analyses, $p < 0.05$ was taken to indicate significance. However, a significant linear correlation between two variables was defined as that meeting both $p < 0.05$ and correlation coefficient (r-value) > 0.2 or < − 0.2 [28].

Results

Demographic characteristics of participants

The demographic characteristics of the healthy pregnant women and non-pregnant women are summarized in Table 1. Between pregnant and non-pregnant women were similar in age (33 ± 4 and 31 ± 3 years, $p = 0.126$), body mass index (BMI) (19.3 ± 0.7 and 20.2 ± 1.5 kg/m^2, $p = 0.067$), and BSA (1.50 ± 0.09 and 1.49 ± 0.09 m^2, $p = 0.848$). However, the proportion of nulliparous women was significantly different (5 (42%) and 14 (93%) respectively, p < 0.05, Fisher's exact test).

CMR examination and blood tests were performed at gestational week 25.3 ± 0.6 (26.4 to 24.0) and 33.7 ± 0.7 (34.9 to 33.1) for the 2nd and 3rd trimesters of pregnancy, respectively, and on postpartum day 35 ± 4 (41 to 31).

Hemoglobin concentrations were significantly higher 1 month postpartum than in the 2nd, 3rd trimesters and in non-pregnant women. The BNP concentration was significantly higher in the 2nd trimester than at 1 month postpartum and in non-pregnant women.

LV and RV parameters on cine CMR

The structural and systolic functional parameters of the LV and RV determined by cine CMR, including peak global longitudinal strain (GLS), in the pregnant women and in the non-pregnant women are summarized in Tables 2 and 3, respectively. In pregnant women, LV stroke volume (SV) was not substantially altered during pregnancy compared to 1 month postpartum, but heart rate (HR) was significantly higher in the 2nd trimester than at 1 month postpartum (76 ± 8 vs 64 ± 8 bpm; $p < 0.05$), resulting in significantly greater cardiac output (CO) and cardiac index (CI) in the 2nd trimester (5.7 ± 1.6 L/min

Table 1 Demographic characteristics of the participating women

	Pregnant	Non-pregnant
Number of women	12	15
Number of nulliparous women	5 (42%)†	14 (93%)
Age (y)	33 ± 4	31 ± 3
Pre-pregnancy BMI (kg/m^2)	19.3 ± 0.7	20.2 ± 1.5
Pre-pregnancy BSA (m^2)	1.50 ± 0.09	1.49 ± 0.09
Pre-pregnancy Hb (g/dL)	NA	13.0 ± 0.9
Pre-pregnancy BNP (pg/mL)	NA	13 ± 5
BSA (m^2) at CMR		
2nd trimester	1.53 ± 0.10	NA
3rd trimester	1.57 ± 0.11	NA
Postpartum 1 month (PP1M)	1.52 ± 0.11	NA
Hb (g/dL) at CMR		
2nd trimester	11.2 ± 1.0 *†	NA
3rd trimester	11.2 ± 0.8*†	NA
Postpartum 1 month (PP1M)	12.3 ± 1.0	NA
BNP (pg/mL) at CMR		
2nd trimester	20 ± 1 *†	NA
3rd trimester	14 ± 6	NA
Postpartum 1 month (PP1M)	11 ± 8	NA
Gestational week at delivery	39.3 ± 1.4	NA

BMI Body mass index, BSA Body surface area, CMR Cardiovascular magnetic resonance,
[Hb]/[BNP] Blood concentration of hemoglobin/brain type natriuretic peptide, NA Not applicable
*, P < 0.05 vs. postpartum 1 month; †, P < 0.05 vs. non-pregnant women

and 3.7 ± 0.9 L/min/m^2) than at 1 month postpartum (4.3 ± 1.1 L/min and 2.8 ± 0.7 L/min/m^2, $p < 0.05$) and in non-pregnant women (4.3 ± 0.7 L/min and 2.9 ± 0.4 L/min/m^2, $p < 0.05$), respectively. As with LV, RV CO (6.2 ± 1.3 mL/min) and CI (4.0 ± 0.7 mL/min/m^2) were significantly greater in the 2nd trimester than at 1 month postpartum (4.9 ± 0.9 mL/min, $p < 0.05$ and 3.2 ± 0.5 mL/min/m^2, $p < 0.05$) and in non-pregnant women (4.8 ± 0.6 mL/min, $P < 0.05$ and 3.2 ± 0.3 mL/min/m^2, p < 0.05), respectively. LV end-diastolic volume (EDV) was significantly greater in the 3rd trimester (126 ± 22 mL) than in non-pregnant women (108 ± 14 mL, p < 0.05). LVM and LVM index were significantly greater in the 3rd trimester (88.7 ± 11.8 g and 56.5 ± 6.5 g/m^2) than at 1 month postpartum (72.0 ± 9.8 g, p < 0.05 and 47.5 ± 6.0 g/m^2, p < 0.05) and in non-pregnant women (66.3 ± 13.9 g, p < 0.05 and 44.5 ± 8.0 g/m^2, p < 0.05), respectively (Fig. 3). Mean LV wall thickness was also significantly greater in the 3rd trimester (5.09 ± 0.57 mm) than at 1 month postpartum (4.53 ± 0.50 mm, p < 0.05) and in non-pregnant women (4.57 ± 0.63 g, p < 0.05). Pearson's linear correlation coefficients were 0.76 ($p < 0.001$), 0.75 (p < 0.001), and 0.56 (p < 0.001) for LVEDV, LV

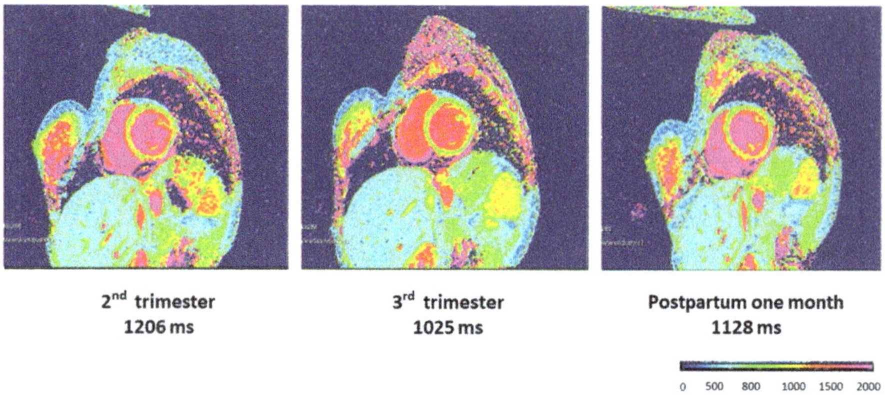

Fig. 2 Native T1 mapping using MOLLI in a representative pregnant woman, with a native T1 of 1206 ms in the 2nd trimester, 1025 ms in the 3rd trimester, and 1128 ms at 1 month postpartum

end-systolic volume (ESV), and LVM, respectively, against actual body weight.

LV strain by feature tracking

LV GLS showed no significant difference among the 2nd and 3rd trimesters, 1 month postpartum, and in non-pregnant women (− 19.5 ± 1.8, − 19.7% ± 2.2, − 19.0% ± 2.0%, and − 19.3 ± 1.9%, respectively, $p = 0.66$) (Fig. 4). RV GLS also showed no significant difference among the 2nd and 3rd trimesters, 1 month postpartum, and non-pregnant women (− 28.0 ± 3.1, − 25.6% ± 3.4, − 25.7% ± 3.9%, and − 26.0% ± 5.0%, respectively, $p = 0.42$) (Fig. 4).

Native myocardial T1 determined by the MOLLI sequence

Native myocardial T1 in pregnant women was 1133 ± 55 ms (95%CI 1095.8 to 1169.4 ms), 1138 ± 86 ms (95%CI 1081 to 1194 ms), and 1105 ± 45 ms (95% CI 1075 to 1134 ms) in the 2nd trimester, the 3rd trimester, and at 1 month postpartum, respectively, whereas native myocardial T1 in non-pregnant women was 1129 ± 52 ms (95% CI 1100 to 1159 ms) (Fig. 5). Thus, no significant difference was noted in native myocardial T1 among the 2nd and 3rd trimesters, 1 month postpartum, and non-pregnant women ($p = 0.59$). Pearson's linear correlation analysis demonstrated that native myocardial

Table 2 Left ventricular parameters on CMR

	Pregnant women			
	2nd (n = 12)	3rd (n = 12)	Postpartum (n = 12)	Non-pregnant women (n = 15)
LVSV (mL)	74.0 ± 18.1†	71.1 ± 13.7	66.0 ± 13.1	62.2 ± 9.8
LVSVI (mL/m²)	48.1 ± 10.4	45.3 ± 7.6	43.4 ± 7.9	41.7 ± 6.5
LVCO (L/min)	5.7 ± 1.6*†	5.2 ± 1.2†	4.3 ± 1.1	4.3 ± 0.7
LVCI (L/min/m²)	3.7 ± 0.9*†	3.3 ± 0.7	2.8 ± 0.7	2.9 ± 0.4
LVEF (%)	60.2 ± 8.7	56.7 ± 5.0	57.7 ± 4.5	57.4 ± 4.6
LVEDV (mL)	123 ± 21	126 ± 22†	115 ± 21	108 ± 14
LVEDVI (mL/m²)	79.8 ± 9.8	80.0 ± 11.1	75.0 ± 10.4	73.2 ± 9.3
LVESV (mL)	48.7 ± 13.5	54.5 ± 11.5†	48.6 ± 10.4	46.4 ± 8.3
LVESVI (mL/ m²)	31.7 ± 8.0	34.6 ± 5.8	31.7 ± 4.9	31.4 ± 5.3
LVM (g)	82.6 ± 18.2†	88.7 ± 11.8*†	72.0 ± 9.8	66.3 ± 13.9
LVMI (g/m²)	53.7 ± 10.2†	56.5 ± 6.5*†	47.5 ± 6.0	44.5 ± 8.0
LVM/EDV (g/mL)	0.68 ± 0.13	0.72 ± 0.13	0.65 ± 0.14	0.61 ± 0.14
Heart rate (bpm)	76 ± 8*†	73 ± 7*	64 ± 8	69 ± 9
LV peak strain (%)	−19.5 ± 1.8	−19.7 ± 2.2	−19.0 ± 2.0	−19.3 ± 1.9
LV mean wall thickness (mm)	4.8 ± 0.7	5.1 ± 0.5*†	4.5 ± 0.5	4.6 ± 0.6
LV mean wall thickness index (mm/m²)	3.1 ± 0.4	3.2 ± 0.3	3.0 ± 0.3	3.0 ± 0.4

2nd and 3rd Trimesters of pregnancy, *BSA* Body surface area;
LV Left ventricular, *LVM* LV mass, *SV* Stroke volume, *CO* Cardiac output, *EF* Ejection fraction,
EDV End-diastolic volume, *ESV* End-systolic volume
*, $P < 0.05$ vs. data for postpartum one month; †, $P < 0.05$ vs. data for non-pregnant women

Table 3 Right ventricular parameters on CMR

| | Pregnant women (n = 12) | | | |
	2nd (n = 12)	3rd (n = 12)	Postpartum (n = 12)	Non-pregnant women (n = 15)
RVSV (mL)	80.8 ± 13.5	78.8 ± 12.2	75.8 ± 13.1	71.1 ± 10.3
RVSVI (mL/m^2)	52.6 ± 6.8	50.5 ± 4.7	49.7 ± 6.8	47.5 ± 5.4
RVCO (L/min)	6.2 ± 1.3*†	5.7 ± 1.1†	4.9 ± 0.9	4.8 ± 0.6
RVCI (L/min/m^2)	4.0 ± 0.7*†	3.6 ± 0.6†	3.2 ± 0.5	3.2 ± 0.3
RVEF (%)	60.3 ± 3.8†	60.2 ± 3.9†	59.3 ± 6.3	56.2 ± 5.2
RVEDV (mL)	133 ± 19	129 ± 18	126 ± 20	126 ± 18
RVEDVI (mL/m^2)	86.3 ± 9.7	82.2 ± 8.3	82.9 ± 10.2	84.2 ± 9.5
RVESV (mL)	53.3 ± 9.7	52.3 ± 10.0	50.5 ± 11.4	55.0 ± 12.5
RLVESVI (mL/ m^2)	34.7 ± 5.3	33.3 ± 5.5	33.2 ± 6.7	36.8 ± 7.8
RV peak strain (%)	−28.0 ± 3.1	−25.6 ± 3.4	−25.7 ± 3.9	−26.0 ± 5.0

2nd and 3rd Trimesters of pregnancy, BSA Body surface area,
RV Right ventricular, SV Stroke volume, CO Cardiac output, EF Ejection fraction,
EDV End-diastolic volume, ESV End-systolic volume; *, P < 0.05 vs. data for postpartum 1 month;
†, P < 0.05 vs. data for non-pregnant women

T1 was not correlated with LVM, with r of 0.16 and p = 0.27 (Fig. 6).

Discussion

In this study, reference values of CMR parameters including native myocardial T1 and LV GLS in normal pregnancy were determined in 12 Japanese normal pregnant women. It was found that, in normal pregnancy, LV remodeling occurs without significant alterations of native myocardial T1 and LV GLS, despite the significant increase in LVM. These results observed in normal

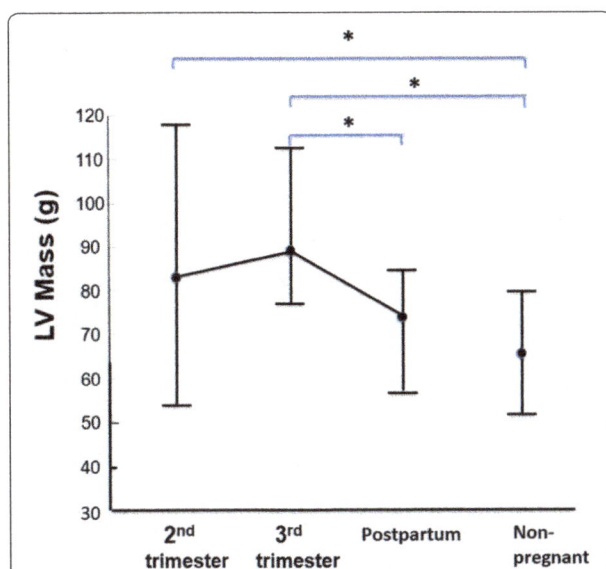

Fig. 3 LVM by the stages of pregnancy in healthy pregnant women and in non-pregnant women. Mean LVM is 82.6 ± 18.2 g in the 2nd trimester, 88.7 ± 11.8 g in the 3rd trimester, 72.0 ± 9.8 g at 1 month postpartum, and 66.3 ± 13.9 g in non-pregnant women. *, P < 0.05

pregnancy will serve as an important basis for identifying myocardial abnormalities in patients with PPCM and other pregnancy-related myocardial diseases.

LVM increased significantly during pregnancy in the normotensive pregnant women in the current study. This finding is consistent with the results in previous studies using echocardiography and CMR [4, 21–23]. In the present study, native T1 in healthy pregnant women showed no significant changes throughout pregnancy and postpartum and as compared with non-pregnant women. The finding that native T1 in normal pregnancy is comparable to that in non-pregnant women confirmed that measurement of native T1 can be as useful to diagnose cardiomyopathy or myocarditis in normal pregnancy as in non-pregnant patients [14]. This finding also suggests that interstitial water retention does not occur in the myocardium of uncomplicated pregnant women.

The myocardium consists of cellular and extracellular interstitial compartments. Therefore, increased LVM without myocardial edema in normal pregnancy in the present study is attributable to an increase in cardiomyocyte volume or increase of the intravascular compartment. Eghbali et al. demonstrated in their animal study that mouse cardiomyocyte volume increased by approximately 70% in pregnancy [29]. In athletes' hearts, which show the cardiac adaptive response to regular athletic training, cardiac adaptation is characterized by an increase in LVM and, as a consequence, eccentric hypertrophy [30]. As in the case of increased LVM in normal pregnant women that was observed in the present study, McDiarmid et al. recently showed, using CMR T1 mapping technique, that increased LVM in athletes' hearts occurs because of an expansion of the cellular compartment rather than of extracellular volume [30]. However, blood volume alteration has not been observed in

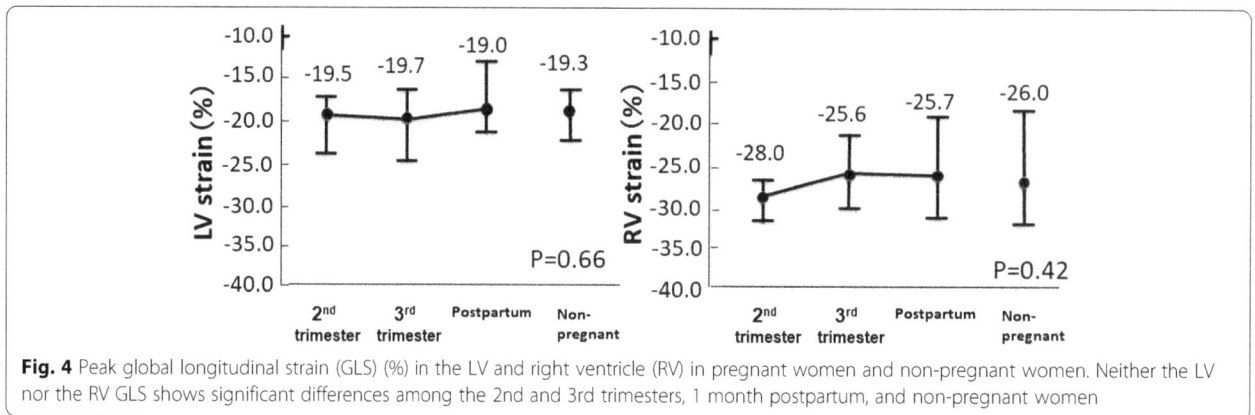

Fig. 4 Peak global longitudinal strain (GLS) (%) in the LV and right ventricle (RV) in pregnant women and non-pregnant women. Neither the LV nor the RV GLS shows significant differences among the 2nd and 3rd trimesters, 1 month postpartum, and non-pregnant women

pregnancy-related physiological heart hypertrophy in mice [24, 29, 30].

In the current study, LV remodeling in healthy pregnant women was not associated with impairment of LV GLS. LV hypertrophy is observed in a variety of LV myocardial conditions such as hypertension, aortic stenosis, hypertrophic cardiomyopathy, amyloidosis, Fabry disease, etc., [31] and in patients with heart failure with preserved ejection fraction [32]. A recent study demonstrated that LV hypertrophy in Fabry disease was associated with significant impairment of LV GLS, even though LV ejection fraction was preserved [33]. Another study showed that GLS is impaired in patients with heart failure with preserved ejection fraction (HFpEF) [34]. The present results suggest that increased LVM in healthy pregnant women is the adaptive response to an increased heart workload.

Significant positive correlations between body weight and LV volume and LVM were observed in the present study. It is known that LV volume and LVM increase along with the increase of body weight even in non-pregnant women [35]. However, pregnancy-related cardiac remodeling can be a complex process that

involves many factors, including changes in the signaling pathways and composition of extracellular matrix, as well as the levels of sex hormones. Underlying molecular mechanisms of cardiac remodeling during human pregnancy remain unknown. In mouse experiments, pregnancy-related physiologic heart hypertrophy was different from pathologic hypertrophy in terms of gene expression. It is supposed that the increase in estrogen toward the end of pregnancy plays a substantial role in the expressions of certain genes, which contributes to pregnancy-related heart hypertrophy [29]. Furthermore, some animal studies reported that fibrosis is minimal or absent in the pregnant heart in the rat [24]. The results of the current study are in line with these findings of previous animal studies [24, 29]. Thus, LV remodeling may not simply be attributable to the overweight and the natural volume overload during pregnancy.

The second and third trimesters of pregnancy and 1 month postpartum were selected to observe the time course of the CMR parameters. The first trimester was omitted because performing CMR in this period is still

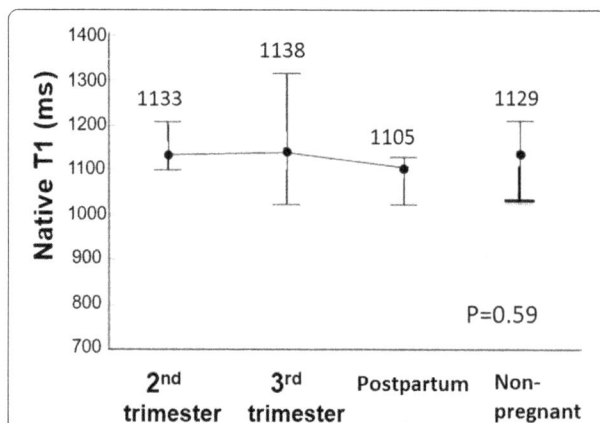

Fig. 5 Native T1 determined using MOLLI. Change in the native T1 using MOLLI by the stage of pregnancy and in non-pregnant women. Native T1 shows no significant differences among the 2nd and 3rd trimesters, 1 month postpartum, and non-pregnant women

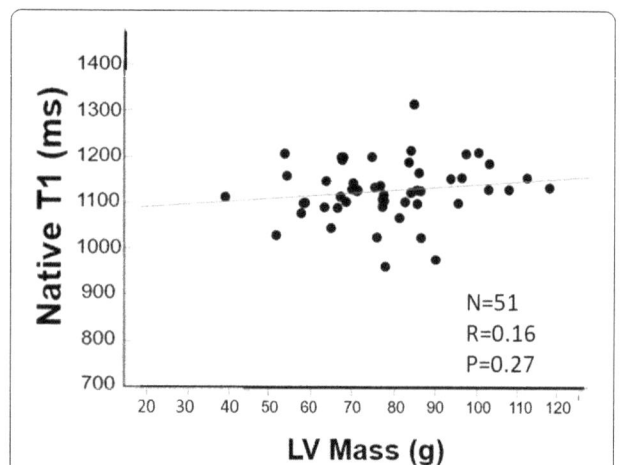

Fig. 6 Association between LVM and native T1 during pregnancy and in non-pregnant women. N = number of samples, R = correlation efficient, P=P value

controversial in normal pregnant women. The reason why 24–28 weeks was selected in the 2nd trimester is that circulating blood volume starts to increase in the 1st trimester and reaches almost its peak during this period [7, 36, 37]. The period of 32–36 weeks was selected in the 3rd trimester because circulating blood volume maintains its peak, and the heart overload is the greatest in this period [7, 36, 37]. Postpartum 3 months would be preferred to confirm that CMR parameters return to the baseline because the decrease in cardiac output toward baseline typically occurs between 6 and 12 weeks postpartum [7, 38]. However, it is almost impossible in Japan to obtain consent from all participants to perform CMR examinations or laboratory tests other than at postpartum 1 month, because all women and neonates in Japan see a doctor at postpartum 1 month as a routine visit. Therefore, 1 month postpartum was selected.

Early diagnosis of PPCM is important for better outcomes, because delay in the diagnosis of PPCM is associated with worse outcomes, such as death or heart transplantation [2, 39]. Myocardial tissue characterization by CMR in patients with PPCM has been only sporadically described, mainly using LGE CMR. However, the prevalence of LGE in PPCM varies substantially, ranging from 5 to 71% in those previous studies [15–19]. Although LGE CMR is a robust technique for identifying focally abnormal regions such as myocardial damage and fibrosis, LGE CMR is not sufficiently sensitive to detect diffuse myocardial disease. Furthermore, LGE CMR requires the administration of gadolinium contrast medium, which is recommended to be avoided until after delivery unless absolutely necessary [40]. Therefore, native T1 mapping, which is obtained without gadolinium contrast injection, may play an important role for the diagnosis of PPCM and the clinical management of PPCM patients.

In the present study, RVEDV showed an increasing trend during pregnancy. RV parameters are more easily accessible by CMR than by echocardiography, since CMR is not limited by variations of ventricular geometry, body habitus etc., which are major limiting factors of echocardiography. A previous study by Ducas et al. demonstrated that RVEDV was significantly increased from baseline during pregnancy [4]. The present findings are in accordance with the result from the previous study. More importantly, RVEF and RV GLS during pregnancy were not significantly altered compared with those at 1 month postpartum in the current study. This might represent the adaptive response of the RV to the increased heart workload, as in the LV. In the current study, some deviation was noted in LVEF and RVEF, and the standard deviations for LVEF were slightly higher than those for RVEF. However, they might occur because, even in the study of reference ranges for CMR in Korean population cohort, such differences were observed in male [41]. The considerably large standard deviation

values for LVESV compared to the mean LVESV (i.e. 48.7 ± 13.5 mL) might be within the same range for LVESV as in the normal Chinese population (60 ± 12 ml) [42].

Clinical implications
In this study, reference values of myocardial T1 relaxation time and GLS were determined in 12 Japanese normal pregnant women. These data are useful to determine if these CMR parameters are abnormal in patients with suspected PPCM. The current results can also serve as an important baseline not only in PPCM patients, but also in other pregnancy-related cardiac diseases, for example, in identifying myocardial edema or inflammation in pregnant patients with acute myocarditis.

Limitations
There are three limitations in this study. First, there was a small number of participants. The age distribution of the pregnant women is an important issue since it pertains to the age range of 20–35 years and the age range of 35–39 years. In the present study population, the numbers of subjects in the age range of 20–35 years and the age range of 35–39 years were 8 and 4 in pregnant women and 12 and 3 in non-pregnant controls, respectively. However, because of the small sample size, it was not possible to show any significant age-related differences among the group and between groups. Future studies with a larger number of participants are warranted. Second, there was a difference in parity between pregnant women and non-pregnant controls. Third, no CMR findings were compared to the results of cardiac biopsy or heart catheterization as the gold standard technique for tissue characterization or functional assessment of the heart.

Conclusion
Despite the presence of LV hypertrophy during pregnancy, T1 relaxation time measured by the CMR MOLLI method and myocardial strain by feature-tracking CMR were not different from those in non-pregnant women. These results observed in normal pregnancy will serve as an important basis for identifying myocardial abnormalities in patients with PPCM and other pregnancy-related myocardial diseases.

Abbreviations
BMI: Body mass index; BNP: Brain type natriuretic peptide; BSA: Body surface area; CI: Cardiac index; CMR: Cardiovascular magnetic resonance; CO: Cardiac output; DICOM: Digital Imaging and Communication in Medicine; EDV: End-diastolic volume; EF: Ejection fraction; ESV: End-systolic volume; FA: Flip angle; FOV: Field of view; GLS: Global longitudinal strain; Hb: Hemoglobin; HFpEF: Heart failure with preserved ejection fraction; HR: Heart rate; LA: Left atrium/left atrial; LGE: Late gadolinium enhancement; LV: Left ventricle/left ventricular; LVM: Left ventricular mass; MOLLI: Modified Look Locker inversion recovery; PPCM: Peripartum cardiomyopathy; RV: Right ventricle/right ventricular; SV: Stroke volume; TE: Echo time; TR: Repetition time

Acknowledgements
The authors would like to thank Prof. Philip J. Steer (Emeritus Professor, Imperial College London) for providing technical advice regarding this manuscript. The authors also thank Shinichi Takase (Radiologic Technologist, Mie University Hospital) for acquiring CMR images for all participants of this study and providing technical support regarding this study.

Authors' contributions
MN participated in study design, scored the studies, conducted the statistical analysis, interpreted the data, and drafted the manuscript. MI participated in study design, scored the studies, interpreted the data, and revised the manuscript. KD participated in study design and interpreted the data. HT and EK interpreted the data. MI and HS participated in study design, interpreted the data, and revised the manuscript. TI conceived the study, participated in its design, interpreted the data, and revised the manuscript. All authors read and approved the final manuscript.

Competing interests
Dr. Sakuma and Dr. Ishida received a departmental research grant from Fuji Pharma Co., Ltd., Daiichi Sankyo Co., Ltd., and FUJIFILM RI Pharma Co., Ltd.. Dr. Ito and Dr. Dohi received a departmental research grant from MSD K.K., Daiichi Sankyo Co, Ltd., Astellas Pharma Inc., Otsuka Pharmaceutical Co., Ltd., and Takeda Pharmaceutical Co, Ltd.. Dr. Sakuma received lecture fees from Bayer Yakuhin, Ltd. Dr. Ito received lecture fees from Daiichi Sankyo Co, Ltd., Mitsubishi Tanabe Pharma Corporation, and Bayer Yakuhin, Ltd. Dr. Dohi received lecture fees from Otsuka Pharmaceutical Co.. All other authors have no conflicts of interest to declare. No relevant conflicts of interest related to the article were disclosed by the authors.

Author details
[1]Department of Obstetrics and Gynecology, Mie University Hospital, 2-174 Edobashi, Tsu, Mie 514-8507, Japan. [2]Department of Radiology, Mie University Hospital, 2-174 Edobashi, Tsu, Mie 514-8507, Japan. [3]Department of Cardiology and Nephrology, Mie University Hospital, 2-174 Edobashi, Tsu, Mie 514-8507, Japan.

References
1. Ersbøll AS, Damm P, Gustafsson F, Vejlstrup NG, Johansen M. Peripartum cardiomyopathy: a systematic literature review. Acta Obstet Gynecol Scand. 2016;95:1205–19.
2. Kamiya CA, Yoshimatsu J, Ikeda T. Peripartum cardiomyopathy from a genetic perspective. Circ J. 2016;80:1684–8.
3. Sliwa K, Hilfiker-Kleiner D, Petrie MC, Mebazaa A, Pieske B, Buchmann E, et al. Heart failure Association of the European Society of cardiology working group on Peripartum cardiomyopathy. Current state of knowledge on aetiology, diagnosis, management, and therapy of peripartum cardiomyopathy: a position statement from the heart failure Association of the European Society of cardiology working group on peripartum cardiomyopathy. Eur J Heart Fail. 2010;12:767–78.
4. Ducas RA, Elliott JE, Melnyk SF, Premecz S, daSilva M, Cleverley K, et al. Cardiovascular magnetic resonance in pregnancy: insights from the cardiac hemodynamic imaging and remodeling in pregnancy (CHIRP) study. J Cardiovasc Magn Reson. 2014;16:1.
5. Kanal E, Barkovich AJ, Bell C, Borgstede JP, Bradley WG Jr, Froelich JW, et al. ACR blue ribbon panel on MR safety. ACR guidance document for safe MR practices: 2007. ARJ Am J Roentgenol. 2007;188:1447–74.
6. ACOG Committee Opinion. Number 299, September 2004 (replaces no. 158, September 1995). Guidelines for diagnostic imaging during pregnancy. Obstet Gynecol. 2004;104:647–51.
7. Stewart RD, Nelson DB, Matulevicius SA, Morgan JL, McIntire DD, Drazner MH, et al. Cardiac magnetic resonance imaging to assess the impact of maternal habitus on cardiac remodeling during pregnancy. Am J Obstet Gynecol. 2016;214:640.e1–6.
8. Amano Y, Takeda M, Tachi M, Kitamura M, Kumita S. Myocardial fibrosis evaluated by look-locker and late gadolinium enhancement magnetic resonance imaging in apical hypertrophic cardiomyopathy: association with ventricular tachyarrhythmia and risk factors. J Magn Reson Imaging. 2014;40:407–12.
9. Wong TC, Piehler KM, Zareba KM, Lin K, Phrampus A, Patel A, et al. Myocardial damage detected by late gadolinium enhancement cardiovascular magnetic resonance is associated with subsequent hospitalization for heart failure. J Am Heart Assoc. 2013;18:2.
10. Cannaò PM, Altabella L, Petrini M, Alì M, Secchi F, Sardanelli F. Novel cardiac magnetic resonance biomarkers: native T1 and extracellular volume myocardial mapping. Eur Heart J Suppl. 2016;18(Suppl E):E64–71.
11. Moon JC, Messroghli DR, Kellman P, Piechnik SK, Robson MD, Ugander M, et al. Society for Cardiovascular Magnetic Resonance Imaging; cardiovascular magnetic resonance working Group of the European Society of cardiology. Myocardial T1 mapping and extracellular volume quantification: a Society for Cardiovascular Magnetic Resonance (SCMR) and CMR working Group of the European Society of cardiology consensus statement. J Cardiovasc Magn Reson. 2013;15:92.
12. Ferreira VM, Piechnik SK, Dall'Armellina E, Karamitsos TD, Francis JM, Ntusi N, et al. T(1) mapping for the diagnosis of acute myocarditis using CMR: comparison to T2-weighted and late gadolinium enhanced imaging. JACC Cardiovasc Imaging. 2013;6:1048–58.
13. Goto Y, Ishida M, Takase S, Sigfridsson A, Uno M, Nagata M, et al. Comparison of displacement encoding with stimulated echoes to magnetic resonance feature tracking for the assessment of myocardial strain in patients with acute myocardial infarction. Am J Cardiol. 2017;119:1542–7.
14. Haaf P, Garg P, Messroghli DR, Broadbent DA, Greenwood JP, Plein S. Cardiac T1 mapping and extracellular volume (ECV) in clinical practice: a comprehensive review. J Cardiovasc Magn Reson. 2016;18:89.
15. Mouquet F, Lions C, de Groote P, Mouquet F, Lions C, de Groote P, et al. Characterisation of peripartum cardiomyopathy by cardiac magnetic resonance imaging. Eur Radiol. 2008;18:2765–9.
16. Renz DM, Röttgen R, Habedank D, Wagner M, Böttcher J, Pfeil A, et al. New insights into peripartum cardiomyopathy using cardiac magnetic resonance imaging. Rofo. 2011;183:834–41.
17. Arora NP, Mohamad T, Mahajan N, Danrad R, Kottam A, Li T, et al. Cardiac magnetic resonance imaging in peripartum cardiomyopathy. Am J Med Sci. 2014;347:112–7.
18. Haghikia A, Röntgen P, Vogel-Claussen J, Schwab J, Westenfeld R, Ehlermann P, et al. Prognostic implication of right ventricular involvement in peripartum cardiomyopathy: a cardiovascular magnetic resonance study. ESC Heart Fail. 2015;2:139–49.
19. Schelbert EB, Elkayam U, Cooper LT, Givertz MM, Alexis JD, Briller J, et al. Investigations of Pregnancy Associated Cardiomyopathy (IPAC) investigators. Myocardial damage detected by late gadolinium enhancement cardiac magnetic resonance is uncommon in peripartum cardiomyopathy. J Am Heart Assoc. 2017;6. https://doi.org/10.1161/JAHA.117.005472.
20. Pritchard JA. Changes in blood volume during pregnancy. Anesthesiology. 1965;26:393–9.
21. Cong J, Yang X, Zhang N, Shen J, Fan T, Zhang Z. Quantitative analysis of left atrial volume and function during normotensive and preeclamptic pregnancy: a real-time three-dimensional echocardiography study. Int J Cardiovasc Imaging. 2015;31:805–12.
22. Estensen ME, Beitnes JO, Grindheim G, Aaberge L, Smiseth OA, Henriksen T, et al. Altered maternal left ventricular contractility and function during normal pregnancy. Ultrasound Obstet Gynecol. 2013;41:659–66.
23. Simmons LA, Gillin AG, Jeremy RW. Structural and functional changes in left ventricle during normotensive and preeclamptic pregnancy. Am J Physiol Heart Circ Physiol. 2002;283:H1627–33.
24. Li J, Umar S, Amjedi M, Iorga A, Sharma S, Nadadur RD, et al. New frontiers in heart hypertrophy during pregnancy. Am J Cardiovasc Dis. 2012;2:192–207.
25. Messroghli DR, Radjenovic A, Kozerke S, Higgins DM, Sivananthan MU, Ridgway JP. Modified look-locker inversion recovery (MOLLI) for high-resolution T1 mapping of the heart. Magn Reson Med. 2004;52:141–6.
26. Vinnakota KC, Bassingthwaighte JB. Myocardial density and composition: a basis for calculating intracellular metabolite concentrations. Am J Physiol Heart Circ Physiol. 2004;286:H1742–9.
27. Taylor AJ, Salerno M, Dharmakumar R, Jerosch-Herold M. T1 mapping: basic techniques and clinical applications. JACC Cardiovasc Imaging. 2016;9:67–81.
28. Guilford JP. Fundamental statistics in psychology and education. New York: McGraw Hill; 1956.

29. Eghbali M, Deva R, Alioua A, Minosyan TY, Ruan H, Wang Y, et al. Molecular and functional signature of heart hypertrophy during pregnancy. Circ Res. 2005;96:1208–16.

30. McDiarmid AK, Swoboda PP, Erhayiem B, Lancaster RE, Lyall GK, Broadbent DA, et al. Athletic cardiac adaptation in males is a consequence of elevated myocyte mass. Circ Cardiovasc Imaging. 2016;9:e003579.

31. Sado DM, White SK, Piechnik SK, Banypersad SM, Treibel T, Captur G, et al. Identification and assessment of Anderson-Fabry disease by cardiovascular magnetic resonance noncontrast myocardial T1 mapping. Circ Cardiovasc Imaging. 2013;6:392–8.

32. Shah AM, Pfeffer MA. The many faces of heart failure with preserved ejection fraction. Nat Rev Cardiol. 2012;9:555–6.

33. Pica S, Sado DM, Maestrini V, Fontana M, White SK, Treibel T, et al. Reproducibility of native myocardial T1 mapping in the assessment of Fabry disease and its role in early detection of cardiac involvement by cardiovascular magnetic resonance. J Cardiovasc Magn Reson. 2014;16:99.

34. Hayashi T, Yamada S, Iwano H, Nakabachi M, Sakakibara M, Okada K, et al. Left ventricular global strain for estimating relaxation and filling pressure - a multicenter study. Circ J. 2016;80:1163–70.

35. Woodiwiss AJ, Libhaber CD, Majane OH, Libhaber E, Maseko M, Norton GR. Obesity promotes left ventricular concentric rather than eccentric geometric remodeling and hypertrophy independent of blood pressure. Am J Hypertens. 2008;21:1144–51.

36. Savu O, Jurcuţ R, Giuşcă S, van Mieghem T, Gussi I, Popescu BA, et al. Morphological and functional adaptation of the maternal heart during pregnancy. Circ Cardiovasc Imaging. 2012;5:289–97.

37. Sanghavi M, Rutherford JD. Cardiovascular physiology of pregnancy. Circulation. 2014;130:1003–8.

38. Melchiorre K, Sharma R, Khalil A, Thilaganathan B. Maternal cardiovascular function in normal pregnancy: evidence of maladaptation to chronic volume overload. Hypertension. 2016;67:754–62.

39. Goland S, Modi K, Bitar F, Janmohamed M, Mirocha JM, Czer LS, et al. Clinical profile and predictors of complications in peripartum cardiomyopathy. J Card Fail. 2009;15:645–50.

40. Thomsen HS, Morcos SK, Almén T, Bellin M-F, Bertolotto M, Bongartz G, et al. Nephrogenic systemic fibrosis and gadolinium-based contrast media: updated ESUR contrast medium safety committee guidelines. Eur Radiol. 2013;23:307–18.

41. Chang SA, Choe YH, Jang SY, Kim SM, Lee SC, Oh JK. Assessment of left and right ventricular parameters in healthy Korean volunteers using cardiac magnetic resonance imaging: change in ventricular volume and function based on age, gender and body surface area. Int J Cardiovasc Imaging. 2012;28:141–7.

42. Le TT, Tan RS, De Deyn M, Goh EP, Han Y, Leong BR, et al. Cardiovascular magnetic resonance reference ranges for the heart and aorta in Chinese at 3T. J Cardiovasc Magn Reson. 2016;18:21.

18

Importance of operator training and rest perfusion on the diagnostic accuracy of stress perfusion cardiovascular magnetic resonance

Adriana D. M. Villa[1†], Laura Corsinovi[1,2†], Ioannis Ntalas[1,3], Xenios Milidonis[1], Cian Scannell[1], Gabriella Di Giovine[1], Nicholas Child[1], Catarina Ferreira[4], Muhummad Sohaib Nazir[1], Julia Karady[1], Esmeralda Eshja[5], Viola De Francesco[1], Nuno Bettencourt[6], Andreas Schuster[7,8,9], Tevfik F. Ismail[1], Reza Razavi[1] and Amedeo Chiribiri[1*]

Abstract

Background: Clinical evaluation of stress perfusion cardiovascular magnetic resonance (CMR) is currently based on visual assessment and has shown high diagnostic accuracy in previous clinical trials, when performed by expert readers or core laboratories. However, these results may not be generalizable to clinical practice, particularly when less experienced readers are concerned. Other factors, such as the level of training, the extent of ischemia, and image quality could affect the diagnostic accuracy. Moreover, the role of rest images has not been clarified.
The aim of this study was to assess the diagnostic accuracy of visual assessment for operators with different levels of training and the additional value of rest perfusion imaging, and to compare visual assessment and automated quantitative analysis in the assessment of coronary artery disease (CAD).

Methods: We evaluated 53 patients with known or suspected CAD referred for stress-perfusion CMR. Nine operators (equally divided in 3 levels of competency) blindly reviewed each case twice with a 2-week interval, in a randomised order, with and without rest images. Semi-automated Fermi deconvolution was used for quantitative analysis and estimation of myocardial perfusion reserve as the ratio of stress to rest perfusion estimates.

Results: Level-3 operators correctly identified significant CAD in 83.6% of the cases. This percentage dropped to 65.7% for Level-2 operators and to 55.7% for Level-1 operators ($p < 0.001$). Quantitative analysis correctly identified CAD in 86.3% of the cases and was non-inferior to expert readers ($p = 0.56$). When rest images were available, a significantly higher level of confidence was reported ($p = 0.022$), but no significant differences in diagnostic accuracy were measured ($p = 0.34$).

Conclusions: Our study demonstrates that the level of training is the main determinant of the diagnostic accuracy in the identification of CAD. Level-3 operators performed at levels comparable with the results from clinical trials. Rest images did not significantly improve diagnostic accuracy, but contributed to higher confidence in the results. Automated quantitative analysis performed similarly to level-3 operators. This is of increasing relevance as recent technical advances in image reconstruction and analysis techniques are likely to permit the clinical translation of robust and fully automated quantitative analysis into routine clinical practice.

Keywords: Cardiovascular magnetic resonance, Stress perfusion imaging, Coronary artery disease, Quantitative assessment, Myocardial ischemia, Diagnostic accuracy, Training

* Correspondence: amedeo.chiribiri@kcl.ac.uk
†Adriana D. M. Villa and Laura Corsinovi contributed equally to this work.
[1]School of Biomedical Engineering & Imaging Sciences, King's College London, King's Health Partners, 4th Floor Lambeth Wing, St Thomas' Hospital, London SE1 7EH, UK
Full list of author information is available at the end of the article

Background

Stress perfusion cardiovascular magnetic resonance (CMR) is increasingly used for the evaluation of patients with known or suspected coronary artery disease (CAD) and has a class I indication for patients at intermediate risk of CAD according to recent guidelines [1, 2].

Stress perfusion CMR has been shown to be highly accurate for the detection of CAD, with sensitivity ranging from 75 to 91% and specificity ranging from 59 to 87% [3–5]. It should be noted that in most of these studies, visual assessment has been carried out either by a core laboratory or by expert readers, and therefore the findings may not be generalizable to routine clinical practice. As stress perfusion CMR gains acceptance and becomes more available, it will inevitably be performed in lower volume and less experienced centers.

Stress perfusion CMR is typically evaluated by visual assessment. This can be influenced by the extent of ischemia and the presence of areas of relatively preserved perfusion, which can be used as reference [6]. Moreover, image artefacts can complicate the interpretation of the images. Dark rim artefacts, which are commonly observed during stress perfusion, can be misdiagnosed as subendocardial perfusion abnormalities [7], in particular when relatively long acquisition times are used and spatial resolution is low. Moreover, areas of infarction are frequently associated with delayed perfusion [8, 9]. The simultaneous evaluation of stress and rest perfusion CMR and late gadolinium enhancement (LGE) images is recommended to identify areas of myocardial infarction and improve the specificity of the interpretation [10, 11], and to exclude imaging artefacts [10].

Additionally, it has been suggested that rest perfusion images could play an important role in improving the identification of imaging artefacts when signal abnormalities are present on both stress and rest images [10]. The acquisition of rest images enables quantification of perfusion reserve, but prolongs scan times and requires additional contrast dosing.

Stress perfusion CMR is complex to read and requires significant training and experience. However, the impact of training and experience has not been formally studied and as yet, there are no specific recommendations in current guidelines, apart from stating that stress perfusion CMR should be part of the training program for Level-2 readers [12]. It is hoped that fully quantitative automated methods may help bridge training gaps and support clinical decision making.

We sought to determine the importance of the level of training of the operator on the diagnostic accuracy of stress perfusion CMR; the role of rest perfusion images in the identification of imaging artefacts and in the correct detection of CAD; and to systematically compare the results of visual assessment with semi-automated quantitative analysis to determine its additional value.

Methods

Consecutive patients ($n = 53$) referred for stress perfusion CMR for suspected CAD were retrospectively included in the study. All patients had invasive coronary angiography on the basis of the clinical indication within 1 month of the CMR examination. Exclusion criteria were contraindications to CMR, gadolinium-based contrast agents or adenosine. Patients with previous coronary artery bypass grafting, hypertrophic cardiomyopathy, aortic stenosis, or other primary myopathic or valvular disease were excluded. All subjects gave written informed consent in accordance with ethical approval. This study complies with the Declaration of Helsinki.

Image acquisition

CMR images were acquired using a 3T scanner (Achieva, Philips Healthcare, Best, The Netherlands) equipped with 32-channel phased-array cardiac coil. The protocol included functional assessment, adenosine stress and rest first pass perfusion imaging, and LGE. The images were acquired using standard acquisition protocols and in end-expiratory breath-hold. For stress imaging, 140 µg/kg/min of adenosine was administered. Imaging commenced at least 3 minutes after infusion initiation. A dual bolus (equal volumes of 0.0075 mmol/kg followed by 0.075 mmol/kg after a 20-s pause) of contrast agent (gadobutrol/Gadovist, Schering, Germany) was injected at 4 ml/s by a power injector [13]. For perfusion, a saturation recovery prepared gradient echo pulse sequence accelerated with k–t sensitivity encoding acceleration with 11 training profiles was used. Typical imaging parameters were: 3 short-axis slices covering standard American Heart Association (AHA) segments [14], 120 acquired dynamics/slice, flip angle 20°, TR 2.5 ms, TE 1.25 ms, saturation pre-pulse recovery time 100 ms, pixel size 1.9 × 1.9 mm, slice thickness 10 mm.

Typical imaging parameters for LGE imaging were: long and short axis to fully cover the left ventricle, inversion recovery turbo field echo, flip angle 25°, TR 6 ms, TE 3 ms, pixel size 0.7 × 0.7 mm, slice thickness 10 mm.

Operator selection

Nine operators were chosen amongst the physicians working in our unit and in other European institutions, on the basis of their level of competency, according to the European Society of Cardiology (ESC)/European Association of Cardiovascular Imaging (EACVI) training guidelines [12]. A total of 9 operators, 3 for each competency level, were chosen; all operators had recently obtained the ESC/EACVI certification (within 2 months) for the appropriate level. In brief, level-1 competency ESC certification requires 20 continuous medical education (CME) hours, involvement in 50 CMR cases and 1-month fellowship; level-2 requires at least 50 CME hours, involvement in 150 clinical cases of which 25 must be perfusion studies, a minimum of 3-months fellowship and the European CMR exam; level-3 requires at least 50 CME hours, involvement in 300 clinical cases of which a minimum of 50 must be perfusion studies, at least 12-months training and the European CMR exam. Level-1 competency reflects core CMR training, level-2 is required to report CMR studies with support from a Level-3 operator and Level-3 is required to perform, interpret and report CMR studies fully independently [12].

Image analysis – Visual assessment

Each operator was asked to report each of the 53 scans twice over a 4-week period, with a minimum interval of 2 weeks between first and second read. The scans were anonymized and presented to the operator as a full dataset, including stress and rest perfusion and LGE, or as reduced datasets, including stress perfusion and LGE only. The full and reduced datasets were analysed blinded to clinical and angiographic data and in a randomized order on different days. The study flowchart can be seen in Fig. 1.

Visual assessment of adenosine stress perfusion CMR and LGE images, displayed side-by-side, was performed as per clinical practice, in accordance with standardized CMR protocols [15]. A perfusion defect was defined as a regional reduction in myocardial signal during LV first-pass of contrast agent, not related to artefacts and not corresponding to an area of scar on LGE images.

Operators were asked to fill an on-line standardized form and to identify segments with inducible ischemia, to identify the presence and transmurality of LGE [16], to identify the most likely culprit coronary artery based on the standard AHA segmentation [14], and to grade their confidence in the diagnosis and the perceived image quality.

The confidence was graded as: 0- very unconfident, 1- unconfident, 2- confident, 3- very confident. The perceived image quality was graded as: 0- poor, 1- moderate, 2- good, 3- excellent.

Coronary angiography results have been used as reference standard. The threshold for coronary artery lumen stenosis was 70% diameter stenosis for epicardial vessels. All invasive angiographic images have been reviewed by consensus of expert operators.

Image analysis – Quantitative assessment

A different operator, blinded to results of visual perfusion assessment and other clinical/angiographic data, performed the segmentation of the images for semi-automated quantitative analysis using software and methods previously developed and validated by our group. Respiratory motion was corrected using affine image registration by maximization of the joint correlation between consecutive dynamics within an automatically determined region of interest [17]. A temporal maximum intensity projection was calculated to serve as a feature image for automatic contour delineation method. The operator then manually optimized the automatically generated contours to avoid partial volume effects at the endocardial and epicardial borders [17]. The intervention of the operator was limited to image segmentation. Quantitative perfusion analysis was then automatically performed by Fermi-constrained deconvolution according to the methods described by Wilke et al. [18] and Jerosch-Herold et al. [19], optimised for high-resolution pixel-wise analysis [20, 21]. Myocardial perfusion reserve (MPR) was calculated as the ratio between stress and rest myocardial blood flow (MBF) estimates. Ischemia was defined as segments with MPR < 1.5, according to previously validated criteria [22, 23].

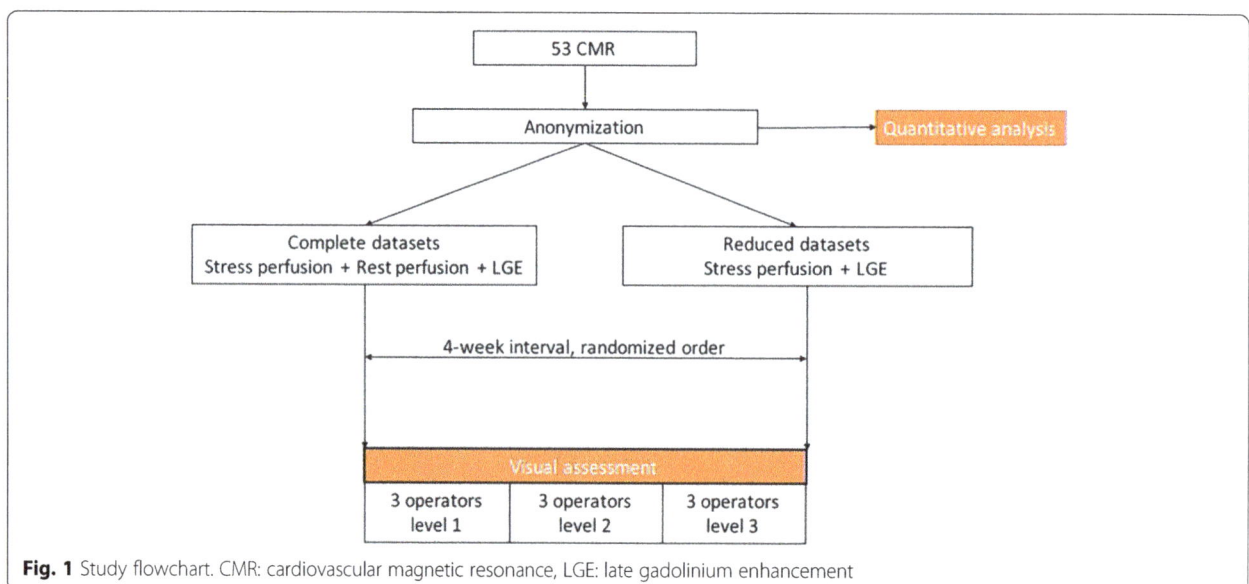

Fig. 1 Study flowchart. CMR: cardiovascular magnetic resonance, LGE: late gadolinium enhancement

Statistical analysis

Continuous variables are presented as mean ± standard deviation for normally distributed variables and as median with interquartile range for non-parametric data. Normality was assessed with Q-Q plots and the Kolmogorov-Smirnov test. Continuous variables were compared using an unpaired Student *t test* or the Wilcoxon rank-sum test, as appropriate, and categorical data were compared between groups using the Fisher exact test and Pearson chi-square test. The McNemar test was used for paired dichotomous data. Two-tailed values of $p < 0.05$ were considered to be statistically significant. One-way ANOVA was used to determine differences between multiple groups. Bonferroni correction was used to account for multiple testing.

Results

Characteristics of the population

The mean age of the population ($n = 53$) was 60.6 ± 12.7 years. Demographic data are shown in Table 1. The prevalence of CAD in the group of patients included in the analysis was 30.2%, with 16/53 patients positive for CAD on invasive coronary angiography. Left anterior descending (LAD) lesions were identified in 9 (17%) of the cases, left circumflex (LCX) lesions in 8 (15.1%) of the cases, and right coronary artery (RCA) in 13 (24.5%) of the cases. Within the group of patients with CAD, 8 patients had 1-vessel disease (50%), 5 patients 2-vessel disease (31.3%) and 3 patients 3-vessel disease (18.8%).

Impact of operator training on correct CAD identification

There was a significant correlation between an operator's training level and the rate of correct identification of CAD on a per patient level on visual assessment. The diagnosis of Level-3 operators agreed with invasive coronary angiography in 83.6 ± 2.3% of the cases, while this percentage dropped to 65.7 ± 4.3% for Level-2 operators and to 55.7 ± 5.3% for Level-1 operators ($p < 0.001$ between the 3 groups) (Fig. 2). A significant difference in the agreement with angiography between different levels of training was also observed in a sub-analysis per

Table 1 Demographic characteristics of the population

	All ($n = 53$)
Age (years)	60.6 ± 12.7
Male gender	36 (67.9%)
Hypertension	30 (56.6%)
Dyslipidaemia	23 (43.4%)
Diabetes	10 (18.9%)
Current smoker	13 (24.5%)
Previous PCI	9 (17%)
Family history of CAD	12 (22.6%)

PCI percutaneous coronary artery intervention, *CAD* coronary artery disease

coronary territory ($p < 0.001$) (Fig. 3). When different perfusion territories were compared, the agreement between CMR and coronary angiography was higher for the LAD territory, followed by the LCX and by the RCA territories. The same trend was observed in all groups of operators, regardless of the level of training ($p < 0.001$).

The sensitivity and specificity for operators of different levels of training are reported in Fig. 4. Level-1 operators showed high sensitivity (86.5 ± 6.1%) and low specificity (41.9 ± 10.9%). Level-2 operators had a sensitivity of 57.3 ± 4.7% and a specificity of 69.4 ± 9.9%. Level-3 operators showed a sensitivity of 71.9 ± 13% and a specificity of 88.7 ± 6.7% respectively. There was a statistically significant difference for both sensitivity and specificity between different levels of training ($p < 0.001$) (Fig. 4).

Impact of rest perfusion on correct identification of CAD

When rest images were available, there was no statistically significant difference at all levels of training (Fig. 5) and in the overall analysis (69.6 ± 14.3% vs 67.1 ± 13.1%; $p = 0.34$). However, when rest images were available, a significantly higher level of confidence was reported by the operators ($p = 0.022$) and subjective image quality was scored at a higher level ($p = 0.012$).

CAD classification

Figure 6 shows a comparison between the extent of CAD identified by the operators on CMR images in comparison with invasive coronary angiography. An overestimation of the severity of CAD was observed in Level-1 operators, regardless of the number of vessels with CAD. Despite being more accurate, Level-2 and Level-3 operators significantly underestimated the number of positive perfusion territories in patients with multi-vessel CAD.

Impact of quantitative analysis on correct CAD identification

Quantitative analysis was successfully performed in 51 patients. In 2 cases of patients without CAD, the automated algorithms failed and no results could be calculated. In both cases, this was due to the low quality of the diluted pre-bolus used for the estimation of the arterial input function. Level-3 visual assessment of the 2 cases where quantification failed yielded the correct diagnosis in both cases when both stress and rest images were made available to the readers, and in 66% of interpretations when only stress perfusion was made available to the readers. Quantitative stress perfusion CMR analysis agreed with the results of invasive angiography in 86.3% of the cases, performing significantly better than Level-1 and Level-2 operators ($p < 0.001$). Level-3 visual assessment and quantitative analysis were not significantly different ($p = 0.56$) (Fig. 2). Quantitative analysis had a sensitivity of 68.8% and specificity of 94.3%. When

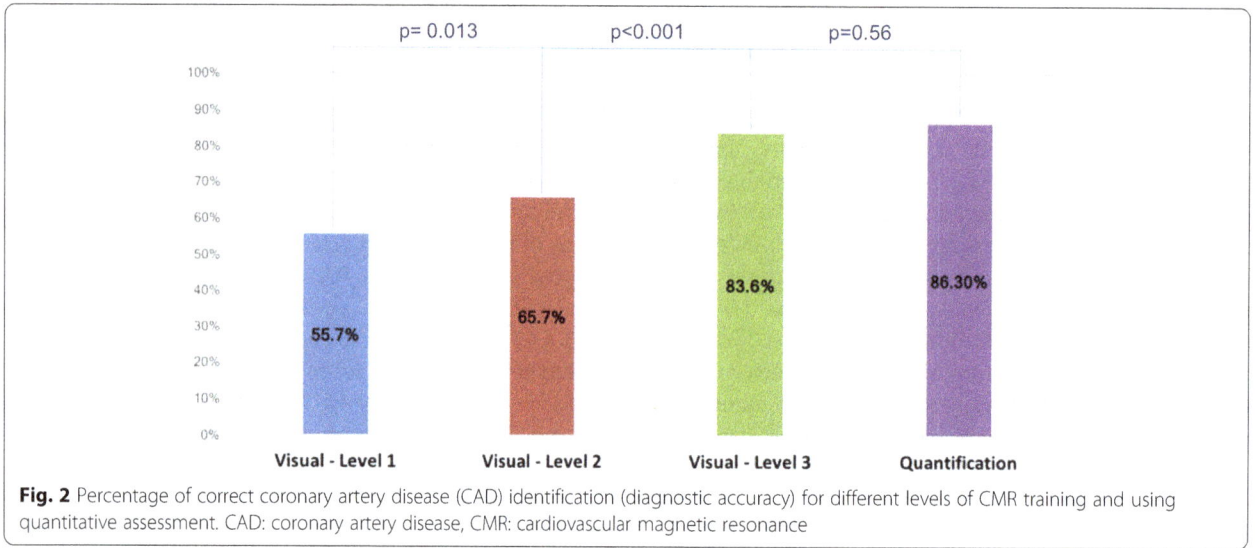

Fig. 2 Percentage of correct coronary artery disease (CAD) identification (diagnostic accuracy) for different levels of CMR training and using quantitative assessment. CAD: coronary artery disease, CMR: cardiovascular magnetic resonance

the 2 cases in which quantitative analysis failed are considered as a missed diagnosis, the concordance of quantitative analysis with invasive angiography was 83%, with a sensitivity of 68.8% and a specificity of 89.2%.

Discussion

This study has several important findings. Operator training and experience had a significant impact on diagnostic accuracy. Only Level-3 trained operators had an accuracy comparable with the results reported by large clinical trials [3–5]. Rest images did not significantly improve the diagnostic accuracy of stress perfusion CMR but, when available, contributed to a significantly higher confidence of the operators in their reports and to a higher perceived image quality, regardless of the level of training. Finally, semi-automated quantitative analysis performed better than Level-1 and Level-2 operators,

but similarly to a Level-3 operator. Quantitative analysis however failed in 2/53 cases due to technical reasons related to the administration of the diluted pre-bolus. However, the same cases could be analysed visually.

Stress perfusion CMR plays an increasingly important role in the evaluation of patients with known or suspected CAD. Recent European guidelines recommend the use of stress perfusion CMR in patients with suspected CAD and intermediate pre-test probability, with a class 1 indication and level of evidence A, similarly to stress echocardiography and nuclear imaging [1, 2]. US guidelines recommend stress perfusion CMR with 2A indication [24], particularly in specific subgroups of patients [25]. These indications are based on the assumption that stress perfusion CMR is highly accurate for the identification of CAD and compares favorably with other functional modalities. In large trials and meta-analyses, the sensitivity ranged

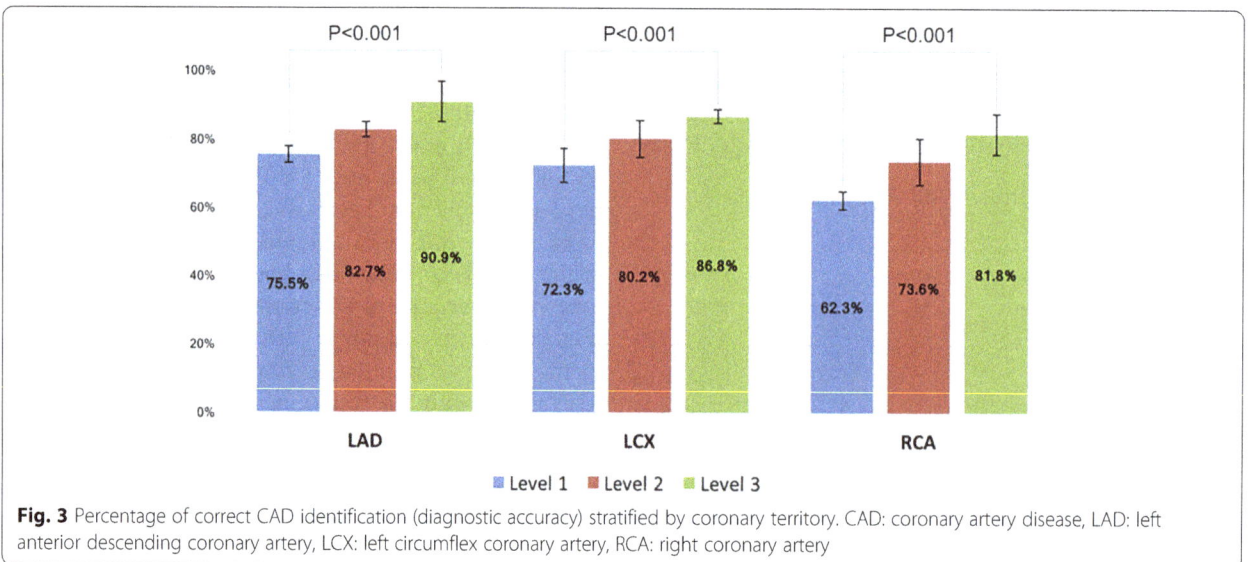

Fig. 3 Percentage of correct CAD identification (diagnostic accuracy) stratified by coronary territory. CAD: coronary artery disease, LAD: left anterior descending coronary artery, LCX: left circumflex coronary artery, RCA: right coronary artery

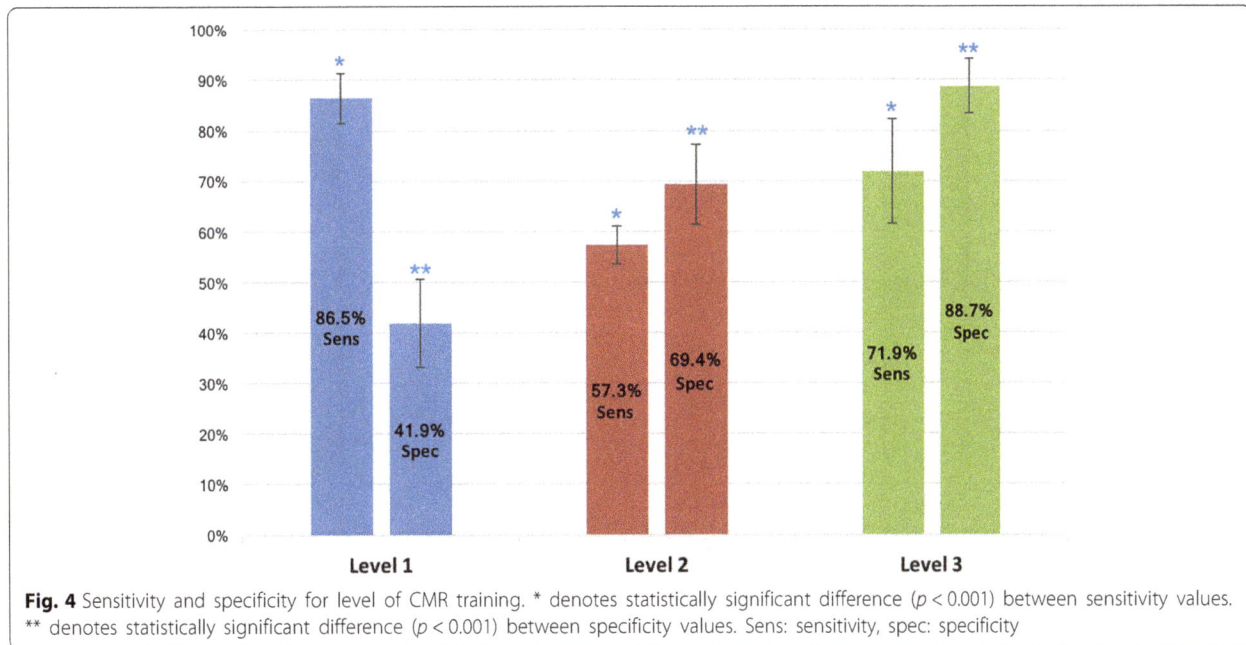

Fig. 4 Sensitivity and specificity for level of CMR training. * denotes statistically significant difference ($p < 0.001$) between sensitivity values. ** denotes statistically significant difference ($p < 0.001$) between specificity values. Sens: sensitivity, spec: specificity

from 75% [3] to 91% [4] and specificity ranged from 59% [3] to 87% [5]. In the CE-MARC study [26], sensitivity was 86.5% and specificity was 83.4%, and the MR-IMPACT 2 trial [27] reported a sensitivity of 75% and a specificity of 59%. These wide intervals most likely represent the variability in study design, the different prevalence of disease in different populations, and variability in the criteria used for visual assessment.

The diagnostic accuracy of stress perfusion CMR reported in the literature is often the result of visual assessment carried out by expert readers, which are usually Level-3 operators and often are internationally recognized experts.

Our study demonstrates that the diagnostic accuracy varied significantly amongst groups of readers with different levels of training, and reached values comparable with those of large studies only in the group of Level-3 operators. These results confirm the high diagnostic accuracy of stress perfusion CMR in comparison with coronary angiography, however clearly indicate the need for Level-3 supervision when stress perfusion scans are reported.

From the analysis of the sensitivity and specificity for the detection of CAD in different groups, it emerges that Level-1 operators had high sensitivity (86.5%). This came however at the cost of a reduced specificity (41.9%) and rate of overall correct CAD detection (55.7%). Factors such as

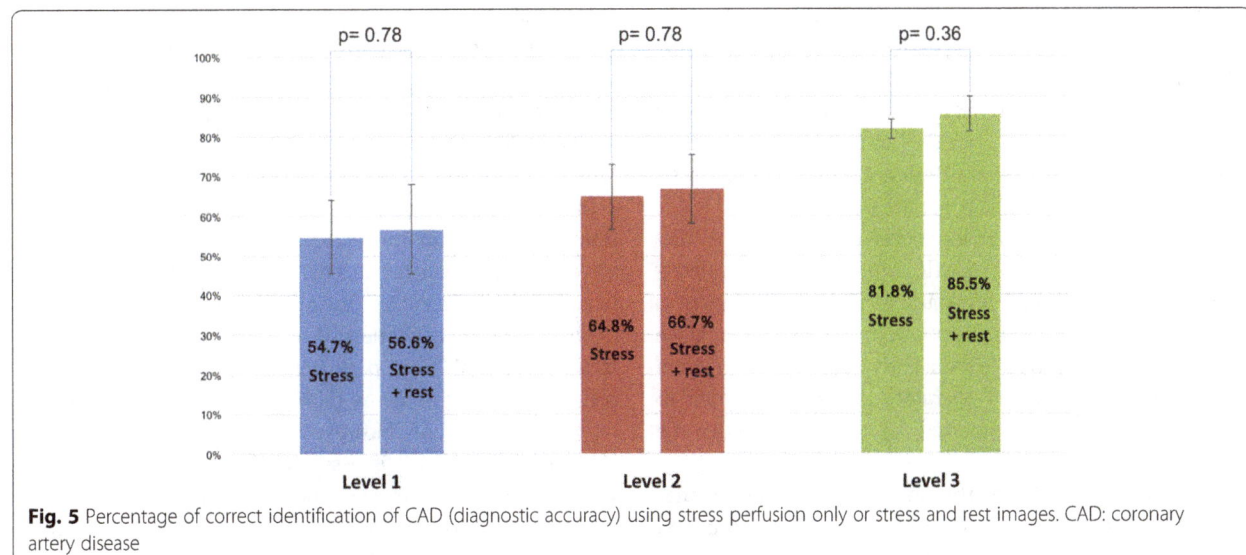

Fig. 5 Percentage of correct identification of CAD (diagnostic accuracy) using stress perfusion only or stress and rest images. CAD: coronary artery disease

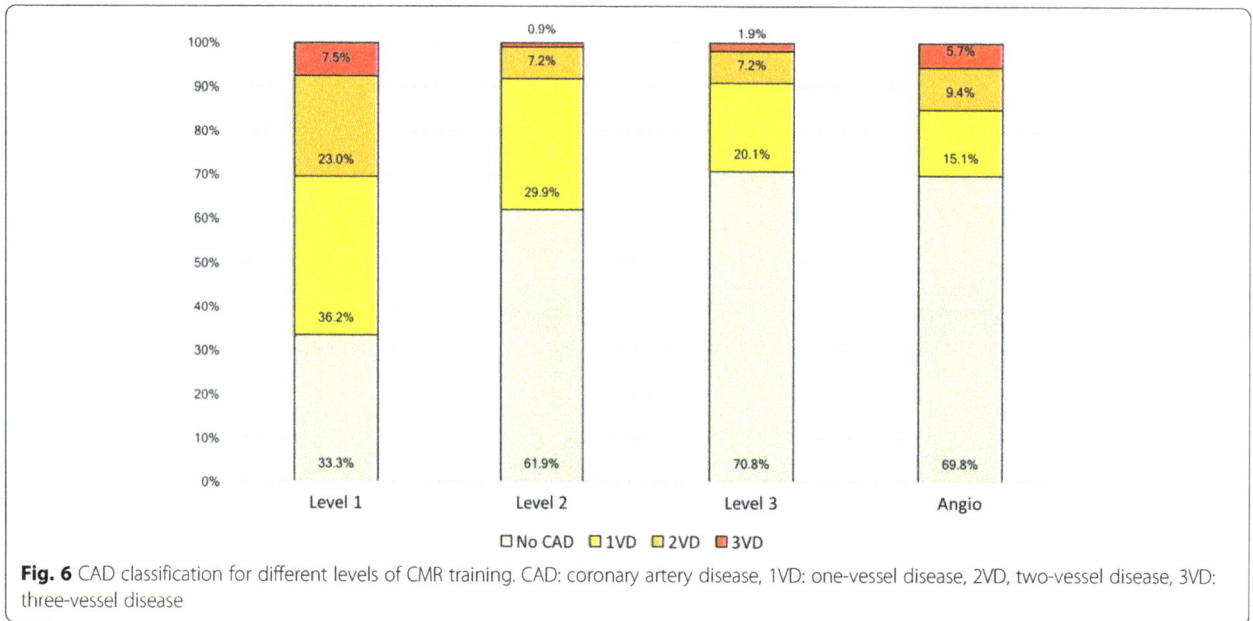

Fig. 6 CAD classification for different levels of CMR training. CAD: coronary artery disease, 1VD: one-vessel disease, 2VD, two-vessel disease, 3VD: three-vessel disease

image quality and the prevalence of dark rim artefacts, which can mimic the presence of subendocardial perfusion defects, could have played a role. In comparison, Level-3 operators under-called the disease (sensitivity 71.9%), but had a high specificity (88.7%). All diagnostic investigations involve a trade-off between sensitivity and specificity. At a population level and from a health-economic perspective, we feel that the results achieved by Level 3 operators represent a reasonable balance between the need to identify significant coronary disease and the high specificity required to avoid increasing down-stream investigation costs through increased referral for invasive coronary angiography. The work of Patel et al. [28] highlights the need for better selection of patients for invasive investigation given the costs and potential morbidity incurred by this.

Our results support the recommendations from the ESC [12], which state that Level-1 operators hold the basic knowledge in CMR sufficient to select appropriate CMR indications and interpret CMR reports, but are not cleared to report CMR scans. This is reflected in our result by the fact that Level-1 operators demonstrated a very low diagnostic accuracy, with poor specificity for the presence of CAD. According to the ESC guidelines, Level-2 operators may actively perform and report CMR, but are not completely independent and should work under the supervision of a Level-3 expert. This is also supported by our results, since Level-2 operators were significantly less accurate than Level-3 operators. Level-3 operators instead performed to levels similar to those reported by studies such as the CE-MARC [26].

It should be noted that the Society for Cardiovascular Magnetic Resonance (SCMR) guidelines on training [29] differ slightly from the ESC guidelines used in this study

to define the level of training of the operators. According to the SCMR guidelines, Level-2 operators can independently report CMR scans, whereas Level-3 certification has more to do with being able to lead a CMR unit and perform research in the field. Both guidelines agree that Level-1 training is not sufficient to practice CMR.

It has been suggested that rest perfusion images play an important role in improving the identification of imaging artefacts when signal abnormalities are present on both stress and rest images [10]. When assessing stress perfusion CMR visually, guidelines advise displaying both rest and stress images side-by-side to identify correctly inducible perfusion defect and artefacts [10, 11].

In our study, we did not find any significant difference in the diagnostic accuracy when rest images were available. Our findings mirror those of Biglands et al. [30]. However, when testing the operator confidence and the perceived image quality, a statistically significant difference was noted when both stress and rest images were available. The increased confidence was more evident for Level-1 and Level-2 operators.

Interestingly, Level-1 operators reported a higher confidence score than more experienced operators, despite lower overall accuracy. This could reflect a cognitive bias, also known as the Dunning-Kruger effect [31].

The diagnostic usefulness of rest perfusion imaging resides in the finding of "fixed perfusion defect" on both stress and rest images, which may be related to artefacts or to areas of myocardial infarction. However, this may be overcome when stress perfusion CMR is assessed visually side-by-side with LGE, as per guidelines [11] and as in our study. Nevertheless, rest perfusion imaging remains a fundamental requirement for perfusion quantification and MPR estimation.

Semi-automated quantitative assessment performed better than Level-1 and Level-2 operators and similarly to Level-3 operators for the detection of CAD. The latter is in keeping with the results of several other studies that reported high sensitivity and specificity for quantitative analysis, with sensitivity ranging from 80% [22] to 94.4% [32] and specificity ranging from 81% [33] to 100% [34]. Previous studies from Patel et al. [6] and Mordini et al. [35] compared quantitative with visual and semi-quantitative analysis and demonstrated that quantitative analysis is superior to visual assessment and semi-quantitative assessment in the detection of ischemia, and that quantitative analysis is the most accurate method to measure the total ischemic burden.

In the present study, quantitative analysis was performed using a semi-automated method which requires user input to confirm the automated segmentation of the images, but eliminates inter-observer variability for what concerns the quantification procedure. This is of increasing relevance as recent technical advances in image reconstruction and analysis techniques are likely to permit the clinical translation of robust and fully automated quantitative analysis into routine clinical practice [36–39]. In our study however, the dual bolus approach used for arterial input function measurements failed in 2 subjects, impeding quantitative analysis. The advent of dual sequences capable of a more accurate assessment of the concentration of gadolinium in the main bolus input function may make the use of dual bolus redundant in the near future [37, 40].

Limitations

This study included a selected population with suspected CAD and we excluded patients with primary cardiomyopathy. Thus, our results on diagnostic accuracy do not include other patterns of perfusion abnormalities, which may require even more experience to discern (e.g., microvascular dysfunction).

Moreover, we used an anatomical reference standard (invasive coronary angiography) to compare operators' performances in interpreting a functional test, while a functional reference standard (e.g., fractional flow reserve) may be more appropriate.

Our results demonstrate that similarly accurate detection of CAD can be achieved by Level-3 operators and by automated perfusion quantification. Although our study was not powered to demonstrate the superiority of quantitative analysis, this has been the subject of a recent study which has reported very similar findings [30]. The non-inferiority of automated quantification to expert visual reads, in combination with the prognostic value of quantitative analysis [23] will facilitate more widespread adoption of stress perfusion CMR by less experienced readers.

Finally, all stress perfusion CMR were acquired in a single center, using a 3 T Philips scanner and a high-resolution k-t sequence. This may not reflect the standard clinical acquisition in other centres.

Conclusions

This study demonstrates that visual assessment of stress perfusion CMR is challenging for Level-1 and Level-2 operators but accurate in the hands of Level-3 operators. Our results highlight the importance of the recommendations of the ESC/EACVI training guidelines in CMR, which recommend independent reporting for Level-3 operators only and supervised reporting for Level-2 trained operators. The availability of rest perfusion images was associated with significantly higher confidence and higher perceived image quality, regardless of the level of training of the operator. Quantitative analysis performed similarly to Level-3 trained operators and could represent, in the future, a valid alternative to visual assessment.

Abbreviations
AHA: American Heart Association; CAD: Coronary artery disease; CME: Continuous medical education; CMR: Cardiovascular magnetic resonance; EACVI: European Association of Cardiovascular Imaging; ESC: European Society of Cardiology; LAD: Left anterior descending coronary artery; LCX: Left circumflex coronary artery; LGE: Late gadolinium enhancement; MBF: Myocardial blood flow; MPR: Myocardial perfusion reserve; RCA: Right coronary artery; SCMR: Society for Cardiovascular Magnetic Resonance

Acknowledgements
This work was supported by the National Institute for Health Research (NIHR) Cardiovascular Health Technology Cooperative (HTC) and Biomedical Research Centre (BRC) awarded to Guy's & St Thomas' NHS Foundation Trust in partnership with King's College London. The views expressed are those of the author(s) and not necessarily those of the NHS, the NIHR or the Department of Health. This work was additionally supported by the Wellcome/EPSRC Centre for Medical Engineering at King's College London [WT 203148/Z/16/Z].
We are grateful to the radiographers at the School of Biomedical Engineering and Imaging Sciences at King's College London for their support in the acquisition of the images.
MSN was funded through a fellowship from the Medical Research Council [MR/P01979X/1].

Funding
This work was supported by the National Institute for Health Research (NIHR) Cardiovascular Health Technology Cooperative (HTC) and Biomedical Research Centre (BRC) awarded to Guy's & St Thomas' NHS Foundation Trust in partnership with King's College London. This work was additionally supported by the Wellcome/EPSRC Centre for Medical Engineering at King's College London [WT 203148/Z/16/Z]. MSN was funded through a fellowship from the Medical Research Council [MR/P01979X/1]. All funding bodies equally contributed to the collection, analysis, and interpretation of the data and to the investigators' salaries during the study.

Authors' contributions
ADMV, LC, NB and AC conceived the study and participated in the study design and coordination. IN, GDG, NC, CF, MSN, JK, ES, VDF and AS analysed the data. ADMV, LC, XM, CS and TFI performed the data analysis. AC segmented the data for quantitative analysis. ADMV and LC drafted the manuscript. All authors critically revised the manuscript for important intellectual content, read and approved the final manuscript.

Competing interests
The authors declare that they have no competing interests.

Author details
[1]School of Biomedical Engineering & Imaging Sciences, King's College London, King's Health Partners, 4th Floor Lambeth Wing, St Thomas' Hospital, London SE1 7EH, UK. [2]Cardiology Department of the Basingstoke and North Hampshire Hospital, Basingstoke, UK. [3]Cardiology Department, St. Thomas' Hospital, Guy's and St Thomas' NHS Foundation Trust, London, UK. [4]Faculdade de Ciências da Saúde CICS, UBI, Covilhã, Portugal. [5]Radiology Department, ICS Maugeri IRCCS, Porto, Italy. [6]Cardiovascular R&D Unit, Faculty of Medicine, University of Porto, Porto, Portugal. [7]Department of Cardiology, Royal North Shore Hospital, The Kolling Institute, Northern Clinical School, University of Sydney, Sydney, Australia. [8]Department of Cardiology and Pneumology, University Medical Center Göttingen, Georg-August University, Göttingen, Germany. [9]German Center for Cardiovascular Research (DZHK), Partner Site Göttingen, Göttingen, Germany.

References

1. Task Force Members, Montalescot G, Sechtem U, Andreotti F, Arden C, Budaj A, et al. ESC guidelines on the management of stable coronary artery disease: The Task Force on the management of stable coronary artery disease of the European Society of Cardiology. Eur Heart J. 2013;34:2949–3003.
2. Authors Task Force members, Kolh P, Alfonso F, Collet J-P, Cremer J, Falk V, et al. ESC/EACTS Guidelines on myocardial revascularization. Eur Heart J. 2014;35:ehu278–619 The Oxford University Press.
3. Schwitter J, Wacker CM, Wilke N, Al-Saadi N, Sauer E, Huettle K, et al. Superior diagnostic performance of perfusion-cardiovascular magnetic resonance versus SPECT to detect coronary artery disease: the secondary endpoints of the multicenter multivendor MR-IMPACT II (magnetic resonance imaging for myocardial perfusion assessment in coronary artery disease trial). J Cardiovasc Magn Reson. 2012;14:1.
4. Nandalur KR, Dwamena BA, Choudhri AF, Nandalur MR, Carlos RC. Diagnostic performance of stress cardiac magnetic resonance imaging in the detection of coronary artery disease. J Am Coll Cardiol. 2007;50:1343–53.
5. Li M, Zhou T, Yang L-F, Peng Z-H, Ding J, Sun G. Diagnostic accuracy of myocardial magnetic resonance perfusion to diagnose ischemic stenosis with fractional flow reserve as reference: systematic review and meta-analysis. JACC Cardiovasc Imaging. 2014;7:1098–105.
6. Patel AR, Antkowiak PF, Nandalur KR, West AM, Salerno M, Arora V, et al. Assessment of advanced coronary artery disease: advantages of quantitative cardiac magnetic resonance perfusion analysis. J Am Coll Cardiol. 2010;56: 561–9.
7. Ferreira PF, Gatehouse PD, Mohiaddin RH, Firmin DN. Cardiovascular magnetic resonance artefacts. J Cardiovasc Magn Reson. 2013;15:41.
8. Chiribiri A, Leuzzi S, Conte MR, Bongioanni S, Bratis K, Olivotti L, et al. Rest perfusion abnormalities in hypertrophic cardiomyopathy: correlation with myocardial fibrosis and risk factors for sudden cardiac death. Clin Radiol. 2015;70:495–501.
9. Villa ADM, Sammut E, Zarinabad N, Carr-White G, Lee J, Bettencourt N, et al. Microvascular ischemia in hypertrophic cardiomyopathy: new insights from high-resolution combined quantification of perfusion and late gadolinium enhancement. J Cardiovasc Magn Reson. 2016;18:4.
10. Klem I, Heitner JF, Shah DJ, Sketch MH, Behar V, Weinsaft J, et al. Improved detection of coronary artery disease by stress perfusion cardiovascular magnetic resonance with the use of delayed enhancement infarction imaging. J Am Coll Cardiol. 2006;47:1630–8.
11. Schulz-Menger J, Bluemke DA, Bremerich J, Flamm SD, Fogel MA, Friedrich MG, et al. Standardized image interpretation and post processing in cardiovascular magnetic resonance: Society for Cardiovascular Magnetic Resonance (SCMR) Board of Trustees Task Force on Standardized Post Processing. J Cardiovasc Magn Reson. 2013;15:35 BioMed Central Ltd.
12. Plein S, Schulz-Menger J, Almeida A, Mahrholdt H, Rademakers F, Pennell D, et al. Training and accreditation in cardiovascular magnetic resonance in Europe: a position statement of the working group on cardiovascular magnetic resonance of the European Society of Cardiology. Eur Heart J. 2011;32:793–8 Oxford University Press.
13. Ishida M, Schuster A, Morton G, Chiribiri A, Hussain ST, Paul M, et al. Development of a universal dual-bolus injection scheme for the quantitative assessment of myocardial perfusion cardiovascular magnetic resonance. J Cardiovasc Magnetic Resonance. 2011;13:28.
14. Cerqueira MD, Weissman NJ, Dilsizian V, Jacobs AK, Kaul S, Laskey WK, et al. Standardized myocardial segmentation and nomenclature for tomographic imaging of the heart a statement for healthcare professionals from the cardiac imaging committee of the council on clinical cardiology of the American heart association. Int J Cardiovasc Imaging. 2002;18:539–42. Lippincott Williams & Wilkins. Available from: http://circ.ahajournals.org/cgi/doi/10.1161/hc0402.102975.
15. Kramer CM, Barkhausen J, Flamm SD, Kim RJ, Nagel E. Standardized cardiovascular magnetic resonance (CMR) protocols 2013 update. J Cardiovasc Magnetic Resonance. 2013;15:91.
16. Kim RJ, Wu E, Rafael A, Chen E-L, Parker MA, Simonetti O, et al. The use of contrast-enhanced magnetic resonance imaging to identify reversible myocardial dysfunction. N Engl J Med. 2000;343:1445–53.
17. Hautvast G, Chiribiri A, Zarinabad N, Schuster A, Breeuwer M, Nagel E. Myocardial blood flow quantification from MRI by deconvolution using an exponential approximation basis. IEEE Trans Biomed Eng. 2012;59:2060–7.
18. Wilke N, Jerosch-Herold M, Wang Y, Huang Y, Christensen BV, Stillman AE, et al. Myocardial perfusion reserve: assessment with multisection, quantitative, first-pass MR imaging. Radiology. 1997;204:373–84.
19. Jerosch-Herold M, Wilke N, Stillman AE. Magnetic resonance quantification of the myocardial perfusion reserve with a Fermi function model for constrained deconvolution. Med Phys. 1998;25:73–84.
20. Zarinabad N, Chiribiri A, Hautvast GLTF, Ishida M, Schuster A, Cvetkovic Z, et al. Voxel-wise quantification of myocardial perfusion by cardiac magnetic resonance. Feasibility and methods comparison. Magn Reson Med. 2012;68:1994–2004.
21. Sammut E, Zarinabad N, Wesolowski R, Morton G, Chen Z, Sohal M, et al. Feasibility of high-resolution quantitative perfusion analysis in patients with heart failure. J Cardiovasc Magn Reson. 2015;17:13.
22. Lockie T, Ishida M, Perera D, Chiribiri A, De Silva K, Kozerke S, et al. High-resolution magnetic resonance myocardial perfusion imaging at 3.0-Tesla to detect hemodynamically significant coronary stenoses as determined by fractional flow reserve. J Am Coll Cardiol. 2011;57:70–5.
23. Sammut EC, Villa ADM, Di Giovine G, Dancy L, Bosio F, Gibbs T, et al. Prognostic value of quantitative stress perfusion cardiac magnetic resonance. JACC Cardiovasc Imaging. 2018;11(5):686–94. https://doi.org/10.1016/j.jcmg.2017.07.022.
24. Fihn SD, Gardin JM, Abrams J, Berra K, Blankenship JC, Dallas AP, et al. ACCF/AHA/ACP/AATS/PCNA/SCAI/STS guideline for the diagnosis and management of patients with stable ischemic heart disease: a report of the American College of Cardiology Foundation/American Heart Association task force on practice guidelines, and the American College of Physicians, American Association for Thoracic Surgery, Preventive Cardiovascular Nurses Association, Society for Cardiovascular Angiography and Interventions, and Society of Thoracic Surgeons. Circulation. 2012;126(25):e354–471. https://doi.org/10.1161/CIR.0b013e318277d6a0.
25. American College of Cardiology Foundation Task Force on Expert Consensus Documents, Hundley WG, Bluemke DA, Finn JP, Flamm SD, Fogel MA, et al. ACCF/ACR/AHA/NASCI/SCMR expert consensus document on cardiovascular magnetic resonance: a report of the American College of Cardiology Foundation task force on expert consensus documents. J Am Coll Cardiol. 2010;55(23):2614–62. https://doi.org/10.1016/j.jacc.2009.11.011.
26. Greenwood JP, Maredia N, Younger JF, Brown JM, Nixon J, Everett CC, et al. Cardiovascular magnetic resonance and single-photon emission computed tomography for diagnosis of coronary heart disease (CE-MARC): a prospective trial. Lancet. 2012;379:453–60.
27. Schwitter J, Wacker CM, Wilke N, Al-Saadi N, Sauer E, Huettle K, et al. MR-IMPACT II: magnetic resonance imaging for myocardial perfusion assessment in coronary artery disease trial: perfusion-cardiac magnetic resonance vs. single-photon emission computed tomography for the detection of coronary artery disease: a comparative multicentre, multivendor trial. Eur Heart J. 2013;34:775–81.
28. Patel MR, Peterson ED, Dai D, Brennan JM, Redberg RF, Anderson HV, et al. Low diagnostic yield of elective coronary angiography. N Engl J Med. 2010; 362:886–95. Massachusetts Medical Society.

29. Kim RJ, De Roos A, Fleck E, Higgins CB, Pohost GM, Prince M, et al. Guidelines for training in Cardiovascular Magnetic Resonance (CMR). J Cardiovasc Magn Reson. 2007;9:3–4. https://doi.org/10.1080/10976640600778064.

30. Biglands JD, Ibraheem M, Magee DR, Radjenovic A, Plein S, Greenwood JP. Quantitative myocardial perfusion imaging versus visual analysis in diagnosing myocardial ischemia: a CE-MARC substudy. JACC: Cardiovascular Imaging. 2018;11:711–8.

31. Kruger J, Dunning D. Unskilled and unaware of it: how difficulties in recognizing one's own incompetence lead to inflated self-assessments. J Pers Soc Psychol. 1999;77:1121–34.

32. Biglands JD, Magee DR, Sourbron SP, Plein S, Greenwood JP, Radjenovic A. Comparison of the diagnostic performance of four quantitative myocardial perfusion estimation methods used in cardiac MR imaging: CE-MARC substudy. Radiology. 2015;275:393–402 Radiological Society of North America.

33. Morton G, Chiribiri A, Ishida M, Hussain ST, Schuster A, Indermuehle A, et al. Quantification of Absolute Myocardial Perfusion in Patients With Coronary Artery Disease: Comparison Between Cardiovascular Magnetic Resonance and Positron Emission Tomography. J Am Coll Cardiol. 2012;60:1546–55.

34. Bernhardt P, Walcher T, Rottbauer W, Wöhrle J. Quantification of myocardial perfusion reserve at 1.5 and 3.0 tesla: a comparison to fractional flow reserve. Int J Cardiovasc Imaging. 2012;28:2049–56.

35. Mordini FE, Haddad T, Hsu LY, Kellman P, Lowrey TB, Aletras AH, et al. Diagnostic accuracy of stress perfusion CMR in comparison with quantitative coronary angiography: fully quantitative, semiquantitative, and qualitative assessment. JACC Cardiovasc Imaging. 2014;7:14–22.

36. Zarinabad N, Hautvast GLTF, Sammut E, Arujuna A, Breeuwer M, Nagel E, et al. Effects of tracer arrival time on the accuracy of high-resolution (voxel-wise) myocardial perfusion maps from contrast-enhanced first-pass perfusion magnetic resonance. Biomedical engineering, IEEE transactions on IEEE. 2014;61:2499–506.

37. Kellman P, Hansen MS, Nielles Vallespin S, Nickander J, Themudo R, Ugander M, et al. Myocardial perfusion cardiovascular magnetic resonance: optimized dual sequence and reconstruction for quantification. J Cardiovasc Magn Reson. 2017;19:43.

38. Jacobs M, Benovoy M, Chang L-C, Arai AE, Hsu LY. Evaluation of an automated method for arterial input function detection for first-pass myocardial perfusion cardiovascular magnetic resonance. J Cardiovasc Magn Reson. 2016;18:17.

39. Hsu LY, Jacobs M, Benovoy M, Ta AD, Conn HM, Winkler S, et al. Diagnostic performance of fully automated pixel-wise quantitative myocardial perfusion imaging by cardiovascular magnetic resonance. JACC: Cardiovascular Imaging. 2018;11:697–707.

40. Gatehouse P, Lyne J, Smith G, Pennell D, Firmin D. T2* effects in the dual-sequence method for high-dose first-pass myocardial perfusion. J Magn Reson Imaging. 2006;24:1168–71.

19

Myocardial native T2 measurement to differentiate light-chain and transthyretin cardiac amyloidosis and assess prognosis

Fourat Ridouani[1*] ⓘ, Thibaud Damy[2,3], Vania Tacher[1], Haytham Derbel[1], François Legou[1], Islem Sifaoui[1], Etienne Audureau[4], Diane Bodez[2,3], Alain Rahmouni[1] and Jean-François Deux[1,3]

Abstract

Background: To assess the diagnostic and prognosis value of myocardial native T2 measurement in the distinction between Light-chain (AL) and Transthyretin (ATTR) cardiac amyloidosis (CA).

Methods: Forty-four patients with CA (24 AL; 20 ATTR) and 40 healthy subjects underwent 1.5 T cardiovascular magnetic resonance (CMR). They all underwent T1 and T2 mapping (modified Look-Locker inversion recovery), cine and late gadolinium enhancement (LGE) imaging. The Query Amyloid Late Enhancement (QALE) score, myocardial native T2, T1 and extra cellular volume fraction (ECV) were calculated for all patients.

Results: Of the 44 patients, 36 (82%) exhibited enhancement on LGE images. Mean QALE score of AL (7.9 ± 6) and ATTR (10.5 ± 5) patients were similar ($p = 0.6$). Myocardial native T2 was significantly ($p < 0.0001$) higher in AL (63.2 ± 4.7 ms) than in ATTR (56.2 ± 3.1 ms) patients, and both higher ($p < 0.001$) than healthy subjects (51.1 ± 3.1 ms). Myocardial native T2 was highly correlated with myocardial native T1 (Spearman's rho $= 0.79$; $p < 0.001$) and exhibited higher diagnostic performance than T1 to separate AL and ATTR patients: the area under curve (AUC) of T2 was 0.94 (95% CI: 0.86–1, $p < 0.001$) and the AUC of T1 was 0.77 (95% CI: 0.62–0.91, $p = 0.03$). Myocardial native T2 did not impact overall survival in patients (HR 1.03 (0.94–1.12); $p = 0.53$) in contrast to ECV that was the best predictor of outcome (HR 1.66 per 0.1 increase in ECV (1.24–2.22); $p = 0.0006$).

Conclusions: Myocardial native T2 significantly is increased in CA, especially in AL patients in comparison to ATTR patients. Myocardial native T2 does not impact survival in CA patients in contrast to ECV that was the best predictor of outcome.

Keywords: Amyloidosis, CMR, T2 mapping

Background

Cardiac amyloidosis (CA) is characterized by interstitial amyloid infiltration which leads to progressive thickening of cardiac walls, diastolic dysfunction, and restrictive cardiomyopathy [1–3]. Cardiac involvement in systemic amyloidosis leads to a progressive, fatal, cardiac failure and is an important factor in treatment options and prognosis [4]. Diagnosis of CA may be challenging because clinical symptoms, cardiac biomarkers, and transthoracic echocardiographic abnormalities are nonspecific, especially when other causes of hypertrophy exist [5–7]. Moreover, they often appear at a late stage of the disease. Cardiovascular magnetic resonance (CMR) imaging has been reported a promising tool to detect cardiac involvement [8]. Late gadolinium enhanced (LGE) sequence shows either diffuse or circumferential enhancement after gadolinium injection that is highly specific to CA [9–11]. The measurement of myocardial native T1 and extracellular volume fraction (ECV) using parametric sequences can also provide useful

* Correspondence: ridouanifourat@gmail.com
[1]Radiology Department, Henri Mondor Hospital, University Paris Est Créteil, Assistance Publique-Hôpitaux de Paris, 51 av Mal de Lattre de Tassigny, 94000 Créteil, France
Full list of author information is available at the end of the article

additive insights for the diagnosis [12] that could be very useful when gadolinium infusion is contra-indicated. Therefore, CA is associated with a significant rise in myocardial native T1 and ECV [13, 14]. These parameters could be considered as early diagnostic markers [15] useful to predict mortality [16]. In contrast to myocardial native T1, myocardial T2 relaxation time variations have been less often evaluated in CA, and controversial findings were reported [17–19].

Although CMR consistently detects CA, diagnosis of the types of amyloidosis, in particular the distinction between light chain (AL) and transthyretin (ATTR) amyloidosis, may be challenging [20]. In most cases, ATTR had a more increased left ventricular (LV) mass, a thicker interventricular septum (IVS), larger atrial areas, smaller cavity volumes and a lower LV ejection fraction (LVEF) than AL amyloidosis [8]. Myocardial enhancement on LGE sequence is reported to be more intense in ATTR than in AL amyloidosis, with predominant transmural enhancement and frequent right ventricular (RV) involvement [21]. More recently, using parametric imaging, Fontana et al. reported that ATTR amyloid deposits were larger than AL amyloid deposits and were associated with a ~ 20% increase in cell volume [22], suggesting a concomitant myocyte hypertrophy. AL amyloidosis was associated with a greater elevation of myocardial native T1 and a smaller ECV suggests myocardial edema. However, T2 mapping sequences were not performed to confirm this hypothesis. In this study, we hypothesized that in CA the myocardial edema represented a significant component of cardiac involvement with a different intensity between AL and ATTR patients. We used native T1 and T2 mapping parametric sequences to detect edema in those patients, and to evaluate relationships between parametric data and biological parameters, as well as patients' survival.

Materials and methods
Study population
The study was approved by our local Research Ethics Committee and included written informed consent from each subject. Forty-four consecutive patients with CA (AL, n = 24, ATTR, n = 20, 9 mutant and 11 wild type) who underwent CMR between January 2013 and December 2014 at our center were retrospectively identified. Diagnosis and the type of systemic amyloidosis was biopsy-proven for all patients (labial or endomyocardial biopsy (EMB)). For patients with AL amyloidosis, cardiac involvement was histologically confirmed by EMB performed 1.2 (0–6) months after CMR. For the patients with ATTR amyloidosis, diagnosis of CA was based on significant heart retention of 99mTc-HMDP bone tracer on scintigraphy (n = 20; 100%) as recently proposed in the literature [23]. TTR genetic testing was obtained for

all ATTR amyloidosis individuals: 5 (56%) patients carried Val30Met TTR mutation and the remaining 4 (44%) mutant ATTR patients carried other mutations; wild-type ATTR amyloidosis patients had no TTR mutation.

For all patients, NT-proBNP, troponin T and creatinine (µmol/L) levels, and echocardiography parameters (IVS thickness, LVEF, transmitral E/E' ratio and global longitudinal strain) were recorded at the time of CMR as previously described [24]. A control group of 40 healthy subjects (20 males; 40 ± 12 years) was also included in the study and explored with CMR. Echocardiography parameters (IVS thickness, LVEF and global longitudinal strain) and levels of creatinine were recorded for all healthy subjects as well.

CMR imaging
Acquisition protocol
All patients and healthy subjects were explored using the same CMR protocol except for post contrast imaging sequences that were not performed for the latter. CMR imaging was performed with a 1.5 T CMR system (Magnetom Avanto, Siemens Healthineers, Erlangen, Germany) equipped with a high-performance gradient sub-system (maximum amplitude, 40 mT/m; minimum rise, 200 µs), and an 8-channel phased-array cardiac coil. Unenhanced cine balanced steady state free precession (bSSFP) sequences, acquired in the LV short-axis section and encompassing the entire LV were performed on all patients. The following parameters were used: TR/TE, 2.8/1.4 (apparent TR, 31.4 ms; 11 segments); flip angle, 82°; matrix size, 192 × 192; FOV, 300 × 270 mm; slice thickness, 8 mm. Retrospective electrocardiogram (ECG) gating was used with 25 phases per section.

T1 maps were acquired before injection (myocardial native T1) and 15 min after gadolinium administration (0.2 mmol/Kg of gadolinium (Dotarem; Guerbet; Aulnay-sous-Bois; France)) in all the patients in a middle short-axis and in the four-chamber planes using the modified Look-Locker inversion recovery (MOLLI) sequence [25]. The following parameters were used: 3 inversion sets of 3/3/5 images, TE/TR = 1.06/2.5 ms, nominal flip angle = 35°, TI_1 = 100 ms, DTI = 80 ms, matrix = 192 × 154, FOV = 340 × 274 mm^2, BW = 930 Hz/pixels, slice thickness = 8 mm, generalized autocalibrating partially parallel acquisition (GRAPPA) 2 with 36 separated reference lines, 75% of partial Fourier, 3 R-R cycles recovery period and an acquisition time = 17 R-R cycles. T2 maps were generated using a non-product bSSFP sequence with an adiabatic T2 preparation, and acquired at the same location as T1 maps. The following parameters were used: TE/TR = 1.12/2.6 ms, 3 T2-preparation times = 0/25/55 ms, matrix = 192 × 154, FOV = 340 × 154, BW = 930 Hz/pixels, slice thickness = 6 mm, GRAPPA 2 with 36 separated reference lines, 75% of partial Fourier, acquisition time = 12 R-R cycles. All images were acquired within a single breath hold. A fast variational non-rigid registration algorithm was used to correct for residual cardiac and respiratory motion between images, aligning all T1- and T2-prepared frames to the center frame. Finally, T1 and T2 maps were generated from these motion-corrected images by fitting a mono-exponential decay curve at each pixel. A short Tau inversion recovery (STIR) T2-weighted image was acquired in the middle short axis section at the same level as T1 and T2 maps using the following parameters: TE/TR = 49/1500 to 2500 ms (depending on the heart rate), matrix = 192 × 154; field-of-view (FOV) = 340 × 154, BW = 255 Hz/pixel, slice thickness = 8 mm, turbo factor 15 and TI 150 ms. A surface coil intensity correction algorithm was used to compensate the myocardial intensity inhomogeneity.

LGE images covering the LV in short-axis and long-axis views were obtained 10 min after injection of 0.2 mmol/Kg of gadolinium (Dotarem; Guerbet; Aulnay-sous-Bois; France) in all the patients. A segmented 3D IR gradient-echo T1-weighted sequence was used with the following parameters: repetition time of 3.9 ms, echo time of 1.4 ms, flip angle of 10°, matrix size of 192 × 192, FOV 300 × 270 mm, 12 sections, and 6 mm slice thickness. Image acquisition lasted between [12 to 20 s] depending on the heart rate. A dedicated inversion recovery time (TI) scouting sequence was used before acquisition of LGE images to adjust the optimal TI. Phase sensitive inversion recovery (PSIR) images were systematically acquired after acquisition of LGE images because suboptimal nulling of the myocardial signal may be encountered in CA [26]. Sequence parameters of the PSIR sequence were as follows: repetition time of 835 ms, echo time of 3.3 ms, flip angle of 10°, matrix size of 256 × 156, FOV 300 × 270 mm, and 8 mm slice thickness. Image acquisition lasted between 8 to 12 s, depending on the heart rate. Five PSIR images were acquired in the short-axis plane encompassing the LV. One slice was also acquired in the 4-chamber and in the 2-chamber view.

Image analysis
Qualitative analysis
Two reviewers, with 15 (JFD) and 3 (FR) years of experience in cardiovascular imaging, analyzed anonymously CMR images of all patients in consensus on a dedicated acquisition platform (Leonardo; Siemens Healthineers). The readers were blinded to the clinical data. LGE were scored on a five-point scale: 0: no abnormal enhancement detected within cardiac chambers, 1: doubtful enhancement within LV, 2: subendocardial enhancement of LV, 3: diffuse enhancement of LV, 4: patchy enhancement. Abnormal enhancement of RV and atria was also

noted. Myocardial enhancement was also evaluated using the Query Amyloid Late Enhancement (QALE) score as previously reported [21]. The QALE score was performed on LGE images at the base, mid ventricle and apex in the LV and RV. Each LV level is scored according to the degree of LGE, with the highest score for circumferential and transmural LV LGE. The QALE score range for the whole heart in each patient is from 0 (no detectable LGE in the LV or RV) to 18 (global transmural LV LGE at all 3 levels plus RV involvement).

Quantitative analysis
The IVS was measured for all subjects on the end-diastolic short-axis cine image acquired at the middle part of the LV. LV indexed end-diastolic volume, indexed end-systolic volume, LVEF and indexed cardiac mass were calculated on cine short-axis images using a dedicated software (cmr42; Circle Cardiovascular Imaging Inc.; Calgary; Alberta; Canada). For myocardial native T1 and T2 measurements, the mid-ventricular short-axis and the 4 chamber images were manually contoured to outline the endocardium and epicardium, and the average T1 and T2 values were calculated for all patients using a dedicated software (cmr42). Same measurements were performed on post contrast T1 mapping images. In addition, T1 values of blood pool before and after contrast administration were calculated from a region-of-interest (ROI) placed in the blood pool cavity on the middle short-axis section. ECV was calculated using the following formula: ECV = λ (1- hematocrit), where λ = [(1/T1 myocardium $_{post-Gd}$) − (1/T1 myocardium $_{pre-Gd}$)] / [(1/T1 blood pool $_{post-Gd}$) − (1/T1 blood pool $_{pre-Gd}$)]. Intra cellular volume (ICV) was calculated as follows: ICV = 1 − ECV. Lastly, Total amyloid volume and Total cell volume were calculated using the following formulas:

Total amyloid volume (mL/m^2) = ECV x LV volume.
Total cell volume (mL/m^2) = ICV x LV volume.

T2 ratio was calculated by dividing signal intensity of LV myocardium (obtained from manual contouring of endocardial and epicardial LV boundaries of short-axis T2 STIR image) and signal intensity of chest wall muscle.

Follow up and survival
Follow-up began at completion of the CMR. Dates and status of death were obtained from the medical records; as needed, details were obtained by contacting the referring physician.

Statistical analysis
Quantitative data are expressed as means ± SD or medians and interquartile (IQR) depending on the normality of the data. Categorical variables were described as number (%)

Table 1 Population characteristics

Characteristics	AL (n = 24)	ATTR (n = 20)	Healthy subjects (n = 40)	p*
Clinical				
Age (years)	65 ± 12	73 ± 15	40 ± 12	0.04$^\$$
Male (%)	14 (58)	17 (85)	20 (50)	0.04
BMI (kg/m²)	24.7 ± 3	24.5 ± 4	22.1 ± 3	0.2
Diabetes	2	5	–	0.1
NYHA(I/II/III/IV)	3/9/9/3	2/8/9/1	–	0.6
Hypertension	9	13	–	0.1
Hyperlipidemia	9	9	–	0.9
NT-pro BNP (pg/mL)	6317 (340–18,908)	2384 (542–9129)	–	0.3
Troponin T (pg/mL)	52 (14–112)	38 (8–54)	–	0.5
Creatinine (µmol/L)	110 (78–275)	101 (89–167)	63 (55–77)	0.6$^\$$
Echocardiography				
Septal thickness (mm)	17 ± 5	18 ± 9	8 ± 4	0.4$^\$$
LVEF (%)	57 ± 15	50 ± 16	66 ± 15	0.2$^\$$
Transmitral E/A	3.6 ± 8	2.6 ± 8	–	0.2
E/E'	16.3 ± 8	15.5 ± 8	–	0.9
GLS (−%)	12 (6–17)	9 (8–15)	18 (15–22)	0.8$^\$$

AL light chain amyloidosis; *ATTR* Transthyretin amyloidosis; *BMI* Body Mass Index; *GLS* Global longitudinal strain; *LVEF* left ventricular ejection fraction; *NT-proBNP* N-terminal pro-B-type natriuretic peptide; *NYHA* New York Heart Association

*: AL vs. ATTR patients; $: $p < 0.001$: Healthy subjects vs. CA patients

and compared using the χ^2 or the Fisher's exact test, as appropriate. Differences between continuous data were tested using unpaired t-test or Mann–Whitney rank sum test for two groups comparisons, and analysis of variance (ANOVA) or Kruskal-Wallis for three groups comparisons followed by post-hoc pairwise comparisons with Bonferroni correction in case of global significance, as appropriate. Spearman's rank correlation coefficients were calculated to assess correlation between continuous variables. Receiver operating characteristic (ROC) analysis, with corresponding measures of statistical uncertainty (i.e., 95% confidence intervals), was applied to myocardial native T1 and T2 and QALE score to identify optimal cut-off values for cardiac involvement based on the highest Youden index. Sensitivity and specificity were calculated using the thresholds previously defined. Overall

Table 2 Comparison of cardiac MRI parameters between groups

MRI parameters	AL (n = 24)	ATTR (n = 20)	Healthy subjects (n = 40)	p*
LV EDV (mL/m²)	74 ± 23	89 ± 27	77 ± 16	0.06$^\£$
LV ESV (mL/m²)	35 ± 21	47 ± 28	27 ± 9	0.1$^\$$
IVS (mm)	17 ± 3	18 ± 3	9 ± 2	0.3
LV mass (g/m²)	97 ± 28	115 ± 31	63 ± 11	0.04$^\$$
LVEF (%)	56 ± 18	50 ± 19	65 ± 8	0.3$^\$$
Native T1 (ms)	1104 ± 54	1066 ± 42	975 ± 26	0.01$^\$$
Native T2 (ms)	63.2 ± 4.7	56.2 ± 3.1	51.1 ± 3.1	0.0001$^\$$
T2 ratio	1.31 ± 0.4	1.41 ± 0.2	1.44 ± 0.3	0.2
Post contrast T1 (ms)	378 ± 73	363 ± 69	NA	0.9
ECV	0.53 ± 0.17	0.46 ± 0.11	NA	0.2
ICV	0.47 ± 0.17	0.54 ± 0.11	NA	0.2
T. amyloid vol. (mL/m²)	57 ± 27	53 ± 22	NA	0.7
T. cell vol. (mL/m²)	47 ± 15	61 ± 19	NA	0.04

*: AL vs. ATTR patients

$: $p < 0.005$: Healthy subjects and CA patients

£: $p = 0.4$: Healthy subjects and CA patients

survival was measured from the date of CMR to the date of death or last follow-up. Unadjusted survival curves were plotted by the Kaplan-Meier method, using log-rank tests to assess significance for group comparison. Unadjusted Cox proportional hazards regression models were performed to compute hazard ratios (HR) along with their 95% confidence intervals. Based on Schoenfeld residuals, all predictors were tested for the proportional-hazards assumption which was not found to be violated. For continuous variables, optimal thresholds for overall survival were determined using recursive partitioning analysis (RPA), based on the martingale residuals from a Cox model to determine the optimal value among all possible cut-points. Data were considered significant if $p < 0.05$. Analyses were performed using SPSS 25.0 (International

Business Machines, Armonk, New York, USA) and Stata v14.1 (StataCorp, College Station, Texas, USA), using an implementation of RPA for Stata by Wim van Putten [27].

Results
Population characteristics
Patients with ATTR amyloidosis were older compared with AL amyloidosis patients (73 vs. 65 years; $p = 0.04$) and predominantly male (85% vs. 58%; p = 0.04). No significant differences were detected between AL and ATTR patients regarding biological and echocardiographic parameters. Healthy subjects were significantly younger than AL ($p < 0.001$) and ATTR ($p < 0.001$) patients and did not exhibit cardiac hypertrophy. They had

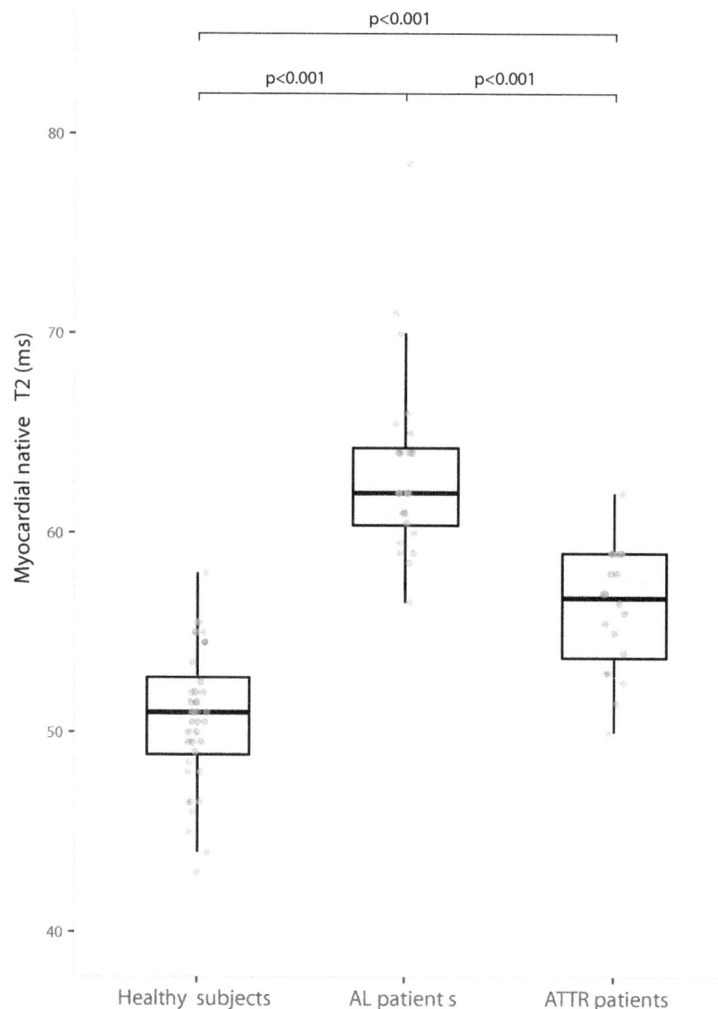

Fig. 1 Graph shows myocardial native T2 values in healthy subjects, patients with AL amyloidosis and patients with ATTR amyloidosis. Results are shown as boxplots, with each box representing the interquartile range (1st to 3rd quartile, IQR), the line within the box indicating the median, and the whiskers extending to 1.5 times the IQR above and below the box; the dots represent individual values for each patient. Myocardial native T2 is significantly ($p < 0.0001$) higher in patients than in healthy subjects. Among patients, myocardial native T2 is significantly ($p < 0.001$) higher in AL than in ATTR patients

higher LVEF than AL ($p < 0.001$) and ATTR ($p < 0.001$) patients. All data are reported in the Table 1.

CMR images analysis
Qualitative analysis
Thirty-six (82%) patients exhibited enhancement of the LV on LGE images, described as subendocardial (grade 2) in 10 patients (23%; 5 AL and 5 ATTR), diffuse (grade 3) in 22 patients (50%; 10 AL and 12 ATTR) and patchy (grade 4) in 4 patients (9%; 3 AL and 1 ATTR). Six patients (14%; 4 AL and 2 ATTR) were considered as doubtful (grade 1) and 2 patients (4.5%; 2 AL) were considered negative (grade 0). RV involvement was suspected in 21 patients (48%; 11 AL and 10 ATTR) and atrial involvement was suspected in 21 patients (48%; 14

AL and 7 ATTR). Mean QALE score of AL (7.9 ± 6) and ATTR (10.5 ± 5) patients did not exhibit significant difference ($p = 0.6$).

Quantitative analysis
LV mass was significantly ($p < 0.05$) higher in ATTR than in AL patients. Healthy subjects had significantly ($p < 0.001$) higher LVEF than AL and ATTR patients, and did not exhibit cardiac hypertrophy. All data are reported in the Table 2.

Mapping images
Myocardial native T2 was significantly higher in AL and ATTR patients than in healthy subjects $p < 0.001$ for both). A significant raise of myocardial native T1 was

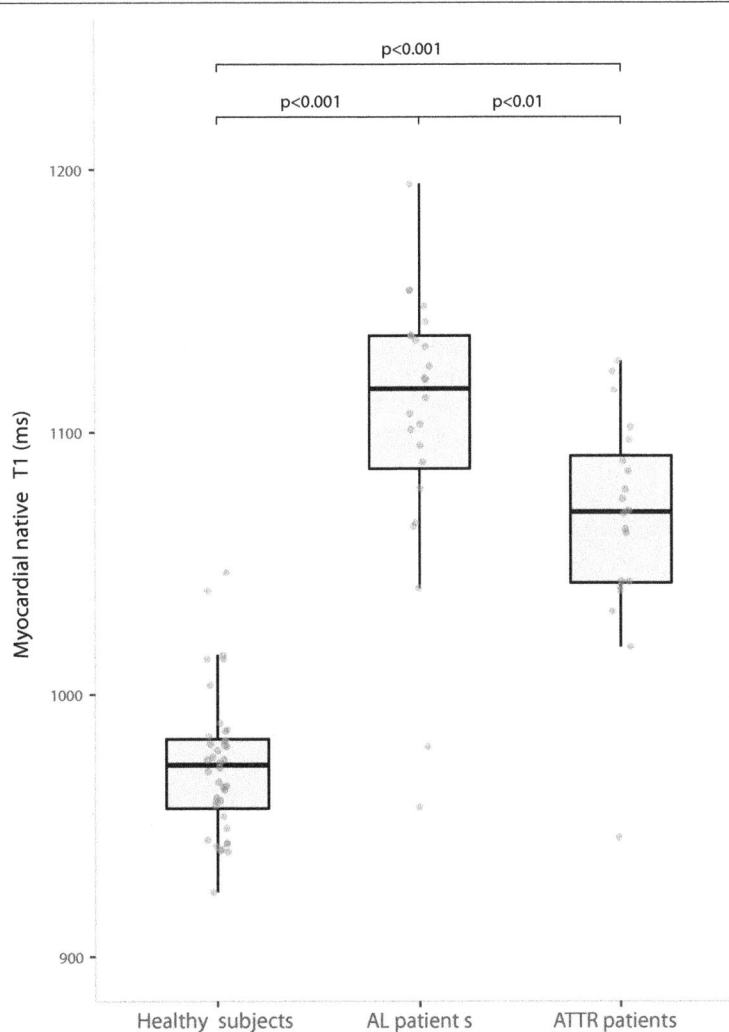

Fig. 2 Graph shows myocardial native T1 values in healthy subjects, patients with AL amyloidosis and patients with ATTR amyloidosis. Results are shown as boxplots, with each box representing the interquartile range (1st to 3rd quartile, IQR), the line within the box indicating the median, and the whiskers extending to 1.5 times the IQR above and below the box; the dots represent individual values for each patient. Myocardial native T1 is significantly (p < 0.001) higher in patients than in healthy subjects. Among patients myocardial native T1 is significantly (p < 0.01) higher in AL than in ATTR patients

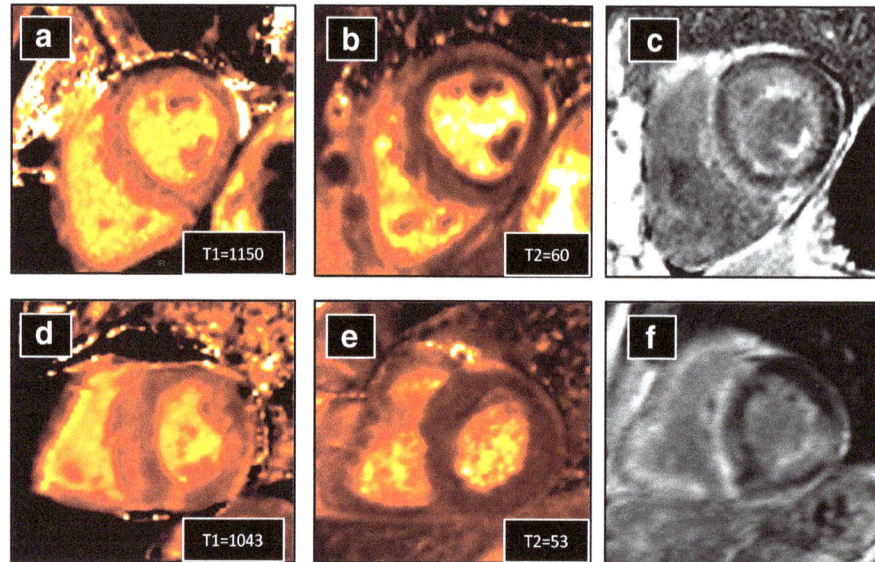

Fig. 3 Examples of MOLLI native T1 maps (**a**, **d**), T2 maps (**b**, **e**) and LGE images (**c**, **f**) obtained in one patient with AL amyloidosis (first line) and one patient with ATTR amyloidosis (second line). AL patient exhibited higher values of myocardial native T1 and T2 (1150 and 60 ms, respectively for T1 and T2) than ATTR patient (1043 and 53 ms, respectively for T1 and T2). Both patients exhibited diffuse myocardial enhancement of left and right ventricles on LGE images

also noticed in CA patients (AL (1104 ± 54 ms); ATTR (1066 ± 42 ms)) compared to healthy subjects (975 ± 26 ms; $p < 0.001$) (Figs. 1 and 2). Examples of patients are reported in the Fig. 3. When considering the difference between AL and ATTR patients, we reported that T2 was significantly ($p < 0.001$) higher in AL (63.2 ± 4.7 ms) than in ATTR (56.2 ± 3.1 ms) patients. A raise of myocardial native T1 was also observed in AL patients (1104 ± 54 ms) in comparison to ATTR patients (1066 ± 42 ms), but in a less significant manner ($p < 0.01$). AL and ATTR patients did not exhibit significant difference regarding other mapping parameters (post

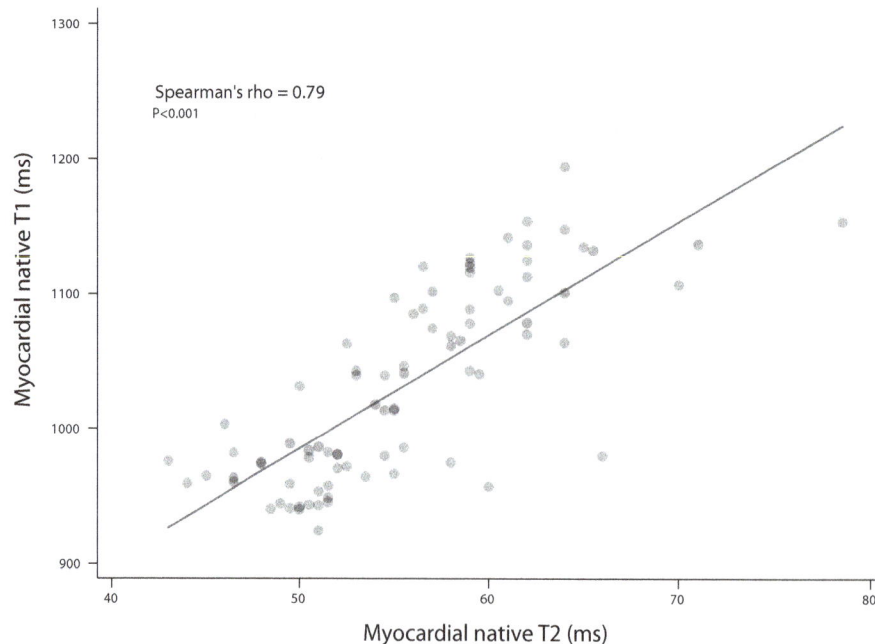

Fig. 4 Graph shows the relationship between myocardial native T1 and myocardial native T2 in the overall population (Spearman's rho = 0.79; $p < 0.001$). The dots represent individual values for each patient. The solid line represents the fitted regression line along with its 95% confidence interval

contrast myocardial T1, ECV, ICV and Total amyloid volume) except for total cell volume that was significantly higher in ATTR (61 ± 19 mL/m^2) than in AL patients (47 ± 15 mL/m^2; $p = 0.04$). T2 ratio did not exhibit significant differences ($p = 0.2$) between groups (1.31 ± 0.4, 1.41 ± 0.2 and 1.44 ± 0.3, respectively for AL patients, ATTR patients and healthy subjects). All data are reported in Table 2.

Relationship between myocardial native T2 and other parameters

Myocardial native T2 was strongly correlated with myocardial native T1 (Spearman's rho = 0.79; p < 0.001) (Fig. 4) and less markedly correlated with indexed LV mass (Spearman's rho = 0.36; $p = 0.001$), Total cell volume (Spearman's rho = -0.38; $p = 0.03$) and LVEF (Spearman's rho = -0.26; $p = 0.02$).

ROC-curve analysis

AL patients formed the positive case group and ATTR patients were considered as negative cases. Healthy subjects were excluded to reflect clinical practice. The area under curve (AUC) of myocardial native T2 for diagnosed AL patients as opposed to ATTR patients was 0.94 (95% CI: 0.86–1, $p < 0.001$), higher than that of T1 (0.77 (95% CI: 0.62–0.91, $p = 0.03$)) (Fig. 5). For QALE score, the AUC to distinguish between ATTR and AL patients was 0.64 (95% CI: 0.48–0.81, $p = 0.1$) With a cut-off of 59.2 ms, the sensitivity and specificity of myocardial native T2 were 83 and 95%, respectively. One hundred percent of specificity was obtained with a cut-off of 63 ms (sensitivity 42%). Lower performances were obtained using T1: with a cut-off of 1092 ms, the sensitivity and specificity of myocardial native T1 to diagnose AL patients were 71 and 75%, respectively. One hundred percent of specificity was obtained with a cut-off of 1130 ms (sensitivity 37%). Myocardial native T1 and T2 exhibited similar performances to distinguish between patients and healthy subjects (AUC = 0.95, (95% CI: 0.90–1, $p < 0.001$).

Survival analysis

Survival analysis was performed in the cohort of 42 patients with CA. In total, 18 of 42 patients died during a median follow-up of 27 months (interquartile range: 14–40 months). Myocardial native T2 was not significantly associated with overall survival in patients with CA (HR 1.03 (0.94–1.12); $p = 0.53$). Univariate Cox regression identified the following predictors: ECV (HR 1.66 per 0.1 increase in ECV (1.24–2.22); $P = 0.0006$), IVS thickness (HR 1.18 per 1 mm increase in IVS thickness (1.02–1.37); $P = 0.02$), LVEF (HR 0.64 per 10% increase in LVEF (0.47–0.87); $p = 0.005$) and post contrast myocardial T1 (HR 0.89 per 10 units increase in T1 value (0.84–0.95); $p = 0.0005$). For ECV, a value of 0.59 was identified by recursive partitioning as the optimal cutoff to predict overall survival: HR 5.33 (1.70–16.71), $p = 0.004$. Kaplan-Meier curve for patients according to ECV level is shown in Fig. 6.

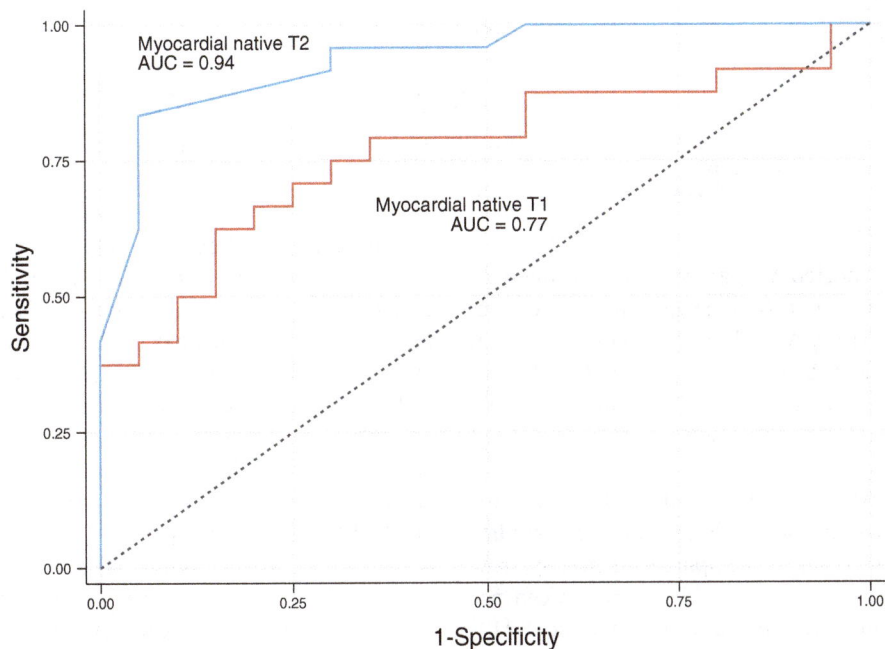

Fig. 5 Receiver operating characteristic curves for myocardial native T2 and T1

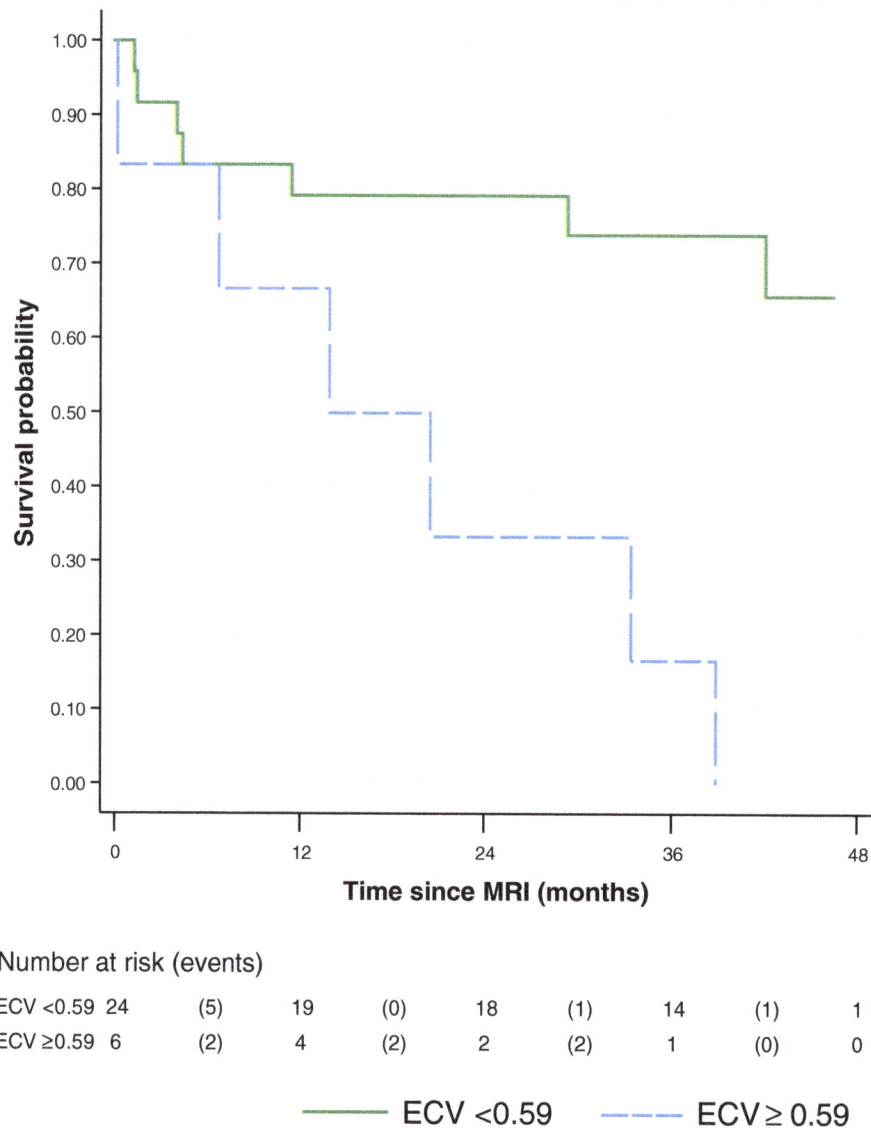

Fig. 6 Kaplan-Meier curve for overall survival according to ECV value. A median value of 0.59 was the best predictor of survival: log-rank test $p = 0.004$; Unadjusted HR 5.33 (1.70–16.71)

Discussion

In this study, we reported a significant raise of myocardial native T2 relaxation time suggesting myocardial edema in patients with CA, and more pronounced in AL compared to ATTR patients. Myocardial native T2 exhibited higher performances than T1 to differentiate AL and ATTR amyloidosis but was not a predictor of survival.

The question of variation of myocardial T2 in CA remains controversial in the literature with few studies addressing this topic. Using T2 mapping sequence, Sparrow et al. [18] did not find significant differences between patients with CA and controls whereas Wassmuth et al. [19] and our team [17] reported that the T2 ratio was lower in patients with CA and independently associated with

shortened survival. Recently Fontana et al. showed a greater elevation of T1 (and lower ECV) in AL than in ATTR patients suggesting that myocardial edema, induced by the toxic effect of AL amyloid fibrils on cardiomyocytes, may explain this difference [22]. The significant raise of myocardial native T2 that we reported here confirms this hypothesis of myocardial edema in AL patients. Interestingly, we also detected a less intense but significant myocardial edema in ATTR patients, suggesting that the toxic effect of amyloid fibrils is probably a general phenomenon in amyloidosis. However, we did not detect a significant correlation between T2 and troponin level in favor of a direct toxicity of amyloid proteins on cardiomyocytes. From a clinical point of view, myocardial native T2 exhibited good performances to separate AL and ATTR amyloidosis in our study

(AUC = 0.94), higher than T1 (AUC = 0.77) and QALE LGE score (AUC = 0.65), suggesting that it could be used as an additional marker to differentiate these 2 types of CA whose management is different. Although potentially performant to differentiate AL and ATTR, T2 does not seem to be a good marker of survival in our study, in contrast to ECV that deeply influences survival. The prognostic impact of ECV in amyloidosis was reported in several studies [16, 28, 29].

Surprisingly, we did not find in this study a significant reduction of T2 ratio in CA patients in comparison to healthy subjects, as previously reported by our group [17] and others [19]. We have no formal explanation for these results. It is possible that diffuse skeletal muscular edema exists in amyloidosis and may alter the relevance of T2 ratio by balancing more or less the increase of myocardial signal on T2 images [30]. In addition, the T2 STIR sequence is known to be sensitive to artifacts and is accompanied by a lower level of diagnostic confidence than T2 mapping as previously reported. In this work, the significance of the T2 map was higher than those observed in the previous studies on the T2 ratio supporting the impression of reliability of the T2 mapping.

In the light of our results, one can also deduce that the raise of myocardial T1 in cardiac amyloidosis is not only a simple consequence of passive amyloid proteins deposit, but is also driven by myocardial edema. The high correlation between myocardial native T1 and T2 that we noticed suggests a reciprocal influence and reinforces this idea. Therefore, because of the dual origin of its signal (interstitium and myocytes), caution should be taken to use solely T1 as a direct marker of amyloid burden and as a surrogate endpoint in drug development [31]. Its variations should be analyzed at the light of ECV value that is the purest measure of amyloid burden [8].

ATTR patients exhibited higher indexed LV mass and total cell volume in comparison to AL patients in our report, suggesting that extracellular deposition of amyloid proteins was associated with a concomitant cell hypertrophy in ATTR. These results are in line with Fontana et al. who reported a 18% increase of the intracellular space in ATTR vs. AL patients [22]. Nevertheless, we did detect significant difference of ECV and total amyloid volume between AL and ATTR in contrast to the aforementioned study that reported a significant raise of these values in ATTR patients, suggesting a more extensive amyloid deposition. We also failed to reproduce the results of Dungu et al. regarding differentiation of AL and ATTR using LGE sequences [21]. The QALE score was slightly higher in ATTR than in AL patients but did not exhibit significant difference as previously reported. Similarly, we did not observe systematic RV involvement in ATTR patients, as described by Dungu et al. [21].

Study limitation

First, the number of subjects included in this work was relatively limited and control group was younger than AL and ATTR patients, a difference that may influence (weakly) measurements of myocardial native T1 with the MOLLI sequence [32]. Second, we did not include other causes of LV wall thickening such as hypertrophic cardiomyopathies, aortic stenosis or hypertensive cardiomyopathies. Third, calculation of myocardial T1 and T2 was not performed on the entire LV. The basal part of the LV, more commonly affected in CA, was also not measured specifically using a short-axis basal section. Finally, the measurements of myocardial T1 and T2 included both LGE + and LGE- myocardial areas; focal variations of T1 and T2 maps related to amyloid proteins deposit were not studied.

Conclusion

In this study, we reported a significant raise of myocardial native T2 in AL patients in comparison to ATTR patients. T2 separated effectively AL and ATTR patients and could be considered as an additional marker to distinguish these 2 types of CA. Although more intense than in AL amyloidosis, myocardial edema was also detected in ATTR patients suggesting that myocardial edema plays a role in the raise of myocardial native T1 in CA. As opposed to ECV, T2 did not seem to impact survival of CA patients.

Abbreviations

AL: Light chain; ANOVA: Analysis of variance; ATTR: Transthyretin; AUC: Areas under curve; bSSFP: Balanced steady state free precession; CA: Cardiac amyloidosis; CMR: Cardiovascular magnetic resonance; ECG: Electrocardiogram; ECV: Extracellular volume fraction; EMB: Endomyocardial biopsy; HR: Hazard ratios; ICV: Intracellular volume; IVS: Interventricular septum; LGE: Late gadolinium enhanced; LV: Left ventricle/left ventricular; LVEF: Left ventricular ejection fraction; MOLLI: Modified Look-Locker inversion recovery; PSIR: Phase sensitive inversion recovery; QALE: Query amyloid late enhancement; ROC: Receiver operating characteristic; ROI: Region-of-interest; RPA: Recursive partitioning analysis; RV: Right ventricle/right ventricular; STIR: Short tau inversion recovery; TI: Inversion time

Funding

The funding is provided by our department association (ARIM).

Authors'

All authors made contribution to the study and reviewed the manuscript. FR and JFD analyzed and interpreted the data, and were the major contributor in writing the manuscript. TD and DB were of a major collaboration in the clinical follow up. VT, FL, HD, IS and AR participated in the analysis and the interpretation of the MRI data. EA performed all the statistical analysis. All authors read and approved the final manuscript.

Competing interests

Author(s) declare(s) that they have no competing interests.

Author details

[1]Radiology Department, Henri Mondor Hospital, University Paris Est Créteil, Assistance Publique-Hôpitaux de Paris, 51 av Mal de Lattre de Tassigny, 94000 Créteil, France. [2]Cardiology Department, Henri Mondor Hospital, University Paris Est Créteil, Assistance Publique-Hôpitaux de Paris, Créteil, France. [3]National Referal Centre for Cardiac Amyloidoses, Henri Mondor Hospital, Créteil, France. [4]Public Health Department, Henri Mondor Hospital, CEpiA EA7376, University Paris Est Créteil, Assistance Publique-Hôpitaux de Paris, Créteil, France.

References

1. Alkhawam H, Patel D, Nguyen J, et al. Cardiac amyloidosis: pathogenesis, clinical context, diagnosis and management options. Acta Cardiol. 2017;72:380–9.
2. Falk RH, Alexander KM, Liao R, Dorbala S. AL (light-chain) cardiac amyloidosis: a review of diagnosis and therapy. J Am Coll Cardiol. 2016;68:1323–41.
3. Gertz MA, Benson MD, Dyck PJ, et al. Diagnosis, prognosis, and therapy of transthyretin amyloidosis. J Am Coll Cardiol. 2015;66:2451–66.
4. Rapezzi C, Merlini G, Quarta CC, et al. Systemic cardiac amyloidoses: disease profiles and clinical courses of the 3 main types. Circulation. 2009;120:1203–12.
5. Damy T, Costes B, Hagege AA, et al. Prevalence and clinical phenotype of hereditary transthyretin amyloid cardiomyopathy in patients with increased left ventricular wall thickness. Eur Heart J. 2016;37:1826–34.
6. Galat A, Guellich A, Bodez D, et al. Aortic stenosis and transthyretin cardiac amyloidosis: the chicken or the egg. Eur Heart J. 2016;37:3525–31.
7. Laptseva N, Zuber M, Bode PK, Flammer AJ. Cardiac amyloidosis: still challenging. Eur Heart J. 2017;38:122.
8. Fontana M, Chung R, Hawkins PN, Moon JC. Cardiovascular magnetic resonance for amyloidosis. Heart Fail Rev. 2015;20:133–44.
9. Maceira AM, Prasad SK, Hawkins PN, Roughton M, Pennell DJ. Cardiovascular magnetic resonance and prognosis in cardiac amyloidosis. J Cardiovasc Magn Reson. 2008;10:54.
10. Ruberg FL, Appelbaum E, Davidoff R, et al. Diagnostic and prognostic utility of cardiovascular magnetic resonance imaging in light-chain cardiac amyloidosis. Am J Cardiol. 2009;103:544–9.
11. Syed IS, Glockner JF, Feng D, et al. Role of cardiac magnetic resonance imaging in the detection of cardiac amyloidosis. JACC Cardiovasc Imaging. 2010;3:155–64.
12. Karamitsos TD, Piechnik SK, Banypersad SM, et al. Noncontrast T1 mapping for the diagnosis of cardiac amyloidosis. JACC Cardiovasc Imaging. 2013;6:488–97.
13. Liu JM, Liu A, Leal J, et al. Measurement of myocardial native T1 in cardiovascular diseases and norm in 1291 subjects. J Cardiovasc Magn Reson. 2017;19:74.
14. Mongeon FP, Jerosch-Herold M, Coelho-Filho OR, Blankstein R, Falk RH, Kwong RY. Quantification of extracellular matrix expansion by CMR in infiltrative heart disease. JACC Cardiovasc Imaging. 2012;5:897–907.
15. Fontana M, Banypersad SM, Treibel TA, et al. Native T1 mapping in transthyretin amyloidosis. JACC Cardiovasc Imaging. 2014;7:157–65.
16. Banypersad SM, Fontana M, Maestrini V, et al. T1 mapping and survival in systemic light-chain amyloidosis. Eur Heart J. 2015;36:244–51.
17. Legou F, Tacher V, Damy T, et al. Usefulness of T2 ratio in the diagnosis and prognosis of cardiac amyloidosis using cardiac MR imaging. Diagn Interv Imaging. 2017;98:125–32.
18. Sparrow P, Amirabadi A, Sussman MS, Paul N, Merchant N. Quantitative assessment of myocardial T2 relaxation times in cardiac amyloidosis. J Magn Reson Imaging. 2009;30:942–6.
19. Wassmuth R, Abdel-Aty H, Bohl S, Schulz-Menger J. Prognostic impact of T2-weighted CMR imaging for cardiac amyloidosis. Eur Radiol. 2011;21:1643–50.
20. Di Bella G, Pizzino F, Minutoli F, et al. The mosaic of the cardiac amyloidosis diagnosis: role of imaging in subtypes and stages of the disease. Eur Heart J Cardiovasc Imaging. 2014;15:1307–15.
21. Dungu JN, Valencia O, Pinney JH, et al. CMR-based differentiation of AL and ATTR cardiac amyloidosis. JACC Cardiovasc Imaging. 2014;7:133–42.
22. Fontana M, Banypersad SM, Treibel TA, et al. Differential myocyte responses in patients with cardiac transthyretin amyloidosis and light-chain amyloidosis: a cardiac MR imaging study. Radiology. 2015;277:388–97.
23. Gillmore JD, Maurer MS, Falk RH, et al. Nonbiopsy diagnosis of cardiac transthyretin amyloidosis. Circulation. 2016;133:2404–12.
24. Bodez D, Ternacle J, Guellich A, et al. Prognostic value of right ventricular systolic function in cardiac amyloidosis. Amyloid. 2016;23:158–67.
25. Messroghli DR, Radjenovic A, Kozerke S, Higgins DM, Sivananthan MU, Ridgway JP. Modified look-locker inversion recovery (MOLLI) for high-resolution T1 mapping of the heart. Magn Reson Med. 2004;52:141–6.
26. vanden Driesen RI, Slaughter RE, Strugnell WE. MR findings in cardiac amyloidosis. AJR Am J Roentgenol. 2006;186:1682–5.
27. van Putten W. CART: Stata module to perform Classification And Regression Tree analysis. In: Components SS, ed. Economics. BCDo. 2006:S456776.
28. Martinez-Naharro A, Treibel TA, Abdel-Gadir A, et al. Magnetic resonance in transthyretin cardiac amyloidosis. J Am Coll Cardiol. 2017;70:466–77.
29. Wong TC, Piehler K, Meier CG, et al. Association between extracellular matrix expansion quantified by cardiovascular magnetic resonance and short-term mortality. Circulation. 2012;126:1206–16.
30. Thavendiranathan P, Walls M, Giri S, et al. Improved detection of myocardial involvement in acute inflammatory cardiomyopathies using T2 mapping. Circ Cardiovasc Imaging. 2012;5:102–10.
31. Hur DJ, Dicks DL, Huber S, et al. Serial native T1 mapping to monitor cardiac response to treatment in light-chain amyloidosis. Circ Cardiovasc Imaging. 2016;9
32. Kellman P, Hansen MS. T1-mapping in the heart: accuracy and precision. J Cardiovasc Magn Reson. 2014;16:2.

Society for Cardiovascular Magnetic Resonance (SCMR) expert consensus for CMR imaging endpoints in clinical research: part I - analytical validation and clinical qualification

Valentina O. Puntmann[1,2], Silvia Valbuena[3], Rocio Hinojar[4], Steffen E. Petersen[5], John P. Greenwood[6], Christopher M. Kramer[7], Raymond Y. Kwong[8], Gerry P. McCann[9,10], Colin Berry[11,12], Eike Nagel[1*] and on behalf of SCMR Clinical Trial Writing Group

Abstract

Cardiovascular disease remains a leading cause of morbidity and mortality globally. Changing natural history of the disease due to improved care of acute conditions and ageing population necessitates new strategies to tackle conditions which have more chronic and indolent course. These include an increased deployment of safe screening methods, life-long surveillance, and monitoring of both disease activity and tailored-treatment, by way of increasingly personalized medical care. Cardiovascular magnetic resonance (CMR) is a non-invasive, ionising radiation-free method, which can support a significant number of clinically relevant measurements and offers new opportunities to advance the state of art of diagnosis, prognosis and treatment. The objective of the SCMR Clinical Trial Taskforce was to summarizes the evidence to emphasize where currently CMR-guided clinical care can indeed translate into meaningful use and efficient deployment of resources results in meaningful and efficient use. The objective of the present initiative was to provide an appraisal of evidence on *analytical validation*, including the accuracy and precision, and *clinical qualification* of parameters in disease context, clarifying the strengths and weaknesses of the state of art, as well as the gaps in the current evidence This paper is complementary to the existing position papers on standardized acquisition and post-processing ensuring robustness and transferability for widespread use. Themed imaging-endpoint guidance on trial design to support drug-discovery or change in clinical practice (part II), will be presented in a follow-up paper in due course. As CMR continues to undergo rapid development, regular updates of the present recommendations are foreseen.

Keywords: Cardiac magnetic resonance, Imaging, Biomarker, Position paper, SCMR

* Correspondence: eike.nagel@cardiac-imaging.org
[1]Institute of Experimental and Translational Cardiovascular Imaging, Goethe University Hospital Frankfurt, Frankfurt, Germany
Full list of author information is available at the end of the article

Outline

1. Rationale

Cardiovascular disease (CVD) remains the greatest cause of morbidity and mortality globally. The changing natural history of CVD due to improved care of acute conditions and ageing population necessitates new strategies to tackle conditions with a more chronic and indolent course. These include an increased deployment of safe screening methods, life-long surveillance, and monitoring of both disease activity and tailored-treatment, by way of increasingly personalised medical care. Cardiovascular magnetic resonance (CMR), is a non-invasive, radiation-free method, which can support a significant number of clinically relevant measurements, offers many new opportunities to advance the state of art of diagnosis, prognosis and treatment of patients with CVD. Several key CMR measurements are highly accurate and reproducible, providing gold-standard measures in cardiovascular imaging. Published agreements on standardized acquisition and post-processing ensure robustness and transferability for widespread use [1, 2]. With the growing evidence on diagnostic and prognostic role, CMR measurements may be well-suited as imaging biomarkers for assessment of novel clinical management pathways and therapies. Yet, despite the enthusiasm, the body of evidence, and the overt potential to improve patients care, the impact of CMR towards clinical cardiology practice remains limited, by way of access to the technology (scanner, scan-time), operational imaging skill and allocation of the healthcare

resources. Hence, the objective of this taskforce is to emphasize the evidence where CMR-guided clinical care indeed means that deployment of resources results in meaningful and efficient use, by providing an appraisal of evidence on *analytical validation*, including the accuracy and precision, and *qualification* of parameters in disease context (part I). The manuscript structure, preparation and evidence appraisal procedures were based on a prior agreement within the SCMR CT Writing Group (WG) (Fig. 1- Flowchart), as well as general guidance of the SCMR on Expert Consensus publications. This included the assignment of themed subsection to a minimum of 2 and a maximum of 5 authors with background of contribution to the field, which are included in the authors' list (Table 1). The resulting material was subsequently reviewed and edited to adopt a common reporting format of a summary-text and evidence-rich tables. As per SCMR CT WG consensus, the studies were included, if providing a robust independent (non-CMR) comparator (validation) or including > 50 subjects (normal values) or > 25 in patient group (proof of concept), and > 100 for outcome study. Smaller studies were included if no other evidence was available and with consensus of the writing group. We strived to set out qualified recommendations for appropriate surrogate use of imaging measures biomarkers using consensus statements produced by the SCMR CT WG upon the presentation of summarised data. The weighing of evidence was based on consensus criteria of the SCMR CT WG, and assigned as promising, if multiple (3 or more) publications from independent groups existed, and favourable, if also cited by the practice guidelines. The final steps included a review and approval by all co-authors, followed by 3 independent external reviewers, commissioned by the SCMR Board of Trustees, in line with the societal rules on consensus statements. This report clarifies the strengths and weaknesses of the state of art, as well as the gaps in the current evidence (Table 2). The SCMR CT WG statements are based on the available evidence up to and including April 2017. The target audience includes clinical investigators considering the application of CMR-imaging endpoints in clinical studies and trials involving human subjects. Themed imaging-endpoint guidance on trial design to support drug-discovery or change in clinical practice (part II), will be presented in a follow-up paper in due course. As CMR continues to undergo rapid development, regular updates of the present recommendations are foreseen.

2. Imaging parameters as biomarkers and endpoints

A biomarker is a characteristic that can be objectively measured and evaluated as an indicator of normal biological processes, pathogenic processes or pharmacological response to a therapeutic intervention [3]. They

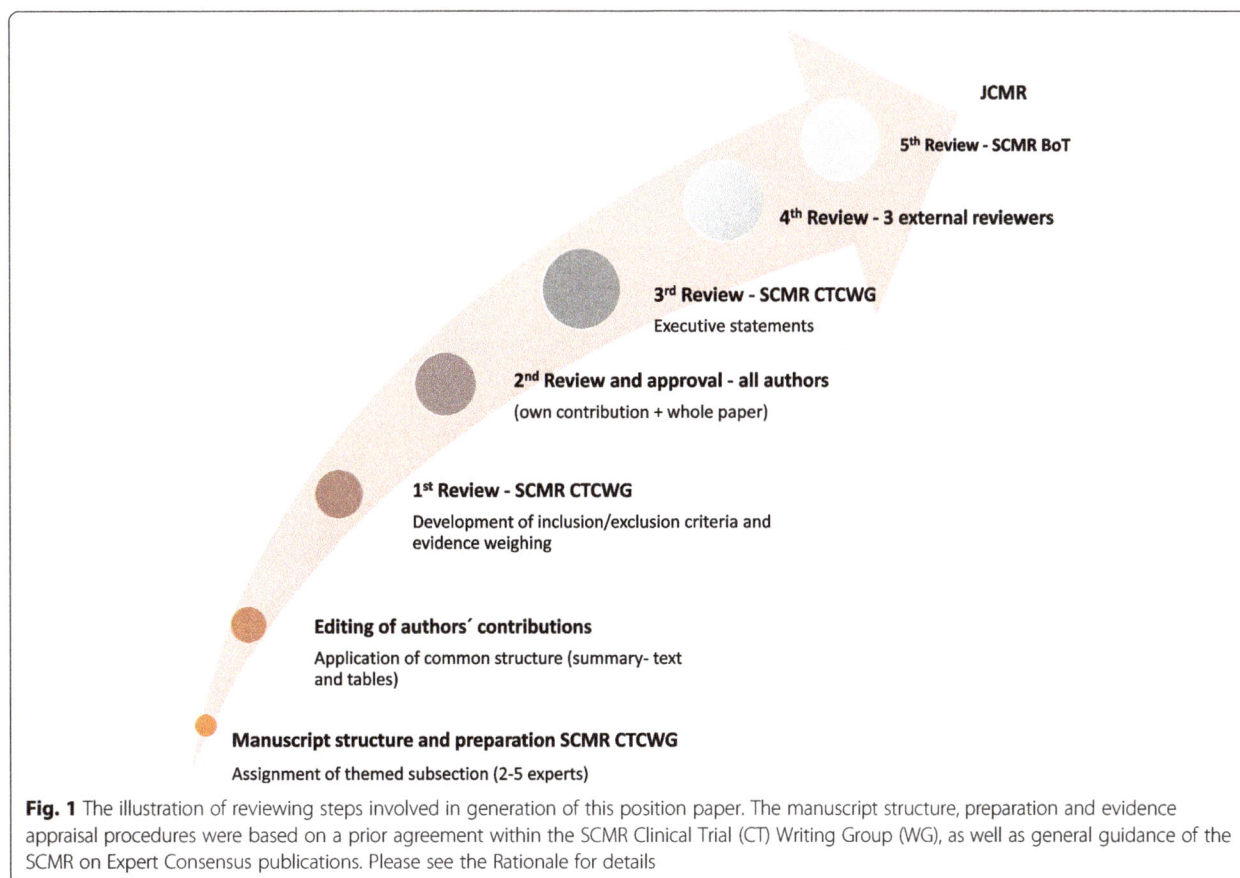

Fig. 1 The illustration of reviewing steps involved in generation of this position paper. The manuscript structure, preparation and evidence appraisal procedures were based on a prior agreement within the SCMR Clinical Trial (CT) Writing Group (WG), as well as general guidance of the SCMR on Expert Consensus publications. Please see the Rationale for details

Table 1 Characteristics of contributing authors

Contributing authors' characteristics	Count (%); Median(IQR)
MR Vendors	
Siemens	26 (53)
Philips	17(35)
General Electrics	6(12)
Field Strength	
1.5 Tesla	37(76)
3.0 Tesla	17(35)
Both	15(31)
Specialty	
Cardiology	25(51)
Radiology	18(38)
Other	5(10)
Number of previously co-authored Societal consensus papers (any)	3(1–4.5)
Number of previously co-authored SCMR Consensus papers	2(1–3)
[a]Number of previously co-authored papers in the CMR field	86(57–141)
[b]Number of previously co-authored papers in the author's themed field	44(23–68)

Search criteria (Pubmed): [a]Surname, First initial + cardiac + magnetic; [b]Surname, First initial + magnetic+ theme

can serve as indicators of a disease presence or activity and reflect the rate of disease progression and response to treatment. Reliable biomarker's characteristics include an accurate measurement, which is reproducible across multiple laboratories, and in a clinical setting, an adequate sensitivity and specificity for disease detection, severity and prognostic outcome. The biomarker evaluation framework foresees the following steps of biomarker characterisation: analytical validation, clinical qualification and utilization, and subsequently, a constant re-evaluation of the preceding steps [3]. It is also a sequence of interdependent steps, which continually inform each other. This process clarifies the biomarker's application within a defined disease context and possible roles, from exploratory use to surrogate endpoint. ***Analytical validation*** involves assessment of assays or techniques supporting the acquisition of measurements, as well as establishing the range of conditions, under which the measurement will give reproducible and accurate data. Important performance metrics include precision, accuracy, lab-to-lab reproducibility, limits of detection and signal-to-noise, as well as determination of the reference values. ***Qualification*** refers to summation of the available evidence about the biomarker-disease-relationship, including its relevance, diagnostic and prognostic value. Also, causal relationships

Table 2 Summary table for Executive statements for CMR endpoints

		Number of studies	Total number of subjects
Ventricular volumes and function			
CMR is the reference standard for quantification of LV and RV volumes, function and mass. CMR should be considered as the first line technique in clinical trials requiring one of these parameters for in- or exclusion or as an endpoint. The evidence for the use of quantification of cardiac function and volumes is favourable.			
Analytical validation	Excellent validation of LV mass and volumes	7	121
Precision	Large body of evidence on interstudy, inter- and intraobserver reproducibility	2*	32
Normal values	Available for various field strengths, imaging sequences, post-processing approaches, age-, sex- and ethnicity groups	9	6895
Qualification/ Utilisation	The original evidence base by transthoracic echocardiography has been revalidated and expanded upon by CMR	7	14,711
Regional wall motion, deformation and dyssynchrony			
CMR-based strain-imaging techniques seem similarly suited as echocardiographic techniques for assessing longitudinal motion and strain. The evidence for the use of CMR-based strain imaging techniques is promising.			
Analytical validation	CMR tagging techniques have been well validated. Other MR based strain imaging techniques have been either directly compared with tagging or indirectly against a technique originally compared to tagging.	11	600
Precision	Limited data on inter-study reproducibility	9	168
Normal values	Normal values are available, but show considerable regional variation as well as variation between different studies	11	3191
Qualification/ Utilisation	Outcome data suggest utility in addition to standard measures of care in clinical management.	5	2462
Diastolic function			
CMR may have advantages over other techniques by direct assessment of myocardial tissue. The evidence for the use of CMR-based assessment of diastolic function is promising.			
Analytical validation	Reasonably well validated versus PV loops and echocardiography for diastolic filling, atrial volumes and function and transmitral and pulmonary venous flow	4	212
Late gadolinium enhancement			
CMR based LGE should be used as the first line technique in clinical trials requiring the assessment of regional scar or fibrosis for inclusion or exclusion or as an endpoint. CMR should also be employed for optimal risk-classification of trial subjects with ischemic or non-ischemic cardiomyopathies. The evidence for the use of LGE imaging for visual detection of regional myocardial fibrosis and quantification of ischaemic scar is favourable. The quantification of non-ischaemic scar remains promising.			
Analytical validation	Extensively validated as a marker of irreversible damage post myocardial infarction in animals as well as versus biopsies, in explanted hearts and versus other imaging techniques	8	406
Precision	Strong data on inter-study reproducibility	7	200
Qualification/ Utilisation	Strong parameter to predict outcome, superior to volumes and function.	37	12,562
T2-weighted imaging			
Due to the availability of many different sequences no generally accepted standard has been defined. For clinical trials, it is important to use a validated and standardized approach amongst different centres and vendors and use normal values and effect sizes specifically for these sequences. The evidence for the use of T2W imaging of AAR is promising.			
Analytical validation	Well validated in animals, phantoms and humans	15	817

Table 2 Summary table for Executive statements for CMR endpoints (Continued)

		Number of studies	Total number of subjects
Precision	Scarce data on inter-study reproducibility in acute myocardial infarction. Lack of reproducibility data and outcome studies for T2W-oedema imaging in inflammatory cardiac conditions	4	234
Qualification/Utilisation	Small number of outcome studies using AAR	17	1509

T1 mapping

Due to the availability of many different sequences, no generally accepted standard has been defined. To employ T1 mapping in clinical trials, the use of validated (well understood sequence) and standardised approach amongst different centres and vendors is mandatory, due to the different normal values and effect sizes between various sequences. CMR T1-mapping may be considered as a standard for adequate risk-assessment of patients with non-ischemic dilated cardiomyopathy in clinical trials. The evidence for the use of T1 mapping is promising.

		Number of studies	Total number of subjects
Analytical validation	Well validated in phantoms, animal models, human biopsies and explanted hearts.	15	267
Precision	Evidence on interstudy, inter- and intraobserver variability	10	270
Normal values	Sequence-specific normal values available	4	1735
Qualification/Utilisation	Strong predictors of outcome in non-ischaemic dilated cardiomyopathies, superior to volumes, function and LGE.	37	6153

T2 mapping

Due to the availability of many different sequences no generally accepted standard has been defined. The use a validated and standardized approaches amongst different centres and vendors is mandatory for the use in clinical trials, due to the different normal values and effect sizes specifically for these sequences. The timing of imaging after an acute event must be highly standardized.
The evidence for the use of T2 mapping is promising.

		Number of studies	Total number of subjects
Analytical validation	Well validated against phantoms, animal models, human biopsies and other imaging biomarkers	11	340
Precision	Evidence on interstudy, inter- and intraobserver variability	1*	73
Normal values	Sequence-specific normal values available	3	205
Qualification/Utilisation	Useful in detecting myocardial oedema and inflammation	12	680

T2* mapping

T2* can be regarded as the clinical reference standard in thalassemia and provide superior outcome data if used for therapy guidance. T2* measurements during or shortly after an acute coronary or vascular event provides important prognostic information in terms of short-term LV remodelling. The evidence for the use of T2* mapping is favourable.

		Number of studies	Total number of subjects
Analytical validation	Excellently validated and standardized in iron-overload	17	1728
Precision	Evidence on interscanner, intercenter, interstudy, inter- and intraobserver variability	4*	59
Normal values	Normal values and established clinically relevant cut-offs available	5	100
Qualification/Utilisation	Outcome data in thalassaemia major. Prognostic information after a coronary event	19	1778

Stress myocardial perfusion

Perfusion imaging should be considered as a first line technique for assessing the presence, extent and localization of inducible ischemia. Its use for full quantification requires locally validated and standardized sequences with specific normal values. The evidence for the use of myocardial perfusion imaging for visual detection of ischaemia is favourable. The quantification remains promising.

Table 2 Summary table for Executive statements for CMR endpoints *(Continued)*

		Number of studies	Total number of subjects
Analytical validation	Well-validated against animal models and alternative techniques	63	10,916
Precision	Limited evidence on interstudy, inter- and intraobserver reproducibility due to need of stress and contrast injection	5*	73
Normal values	Limited data on normal values due to lack of standardization of image acquisition and post-processing	3	42
Qualification/ Utilisation	Large body of evidence showing significant predictive association for the presence/severity of myocardial ischemia with outcome	14	26,494
Vascular			
	CMR vascular imaging is well suited to assess vascular anatomy and function. Aortic and carotid vessel wall imaging, are robust markers of atherosclerotic burden in these vessels and can be used in clinical trials.		
Analytical validation	Validation of PWV against alternative techniques and T2 mapping against histology	7	237
Precision	Limited evidence on interstudy reproducibility of anatomical and tissue measurements. Excellent evidence for PWV	6	95
Normal values	Available for different anatomical and functional measurements	7	4112
Qualification/ Utilisation	Aortic wall imaging and PWV serve robust biomarkers of cardiovascular risk	2	5797

LV left ventricle, *RV* right ventricle, *PV* pressure-volume, *LGE* ate gadolinium enhancement, *AAR* area at risk, *PWV* pulse wave velocity. *Only studies reporting interstudy variability are included

to disease pathogenesis are considered, including the effects of therapeutic intervention on the imaging marker and to the clinical endpoints of interest. **(4)** *Utilization* is a contextual analysis of the above evidence with regards to the definition of the context for the biomarker' proposed clinical use. In addition, factors such as prevalence, heterogeneity, morbidity and mortality of the disease, as well as the risks and benefits of an intervention are considered.

3. Executive statements - SCMR Clinical Trial Writing Group

CMR uniquely provides quantitative information on cardiac function (LV, RV and valves) and myocardial tissue characteristics that are diagnostic of acute and chronic disease. CMR involves contrast- and non-contrast media imaging techniques. CMR does not involve ionising radiation and can be safely repeated.

Ventricular volumes and function

The ability of CMR to assess left ventricular (LV) and right ventricular (RV) volumes and function accurately and precisely has been demonstrated in excellent validation studies with a large body of evidence on inter-study reproducibility. Standardised approach to quantification is available. There are extensive sets of normal values for gradient echo (GRE) sequences, whereas smaller sets support the modern acquisition techniques (balanced steady state free precession (bSSFP)). Thus, the appropriate reference ranges need to be selected for the technique used. The accuracy and reproducibility of novel post-processing algorithms based on signal intensity thresholding remains unknown. CMR is rightly regarded as the reference standard for the assessment of left and right ventricular volumes and left ventricular mass. CMR should be considered as the first line technique in clinical trials requiring one of these parameters for in- or exclusion or as an endpoint. The evidence for the use of quantification of cardiac function and volumes is favourable.

i. Regional wall motion, deformation and dyssynchrony

CMR tagging techniques have been well validated. Other CMR based strain imaging techniques have been either directly compared with tagging or indirectly against a technique originally compared to tagging. Accuracy, precision and normal values are still to be further improved especially for radial strain and strain velocities. While normal values are available they show considerable regional variation as well as variation between different studies. There is very limited data on inter-study reproducibility. CMR-based strain-imaging techniques seem similarly suited as echocardiographic techniques for assessing longitudinal motion and strain. The evidence for the use of CMR-based strain imaging techniques is promising.

Diastolic function

CMR has been reasonably well validated versus pressure volume (PV) loops and echocardiography for diastolic filling, atrial volumes and function and transmitral and pulmonary venous flow. More work is required to fully establish its role based on classic LV inflow (filling) parameters (e.g. E/e'). Although CMR may have advantages over other techniques by direct assessment of myocardial tissue, more evidence to support the use of CMR-based assessment of diastolic function is needed.

Late gadolinium enhancement (LGE)

Late gadolinium enhancement (LGE) has been extensively validated as a marker of irreversible damage post myocardial infarction in animals as well as versus biopsies and in explanted hearts, demonstrating excellent accuracy and precision superior to alternative techniques. There are strong data on inter-study reproducibility. LGE is a strong parameter to predict outcome and has been shown to be superior to volumes and function. CMR based LGE should be used as the first line technique in clinical trials requiring the assessment of regional scar or fibrosis for inclusion or exclusion or as an endpoint. CMR should also be employed for optimal risk-classification of trial subjects with ischemic or non-ischemic cardiomyopathies. The evidence for the use of LGE imaging for visual detection of regional myocardial fibrosis and quantification of ischaemic scar is favourable. The quantification of non-ischaemic scar remains promising.

T2-weighted imaging

T2-weighted imaging (T2W) has been well validated in animals, phantoms and humans and demonstrates an excellent ability to visualize areas of significantly increased tissue water or myocardial haemorrhage. There are scarce data on inter-study reproducibility in acute myocardial infarction. There is a small number of outcome studies in area at risk (AAR), including an application in a clinical trial. There is lack of reproducibility data and outcome studies for T2W-oedema imaging (or Lake-Louise criteria) in inflammatory cardiac conditions. Due to the availability of many different sequences no generally accepted standard has been defined. For clinical trials, it is important to use a validated and standardized approach amongst different centres and vendors and use normal values and effect sizes specifically for these sequences. Timing of imaging after an acute event must be highly standardized. Contrast-enhanced cine bSSFP imaging is emerging as possible time-efficient option for imaging the AAR. The evidence for the use of T2W imaging of AAR is promising.

T1-mapping

Myocardial T1-mapping has been well validated in phantoms, animal models, and human biopsies and explanted hearts. In model diseases, the various acquisition techniques demonstrate the ability to relate to diffuse fibrosis, increased extracellular space and oedema, in a quantifiable fashion. T1-mapping indices have been shown to be strong predictors of outcome in non-ischaemic dilated cardiomyopathies, superior to volumes, function and LGE. Due to the availability of many different sequences, no generally accepted standard has been defined. To employ T1 mapping in clinical trials, the use of validated (well understood sequence) and standardized approach amongst different centres and vendors is mandatory, due to the different normal values and effect sizes between various sequences. CMR T1-mapping may be considered as a standard for adequate risk-assessment of patients with non-ischemic dilated cardiomyopathy in clinical trials. The evidence for the use of T1 mapping is promising.

T2-mapping

Myocardial T2-mapping has been well-validated in phantoms, animal models, and human biopsies. The various techniques demonstrate an excellent ability to relate to myocardial water content/oedema, in a quantifiable fashion. Due to the availability of many different sequences no generally accepted standard has been defined. Similar to T1 mapping above, the use a validated and standardized approaches amongst different centres and vendors is mandatory for the use in clinical trials, due to the different normal values and effect sizes specifically for these sequences. The timing of imaging after an acute event must be highly standardized. The evidence for the use of T2 mapping is promising.

T2* -mapping

Myocardial T2* mapping measurements in thalassemia have been excellently validated and standardized for 1.5 T and provide superior outcome data if used for therapy guidance. As such T2* can be regarded as the clinical reference standard in thalassemia. T2* measurements during or shortly after an acute coronary or vascular event provides important prognostic information in terms of short-term LV remodelling. The evidence for the use of T2* mapping is favourable.

Perfusion imaging

CMR perfusion imaging has been well-validated against animal models, alternative techniques as well as related to outcomes. In various meta-analyses, CMR perfusion imaging has been confirmed as the most accurate technique for non-invasive assessment of myocardial ischemia. However, due to the availability of many different sequences

and post-processing parameters, no generally accepted standard for (semi-) quantification has been defined. While there is good correlation of quantification techniques with microspheres and positron emission tomography (PET), normal values are variable and show high inter-study variability. Perfusion imaging should be considered as a first line technique for assessing the presence, extent and localization of inducible ischemia, its use for full quantification requires locally validated and standardized sequences with specific normal values. Trials assessing reduction in ischaemic burden following intervention are currently lacking. The evidence for the use of myocardial perfusion imaging for visual detection of ischaemia is favourable. Quantitative perfusion imaging is increasingly becoming available. At this stage the various approaches require more validation, especially as large outcome studies have been performed with visual analysis.

Vascular imaging

Vascular imaging provides robust quantifiable data on vessel diameters, vessel wall thickness and vessel distensibility. Vascular stiffness measurements aside, there are limited data on truth validation or interstudy reproducibility for some vascular areas. Limited data supports CMR being non-inferior to computed tomography (CT) for aortic visualization and dimensions. Large databases of normal data are available. CMR vascular imaging is well suited to assess vascular anatomy and function. Aortic and carotid vessel wall imaging, are robust markers of atherosclerotic burden in these vessels and can be used in clinical trials. Coronary vessel wall imaging and tissue characterization is a promising research tool but require further advances in the robustness and simplicity of the methods.

4. Ventricular volumes and mass
i. Global volumes, thickness and function

Quantification of cardiac volumes at end-diastole and end-systole, LV mass and global systolic function represent the measurements of cardiac imaging, which are fundamental to decision making in clinical cardiology. These are obtained using standard cine images by CMR and can be processed by virtually every available post-processing software. Cine imaging also supports assessment of regional wall motion abnormalities, either visually or by strain quantification (presently limited to research).

Acquisition
- Cine imaging (bSSFP sequences)
- Acquisition defined in SCMR Standardized Protocols [1]:
  - complete LV and RV coverage using short axis (SAX) stack of slices
  - long axis LV views.

- Older approaches of cine imaging based on fast gradient recalled echo (GRE) sequences: compared to bSSFP sequences, GRE sequences lead to larger LV mass and smaller LV volumes.

Post-processing
- Standardised approach defined in SCMR Standardized Post-processing recommendations [2]
  - LV mass measurement: inclusion of papillary muscles into LV cavity reduces accuracy compared to autopsy, but results in higher precision (smaller observer variability);
  - LV dimensions and wall thickness: most reproducible in 3-chamber view [4];
  - An early study showed higher reproducibility of RV volumes; measured in a transverse (TRA) stack [5], a later study reaffirmed that both SAX and TRA are similarly reproducible, as long as both ventricles acquired in entirety [6, 7].
  - TRA stack does not support reproducible RV mass measurements [2, 7]. No data available for SAX stack.
  - The accuracy and reproducibility of novel post-processing algorithms based on signal intensity thresholding is unknown

Validation
- LV mass: excellent validation against gold-standard in animals and excised human hearts after transplantation (Additional file 1: Table 3ai.1).
- LV function/cardiac output: limited validation against invasive conductance catheters [8, 9]

Precision
- A large body of evidence exists on interstudy, inter- and intraobserver reproducibility (Additional file 1: Table 3ai.2)
- A body of evidence supports superior precision of CMR-derived measurements compared to:
  - radionuclide ventriculography [10]
  - nuclear medicine techniques (PET, single photon emission computed tomography (SPECT)) [11]
  - transthoracic 2- and 3D echocardiography [12, 13]
  - cardiac CT [14]
- Benchmarking datasets available [15]

Normal values
- Normal values available have been derived for various field strengths, imaging sequences, post-processing approaches, age-, sex- and ethnicity groups (Additional file 1: Table 3ai.3), summarised in [16].
- There is moderate variability in normal ranges depending on the population studied and method of quantification.

- SCMR CT WG members recommend the use of normal values that correspond the mode of acquisition and postprocessing (as per SCMR recommendations for acquisition and postprocessing (1,2).

Qualification and utilisation
- Diagnostic interpretation and clinical decision making underlying practice guidelines is based on evidence derived with echocardiography. The cut-off values (most notably for LV ejection fraction) have been adopted by other imaging modalities, including CMR. The original evidence base by transthoracic echocardiography has been revalidated and expanded upon by CMR (Additional file 1: Table 3ai.4).
- Abnormal changes in cardiac volumes, function and LV mass indicate the presence of disease and relate to worse outcome. LV volumes and function by echocardiography have been described as the strongest predictor of survival in heart failure (HF) [17–20]. Recent data with CMR LGE (Additional file 2: Table 3b-i.4) and T1-mapping indices (Additional file 3: Table 3c-i.6) show consistently better prognostic predictive value in HF and non-ischemic cardiomyopathy (NICM).

ii. Regional wall motion and deformation
Myocardial strain imaging enables time-resolved quantification of myocardial contraction and relaxation, which is less influenced by the ventricular pressure/volume loading conditions. Characterisation of these events in various conditions, with aim to better understanding of tissue architecture and the underlying efficiency of deformation, remains an active research domain. Once a complex and often time-consuming acquisition and post-processing, strain imaging with CMR is now made possible using standard cine imaging. Owing to the issues with the reproducibility and an overall lack of incremental diagnostic and prognostic data, the value of strain imaging in clinical use remains investigational.

Acquisition
- Cine imaging (feature tracking)
- Tagging (spatial modulation of magnetization-SPAMM, complementary –SPAMM (CSPAMM) [21], harmonic phase image analysis [22])
- Displacement ENcoding with Stimulated Echoes (DENSE) [23]
- Strain encoding imaging (SENC) [24]

Post-processing
- Visual segmental analysis [2]
- Regional wall motion score

○ Deformation/strain analysis (tagging, feature tracking [25])
○ Dyssynchrony [26]

Results may be presented either segmental (provided for 17 segments as per AHA/ACC) or global (deformation components: longitudinal, radial, circumferential, torsion) values.

Validation

- Validation in phantoms and animals
  ○ Tagging is referred to as the reference standard for strain imaging [27] [28, 29](Additional file 1: Table 3ii.1)
  ○ DENSE [30]
- Comparative studies to tagging:
  ○ DENSE can provide greater reliability and resolution of segmental analysis [30]
  ○ Feature tracking [25]
- Comparative studies to echocardiography:
  ○ Strain by DENSE, tagging, feature tracking (reviewed in [31, 32])
  ○ Dyssynchrony by feature tracking [33]

Precision

- Wall motion based on visual assessment of each segment, observer dependent on training and experience [34] (Additional file 1: Table 3ii.2.)
- Reproducibility may be improved with automated processing [27]
- Some studies demonstrated superior precision of tagging [35], however, the endocardial border may be obscured by a tag line prohibiting adequate assessment of wall thickening
- The best spatial resolution for strain imaging is currently given by DENSE [36]. Fast processing methods are available for analysis of strain and displacement [37].
- Feature-tracking reproducibility remains problematic, especially for radial strain [38, 39].
  ○ Circumferential strain preforms best, if averaged over the whole slice. Regional estimates are more variable (reviewed in).
  ○ Considerable inter-vendor variability of outputs [39, 40]
- Benchmarking datasets available [41].

Normal values

- Normal values available for global strain components (Additional file 1: Table 3ii.3).
- Several studies available for segmental values [42–44], of note, regional values vary significantly in a given heart complicating the definition of normal values and cut-offs.

- One study reported normal values for strain according to segment, age, sex and ethnicity [27]

Qualification/utilisation

Strain imaging with CMR remains an exploratory research domain, due to complex and often time-consuming post-processing. Outcome data suggest utility in addition to standard measures of care in clinical management. (Additional file 1: Table 3ii.5)

1. Regional wall motion score is used as a single value to describe wall motion abnormalities or changes during stress testing [45];
2. Outcome data for deformation analysis of high dose dobutamine stress testing with SENC [46];
3. Global longitudinal strain is a better predictor of outcome in DCM than volumes or ejection fraction [47];
4. Intervendor variability of outputs for feature tracking implies that various algorithms may not convey equivalent information.

Development directions

1. Standardisation of acquisition and post-processing approaches
2. Development of robust normal values for vendor-specific acquisition/post-processing
3. Establishment of characteristic disease-specific or pathophysiology specific signatures of deformation abnormalities (diagnostic and prognostic relevance)
4. Determination of reversibility of parameters/signatures with treatment
5. Utility in guiding treatment through clinical trials.

iii. Diastolic function

Assessment of diastolic relaxation is an indirect approach to myocardial tissue characterisation and can be done by CMR by employing analogous approaches to those used in echocardiography. Increased myocardial stiffness commonly coincides with the states of increased LV wall thickness, either due to global pathological myocardial processes, such as accumulation of myocardial fibrosis or amyloid, or due to regional myocardial injury, such as ischaemic scar. Because CMR provides means of direct tissue characterisation, by LGE and T1 mapping, assessment of diastolic function by CMR is not commonly used.

Acquisition

- Time resolved curve of left ventricular diastolic filling from cine SAX stack [48, 49]. As in echocardiography, these parameters are dependent on loading conditions.
- 2- and 4-chamber cine views for measurement of left atrial (LA) volume
- Phase-contrast gradient echo sequence acquisitions:

- ○ Through-plane flow measurement across mitral valve, pulmonary venous inflow (velocity encoding 130 cm/sec)
  - ○ Basal SAX slice measurement of mitral flow and annulus velocities (velocity encoding < 30 cm/sec)
- Tagging [50]

Post-processing
- Transmitral E and A waves
- Pulmonary venous inflow S, D and A waves
- Mitral annulus velocity e'
- LA size
- Peak early diastolic strain rate (PEDSR)

Validation
- Against PV loops [51]
- Comparative studies with echo [52–54]

Normal values
- Normal values available for early diastolic velocities

Development directions
1. Standardisation of acquisition and post-processing approaches
2. Development of robust normal values for vendor-specific acquisition/post-processing
3. Establishment of characteristic disease-specific or pathophysiology specific signatures of diastolic abnormalities (diagnostic and prognostic relevance)
4. Determination of reversibility of parameters/signatures with treatment
5. Utility in guiding treatment through clinical trials.

5. Tissue characterisation
i. Late gadolinium enhancement
LGE is a myocardial tissue characterization technique, which demonstrates regional myocardial tissue differences based on differential uptake/washout of gadolinium-based contrast agent (GBCA). LGE is optimally suited to visualize myocardial infarction and scar, as well as areas of regional scar/fibrosis in non-ischaemic cardiomyopathies, such as in hypertrophic and dilated cardiomyopathy, sarcoidosis or myocarditis. In acute myocardial infarction or myocarditis, LGE co-localises with areas of cell-necrosis or oedema. Conversely, LGE can also reveal unenhanced areas in the core of the contrast-enhanced regions, representing either microvascular obstruction (MVO) (a no-(re)flow phenomenon) or intramyocardial haemorrhage (IMH).

Acquisition
- Inversion recovery (IR) prepared T1 weighted gradient echo sequences with either individually adapted prepulse delay ('to achieve myocardial signal nulling') and/or inline Phase-Sensitive Inversion-Recovery (PSIR)-based reconstruction algorithm [1]
- Acquired as in full LV coverage in short axis and long axis views during mid-diastole
- ~ 10 min delay time from administration of GBCA [1]
- GBCAs lead to:
  - ○ shortening of T1 - > increased signal intensity in areas of intense GBCA accumulation compared to areas with quick wash-out, such as normal myocardium;
  - ○ differential distribution between myocardial regions with intact myocardial cells (membranes) and expanded extracellular space due to necrosis, fibrosis or scar;
  - ○ in amyloidosis, there is commonly poor contrast difference between the blood and myocardium due to expansion of the extracellular volume throughout the myocardium, resulting in lower gradient in GBCA concentration between these two tissues, save for the bright endocardial border;
- Evidence of LGE is a marker of expanded extracellular space, most commonly seen due to necrotic myocardium or scar tissue
- Methods to assess microvascular obstruction (MVO) (and IMH) include [55–57]:
  - ○ first pass perfusion imaging,
  - ○ early IR-TFE imaging (app. 1 min, no 'nulling', long prepulse delay > 400 msec)
  - ○ LGE (app. 10–20 min)
  - ○ native T1
  - ○ Contrast-enhanced cine-bSSFP
  - ○ First pass and early hypoenhancement less strongly related to remodelling and clinical outcomes than LGE
- Alternative ways to IMH imaging by T2* (see section Mapping) [58].

Post-processing
- Visual assessment reporting on the presence, type (ischemic/non-ischemic), location, and transmurality [2]
- Quantitative assessment (i.e. LGE extent) can be based on several approaches:
  - ○ Manual approach (i.e. visual delineation)
  - ○ full width half maximum (FHWM)
  - ○ The "n"-SD approach (standard deviations, SD): 2SD (for nonischaemic scar)/5SD of the noise (for infarction) above the signal intensity of normal myocardium [2].
  - ○ LGE extent is reported as % of LV mass

- MVO can be measured manually or by SD-thresholds. The strong contrast between scar and MVO results in a highly reproducible delineation [59].

Validation

- Excellent validation of LGE imaging for the presence, extent and transmurality of LGE against reference standard for ischemic scar and non-ischemic fibrosis (animal experiments, human endomyocardial biopsies (EMB), explanted hearts) (Additional file 2: Tables 3b-i.1 and 3b-i.2)
  - In acute myocardial infarction, LGE overestimates infarct size (see T2 imaging section) reviewed in [60].
  - CMR favourably compares to alternative techniques (SPECT, PET) due to its higher sensitivity and spatial resolution to resolve infarct transmurality (based on better spatial resolution) (Additional file 2: Table 3b-i.3)

Precision

- Large body of evidence on interstudy, inter- and intraobserver variability in acute and chronic ischemic scar as well as in NICMs (Additional file 2: Table 3b-i.2)
- No comparison of precision to SPECT/PET due to the poor interstudy reproducibility of the later methods
- No benchmarking datasets available

Normal values

- Normal reference defined as absence of LGE
- Interpretation by pattern (ischemic, non-ischemic, patchy, diffuse), localization (typical coronary artery territory, mid-wall, epicardial, septal, lateral), transmurality (% of wall thickness).

Qualification and utilisation (Additional file 2: Table 3b-i.4)

- Excellent diagnostic tool for the determination of chronic myocardial infarction and regional fibrosis in cardiomyopathies.
- Stronger predictor of outcome than LVejection fraction (EF) and LV volumes in chronic stable disease (HF, chronic CAD)
- Stronger predictor of outcome than LV-EF and LV volumes in acute myocardial infarction
- Stronger predictor of malignant ventricular arrhythmia, sudden death and lower likelihood of improvement with medical therapy in various patient groups with cardiomyopathy
- LGE transmurality able to inform on reversibility of underlying regional wall motion abnormality

- MVO and IMH - predictors of poor outcome, but uncertainty whether these are independent [61] of infarct size or interrelated [62] (IMH occurs in a subset of MVO)

Development directions

- Standardization of acquisition methods and nulling approaches to achieve similar relative signal-to-noise ratios of fibrotic tissue versus normal myocardium (currently dependent on contrast agent type, dose and time after injection, field strength, type of sequence and other variables including the underlying injury itself).
- Improved definition of transmurality and segmental allocation for visual interpretation
- Standardization of quantification methods for LGE. Studies used the FWHM and the SD-based methods, however, this remains suboptimally standardized in terms of
  - To determine the cut-off value, the method with the best prognostic/ diagnostic value.
  - The different data acquisition techniques and post-processing algorithms may require different post-processing approaches.

ii. T2 weighted imaging

Myocardial tissue characterization using electrocardiogram (ECG)-triggered T2 weighted (T2W) sequences is used to demonstrate the regional differences in myocardial water content. T2W imaging is optimally suited to visualize regional oedema, such as in acute myocardial infarction, supporting assessment of area at risk (AAR)/ myocardial salvage index (MSI). It was also applied in myocarditis imaging, as a part of Lake-Louise Criteria (LLC). Owing to lengthy and artefact-prone acquisitions, T2W imaging is less fit for use in everyday clinical practice, and increasingly replaced by the modern quantifiable acquisition alternatives, T1 and T2-mapping.

Acquisition

Several sequences/approaches are available for T2W cardiac imaging [1]:

- T2W black-blood turbo spin echo (T2W-TSE)
- T2W short tau inversion recovery (STIR),
- T2-prepared SSFP
- Emerging new approach for AAR using contrast-enhanced SSFP (based on T2 and T1 contrast) for AAR assessment based on the acquisition of the cine LV stack [63]

- Technical limitations of T2W CMR pulse sequences are susceptible to various influences causing some limitations as endpoints and in clinical practice:

○ long acquisition time over 2 heart beats result in long breath-holds and artefacts due to cardiorespiratory motion;

○ variations in phase array coil sensitivity

○ high signal from slow moving blood (e.g. at the subendocardium and in the ventricular apex)

○ low contrast-noise ratio in differentiating oedematous vs. normal tissue

Post-processing

- T2W imaging of AAR/myocardial salvage ((Additional file 4: Tables 3b-ii.1–2):
  ○ Myocardial salvage is calculated by subtraction of percent infarct size (by LGE) from percent AAR (by T2W imaging) [64, 65].
  ○ MSI is calculated by dividing the salvage area by the AAR.
  ○ Post processing is subjective (based on 'n'-SD threshold approaches or visual delineation)
  ○ Optimal imaging time for AAR assessment is ideally 4–7 days after acute MI [62].
- T2W imaging in myocarditis (LLC) [66]:
  ○ Visually determined areas of hyperintensity in T2W images
  ○ Global oedema ratio: semi-quantitative analysis by normalizing the signal intensity of the myocardium to that of skeletal muscle: values of more than 1.9 indicate myocarditis

Validation

- Hyperintense signal on T2W CMR has been shown to indicate increased myocardial water content, whereas hypointense signal within the hyperintense injured zone indicates IMH (Additional file 4: Table 3b-ii.1)
- Phantom and Tissue studies
  ○ Proton transverse (T2) relaxation times reflect tissue hydration.
  ○ Alterations in T2 signal enable visualisation of regional myocardial oedema as area of hyperintense signal
- Animal models
  ○ The ischemic AAR consists of oedema and is typically greater than infarct size - > T2W imaging represents a non-invasive approach to AAR estimation.
  ○ T2W imaging enables retrospective determination of the ischaemic area-at-risk
  ○ Comparison of contrast-enhanced bSSFP with myocardial perfusion SPECT
- Human studies
  ○ Dynamic changes of AAR after acute myocardial infarction [65, 67, 68]
  ○ Comparison of T2W AAR by CMR with myocardial perfusion SPECT

○ Comparison of contrast enhanced bSSFP with myocardial perfusion SPECT [63]

○ LLC vs. EMB-criteria for myocarditis (Additional file 4: Table 3b-ii.1)

Precision

- Available data on reproducibility of T2W imaging for AAR [69, 70]
- Comparison of T2W vs. T2 mapping for AAR reveals T2 mapping to be more reproducible [71];
- Comparison of seven post-processing approaches for quantifying oedema in T2W imaging in acute MI (2 SD, 3 SD, 5 SD, Otsu, FWHM, manual threshold, and manual contouring) revealed that manual contouring provided the lowest inter, intraobserver, and interstudy variability for both infarct size and oedema quantification [72].
- The FWHM method for infarct size quantification and the Otsu method for myocardial oedema quantification are acceptable alternatives [72].
- No data available for contrast-enhanced bSSFP
- No data available for oedema ratio in myocarditis

Normal values

- Normal reference = absence of hyperintense signal (poor negative predictive value)
- In myocarditis: semiquantitative 'oedema ratio' of < 1.9 (SI of myocardium/SI of skeletal muscle) [66]

Qualification and utilization

○ Detection of myocardial damage in patients with acute coronary syndrome (ACS) [73]

○ Determination of salvaged myocardium in STEMI patients, prediction of higher revascularisation rate and adverse prognosis (Additional file 4: Table 3b-ii.4).

○ Randomised controlled trials using T2W and contrast-enhanced bSSFP AAR as an endpoint (ischaemic preconditioning [74, 75].

○ T2-oedema ratio variable sensitivity across inflammatory cardiomyopathies with moderate positive and poor negative predictive value (Additional file 4: Table 3b-ii.3)

○ No prognostic or therapeutic studies

Development directions

- Native T2 mapping methods enable quantification of T2 relaxation times and are less susceptible to artefacts (see chapter on T2 mapping)
- The utility of T2W-imaging in excluding ACS in the emergency room has become less prominent since the advent of high-sensitivity troponin assays.

6. Quantitative tissue characterisation

i. T1 mapping

T1 mapping is a quantitative tissue characterization technique, which allows quantifying the rate of longitudinal relaxation of myocardial tissue (and blood). The resulting measurements come as an absolute number (time, ms), which is sequence-specific, requiring standardization of acquisition and calibration of values in health and disease.

Acquisition

Sequences allowing acquisition of a series of images (using increasing time delays) during the evolution of the longitudinal relaxation:

- Acquisition in mid-diastole (owing to a lengthy image acquisition time, systolic acquisition window less robust)
- Magnetisation preparation by inversion (180°) or saturation (90°) prepulses
- Several imaging schemes with differences in number of images, pauses for magnetization recovery (which can be defined as either beats or seconds), flip angles, use of adiabatic prepulses, acceleration techniques (half-scan, partial Fourier)
  - resulting in differences in T1 accuracy (with consequences for precision and diagnostic accuracy, see below).
- Native (without GBCA) and post-contrast T1 mapping (typically ~ 10–15 min after administration of GBCA, dose and type of GBCA not standardized)
- Single (midventricular) short axis slice (– > diffuse myocardial disease) or three short axis slices (apical, midventricular, basal) (– > regional myocardial disease)
- Heart-rate dependency:
  - for myocardial T1 with most sequences not relevant within physiological heart rates < 80 bpm;
  - less important for post-contrast images, more relevant for long T1 values such as native blood, or in very severe myocardial disease (amyloidosis, severe oedema), as more time needed for full relaxation;
  - every other beat acquisition (2RR intervals) may be used in tachycardia
- Extracellular volume fraction (ECV) calculation based on pre- and postcontrast T1 mapping acquisitions and blood values which requires standardization and heart rate correction for each component (unclear: identical

sequences/ different schemes for pre/postcontrast acquisitions)

Post-processing

- Pixel-wise image reconstruction and exponential curve-fitting of signal intensity values (3-parameter fitting model):
  - magnitude image detection: $SMAG(t) = abs(A - B \exp.(-t/T1^*))$
  - phase sensitive inversion recovery (PSIR) detection : $SPSIR(t) = A - B \exp.(-t/T1^*)$.
- T1 value equates with the time at 63% recovery of longitudinal magnetisation
- Post-processing affected by the regional variation due to variable sensitivity of phase array coils and artefacts in the lateral wall (septal region of interest (ROI) more precise compared to SAX ROI, segmental values difficult to normalise)
- Myocardial ROI placement:
  - diffuse (global) myocardial involvement:
    - septal ROI [76] or SAX ROI [77, 78]
    - excluding areas of LGE
    - conservatively within the myocardium [76]
  - regional myocardial T1 values:
    - Segmental ROI placement [79]:
    - Significant regional differences in T1 values - > difficulty in normalising segmental T1 values
    - No significant differences between septal values for basal and midventricular slice, however considerable overestimation in apical slice (due to partial volume)
- Blood ROI placed in the centre of the blood pool using same acquisition as above, avoiding papillary muscles
- Post-contrast T1 blood: less in-flow effect compared to native T1
- T1 indices (Additional file 3: Table 3c-i.1):
  - direct measurements: native T1, post-contrast T1
  - calculated indices based on pre- and post-contrast T1 mapping acquisitions:
    - lambda (partition coefficient of contrast agent distribution between blood and myocardium) = (R1myocardiumnative-R1myocardiumpost-contrast)/ (R1bloodnative- R1bloodpost-contrast), where R1 = 1/T1
    - ECV is partition coefficient lambda, which relates to the extracellular space only, by accounting for intracellular space of blood by haematocrit (requires contemporaneous blood sampling): =(1-Ht)x lambda
    - synthetic ECV calculation

- derived from a relationship between haematocrit and longitudinal relaxation rate of blood (R2 = 0.51)
  - derived for selected sequences and a single vendor only [80, 81]

Validation

- Phantom sequence characterisation (T1 accuracy and precision)
- Histological correlation with collagen volume fraction (Additional file 3: Table 3c-i.2)
  - Correlations vary between reports
  - Differences in staining techniques, inclusion/exclusion of areas of LGE
  - Differences in sequence parameters, type/dose/timing of GBCA, different sequences used in pre/postcontrast acquisitions, post-processing (ROI placement)
- Several components of the measured values do not occur in phantoms, such as magnetisation transfer, water-exchange, T2 sensitivity, inflow effects, making a full validation in phantoms or ex-vivo impossible

Precision

- Evidence on interstudy, inter- and intraobserver variability (Additional file 3: Table 3c-i.3)
- No benchmarking datasets available as variability seems mainly dependent on data acquisition

Normal values

- Some sequences have established normal values (Additional file 3: Table 3c-i.4). Of note, every specific implementation may yield slightly different values and requires standardization.

Qualification and utilisation

Abnormal (raised) myocardial T1 values indicate the presence of diseased myocardium and relate to worse outcome:

- Disease models: myocarditis, non-ischaemic dilated cardiomyopathy, amyloidosis, ischaemic cardiomyopathy, hypertrophic cardiomyopathy (Additional file 3: Table 3c-i.5)
- Outcome data (Additional file 3: Table 3c-i.6): T1 values are stronger predictor of outcome than LV function, volumes and LGE:
  - Amyloidosis
  - Non-ischaemic dilated cardiomyopathy
  - Mixed patient cohorts

Development directions

- Sequence and vendor specific standardization of acquisition, normal values and calibration of values in health and disease

- Outcome data
- Data on guiding management
- Pre- and post-contrast T1 mapping acquisitions
  - unclear whether identical sequences or different schemes for pre/post-contrast acquisitions amount to a justifiable counterpart of pre/post-contrast acquisition, but rather a mix of poorly related diagnostic tests.

ii. T2 mapping

T2 mapping is a quantitative tissue characterization method mainly reflecting the water content of the myocardium. It is based on a series of images with different time delays acquired during the diastolic standstill to map the T2 magnetization decay. Increasing evidence base for T2 mapping supports its utility in detection of myocardial inflammation and oedema, in myocarditis and in assessment of acute myocardial infarction (AMI). Myocardial T2 values were shown to decrease with anti-inflammatory treatment.

Acquisition

- Sequences acquiring separate images during the evolution of the transverse relaxation in diastolic standstill
- T2 prepared spin echo sequences with several different schemes with differences in number of image acquisitions, flip angles, accelerating techniques, single-shot vs. multiecho
  - T2-prepared bSSFP sequence
  - T2-hybrid gradient echo and spin echo (GraSE) sequence
- Native acquisition (no contrast agent)
- Single (midventricular) short axis slice (– > diffuse myocardial disease) or three short axis slices (apical, midventricular, basal) (– > regional myocardial disease)
- No regional variation due to variable sensitivity of phase array coil

Post-processing

- Pixel-wise image reconstruction and exponential curve fitting
- T2 value equates with the time at 63% decay of transverse magnetisation, direct myocardial measurement
- ROI placement:
  - Myocardial septal ROI or SAX ROI (in case of diffuse myocardial disease)
  - Segmental ROI placement (in case regional T2 values are desired)

- No significant difference in segmental values for basal and midventricular slice, overestimation in apical slice (partial volume)

Validation
- Phantom sequence characterisation (T2 accuracy and precision)
- Histological validation (Additional file 5: Table 3c-ii.1).
- in animal models
  - AAR
  - AMI reperfused and non-reperfused
    - Detection of AAR (comparison with T2W/LGE approach as reference standard)
- Model diseases: AMI, myocarditis, transplant rejection
- Validation of water component difficult in animals and biopsies
- Has been shown to be superior to T2W imaging and Lake-Louise Criteria for the diagnosis of acute myocarditis (Additional file 5: Table 3c-ii.2)

Precision
- Interstudy, inter- and intraobserver variability (Additional file 5: Table 3c-ii.3)
- No benchmarking datasets available as variability seems mainly due to data acquisition

Normal values
- Several sequences have established normal values (Additional file 5: Table 3c-ii.4)

Qualification and utilisation
- T2 mapping useful in detecting myocardial oedema and inflammation (Additional file 5: Table 3c-ii.5)
  - Acute myocardial infarction
  - Myocarditis, inflammatory cardiomyopathies, including cardiac involvement in systemic inflammatory diseases, tako-tsubo cardiomyopathy
  - Early detection of ongoing inflammation with the possibility of reversal of myocardial damage using anti-inflammatory intervention may be feasible.
  - Added value to T1 mapping in inflammatory conditions, by informing on active inflammation and reversal upon anti-inflammatory intervention [82–84]

iii. T2* mapping

T2* mapping is a quantitative test for the assessment of myocardial iron load in patients with thalassemia. T2* mapping is also employed for visualisation of IMH, such as during or after an acute ischaemic event.

Acquisition
- As per SCMR protocols:
  - single breath-hold multiecho T2* gradient echo sequences (black-blood prepulse) [1]
  - a single midventricular SAX slice - > septal T2*measurement
  - 3 short axis slices - > global T2* measurement
- Each sequence yields sequence specific "absolute" T2* values (in ms)
- Each sequence requires standardisation (validation, normal values, clinically relevant cut-off values) prior to clinical use
- Only 1.5 T and 3 T datasets are validated for measurement of cardiac iron content [85, 86];

Post-processing
- As per SCMR standardised image interpretation and post-processing [2]
- T2* values = the time delay taken for decay of the myocardial signal by 63%
- ROI placement:
  - Myocardial septal ROI in midventricular slice encompassing both epicardial and endocardial borders, to prevent the epicardium-endocardium heterogeneity of iron deposition (informs on global myocardial iron content)
  - Segmental ROI placement (– > regional T2* values)
  - Complete SAX coverage in basal, midventricular and apical slice generates a global T2* value, however, this is less frequently used.
- Significant differences in segmental values reported. Regional variation most likely due to variable sensitivity of phase array coils to different regions.

Validation
- Validation against myocardial and liver iron content (Additional file 6: Table 3c-iii.1 and 2)
  - Ex vivo histological validation - > good correlation of T2* measurements versus chemically assayed iron
  - Biopsy not useful as reference standard

○ Therapy guidance by T2* imaging is superior to other tests – as such T2* in thalassemia can be regarded as the clinical reference standard

Precision
- Evidence on interscanner, intercenter, interstudy, inter- and intraobserver variability (Additional file 6: Table 3c-iii.3)

Normal values
- Iron loading:
  ○ Normal values for 1.5 T (Additional file 6: Table 3c-iii.4)
  ○ Established clinically relevant cut-offs of significant myocardial iron loading (septal ROI):
    - T2* < 20 ms: clinically relevant myocardial iron loading
    - T2* < 10 ms: severe myocardial iron loading
- IMH - intramyocardial hemorrhage
  ○ A myocardial region of interest with a T2* < 20 ms is taken to represent haemorrhage
  ○ T2* (< 20 ms) is highly discriminative of haemorrhagic transformation within the infarct zone vs. infarct zone without haemorrhage or the remote zone

Qualification and utilisation
- T2* useful in detecting relevant cardiac iron overload involvement in thalassemia major – > at T2* < 20 msec
- In cardiac iron loading T2* correlates closely with
  ○ negative cardiac remodelling (ejection fraction, end-diastolic volume (EDV)) and diastolic dysfunction (Additional file 6: Table 3c-iii.2)
  ○ clinical events (HF, arrhythmia) and
  ○ response to iron-depletion treatment (Additional file 6: Tables 3c-iii.5 and 6)
- Comparison with historical data indicate improve survival of patients at risk of iron overload due to cardiac T2* mapping guided iron-depletion therapy [87]
- Interdisciplinary consensus statements recommend surveillance of patients at risk of cardiac iron overload using cardiac T2* mapping [88]
- Serial changes in myocardial oedema and haemorrhage in ischaemic and remote zone after reperfusion [62]
- IMH detection by T2* core is independently associated with adverse LV remodelling, major adverse cardiac events and mortality [89]

7. Stress myocardial perfusion with CMR

Myocardial perfusion CMR testing under the effect of pharmacological agents (myocardial stress-perfusion) is used to demonstrate regional reduction in myocardial perfusion to assess the presence of hemodynamically significant coronary artery stenosis. Myocardial stress perfusion CMR imaging is a routinely used diagnostic test in patients presenting with symptoms and signs of stable angina. It is also used in patients with medium-to-high pretest likelihood of significant (flow-limiting) coronary artery disease (CAD), patients with known coronary artery stenosis to assess significance of specific lesion(s) and patients with previous revascularization or myocardial infarction. Myocardial stress perfusion CMR imaging can also demonstrate the presence of microvascular disease e.g. in patients with angina and normal coronary arteries. In this case, the imaging abnormality during stress testing is typically hypoperfusion of the sub-endocardium with a circumferential distribution. Myocardial stress perfusion CMR imaging may be useful to demonstrate potential CAD aetiology in patients with HF with or without reduced LV ejection fraction. Quantitative perfusion imaging is increasingly becoming available.

Acquisition
- Acquisition as per SCMR Standardized Protocols [1]
  ○ Dynamic acquisition during the passage of the contrast agent bolus (dose 0.05–0.1 mmol/kg body weight) through the left ventricular cavity and the myocardium;
  ○ First pass acquisition during pharmacological stress;
  ○ Repeat pass acquisition at rest (may be omitted for qualitative assessment, if LGE is available to determine infarction)
  ○ 3 short axis slices (basal, midventricular and apical) every heart beat for a minimum of 40–50 heart beats→ a minimum of 40–50 dynamic measurements);
  ○ 3D whole heart acquisition methods available, currently no demonstrated diagnostic advantage over 2D 3-SAX slice acquisition [90];
- Sequences: various sequences available based on saturation prepulse for preparation of magnetization and acquisition of data with either:
  ○ spoiled fast gradient echo (GrE);
  ○ bSSFP pulse sequences;
  ○ typically combined with acceleration techniques:
    - echo planar imaging (GrE-EPI);
    - spatial undersampling (e.g. sensitivity encoding (SENSE)

- generalized autocalibrating partially parallel acquisitions (GRAPPA),
- spatio-temporal undersampling (e.g. k-t Broad Linear Speed up Technique, k-t BLAST or k-t SENSE);
  - differing in the acquired spatial (3x3x8 mm to 1.3 × 1.3x8mm) resolution.
- Diagnostically relevant is the stress acquisition.
- The rest acquisition is used to:
  - discern possible artefacts
  - to support calculation of parameters based on the change of stress and rest perfusion (e.g. myocardial perfusion reserve index - MPRI or myocardial blood flow – MBF - reserve).
- Pharmacological stress is the standard approach (adenosine, regadenosone, dobutamine); exercise stress has shown feasibility in research settings.

Post-processing/interpretation
- as per SCMR Standardized Postprocessing [2]
  - Visual interpretation is the standard clinical approach:
  - Hypoperfusion is defined as segmentally reduced contrast agent uptake at peak stress persisting for 5 consecutive heart beats
    - not present at rest,
    - outside the enhanced myocardium on LGE images.
  - several diagnostic standards of test positivity proposed demonstrating a reduced increase of flow or reduced peak flow in areas subtended by vessels with significant coronary stenosis (see below)
- The benefits of quantitative and semi-quantitative over qualitative interpretation remain at present investigational. Quantitative and semi-quantitative evaluation require:
  - stress and rest acquisition to calculate perfusion reserve or perfusion reserve indices; peak perfusion can be determined from stress images only
  - dual bolus, dual contrast sequences or other algorithms to correct for the non-linearity of signal intensity and contrast agent at higher doses
  - correction for baseline signal differences
  - efficient motion correction
  - a myocardial perfusion reserve index (MPRI) can be calculated from various parameters, usually using the relative upslope between rest and stress (corrected for changes of upslope of the contrast bolus in the left ventricle)

- full quantification can be achieved with various mathematical algorithms (e.g. Fermi deconvolution, Patlak plot).

Validation
- Excellent validation of technique (Additional file 7: Table 3d.1 and 2):
  - Flow in phantoms and microspheres in animals;
  - Comparative effectiveness diagnostic studies and meta-analyses studies of CMR to PET, SPECT, invasive coronary angiography and invasive flow measurements (fractional flow reserve – FFR; Additional file 7: Table 3d.1). Favorable results in comparison to SPECT due to higher spatial resolution. [91, 92]
  - Outcome studies of stress myocardial perfusion CMR imaging validating predictive association of positive and negative outcome (Additional file 7: Table 3d.3), similar results to SPECT.
  - Quantitative perfusion imaging: many approaches require more validation, especially as large outcome studies have been performed with visual analysis

Precision

- Limited evidence on interstudy, inter- and intraobserver reproducibility due to need of stress and contrast injection (Additional file 7: Table 3d.2)

Normal values
- Limited data on normal values due to lack of standardization of image acquisition and post-processing
- Visual assessment: several diagnostic standards on the interpretation of the presence/severity/ prognostic relevance of myocardial hypoperfusion based on number of affected segments:
  - ESC guidelines on stable CAD (16 segment ACC/AHA segmentation) [93]:
    - ≤2/16 segments indicate a good prognosis with optimal medical therapy (OMT) (negative test)
    - ≥ 3/16 segments defined as prognostically relevant (warrants attempt to revascularize on prognostic grounds (positive test)
  - Subsegmentation into 32 segments (with endo- and epicardial division):
    - ≤ 3/32 segments indicate a good prognosis with OMT
    - ≥4/32 segments defined as prognostically relevant [94]
  - MR-INFORM: prognostically relevant ischaemia [95]:

- Either transmural hypoperfusion defect or perfusion defect affecting 2 slices or > 60% in basal and midventricular slice, > 90% in apical slice.
- (Semi-) quantitative assessment of MBF, MPR or MPRI: experimental data available for different field strengths

Qualification and utilisation
- Data from prospective observational studies using stress myocardial perfusion CMR have shown significant predictive association for the presence/severity of myocardial ischemia with outcome (Additional file 7: Table 3d.3):
  ○ Effective cardiac risk reclassification in patients with known or suspected stable CAD [96].
  ○ Excellent negative predictive value - > low event rate in patients with a negative test
  ○ Excellent positive predictive value substantiating the role for revascularisation following positive test to improve prognosis
  ○ Improvement of MPR after percutaneous coronary intervention (PCI)

Development directions
- Standardization of post processing methods (semi quantitative and quantitative) to allow definition of normal values, effect sizes and improvement of reproducibility. Different post processing methods may apply for different data acquisition techniques.
- Improvement of spatial resolution / coverage based on faster acquisition techniques (e.g. compressed sensing)
- Quantitative perfusion imaging is increasingly becoming available. At this stage the various approaches require more validation, especially as large outcome studies have been performed with visual analysis.

8. Vascular endpoints
CMR allows a comprehensive assessment structure and function of the great vessels by anatomical assessment of vessels dimensions and cross-sectional areas, functional assessment of the vessel wall (aortic strain and distensibility, and central (aortic) pulse wave velocity (PWV)). Tissue characterisation by T1-, T2- and proton density-weighted imaging and, more recently, by T2 mapping allows characterization of tissue composition.

Acquisition
Acquisition as per SCMR standardised protocols
- Anatomy and dimensions:
  ○ cardiac triggered-contrast enhanced CMR angiography

  ○ free-breathing 3D balanced acquisition.
- Wall thickness and wall volume by black blood CMR
- Distensibility and strain: balanced (cine) image acquisitions orthogonal to the vessel of interest;
- PWV: measurement of pulse wave travel time/path between ascending and descending aorta
  ○ 'through plane' flow acquisitions in ascending or descending aorta and an anatomical image of thoracic aorta.
  ○ 'inplane' velocity acquisition of thoracic aortic candy-cane
- Wall tissue characterisation by:
  ○ T2 weighted sequences
  ○ T1 inversion recovery GRE sequences (vessel wall gadolinium enhancement)

Post-processing
- Inner-vessel diameters, cross-sectional areas
- PWV: travelled path divided by time delay.
  ○ Foot-to-foot
  ○ Upslope measurements
- Tissue characterisation
  ○ Visual assessment
  ○ Contrast-to-noise (CNR) measurements

Validation

- Comparative studies for aortic PWV and distensibility with alternative techniques, including invasive and tonometric PWV measurements (Additional file 8: Table 3e.1)
- T2 mapping vs. histology of carotid specimens showing accurate quantification of plaque lipid content and the different plaque composition despite similar grade of stenosis (Additional file 8: Table 3e.1).

Precision
- Limited evidence on interstudy reproducibility of anatomical and tissue measurements
- Excellent evidence for PWV: measurements highly reproducible

Normal values
- CMR data from large healthy populations are available for different anatomical and functional measurements adjusted by age, sex and body mass index (BMI) (Additional file 8: Table 3e2).

Qualification and utilisation
- Guiding management in aortic dilatation and aortic valve replacement (Additional file 8: Table 3e2)

- Aortic wall imaging and PWV serve robust biomarkers of cardiovascular risk

Development directions

- Functional assessment of reactive ischemia (or oximetry after cuff induced limb ischaemia) or exercise-induced blood flow in peripheral artery disease [97, 98]

Conclusion

Not applicable.

Abbreviations

AAR: area at risk; ACS: Acute coronary syndrome; AHA/ACC: American Heart Association/American College of Cardiology; BMI: Body-mass index; CAD: Coronary artery disease; Cardiac CT: Computed tomography; CNR: Contrast-noise-ratio; C-SPAMM: Complementary- spatial modulation of magnetization; CT: Clinical trials; CVD: Cardiovascular disease; DCM: Dilated cardiomyopathy; DENSE: Displacement ENcoding with Stimulated Echoes; ECV: Extracellular volume fraction; EDV: End-diastolic volume; EMB: Endomyocardial biopsy; ESC: European Society of Cardiology; FFR: Fractional flow reserve; FWHM: Full width half maximum; GBCA: Gadolinium-based contrast agent; GRAPPA: Generalized auto-calibrating partially parallel acquisitions; GRaSE: T2-hybrid gradient echo and spin echo; GRE: Fast gradient recalled echo; HF: Heart failure; Ht: Haematocrit; IMH: Intramyocardial haemorrhage; IR: Inversion-recovery; IR-TFE: Inversion-recovery turbo field echo; LA: Left atrium; LGE: Late gadolinium enhancement; LLC: Lake Louise criteria; LV: Left ventricle/left ventricular; LV-EF: Left ventricle ejection fraction; MBF: Myocardial blood flow; MI: Myocardial infarction; MPR: Myocardial perfusion reserve; MPRI: Myocardial perfusion reserve index; MRI: Magnetic resonance imaging; MSI: Myocardial salvage index; MVO: Microvascular obstruction; NICM: Non-ischemic cardiomyopathy; OMT: Optimal medical therapy; PCI: Percutaneous coronary intervention; PEDSR: Peak early diastolic strain rate; PET: Positron emission tomography; PSIR: Phase-Sensitive Inversion-Recovery; PV: Pressure-volume; PWV: Pulse wave velocity; ROI: Region of interest; RV: Right ventricle/right ventricular; SAX: Short axis stack; SCMR: Society for Cardiovascular Magnetic Resonance; SD: Standard deviation; SENC: Strain encoding imaging; SENSE: Sensitivity encoding; SPAMM: Spatial modulation of magnetization; SPECT: Single photon emission computed tomography; SSFP: Steady-state free precession; STEMI: ST-elevation myocardial infarction; STIR: T2-weighted short tau inversion recovery; T2W: T2-weighted imaging; T2W-TSE: T2-weighted black-blood turbo spin echo; TRA: Transverse stack

Acknowledgements

Members of the SCMR Clinical Trial Writing Group are Colin Berry, David Bluemke, Jens Bremerich, Rene Botnar, Chiara Bucciarelli-Ducci, Robin P. Choudhury, Marc Dweck, Ingo Eitel, Vic Ferrari, Matthias Friedrich, John Greenwood, Rocio Hinojar, Greg Hundley, Christopher Kramer, Raymond Y. Kwong, Massimo Lombardi, Teresa Lopez Fernandez, Thomas Marwick, Eike Nagel, Jagat Narula, Stefan Neubauer, Amit Patel, Dudley Pennell, E. Steffen Petersen, Sven Plein, Sanjay Prasad, Valentina O. Puntmann, Frank Rademakers, Subha Raman, Hajime Sakuma, Javier Sanz, Jeannette Schulz-Menger, Orlando Simonetti, Andrew Swift, Andrew J. Taylor, T. Teixeira, Holger Thiele, Martin Ugander, Silvia Valbuena, Jos J. Westenberg and Alistair A. Young

Authors' contributions

All authors contributed to the generation of the present manuscript in line the recommendations of the International committee of medical journal editors. All authors read and approved the final manuscript.

Competing interests

The authors declare that they have no competing interests.

Author details

[1]Institute of Experimental and Translational Cardiovascular Imaging, Goethe University Hospital Frankfurt, Frankfurt, Germany. [2]Department of Cardiology, Goethe University Hospital Frankfurt, Frankfurt, Germany. [3]Department of Cardiology, University Hospital La Paz, Madrid, Germany. [4]Department of Cardiology, University Hospital Ramón y Cajal, Madrid, Spain. [5]William Harvey Research Institute, Queen Mary University of London, Barts and the London NIHR Biomedical Research Centre at Barts, London, UK. [6]Leeds Institute of Cardiovascular and Metabolic Medicine, University of Leeds, Leeds, UK. [7]Department of Medicine (Cardiology) and Radiology, Cardiovascular Imaging Center, University of Virginia Health System, Charlottesville, Virginia, USA. [8]Cardiovascular Division, Department of Medicine, Brigham and Womens' Hospital, Boston, Massachusetts, USA. [9]Department of Cardiovascular Sciences, University of Leicester, Leicester, UK. [10]the NIHR Leicester Cardiovascular Biomedical Centre, University Hospitals of Leicester NHS Trust, Glenfield Hospital, Leicester, UK. [11]British Heart Foundation Glasgow Cardiovascular Research Centre, University of Glasgow, Glasgow, UK. [12]West of Scotland Heart and Lung Centre, Golden Jubilee National Hospital, Clydebank, UK.

References

1. Kramer CM, Barkhausen J, Flamm SD, Kim RJ, Nagel E. Society for Cardiovascular Magnetic Resonance Board of Trustees Task Force on Standardized Protocols. Standardized cardiovascular magnetic resonance (CMR) protocols 2013 update. J Cardiovasc Magn Reson. 2013;15:91.
2. Schulz-Menger J, Bluemke DA, Bremerich J, Flamm SD, Fogel MA, Friedrich MG, et al. Standardized image interpretation and post processing in cardiovascular magnetic resonance: Society for Cardiovascular Magnetic Resonance (SCMR) board of trustees task force on standardized post processing. J Cardiovasc Magn Reson. 2013;1(15):35.
3. Biomarkers and surrogate endpoints: Preferred definitions and conceptual framework. Clinical Pharmacology & Therapeutics [Internet]. 2001;69:89–95. Available from: doi https://doi.org/10.1067/mcp.2001.113989
4. Puntmann VO, Gebker R, Duckett S, Mirelis J, Schnackenburg B, Graefe M, et al. Left ventricular chamber dimensions and wall thickness by cardiovascular magnetic resonance: comparison with transthoracic echocardiography. Eur Heart J Cardiovasc Imaging. 2013;14:240–6.
5. Alfakih K, Plein S, Bloomer T, Jones T, Ridgway J, Sivananthan M. Comparison of right ventricular volume measurements between axial and short axis orientation using steady-state free precession magnetic resonance imaging. J Magn Reson Imaging. 2003 Jul;18(1):25–32.
6. Lyen S, Mathias H, McAlindon E, Trickey A, Rodrigues J, Bucciarelli-Ducci C, et al. Optimising the imaging plane for right ventricular magnetic resonance volume analysis in adult patients referred for assessment of right ventricular structure and function. J Med Imaging Radiat Oncol. 2015;59:421–30.
7. Clarke CJ, Gurka MJ, Norton PT, Kramer CM, Hoyer AW. Assessment of the accuracy and reproducibility of RV volume measurements by CMR in congenital heart disease. JACC Cardiovasc Imaging. 2012;5:28–37.
8. Hundley WG1, Li HF, Hillis LD, Meshack BM, Lange RA, Willard JE, Landau C, Peshock RM. Quantitation of cardiac output with velocity-encoded, phase-difference magnetic resonance imaging. Am J Cardiol. 1995;75:1250–5.
9. Lin H-Y, Freed D, Lee TWR, Arora RC, Ali A, Almoustadi W, et al. Quantitative assessment of cardiac output and left ventricular function by noninvasive phase-contrast and cine MRI: Validation study with invasive pressure-volume loop analysis in a swine model. J Magn Reson Imaging. 2011;34:203–10.

10. AKINBOBOYE O, NICHOLS K, WANG Y, DIM U, REICHEK N. Accuracy of radionuclide ventriculography assessed by magnetic resonance imaging in patients with abnormal left ventricles. J Nuclear Cardiology. 2005;12:418–27.

11. Mistry N, Halvorsen S, Hoffmann P, Muller C, Bohmer E, Kjeldsen SE, et al. Assessment of left ventricular function with magnetic resonance imaging vs. echocardiography, contrast echocardiography, and single-photon emission computed tomography in patients with recent ST-elevation myocardial infarction. Eur J Echocardiogr. 2010;11:793 800.

12. Grothues F, Smith GC, Moon JCC, Bellenger NG, Collins P, Klein HU, et al. Comparison of interstudy reproducibility of cardiovascular magnetic resonance with two-dimensional echocardiography in normal subjects and in patients with heart failure or left ventricular hypertrophy. Am. J. Cardiol. 2002;90:29–34.

13. Hoffmann R, Barletta G, Bardeleben von S, Vanoverschelde J-L, Kasprzak J, Greis C, et al. Analysis of Left Ventricular Volumes and Function: A Multicenter Comparison of Cardiac Magnetic Resonance Imaging, Cine Ventriculography, and Unenhanced and Contrast-Enhanced Two-Dimensional and Three-Dimensional Echocardiography. J Am Soc Echocardiogr. 2014;27:292–301.

14. Sharma A, Einstein AJ, Vallakati A, Arbab-Zadeh A, Mukherjee D, Lichstein E. Meta-Analysis of Global Left Ventricular Function Comparing Multidetector Computed Tomography With Cardiac Magnetic Resonance Imaging. Am. J. Cardiol. 2014;113:731–8.

15. Suinesiaputra A, Bluemke DA, Cowan BR, Friedrich MG, Kramer CM, Kwong R, et al. Quantification of LV function and mass by cardiovascular magnetic resonance: multi-center variability and consensus contours. J Cardiovasc Magn Reson. 2015;17:63.

16. Kawel-Boehm N, Maceira A, Valsangiacomo-Buechel ER, Vogel-Claussen J, Turkbey EB, Williams R, et al. Normal values for cardiovascular magnetic resonance in adults and children. J Cardiovasc Magn Reson. 2015;17:29.

17. White HD, Norris RM, Brown MA, Brandt PW, Whitlock RM, Wild CJ. Left ventricular end-systolic volume as the major determinant of survival after recovery from myocardial infarction. Circulation. 1987;76:44–51.

18. Vasan RS, Larson MG, Benjamin EJ, Evans JC, Levy D. Left Ventricular Dilatation and the Risk of Congestive Heart Failure in People without Myocardial Infarction. N Engl J Med. 1997;336:1350–5.

19. Pfeffer MA, Braunwald E. Ventricular remodeling after myocardial infarction. Experimental observations and clinical implications. Circulation. 1990;81: 1161–72.

20. Lauer MS, Evans JC, Levy D. Prognostic implications of subclinical left ventricular dilatation and systolic dysfunction in men free of overt cardiovascular disease (the framingham heart study). Am. J. Cardiol. 1992;70:1180–4.

21. Fischer SE, McKinnon GC, Maier SE, Boesiger P. Improved myocardial tagging contrast. Magnetic Resonance in Medicine. 1993;30:191–200.

22. Osman NF, Kerwin WS, McVeigh ER, Prince JL. Cardiac motion tracking using CINE harmonic phase (HARP) magnetic resonance imaging. Magnetic Resonance in Medicine. 1999;42:1048–60.

23. Kim D, Gilson WD, Kramer CM, Epstein FH. Myocardial tissue tracking with two-dimensional cine displacement-encoded MR imaging: development and initial evaluation. Radiology. 2004;230:862–71.

24. Osman NF, Sampath S, Atalar E, Prince JL. Imaging longitudinal cardiac strain on short-axis images using strain-encoded MRI. Magnetic Resonance in Medicine. 2001;46:324–34.

25. Hor KN, Gottliebson WM, Carson C, Wash E, Cnota J, Fleck R, et al. Comparison of Magnetic Resonance Feature Tracking for Strain Calculation With Harmonic Phase Imaging Analysis. JACC Cardiovasc Imaging. 2010;3:144–51.

26. Lardo AC, Abraham TP, Kass DA. Magnetic Resonance Imaging Assessment of Ventricular Dyssynchrony. J Am Coll Cardiol. 2005;46:2223–8.

27. Claus P, Omar AMS, Pedrizzetti G, Sengupta PP, Nagel E. Tissue Tracking Technology for Assessing Cardiac Mechanics. JACC: Cardiovascular Imaging. 2015;8:1444–60.

28. Young AA, Axel L, Dougherty L, Bogen DK, Parenteau CS. Validation of tagging with MR imaging to estimate material deformation. Radiology. 1993;188:101–8.

29. Yeon SB, Reichek N, Tallant BA, Lima JAC, Calhoun LP, Clark NR, et al. Validation of in vivo myocardial strain measurement by magnetic resonance tagging with sonomicrometry. J. Am. Coll. Cardiol. 2001;38:555–61.

30. Young AA, Li B, Kirton RS, Cowan BR. Generalized spatiotemporal myocardial strain analysis for DENSE and SPAMM imaging. Magnetic Resonance in Medicine. 2011;67:1590–9.

31. Pedrizzetti G, Claus P, Kilner PJ, Nagel E. Principles of cardiovascular magnetic resonance feature tracking and echocardiographic speckle tracking for informed clinical use. J Cardiovasc Magn Reson. 2016;18:43.

32. Tee M, Noble JA, Bluemke DA. Imaging techniques for cardiac strain and deformation: comparison of echocardiography, cardiac magnetic resonance and cardiac computed tomography. Expert Rev Cardiovasc Ther. 2013;11:221–31.

33. Onishi T, Saha SK, Ludwig DR, Onishi T, Marek JJ, Cavalcante JOL, et al. Feature tracking measurement of dyssynchrony from cardiovascular magnetic resonance cine acquisitions: comparison with echocardiographic speckle tracking. J Cardiovasc Magn Reson. 2013;15:95.

34. Hoffmann R, von S B, Kasprzak JD, Borges AC, ten F C, Firschke C, et al. Analysis of Regional Left Ventricular Function by Cineventriculography, Cardiac Magnetic Resonance Imaging, and Unenhanced and Contrast-Enhanced Echocardiography. J Am Coll Cardiol. 2006;47:121–8.

35. Donekal S, Ambale-Venkatesh B, Berkowitz S, Wu CO, Choi E-Y, Fernandes V, et al. Inter-study reproducibility of cardiovascular magnetic resonance tagging. J Cardiovasc Magn Reson. 2013;15:37.

36. Kim D, Epstein FH, Gilson WD, Axel L. Increasing the signal-to-noise ratio in DENSE MRI by combining displacement-encoded echoes. Magnetic Resonance in Medicine. 2004;52:188–92.

37. Suever JD, Wehner GJ, Haggerty CM, Jing L, Hamlet SM, Binkley CM, et al. Simplified post processing of cine DENSE cardiovascular magnetic resonance for quantification of cardiac mechanics. J Cardiovasc Magn Reson. 2014;16:94.

38. Morton G, Schuster A, Jogiya R, Kutty S, Beerbaum P, Nagel E. Inter-study reproducibility of cardiovascular magnetic resonance myocardial feature tracking. J Cardiovasc Magn Reson. 2012;14:43.

39. Schuster A, Stahnke V-C, Unterberg-Buchwald C, Kowallick JT, Lamata P, Steinmetz M, et al. Cardiovascular magnetic resonance feature-tracking assessment of myocardial mechanics: Intervendor agreement and considerations regarding reproducibility. Clin Radiol. 2015;70:989–98.

40. Singh A, Steadman CD, Khan JN, Horsfield MA, Bekele S, Nazir SA, et al. Intertechnique agreement and interstudy reproducibility of strain and diastolic strain rate at 1.5 and 3 Tesla: a comparison of feature-tracking and tagging in patients with aortic stenosis. J Cardiovasc Magn Reson. 2015;41:1129–37.

41. Fonseca CG, Backhaus M, Bluemke DA, Britten RD, Chung JD, Cowan BR, et al. The Cardiac Atlas Project--an imaging database for computational modeling and statistical atlases of the heart. Bioinformatics. 2011;27:2288–95.

42. Augustine D, Lewandowski AJ, Lazdam M, Rai A, Francis J, Myerson S, et al. Global and regional left ventricular myocardial deformation measures by magnetic resonance feature tracking in healthy volunteers: comparison with tagging and relevance of gender. J Cardiovasc Magn Reson. 2013;15:8.

43. Del-Canto I, Lopez-Lereu MP, Monmeneu JV, Croisille P, Clarysse P, Chorro FJ, et al. Characterization of normal regional myocardial function by MRI cardiac tagging. Journal of Magnetic Resonance Imaging. 2013;41:83–92.

44. Moore CC, Lugo-Olivieri CH, McVeigh ER, Zerhouni EA. Three-dimensional systolic strain patterns in the normal human left ventricle: characterization with tagged MR imaging. Radiology. 2000;214:453–66.

45. Kelle S, Roes SD, Klein C, Kokocinski T, de Roos A, Fleck E, et al. Prognostic value of myocardial infarct size and contractile reserve using magnetic resonance imaging. J Am Coll Cardiol. 2009;54:1770–7.

46. Korosoglou G, Gitsioudis G, Voss A, Lehrke S, Riedle N, Buss SJ, et al. Strain-encoded cardiac magnetic resonance during high-dose dobutamine stress testing for the estimation of cardiac outcomes: comparison to clinical parameters and conventional wall motion readings. J Am Coll Cardiol. 2011;58:1140–9.

47. Buss SJ, Breuninger K, Lehrke S, Voss A, Galuschky C, Lossnitzer D, et al. Assessment of myocardial deformation with cardiac magnetic resonance strain imaging improves risk stratification in patients with dilated cardiomyopathy. Eur Heart J Cardiovasc Imaging. 2015;16:307–15.

48. Caudron J, Fares J, Bauer F, Dacher J-N. Evaluation of Left Ventricular Diastolic Function with Cardiac MR Imaging. Radiographics. 2011;31:239–59.

49. Westenberg JJM. CMR for Assessment of Diastolic Function. Current Cardiovascular Imaging Reports. 2011;4:149–58.

50. Fonseca CG, Oxenham HC, Cowan BR, Occleshaw CJ, Young AA. Aging alters patterns of regional nonuniformity in LV strain relaxation: a 3-D MR tissue tagging study. Am J Physiol Heart Circ Physiol. 2003;285:H621–30.

51. Witschey WRT, Contijoch F, McGarvey JR, Ferrari VA, Hansen MS, Lee ME, et al. Real-Time Magnetic Resonance Imaging Technique for Determining Left Ventricle Pressure-Volume Loops. Ann Thorac Surg. 2014;97:1597–603.

52. Brandts A, Bertini M, van Dijk E-J, Delgado V, Marsan NA, van der Geest RJ, et al. Left ventricular diastolic function assessment from three-dimensional three-directional velocity-encoded MRI with retrospective valve tracking. Journal of Magnetic Resonance Imaging. 2011;33:312–9.

53. Rubinshtein R, Glockner JF, Feng D, Araoz PA, Kirsch J, Syed IS, et al. Comparison of Magnetic Resonance Imaging Versus Doppler Echocardiography for the Evaluation of Left Ventricular Diastolic Function in Patients With Cardiac Amyloidosis. Am J Cardiol. 2009;103:718–23.

54. Hees PS, Fleg JL, Dong SJ. Shapiro EP.MRI and echocardiographic assessment of the diastolic dysfunction of normal aging: altered LV pressure decline or load? Am J Physiol Heart Circ Physiol. 2004 Feb;286(2):H782–8.

55. Mather AN, Lockie T, Nagel E, Marber M, Perera D, Redwood S, et al. Appearance of microvascular obstruction on high resolution first-pass perfusion, early and late gadolinium enhancement CMR in patients with acute myocardial infarction. J Cardiovasc Magn Reson. 2009;11:33.

56. de Waha S, Desch S, Eitel I, Fuernau G, Zachrau J, Leuschner A, et al. Impact of early vs. late microvascular obstruction assessed by magnetic resonance imaging on long-term outcome after ST-elevation myocardial infarction: a comparison with traditional prognostic markers. Eur. Heart J. 2010;31:2660–8.

57. Carrick D, Haig C, Rauhalammi S, Ahmed N, Mordi I, McEntegart M, et al. Prognostic significance of infarct core pathology revealed by quantitative non-contrast in comparison with contrast cardiac magnetic resonance imaging in reperfused ST-elevation myocardial infarction survivors. Eur Heart J. 2016;37:1044–59.

58. Carrick D, Haig C, Ahmed N, McEntegart M, Petrie MC, Eteiba H, et al. Myocardial Hemorrhage After Acute Reperfused ST-Segment-Elevation Myocardial Infarction: Relation to Microvascular Obstruction and Prognostic Significance. Circ Cardiovasc Imaging. 2016;9:e004148.

59. Sirol M, Gzara H, Gayat E, Dautry R, Gellen B, Logeart D, et al. Comparison between visual grading and planimetric quantification of microvascular obstruction extent assessment in reperfused acute myocardial infarction. Eur Radiol. 2016;26:2166–75.

60. Mangion K, Corcoran D, Carrick D, Berry C. New perspectives on the role of cardiac magnetic resonance imaging to evaluate myocardial salvage and myocardial hemorrhage after acute reperfused ST-elevation myocardial infarction. Expert Rev Cardiovasc Ther. 2016;14:843–54.

61. Hamirani YS, Wong A, Kramer CM, Salerno M. Effect of microvascular obstruction and intramyocardial hemorrhage by CMR on LV remodeling and outcomes after myocardial infarction: a systematic review and meta-analysis. JACC Cardiovasc Imaging. 2014;7:940–52.

62. Carrick D, Haig C, Ahmed N, Rauhalammi S, Clerfond G, Carberry J, et al. Temporal Evolution of Myocardial Hemorrhage and Edema in Patients After Acute ST-Segment Elevation Myocardial Infarction: Pathophysiological Insights and Clinical Implications. J Am Heart Assoc. 2016;5:e002834.

63. Sörensson P, Heiberg E, Saleh N, Bouvier F, Caidahl K, Tornvall P, et al. Assessment of myocardium at risk with contrast enhanced steady-state free precession cine cardiovascular magnetic resonance compared to single-photon emission computed tomography. J Cardiovasc Magn Reson. 2010;12:25.

64. Eitel I, Desch S, Fuernau G, Hildebrand L, Gutberlet M, Schuler G, et al. Prognostic Significance and Determinants of Myocardial Salvage Assessed by Cardiovascular Magnetic Resonance in Acute Reperfused Myocardial Infarction. J Am Coll Cardiol. 2010;55:2470–9.

65. Berry C, Kellman P, Mancini C, Chen MY, Bandettini WP, Lowrey T, et al. Magnetic resonance imaging delineates the ischemic area at risk and myocardial salvage in patients with acute myocardial infarction. Circ Cardiovasc Imaging. 2010;3:527–35.

66. Friedrich MG, Sechtem U, Schulz-Menger J, Holmvang G, Alakija P, Cooper LT, et al. Cardiovascular Magnetic Resonance in Myocarditis: A JACC White Paper. J Am Coll Cardiol. 2009;53:1475–87.

67. Ibrahim T, Hackl T, Nekolla SG, Breuer M, Feldmair M, Schömig A, et al. Acute myocardial infarction: serial cardiac MR imaging shows a decrease in delayed enhancement of the myocardium during the 1st week after reperfusion. Radiology. 2010;254:88–97.

68. Dall'Armellina E, Karia N, Lindsay AC, Karamitsos TD, Ferreira V, Robson MD, et al. Dynamic changes of edema and late gadolinium enhancement after acute myocardial infarction and their relationship to functional recovery and salvage index. Circ Cardiovasc Imaging. 2011;4:228–36.

69. Khan JN, Nazir SA, Horsfield MA, Singh A, Kanagala P, Greenwood JP, et al. Comparison of semi-automated methods to quantify infarct size and area at risk by cardiovascular magnetic resonance imaging at 1.5T and 3.0T field strengths. BMC Research Notes. 2015;8:52.

70. Lønborg J, Vejlstrup N, Mathiasen AB, Thomsen C, Jensen JS, Engstrøm T. Myocardial area at risk and salvage measured by T2-weighted cardiovascular magnetic resonance: reproducibility and comparison of two T2-weighted protocols. J Cardiovasc Magn Reson. 2011;13:50.

71. McAlindon EJ, Pufulete M, Harris JM, Lawton CB, Moon JC, Manghat N, et al. Measurement of myocardium at risk with cardiovascular MR: comparison of techniques for edema imaging. Radiology. 2015;275:61–70.

72. McAlindon E, Pufulete M, Lawton C, Angelini GD, Bucciarelli-Ducci C. Quantification of infarct size and myocardium at risk: evaluation of different techniques and its implications. Eur Heart J Cardiovasc Imaging. 2015;16:738–46.

73. Cury RC, Shash K, Nagurney JT, Rosito G, Shapiro MD, Nomura CH, et al. Cardiac magnetic resonance with T2-weighted imaging improves detection of patients with acute coronary syndrome in the emergency department. Circulation. 2008;118:837–44.

74. Engstrøm T, Kelbaek H, Helqvist S, Høfsten DE, Kløvgaard L, Clemmensen P, et al. Effect of Ischemic Postconditioning During Primary Percutaneous Coronary Intervention for Patients With ST-Segment Elevation Myocardial Infarction: A Randomized Clinical Trial. JAMA cardiology. 2017;2:490–7.

75. Lønborg J, Kelbaek H, Vejlstrup N, Jørgensen E, Helqvist S, Saunamäki K, et al. Cardioprotective effects of ischemic postconditioning in patients treated with primary percutaneous coronary intervention, evaluated by magnetic resonance. Circ Cardiovasc Interv. 2010;3:34–41.

76. Rogers T, Dabir D, Mahmoud I, Voigt T, Schaeffter T, Nagel E, et al. Standardization of T1 measurements with MOLLI in differentiation between health and disease – the ConSept study. J Cardiovasc Magn Reson. 2013;15:78.

77. Knobelsdorff-Brenkenhoff v F, Prothmann M, Dieringer MA, Wassmuth R, Greiser A, Schwenke C, et al. Myocardial T1 and T2 mapping at 3 T: reference values, influencing factors and implications. J Cardiovasc Magn Reson. 2013;15:53.

78. Piechnik SK, Ferreira VM, Lewandowski AJ, Ntusi NA, Banerjee R, Holloway C, et al. Normal variation of magnetic resonance T1 relaxation times in the human population at 1.5 T using ShMOLLI. J Cardiovasc Magn Reson. 2013;15:13.

79. Dall'Armellina E, Piechnik SK, Ferreira VM, Le Si Q, Robson MD, Francis JM, et al. Cardiovascular magnetic resonance by noncontrast T1-mapping allows assessment of severity of injury in acute myocardial infarction. J Cardiovasc Magn Reson. 2012;14:15.

80. Treibel TA, Fontana M, Maestrini V, Castelletti S, Rosmini S, Simpson J, et al. Automatic Measurement of the Myocardial Interstitium. JACC Cardiovasc Imaging. 2016;9:54–63.

81. Fent GJ, Garg P, Foley JRJ, Swoboda PP, Dobson LE, Erhayiem B, et al. Synthetic Myocardial Extracellular Volume Fraction. JACC Cardiovasc Imaging. 2017;10:1402–4.

82. Puntmann VO, Isted A, Hinojar R, Foote L, Carr-White G, Nagel E. T1 and T2 Mapping in Recognition of Early Cardiac Involvement in Systemic Sarcoidosis. Radiology. 2017;285:162732–72.

83. Hinojar R, Foote L, Arroyo Ucar E, Jackson T, Jabbour A, Yu C-Y, et al. Native T1 in discrimination of acute and convalescent stages in patients with clinical diagnosis of myocarditis: a proposed diagnostic algorithm using CMR. JACC Cardiovasc Imaging. 2015;8:37–46.

84. Hinojar R, Foote L, Sangle S, Marber M, Mayr M, Carr-White G, et al. Native T1 and T2 mapping by CMR in lupus myocarditis: Disease recognition and response to treatment. Int J Cardiol. 2016;222:717–26.

85. Meloni A, Positano V, Keilberg P, De Marchi D, Pepe P, Zuccarelli A, et al. Feasibility, reproducibility, and reliability for the T*2 iron evaluation at 3 T in comparison with 1.5 T. Magn Reson Med. 2012;68:543–51.

86. Alam MH, Auger D, McGill L-A, Smith GC, He T, Izgi C, et al. Comparison of 3 T and 1.5 T for T2* magnetic resonance of tissue iron. J Cardiovasc Magn Reson. 2016;18:40.

87. Modell B, Khan M, Darlison M, Westwood MA, Ingram D, Pennell DJ. Improved survival of thalassaemia major in the UK and relation to T2* cardiovascular magnetic resonance. J Cardiovasc Magn Reson. 2008;10:42.

88. Pennell DJ, Udelson JE, Arai AE, Bozkurt B, Cohen AR, Galanello R, et al. Cardiovascular Function and Treatment in Thalassemia Major: A Consensus Statement From the American Heart Association. Circulation. 2013;128:281–308.

89. Carrick D, Haig C, Ahmed N, Carberry J, Yue May VT, McEntegart M, et al. Comparative Prognostic Utility of Indexes of Microvascular Function Alone or in Combination in Patients With an Acute ST-Segment-Elevation Myocardial Infarction. Circulation. 2016;134:1833–47.

90. Jogiya R, Morton G, De Silva K, Reyes E, Hachamovitch R, Kozerke S, et al. Ischemic Burden by 3-Dimensional Myocardial Perfusion Cardiovascular Magnetic Resonance: Comparison With Myocardial Perfusion Scintigraphy. Circ Cardiovasc Imaging. 2014;7:647–54.

91. Wagner A, Mahrholdt H, Holly TA, Elliott MD, Regenfus M, Parker M, et al. Contrast-enhanced MRI and routine single photon emission computed tomography (SPECT) perfusion imaging for detection of subendocardial myocardial infarcts: an imaging study. The Lancet. 2003;361:374–9.

92. Greenwood JP1, Maredia N, Younger JF, Brown JM, Nixon J, Everett CC, Bijsterveld P, Ridgway JP, Radjenovic A, Dickinson CJ, Ball SG, Plein S. Cardiovascular magnetic resonance and single-photon emission computed tomography for diagnosis of coronary heart disease (CE-MARC): a prospective trial. The Lancet. 2012;379:453–60.

93. Montalescot G, Sechtem U, Achenbach S, Andreotti F, Arden C, et al. ESC guidelines on the management of stable coronary artery disease: the Task Force on the management of stable coronary artery disease of the European Society of Cardiology. Eur Heart J. 2013, 2013:2949–3003.

94. Shaw LJ, Berman DS, Picard MH, Friedrich MG, Kwong RY, Stone GW, et al. Comparative definitions for moderate-severe ischemia in stress nuclear, echocardiography, and magnetic resonance imaging. JACC Cardiovasc Imaging. 2014;7:593–604.

95. Hussain ST, Paul M, Plein S, McCann GP, Shah AM, Marber MS, et al. Design and rationale of the MR-INFORM study: stress perfusion cardiovascular magnetic resonance imaging to guide the management of patients with stable coronary artery disease. J J Cardiovasc Magn Reson. 2012;14:1–1.

96. Shah R, Heydari B, Coelho-Filho O, Murthy VL, Abbasi S, Feng JH, et al. Stress cardiac magnetic resonance imaging provides effective cardiac risk reclassification in patients with known or suspected stable coronary artery disease. Circulation. 2013;128:605–14.

97. Bajwa A, Wesolowski R, Patel A, Saha P, Ludwinski F, Ikram M, et al. Blood Oxygenation Level-Dependent CMR-Derived Measures in Critical Limb Ischemia and Changes With Revascularization. J Am Coll Cardiol. 2016;67:420–31.

98. Pollak AW, Meyer CH, Epstein FH, Jiji RS, Hunter JR, Dimaria JM, et al. Arterial spin labeling MR imaging reproducibly measures peak-exercise calf muscle perfusion: a study in patients with peripheral arterial disease and healthy volunteers. JACC Cardiovasc Imaging. 2012;5:1224–30.

Blood volume measurement using cardiovascular magnetic resonance and ferumoxytol: preclinical validation

Rajiv Ramasawmy, Toby Rogers, Miguel A. Alcantar, Delaney R. McGuirt, Jaffar M. Khan, Peter Kellman, Hui Xue, Anthony Z. Faranesh, Adrienne E. Campbell-Washburn, Robert J. Lederman[*] and Daniel A. Herzka

Abstract

Background: The hallmark of heart failure is increased blood volume. Quantitative blood volume measures are not conveniently available and are not tested in heart failure management. We assess ferumoxytol, a marketed parenteral iron supplement having a long intravascular half-life, to measure the blood volume with cardiovascular magnetic resonance (CMR).

Methods: Swine were administered 0.7 mg/kg ferumoxytol and blood pool T_1 was measured repeatedly for an hour to characterize contrast agent extraction and subsequent effect on V_{blood} estimates. We compared CMR blood volume with a standard carbon monoxide rebreathing method. We then evaluated three abbreviated acquisition protocols for bias and precision.

Results: Mean plasma volume estimated by ferumoxytol was 61.9 ± 4.3 ml/kg. After adjustment for hematocrit the resultant mean blood volume was 88.1 ± 9.4 ml/kg, which agreed with carbon monoxide measures (91.1 ± 18.9 ml/kg). Repeated measurements yielded a coefficient of variation of 6.9%, and Bland-Altman repeatability coefficient of 14%. The blood volume estimates with abbreviated protocols yielded small biases (mean differences between 0.01–0.06 L) and strong correlations (r^2 between 0.97–0.99) to the reference values indicating clinical feasibility.

Conclusions: In this swine model, ferumoxytol CMR accurately measures plasma volume, and with correction for hematocrit, blood volume. Abbreviated protocols can be added to diagnostic CMR examination for heart failure within 8 min.

Keywords: Heart failure, CMR, MRI, Ferumoxytol, Blood volume, T_1 mapping

Background

The hallmark of heart failure is volume overload [1, 2]. Clinical evaluation includes qualitative auscultatory markers of cardiac wall stress (gallops) and lung water (rales), peptide biomarkers of wall stress (natriuretic peptides), qualitative radiographic markers of interstitial lung fluid (infiltrates and Kerley lines etc.), cardiac imaging and invasive markers of pressure overload. Initial management of decompensated heart failure chiefly consists of diuresis to reduce volume overload. Nevertheless, quantitative measures of blood volume are generally not employed clinically, because they are not conveniently accessible and because their value has not been tested.

Accurate measurement of blood volume, if readily accessible, might impact management of chronic and decompensated chronic heart failure [3]. Previous studies have characterized patients with heart failure to have a total blood volume of 20% above body-weight predicted values [4–6].

Current methods to measure blood volume include controlled inhalation of carbon monoxide to tag circulating hemoglobin, or tracer dilution using Evans blue dye or radiopharmaceuticals [4, 7–10], and are infrequently used clinically because of ionizing radiation, cost, and/or complexity in stand-alone examinations. Cardiovascular magnetic resonance (CMR) dilution measurement of

* Correspondence: lederman@nih.gov
Division of Intramural Research, National Heart Lung and Blood Institute, National Institutes of Health, Building 10, Room 2C713, 10 Center Drive, Bethesda, MD 20892, USA

plasma blood volume has been attempted in rats [11] using gadopentetate dimeglumine (Gd-DTPA), which has a relatively short distribution and elimination kinetics that limit measurement accuracy and feasibility. Gadofosveset trisodium, which reversibly binds plasma albumin, might be an attractive alternative because of its a longer intravascular half-life [12] except but it exhibits significant and rapid extravascular distribution, and has been withdrawn from marketing because of poor sales. Hence, we sought to develop a convenient gadolinium-free method to quantify blood volume by using an agent with longer half-life, ferumoxytol, so that it can possibly be included in a standard CMR examination.

Ferumoxytol is a superparamagnetic iron nanoparticle indicated for iron replacement in iron-deficiency anemia. It is an alternative to gadolinium-based CMR contrast agents, which are associated with nephrogenic systemic fibrosis in patients with renal disease, and which are under scrutiny because of unexpected cerebral gadolinium accumulation [13–15]. Ferumoxytol exhibits marked relaxivity effects [16–18], and is a candidate tracer for blood volume measurement because of its long intravascular half-life of 9–14 h and low extravascular biodistribution [19].

The aim of this study is to assess the in vivo feasibility and repeatability of measuring blood volume using ferumoxytol tracer dilution. The accuracy of this measurement is compared against a reference carbon monoxide hemoglobin binding technique. We characterize measurement stability, in face of ferumoxytol elimination from the blood compartment at reduced doses, over a period of 1 h. We also performed Monte Carlo simulations to minimize the number of T_1 measurements and produce an abbreviated acquisition protocol.

Methods
Animals
All procedures were approved by the institutional Animal Care and Use Committee and performed according to NIH guidelines. Swine ($N = 6$ Yucatan, 35–50 kg, S&S Farms, USA) were pre-medicated with glucocorticoids and anti-histamine [20, 21]. Anesthesia was maintained with mechanical ventilation and inhaled isoflurane, and euvolemia restored after overnight fast using 10–15 ml/kg isotonic saline 20 min before blood volume measurements. Femoral arterial and venous femoral introducer sheaths were placed percutaneously.

Ferumoxytol relaxivity in blood in vitro
CMR was performed at 1.5 T (Aera, Siemens Healthineers, Erlangen, Germany), using two standard body arrays. Longitudinal relaxivity r_1 was characterized prior the repeatability study in a Yorkshire swine sample. A series of dilutions of ferumoxytol (0.10–1.72 mM) in 50 mL heparinized swine blood in a heated water bath

(35–41 °C) were characterized with T_1 measurements using with SAturation-recovery single-SHot Acquisition (SASHA) with 11 exponentially spaced saturation times ranging from 100 to 10,000 ms, and a simulated cardiac interval of 1 s (acquisition parameters below).

Ferumoxytol blood volume measurement in vivo
Two successive imaging sessions tested the repeatability of the blood volume measurement at euvolemia. Based on a target post-contrast T_1 of approximately 300 ms for optimal accuracy and precision in the T_1 measurement [11], animals received 0.7 mg/kg (0.011 mM/kg) ferumoxytol diluted in 50 ml saline infused slowly ~ 0.4 ml/sec. As ferumoxytol elimination from the blood is faster at lower concentrations [19], each animal was imaged for an hour to characterize the resultant change in T_1. Three animals underwent an additional imaging session at a reduced dose of ferumoxytol ($N = 1$ at 10%, 20% or 50% of the 0.7 mg/kg dose). Successive imaging sessions were 3–4 days apart. For each imaging session, total blood volume was compared using both CMR and carbon monoxide (CO) rebreathing techniques [22].

Carbon monoxide blood volume measurement in vivo
A reference blood volume was measured using the absorption of CO through a rebreathing apparatus constructed according to the methods proposed by Schmidt et al. [22]. Three baseline samples were drawn from the femoral artery and analyzed for carboxyhemoglobin (COHb) using a blood-gas analyzer (Avoximeter 4000, Accriva Diagnostics, Werfen Company Bedford, Massachusetts, USA).

Following baseline measurements, a 1 ml/kg (max 50 ml) volume of CO was administered to the rebreathing apparatus, and the reservoir bag squeezed to simulate a single inhalation held for 10 s. The animals were then manually ventilated for 2 min before reverting to normal ventilation using a 3-way stopcock. Blood was sampled to measure COHb at 6, 7 and 8 min following CO administration.

CO rebreathing allows for the estimation of blood volume V_{blood} based on the determination of V_{CO}, the volume of CO administered through rebreathing [22]:

$$V_{blood} = V_{CO} \frac{K * 100}{[Hb] * \Delta\%[COHb] * n_H}, \tag{1}$$

where K is a Boyle's Law volume correction factor for standard temperature and pressure, the concentration of hemoglobin is given by $[Hb]$ in g/L, and the hemoglobin oxygen capacity is given by Hüfner's number, $n_H=1.31$ ml/g [23]. The change in the concentration of COHb, $\Delta\%[COHb]$, is calculated from the average baseline and the average over 6 to 8 min post-administration of CO.

To account for systematic losses in the total volume of carbon monoxide administered (V_{CO}) after rebreathing, the following corrections were made. First, a 1% loss due to the affinity of CO to Hb was assumed. Second, corrections for the volume of CO not administered through rebreathing and the volume expired to the air following rebreathing were applied as detailed by Schmidt et al. [22]. The volume of CO remnant in the spirometer was estimated by the product of the rebreathing apparatus volume and the concentration of CO ([CO]) in the rebreathing bag as determined by a CO monitor (Dräger Pac 3500, Dräger, Lübeck, Germany). The mean measured rebreathing bag volume was 2.7 ± 0.3 L, the spirometer's volume was measured to be 0.04 L, and the lung volume of the swine was assumed to be 1 L [24]. The volume of CO removed by the body was estimated from the average [$HbCO$] over 6–8 min, using a previous finding that the concentration of COHb is related to the expired CO (expired CO $= 5.09[COHb] + 2.34$ ppm [25]), and assuming an alveolar ventilation rate of 5 L/min [22], and the average of the blood sampling times (7 min) as the measurement time.

Quantification of blood volume with ferumoxytol

The total circulating blood volume V_{blood} can be estimated by the plasma blood volume V_{plasma}, using the change in longitudinal relaxation rate $R_1 = 1/T_1$ after administration of contrast agent (CA) in conjunction with hematocrit. The change in relaxation rate in response to the infusion of CA is given by:

$$R_1(t) = R_{1,\varnothing} + r_i[CA] \tag{2}$$

where $R_{1,\varnothing}$ represents the native longitudinal relaxation rate before contrast, r_1 is the agent's relaxivity (mM^{-1} s^{-1}), and [CA] is the concentration in mM. $R_1(t)$ decreases towards $R_{1,\varnothing}$ exponentially as the agent is removed from circulation. As iron concentration is given by [CA] $= n_{Fe}/V$, the plasma volume estimate $V'(t)$ can be calculated thus:

$$V'(t) = \frac{r_1 n_{Fe}}{\Delta R_1(t)}, \tag{3}$$

where $\Delta R_1(t) = R_1(t) - R_{1,\varnothing}$, and n_{Fe} is the amount of iron in millimoles. Though n_{Fe} is time-dependent as the ferumoxytol is extracted from circulation, it is treated as constant, as the changing concentration of CA is measured within $R_1(t)$. The injected amount of iron (n_{Fe}) is given by the product of iron concentration of ferumoxytol (30 mg/ml), the molar mass of iron (55.845 g/mol) and the injected volume of ferumoxytol in ml. Sequential measurements of $R_1(t)$ can be used to calculate $V'(t)$ using Eq. 3. As posited by Pannek et al. for Gd-based agents, V_{plasma} can then be calculated by fitting the

estimated 'time-dependent' plasma volume, $V'(t)$ [11], assuming an exponential elimination:

$$V'(t) = V_{plasma} \exp\left(t/\tau\right), \tag{4}$$

where τ is the time constant for extraction of ferumoxytol from circulation. As physiology is typically reported in terms of half-life, this term shall be reported, with the half-life $t_{1/2} = \tau \times \ln 2$. For the purposes of log-linear regression, Eq. (4) can be expressed as follows:

$$\log(V'(t)) = \log(V_{plasma}) + t/\tau, \tag{5}$$

thus V_{plasma} can be determined from the y-intercept. The total blood volume V_{blood} can be calculated by normalizing V_{plasma} by the hematocrit Hct, the ratio of the volume of red blood cells V_{RBC} to V_{plasma}:

$$V_{blood} = V_{plasma} + V_{RBC} \tag{6}$$

$$V_{blood} = \frac{V_{plasma}}{1 - Hct} \tag{7}$$

Hence, blood T_1 measurements pre- and post-ferumoxytol can be used to estimate V_{blood}.

CMR protocol

All SASHA T_1 measurements were acquired in 4-chamber orientation to maximize the number of blood pool pixels in both the left ventricle (LV) and right ventricle (RV) at end-diastole. To measure the coefficient of variation in R_1, five T_1 maps were acquired pre-contrast, and the average of these were taken for the baseline measurement of $R_{1,\varnothing}$. Post-contrast T_1 maps were subsequently acquired every 2 min up to 60 min, yielding ~ 28 T_1 measurements. Breath-hold SASHA imaging parameters were: TE/TR 1.01/2.02 ms, FOV 360 × 270 cm; acquired resolution 1.88 × 2.50 mm, reconstructed resolution 1.88 × 1.88 mm, slice thickness 8 mm, acceleration factor 3 [26]. A customized SASHA protocol used 17 images for 2-parameter T_1 fitting: an initial 'equilibrium' image with no saturation pulse, followed by saturation preparation and imaging in successive heart beats: 8 each with saturation times of 200 and 400 ms [27].

Image analysis

Regions of interest (ROIs) were manually drawn within the LV and RV for all T_1 maps (typically ~ 150/60 pixels for the LV/RV), and myocardial ROIs were drawn at baseline, 4, 20 and 60 min. Plasma volume and ferumoxytol half-life was fitted from 20 to 60 min using Eq. 5 and estimation of the coefficient of determination (r^2) was performed in Matlab (Mathworks, Natick, Massachusetts, USA). V_{blood} was calculated following Eq. 7 and normalized by the animal weight to yield the final estimate in ml/kg.

Abbreviated protocols

The reference acquisition for the estimation of blood volume acquired 26 measurements (5 pre- and 21 post-contrast) spanning over 60 min. We use this data, along with Monte Carlo simulations to develop 3 optimized abbreviated acquisition strategies differing in amount of data, time span, and accuracy. A single baseline T_1 measurement was used for simulated and in vivo data.

- **Protocol #1** (1 post-contrast T_1 measurement) represents the simplest scheme in which a single T_1 measurement at 4 min post-contrast is used to estimate blood volume (similar to Pannek, et al. [11]). V_{blood} is determined directly from Eq. (3) after correction for hematocrit. Protocol #1 ignores for any time-dependence of the contrast washout and aims to acquire data at the earliest point post-administration, minimizing the overall time span of the measurement.
- **Protocol #2** (4+ post-contrast T_1 measurements) acquires an increasing number of sequential T_1 measurements starting with 20, 22 and 24 min after infusion. The additional data enables fitting, yielding for higher accuracy at the expense of time span.
- **Protocol #3** (4 post-contrast T_1 measurements) used 3 sequential measurements (at 20, 22 and 24 min) anchored by a delayed measurement acquired between 30 and 60 min. Fitting is improved in accuracy by increasing the sampling time span, at the expense of workflow.

We also simulate a protocol with timing suitable for human subjects. The simulated 'human' protocols (3+ post-contrast T_1 measurements) were composed of measurements every 2 min up to 20 min. This model assumed acute measurements would be possible in humans, given the expectation of tolerance to ferumoxytol.

To optimize the three acquisition strategies, Monte Carlo simulations were used. A model T_1 recovery curve spanning 60 min post-contrast was created based on the observations from in vivo experiments (Table 1&2): $T_{1,\ \varnothing}$=1600 ms, immediate post-contrast T_1 = 230 ms, ferumoxytol half-life = 3.4 h, v_{Fe}=1.0 ml, and r_1 = 18 mM^{-1} s^{-1}. Each simulation was performed 10,000 times with a T_1 standard deviation of 0.6% (taken from the experimental coefficient of variation), the resultant curves were sub-sampled and fitted following Eq. (5). The standard deviation of plasma volumes ($\sigma_{V_{plasma}}$) and goodness-of-fit (r^2) were recorded for each protocol.

Three protocols were identified through Monte Carlo modelling, and compared to in vivo plasma volume measurements using correlation and Bland-Altman analysis.

Table 1 T_1 values (mean ± SD, n = 12) at baseline and after administration of a 0.7 mg/kg dose of ferumoxytol, across the measurement protocol duration for the LV blood pool, RV blood pool and myocardial tissue (myo) from the repeatability study

	T_1 Baseline (ms)	T_1 Post-ferumoxytol (ms)		
		4 min	20 min	60 min
LV	1604.2 ± 27.7	232.0 ± 12.3	250.6 ± 15.7	281.4 ± 19.7
RV	1807.9 ± 96.8	235.9 ± 14.5	257.1 ± 20.3	289.0 ± 21.7
myo	1135.0 ± 80.2	837.2 ± 42.9	844.5 ± 63.3	860.1 ± 59.3

Statistical analysis

Coefficients of variation (CV) and repeatability coefficients (RC) were calculated for the differences in normalized blood volumes between the replicate euvolemic sessions, and for the baseline T_1, using the following equations:

$$CV = 100\% \frac{\mu}{\sigma} \tag{8}$$

$$RC = 1.96\sqrt{\frac{\sum (x_i-\mu)^2}{n-1}} \frac{100\%}{\mu} \tag{9}$$

where the data x_i composed of n measurements had mean μ and standard deviation σ. The accuracy of the CMR blood volume technique was compared to reference measurements using CO with a non-parametric paired test (Wilcoxon), in addition to a linear regression and Bland-Altman analysis. Low-dose half-lives and blood volumes were compared against the standard dose using Mann-Whitney U tests.

Results

In vivo summary

The baseline swine weight was 41 ± 6 kg (range 35–49 kg) and mean individual deviation from baseline was 0 ± 1 kg indicating no observable change in rapidly growing animals (p > 0.9, one-way ANOVA) over 19 days. Mean baseline heart rate was 118 ± 7 bpm, and baseline mean arterial pressure was 72 ± 14 mmHg. Ferumoxytol induced no serious adverse reactions and mean arterial pressure and heart rate variations were 4 ± 1 mmHg and 0 ± 1 bpm respectively, averaged over 10 min.

Measurement of Relaxivity and T_1

The relaxivity r_1 of ferumoxytol in swine blood in vitro was 18.0 ± 0.4 mM^{-1}·s^{-1}. In vivo baseline T_1 mapping yielded a CV of 0.58 ± 0.27% and 0.90 ± 0.63% for the LV and RV, respectively, and Bland-Altman repeatability coefficients of 1.0 ± 0.5% and 1.6 ± 1.1% respectively within the LV and RV.

T_1 maps before and after administration (at 4, 20 and 60 min) of ferumoxytol can be seen in Fig. 1a, and the

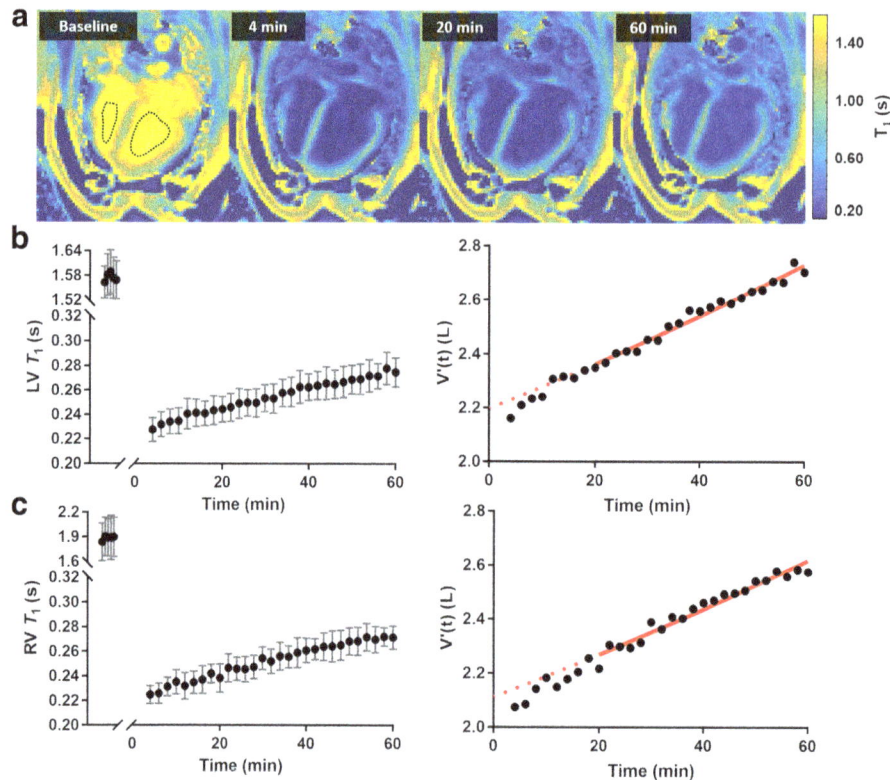

Fig. 1 a Example long-axis T_1 maps and regions-of-interest (ROI) over the duration of a study, and typical T_1 (intra-ROI mean ± SD) recovery profile post-contrast and the corresponding volume $V'(t)$, calculated from Eq. 3, for the (**b**) left-ventricle (LV) and paired (**c**) right-ventricle (RV). A linear fit from 20 to 40 min (solid line) is used to measure the half-life of the contrast agent. The plasma volume can be estimated by extrapolating to the model to 0 min (dotted line)

partial recovery in blood pool T_1 over the hour-long measurement period and the corresponding time-dependent volume estimation, as determined by Eq. 3, is shown for the LV and RV in Figs. 1b and c, respectively. A non-linear rate of contrast extraction was observed until ~ 20 min post-contrast administration, potentially due to a physiological response to ferumoxytol. Thus, fitting was constrained between 20 and 60 min (solid red line), and plasma volume estimated from the intercept (dotted line).

Estimates of blood volume were calculated separately from the LV and RV blood pools. Over the repeatability study, good adherence to the linear model was observed, with $r^2 = 0.97 ± 0.03$ (mean ± SD) for the LV. Fitting was marginally weaker ($r^2 = 0.94 ± 0.10$) for the RV, reflective of the larger intra-ROI variation. The percentage confidence intervals of plasma volume were 0.57% and 0.68% for the LV and RV, respectively. Bland-Altman analysis showed the RV non-significantly over-estimated plasma volume with a mean difference of 0.05 L ($p > 0.27$, paired t-test).

Table 1 shows the T_1 values (mean ± SD) from the repeatability study for the LV and RV blood pools, and myocardium. The LV blood pool T_1 decreased to 14.5%

of baseline after a dose of 0.7 mg/kg ferumoxytol, and over the hour exhibited a 21.3% increase from the immediate post-contrast T_1. Myocardial T_1 reduced to 67% of the baseline and showed only a small amount of recovery at 60 min (2.7%).

Blood volume: repeatability

Over the repeatability study, mean plasma volume (V_{plasma}) was measured as 61.9 ± 4.3 ml/kg, mean blood volume (V_{blood}) was measured as 88.1 ± 9.4 ml/kg using ferumoxytol. Blood hematocrit (*Hct*) was 29.5 ± 3.4% and Hb concentration 9.8 ± 1.1 g/dL. The repeatability of the normalized blood volume from two visits can be seen in Fig. 2a, with a coefficient of variation of 6.9%. The measurements exhibited a mean difference of 8.6 ml/kg (9.8%) between the studies, as can be seen in Fig. 2b. A potential magnitude-dependent bias was observed, and the repeatability coefficient of the technique was calculated to be 14%.

The CO reference measurement yielded a mean blood volume of 90.8 ± 18.9 ml/kg. There was no significant difference between blood volume estimated from ferumoxytol and CO ($p = 0.67$). Bland-Altman comparison (Fig. 2c) between the CMR and CO blood volume

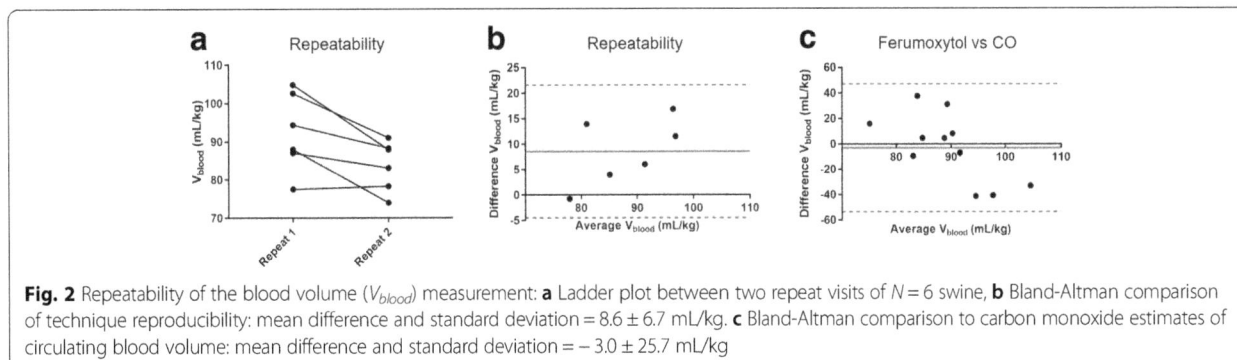

Fig. 2 Repeatability of the blood volume (V_{blood}) measurement: **a** Ladder plot between two repeat visits of $N = 6$ swine, **b** Bland-Altman comparison of technique reproducibility: mean difference and standard deviation = 8.6 ± 6.7 mL/kg. **c** Bland-Altman comparison to carbon monoxide estimates of circulating blood volume: mean difference and standard deviation = − 3.0 ± 25.7 mL/kg

measurements yielded a small mean-difference (carbon monoxide was 2.7 ml/kg larger), though there is a potential trend in this data and a poor correlation $r^2 = 0.13$. The measured CV for the CO blood volume was 18% and the Bland-Altman repeatability coefficient was 32%.

Abbreviated protocols

Monte Carlo modelling of the full protocol yielded a goodness-of-fit r^2 of 0.97, matching the in vivo results, and estimated plasma volume precision as 0.54%. Simulations predicted a more precise measurement of plasma volume with increasing experiment time (Fig. 3). Propagation of error analysis (on Eq. 3) indicates that a 4% error in the measurement of T_1 (based on the observed intra-ROI standard deviation) would result in 4.7% error in the measurement of blood volume. For Protocol #2, though an increased number of acquisitions yielded improved plasma volume precision, a limit of 5 continuous measurements from 20 to 28 min was chosen for practicality, which resulted in error < 3% with a bias of 0 ml. Finally, for Protocol #3, an anchor measurement past 40 min resulted in error < 2%, with a bias of 0 ml. The proposed human protocol achieved ~ 1% error after measuring up to 6 min post-contrast (3 T_1 measurements).

Figure 4 shows the comparison of the three abbreviated protocols based on the simulated precision in blood volume. The simplest scheme - Protocol #1 yielded an r^2 of 0.98 and a Bland-Altman mean under-estimation of 0.06 L (2.4%). Protocol #2, with 5 successive measurements, yielded $r^2 = 0.97$ and a Bland-Altman mean under-estimation of 0.02 L (0.8%). Protocol #3 with 3 early measurements followed by an 'anchor' at 40 min produced an $r^2 = 0.99$ and a Bland-Altman mean under-estimation of 0.01 L (0.4%). These results suggest that all the abbreviated protocols can accurately calculate plasma volume.

Reduced dose ferumoxytol

The effects of a reduced ferumoxytol dose on the normalized change in LV T_1 from baseline, half-life estimated blood volume, and percentage difference from the

blood volume measured in the repeatability study, can all be seen in Table 2. An expected decrease in ΔT_1 was observed with smaller doses, and a significantly shorter half-life was measured across the reduced doses compared to the 0.7 mg/kg dose ($p < 0.02$, Mann-Whitney U). No significant differences in blood volume were calculated using the reduced doses ($p = 0.95$, Mann-Whitney U). Aside from the 50% dose, the estimated blood volumes were within the variability calculated by the repeatability coefficient.

Discussion

We describe a CMR technique to measure total circulating blood volume using injected ferumoxytol and compared it with reference standard carbon monoxide inhalation in swine. We optimized the measurement strategy to propose clinical protocols requiring a maximum of 2–6 additional T_1 measurements. The technique avoids frequent blood tracer sampling, avoids radioactive or dye tracers, and uses a small dose of parenteral iron supplement that can be used for first-pass and steady state CMR angiography.

Measurement of blood volume

We found mean blood volume of 88.1 ± 9.4 ml/kg and 91.1 ± 18.9 ml/kg using ferumoxytol and carbon monoxide respectively. From Monte Carlo modelling, the calculated error in plasma volume was estimated to be 0.54% for the 60-min measurement, which suggests the method is precise. However, the values measured in this study are higher than reported blood volume values of swine (between 35 and 50 kg) range from 56 to 69 ml/kg in Yucatan swine (no weight range given) [28], 61–77 ml/kg in Chester-White [29], in 74–96 ml/kg in Duroc-Jersey swine [30], and between 56 and 68 ml/kg in Hampshire swine [31]. This variability may be in part to age and weights, it has been generally observed that older and larger swine will have a reduced normalized blood volume [31].

Plasma volume was measured using Eq. 3 for both the RV and LV blood pools. Though the baseline RV T_1

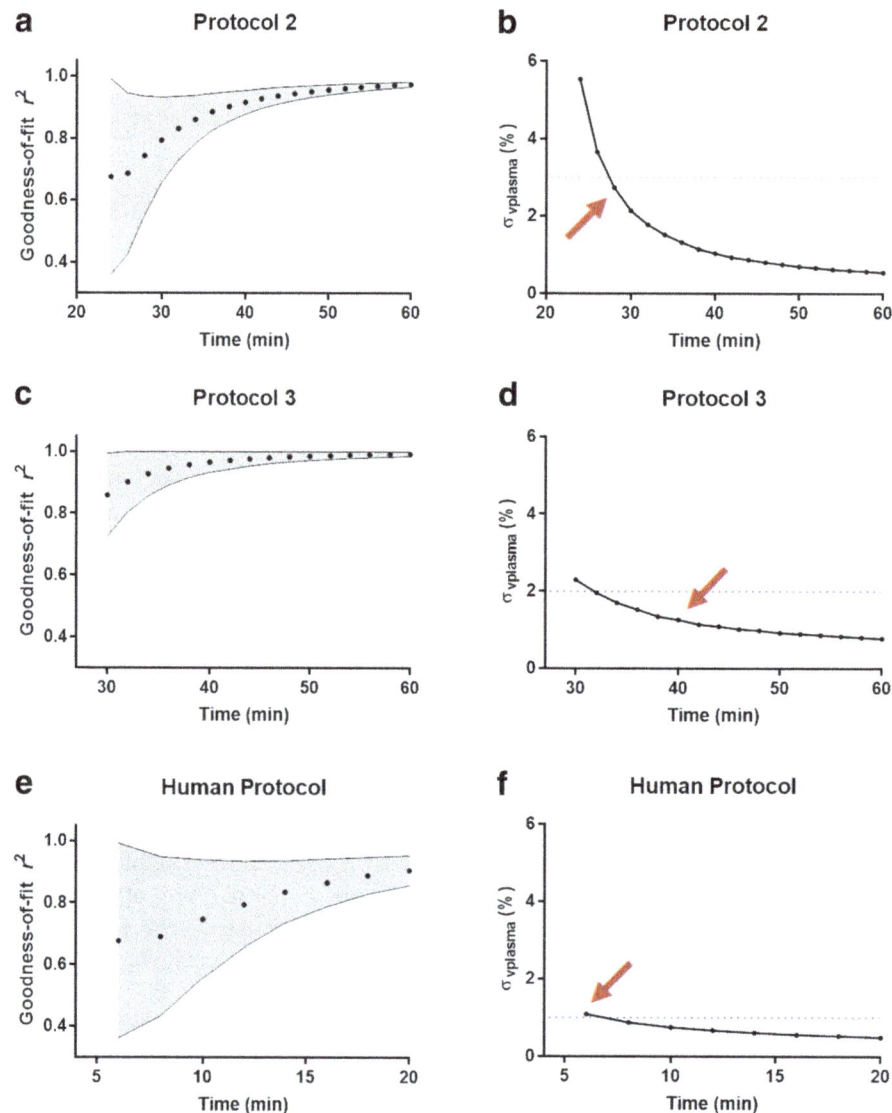

Fig. 3 Results from Monte Carlo simulations ($n = 10,000$) on the effects on goodness-of-fit (r^2) and plasma volume standard deviation ($\sigma_{V_{plasma}}$) as a function of increasing the number of samples from 26 min (Protocol 2) (**a**, **b**) and increasing the time of the 'anchor' point from 30 min (Protocol 3) (**c**, **d**). Shaded regions correspond to the standard deviation of the goodness-of-fit (r^2), and the points selected for in vivo analysis have been marked a red arrow. Dotted lines correspond to a 3, 2 and 1% plasma volume standard deviation in b, d and f respectively. Simulations of a potential 'human protocol' with an increasing number of acute post-contrast sampling (**e**, **f**) reveal that measurements as early as 6 min (red arrow) yield an approximate 1% standard deviation in plasma volume

is higher than LV (13%), both blood pools drop to approximately the same post-contrast T_1 (2% RV/LV ratio). However, the mean difference of blood volume produced a (non-significant) 2% over-estimation, which would suggest that the post-contrast measurement is the dominant factor in volume quantification, and thus a single pre-contrast measurement is sufficient. This is confirmed by propagation of error analysis applied to Eq. 3, which indicated that a 1% error in $T_{1,0}$ and T_1 result in 0.17% and 1.81% errors in blood volume, respectively (data not shown). As the LV ROI had a higher number of pixels and yielded a smaller

intra-ROI variation, this was chosen for the repeatability analysis. Under conditions of hyperoxia, blood hemoglobin T_1 has been reported to increase [32], which is likely to be the source of left-right difference observed in this study at baseline.

In this study, the most accurate measurement of plasma volume required temporal monitoring of blood T_1 as ferumoxytol was extracted from circulation to estimate the agent's half-life through fitting. Since ferumoxytol has been reported to have a dose-dependent extraction rate (ranging from 9 to 14 h in humans) [19], assuming a half-life could lead to errors in the estimation of blood

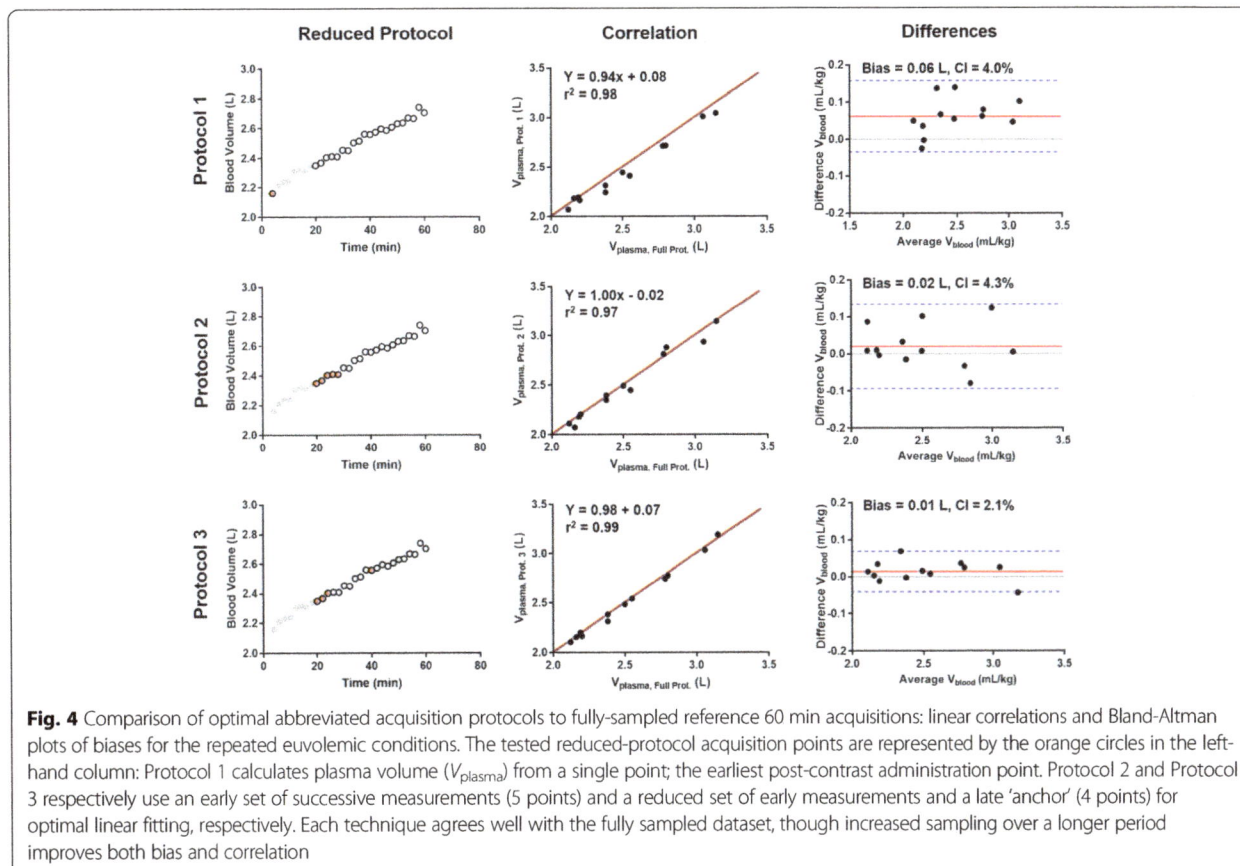

Fig. 4 Comparison of optimal abbreviated acquisition protocols to fully-sampled reference 60 min acquisitions: linear correlations and Bland-Altman plots of biases for the repeated euvolemic conditions. The tested reduced-protocol acquisition points are represented by the orange circles in the left-hand column: Protocol 1 calculates plasma volume (V_{plasma}) from a single point; the earliest post-contrast administration point. Protocol 2 and Protocol 3 respectively use an early set of successive measurements (5 points) and a reduced set of early measurements and a late 'anchor' (4 points) for optimal linear fitting, respectively. Each technique agrees well with the fully sampled dataset, though increased sampling over a longer period improves both bias and correlation

volume. In this study, we found a comparatively short mean half-life of 3.4 ± 0.5 h, potentially due to differences in swine physiology. We measured no significant differences in blood volume at lower doses, but further work is necessary to determine the minimal dose required in humans to achieve sufficient blood volume accuracy.

The V_{plasma} quantification is proportional to the relaxivity of ferumoxytol, r_1. Others report r_1 to be 19.0 ± 1.7 mM^{-1} s^{-1} at 1.5 T [16], in good agreement with our 18.0 ± 0.3 mM^{-1} s^{-1} in blood. Knobloch et al. reported a

Table 2 Comparison of measuring blood volume (V_{blood}) with reduced ferumoxytol doses ($N = 1$, for each dose) in mg/kg of iron (Fe), and percentage of the typical dose used in this study ($N = 12$). Smaller doses resulted in a reduced change in post-contrast LV T_1, and a shorter ferumoxytol half-life, but did not produce a significantly different normalized blood volume ($p = 0.95$, Mann-Whitney U), and except for the 50% dose, the percentage differences from the blood volumes for each subject were within the calculated repeatability coefficient (14%)

Conc. Fe (mg/kg)	ΔT_1 (%)	Half-life (hr)	V_{blood} (mL/kg)	$\%\Delta V_{blood}$
0.69 ± 0.01	-85.5 ± 0.7	3.43 ± 0.49	88.1 ± 9.4	–
0.30 (50%)	-74.6	2.55	79.9	-17.5
0.23 (20%)	-65.9	2.93	95.4	12.1
0.13 (10%)	-53.9	2.51	86.2	-5.7

non-linear behavior of relaxivity in blood, particularly at higher concentrations (> 1 mM), which we avoided to minimize the effect of T_2^* dephasing. As ferumoxytol relaxivity is dependent on field strength, to achieve the same ΔT_1, a higher dose of ferumoxytol would be required at 3 T [16]. Further investigation is required to characterize the accuracy of the blood volume measurements with low doses (< 1 mg/kg) of Ferumoxytol, as some variability was measured here. Additional measurements are required to see any effects on sensitivity at higher, more clinical doses (2–6 mg/kg), particularly due to non-linear effects on relaxivity at higher concentrations.

Sources of error

The repeatability coefficient of porcine blood volume measured by ferumoxytol was 14%, which is higher than previous values of 8% using a ^{131}I tracer [4]. Small inaccuracies in the ferumoxytol-based estimate may be introduced from error in the administered volume and T_1 variation due to heart rate changes over the imaging session.

The calculated Bland-Altman repeatability coefficient of the CO technique (32%) was higher here than previous implementations 0.8–2.7% [8, 33, 34]. The potential sources of error in measuring blood volume with CO have been described [8, 35], but in our lab additional sources of error could include manually rebreathing anesthetized animals, systematic differences in measuring porcine COHb on a human blood-gas analyzer [36], and variability in the CO detector's measurements of the remnant volume in the spirometer (coefficient of variation 25.3 ± 10.2%).

Abbreviated protocols for clinical implementation

Abbreviated protocols yielded small biases (between 0.4–2.4%) and strong correlations ($r^2 = 0.97$–0.99) to the reference 60 min experiment. The chosen abbreviated protocols yielded plasma volume repeatability coefficients of 9%, 14%, and 12% for protocols 1, 2 and 3, respectively.

Each protocol has advantages and disadvantages depending on the time constraints of a CMR exam. The most accurate and precise technique, Protocol #3, requires a 'late' measurement at 40 min post-contrast to improve the fit. This measurement improves as this acquisition moves later in time, but a prolonged measurement becomes unfeasible. The single post-contrast measurement, Protocol #1, is the fastest measurement, but is dependent on an immediate acquisition, and having a very accurate and precise T_1 measurement. A short cluster of five measurements, Protocol #2, combine speed and the accuracy of longitudinal fitting. Protocols #2&3 are not dependent on two-minute interval acquisitions, thus by alternating a post-contrast T_1 acquisition with standard diagnostic scans, these methods can be integrated in to a CMR workflow and could achieve higher accuracy and precision by broadening the measurement period.

The additional imaging time required to measure blood volume with these protocols are minor: one baseline and 1–5 post-contrast T_1 maps. We anticipate that with short, breath-held T_1 scans (~ 11 s), any of the abbreviated protocols, including the contrast administration, will require no more than 5 min of additional time to a CMR exam. A free-breathing T_1 mapping technique (e.g. [37]) may be preferable to avoid repeated breath-held acquisitions, though each may take up to 60 s, and free-breathing techniques may yield an increase in T_1 reproducibility.

Protocol 2 was optimized starting from 20 min given the non-linear acute behavior observed in swine, but we anticipate ferumoxytol will be better tolerated in humans, therefore T_1 measurements could begin earlier. Modelling of this acute 'human' protocol (Fig. 3e-f) predicts that an accurate (0 L bias) and precise (~ 1% error) blood volume measurement could be achieved within a total experiment time (baseline, injection and post-contrast) of 8 min. In addition, as clinical dose of Ferumoxytol yield longer half-lives, a protocol with a few repeats post-contrast may

also be feasible which do not require temporal fitting – however, further work is required to validate this.

Limitations

Ferumoxytol, in higher iron replacement doses, has been associated with reported 0.2% incidence of anaphylactoid reactions and carries a black box warning from the US Food and Drug Administration [38]. The incidence and seriousness appear to be dose- and infusion-rate-dependent, and is probably lower in clinical practice [39–42].

We found Yorkshire and Sinclair mini swine breeds did not tolerate ferumoxytol (data not shown), but that with glucocorticoid and antihistamine premedication and prolonged 2-min infusion, Yucatan mini-swine tolerated ferumoxytol. We studied only healthy swine and not animals exhibiting neurohormonal perturbations characteristic of heart failure.

Finally, the reference CO measurement had much larger variability than previously reported in humans. Though the mean blood volume estimates agreed reasonably with the CMR measurements, there was a low correlation between these values, and therefore difficult to isolate animal variability from the repeatability of each technique.

Conclusion

Ferumoxytol CMR can be used to measure plasma and total blood volume in vivo in swine, with comparable precision and accuracy to reference standard CO rebreathing methods. We design abbreviated acquisition protocols using Monte Carlo simulations and validate in vivo relative to a reference examination. These shorter acquisitions could provide estimates of blood volume in 8 min. Though the clinical value of direct blood volume measurements remains to be established, it may prove useful in the evaluation and management of heart failure and volume overload states as part of standard ferumoxytol-enhanced CMR.

Abbreviations
CA: Contrast agent; CMR: Cardiovascular magnetic resonance; CO: Carbon monoxide; COHb: Carboxyhemoglobin; CV: Coefficient of variation; Fe: Iron; Hb: Hemoglobin; Hct: Hematocrit; LV: Left ventricle/left ventricular; RC: Bland-Altman repeatability coefficient; ROI: Region of interest; RV: Right ventricle/right ventricular; SASHA: SAturation-recovery single-SHot Acquisition; SD: Standard deviation; V_{blood}: Total blood volume; V_{plasma}: Plasma blood volume

Acknowledgements
The authors thank Dr. Benjamin D. Levine of University of Texas Southwestern Medical Center for providing contemporary carbon monoxide rebreathing methodology. We thank Katherine Lucas and Shawn Kozlov from the NHLBI Division of Intramural Research Animal Surgery and Resources Core, and William H. Schenke from the NHLBI Division of Intramural Research Cardiovascular Branch for their assistance with in vivo experiments.

Funding
This work was supported by the Division of Intramural Research, National Heart, Lung, and Blood Institute, National Institutes of Health, Bethesda, Maryland, USA (Z01-HL005062, Z01-HL006061, Z1A-HL006213).

Authors' contributions

The study was conceived by RJL, TR, AZF, RR, ACW, and DAH. RR, MAA, DRM, JMK, AZF and DAH performed data acquisition and analysis. PK and HX provided pulse sequences and in-line quantification toolboxes. Manuscript was drafted by RR and DAH and revised by ACW and RJL. All authors approved the final manuscript.

Competing interests

The authors declare that they have no competing interests.

References

1. Miller WL, Mullan BP. Understanding the heterogeneity in volume overload and fluid distribution in decompensated heart failure is key to optimal volume management: role for blood volume quantitation. JACC Heart Fail. 2014;2(3):298–305.
2. Cody RJ, et al. Sodium and water balance in chronic congestive heart failure. J Clin Invest. 1986;77(5):1441–52.
3. Yancy CW, et al. 2013 ACCF/AHA guideline for the management of heart failure: executive summary: a report of the American College of Cardiology Foundation/American Heart Association Task Force on practice guidelines. Circulation. 2013;128(16):1810–52.
4. Miller WL, Mullan BP. Volume overload profiles in patients with preserved and reduced ejection fraction chronic heart failure: are there differences? A pilot study. JACC Heart Fail. 2016;4(6):453–9.
5. Feldschuh J, Enson Y. Prediction of the normal blood volume. Relation of blood volume to body habitus. Circulation. 1977;56(4 Pt 1):605–12.
6. Eisenberg S. The effect of congestive heart failure on blood volume as determined by radiochromium-tagged red cells. Circulation. 1954;10(6):902–11.
7. Kalra PR, et al. The regulation and measurement of plasma volume in heart failure. J Am Coll Cardiol. 2002;39(12):1901–8.
8. Garvican LA, et al. Carbon monoxide uptake kinetics of arterial, venous and capillary blood during CO rebreathing. Exp Physiol. 2010;95(12):1156–66.
9. Margouleff D. Blood volume determination, a nuclear medicine test in evolution. Clin Nucl Med. 2013;38(7):534–7.
10. Manzone TA, et al. Blood volume analysis: a new technique and new clinical interest reinvigorate a classic study. J Nucl Med Technol. 2007;35(2):55–63. quiz 77, 79
11. Pannek K, et al. Contrast agent derived determination of the total circulating blood volume using magnetic resonance. MAGMA. 2012;25(3):215–22.
12. Aime S, Caravan P. Biodistribution of gadolinium-based contrast agents, including gadolinium deposition. J Magn Reson Imaging. 2009;30(6):1259–67.
13. Kanda T, et al. High signal intensity in the dentate nucleus and globus pallidus on unenhanced T1-weighted MR images: relationship with increasing cumulative dose of a gadolinium-based contrast material. Radiology. 2014;270(3):834–41.
14. Errante Y, et al. Progressive increase of T1 signal intensity of the dentate nucleus on unenhanced magnetic resonance images is associated with cumulative doses of intravenously administered gadodiamide in patients with normal renal function, suggesting dechelation. Investig Radiol. 2014;49(10):685–90.
15. McDonald RJ, et al. Intracranial gadolinium deposition after contrast-enhanced MR imaging. Radiology. 2015;275(3):772–82.
16. Knobloch G, et al. Relaxivity of Ferumoxytol at 1.5 T and 3.0 T. Invest Radiol. 2018;**53**(5):257–63.
17. Reeder SB, Smith MR, Hernando D. Mathematical optimization of contrast concentration for T1-weighted spoiled gradient echo imaging. Magn Reson Med. 2016;75(4):1556–64.
18. Corot C, et al. Recent advances in iron oxide nanocrystal technology for medical imaging. Adv Drug Deliv Rev. 2006;58(14):1471–504.
19. Landry R, et al. Pharmacokinetic study of ferumoxytol: a new iron replacement therapy in normal subjects and hemodialysis patients. Am J Nephrol. 2005;25(4):400–10.
20. Bircher AJ, Auerbach M. Hypersensitivity from intravenous iron products. Immunol Allergy Clin N Am. 2014;34(3):707–23. x-xi
21. Bashir MR, et al. Emerging applications for ferumoxytol as a contrast agent in MRI. J Magn Reson Imaging. 2015;41(4):884–98.
22. Schmidt W, Prommer N. The optimised CO-rebreathing method: a new tool to determine total haemoglobin mass routinely. Eur J Appl Physiol. 2005;95(5–6):486–95.
23. Gorelov V. Theoretical value of Hufner's constant. Anaesthesia. 2004;59(1):97.
24. Holverda S, et al. Measuring lung water: ex vivo validation of multi-image gradient echo MRI. J Magn Reson Imaging. 2011;34(1):220–4.
25. Wald NJ, et al. Carbon monoxide in breath in relation to smoking and carboxyhaemoglobin levels. Thorax. 1981;36(5):366–9.
26. Kellman P, Hansen MS. T1-mapping in the heart: accuracy and precision. J Cardiovasc Magn Reson. 2014;16:2.
27. Kellman P, et al. Optimized saturation recovery protocols for T1-mapping in the heart: influence of sampling strategies on precision. J Cardiovasc Magn Reson. 2014;16:55.
28. Wolfensohn S, Lloyd M. Handbook of laboratory animal management and welfare. 4th ed. Chichester: Wiley-Blackwell. xv; 2013. p. 371.
29. Jensen WN, et al. The kinetics of iron metabolism in normal growing swine. J Exp Med. 1956;103(1):145–59.
30. Burke JD. Blood volume in mammals. Physiol Zool. 1954;27(1):1–21.
31. Hansard SL, Sauberlich HE, Comar CL. Blood volume of swine. Proc Soc Exp Biol Med. 1951;78(2):544–5.
32. Silvennoinen MJ, Kettunen MI, Kauppinen RA. Effects of hematocrit and oxygen saturation level on blood spin-lattice relaxation. Magn Reson Med. 2003;49(3):568–71.
33. Gore CJ, Hopkins WG, Burge CM. Errors of measurement for blood volume parameters: a meta-analysis. J Appl Physiol (1985). 2005;99(5):1745–58.
34. Burge CM, Skinner SL. Determination of hemoglobin mass and blood volume with CO: evaluation and application of a method. J Appl Physiol (1985). 1995;79(2):623–31.
35. Prommer N, Schmidt W. Loss of CO from the intravascular bed and its impact on the optimised CO-rebreathing method. Eur J Appl Physiol. 2007;100(4):383–91.
36. Serianni R, et al. Porcine-specific hemoglobin saturation measurements. J Appl Physiol (1985). 2003;94(2):561–6.
37. Chow K, et al. Robust free-breathing SASHA T1 mapping with high-contrast image registration. J Cardiovasc Magn Reson. 2016;18(1):47.
38. Pharmaceuticals, A., Feraheme package insert. 2018.
39. Nguyen KL, et al. MRI with ferumoxytol: a single center experience of safety across the age spectrum. J Magn Reson Imaging. 2017;45(3):804–12.
40. Ning P, et al. Hemodynamic safety and efficacy of ferumoxytol as an intravenous contrast agents in pediatric patients and young adults. Magn Reson Imaging. 2016;34(2):152–8.
41. Muehe AM, et al. Safety report of Ferumoxytol for magnetic resonance imaging in children and young adults. Investig Radiol. 2016;51(4):221–7.
42. Varallyay CG, et al. What does the boxed warning tell us? Safe practice of using Ferumoxytol as an MRI contrast agent. AJNR Am J Neuroradiol. 2017;38(7):1297–302.

Associations and prognostic significance of diffuse myocardial fibrosis by cardiovascular magnetic resonance in heart failure with preserved ejection fraction

Clotilde Roy[1,2]* (iD), Alisson Slimani[1,2], Christophe de Meester[1,2], Mihaela Amzulescu[1,2], Agnes Pasquet[1,2], David Vancraeynest[1,2], Christophe Beauloye[1,2], Jean-Louis Vanoverschelde[1,2], Bernhard L. Gerber[1,2] and Anne-Catherine Pouleur[1,2]

Abstract

Background: Increased myocardial fibrosis may play a key role in heart failure with preserved ejection fraction (HFpEF) pathophysiology. The study aim was to evaluate the presence, associations, and prognostic significance of diffuse fibrosis in HFpEF patients compared to age- and sex-matched controls.

Methods: We prospectively included 118 consecutive HFpEF patients. Diffuse myocardial fibrosis was estimated by extracellular volume (ECV) quantified by cardiovascular magnetic resonance with the modified Look-Locker inversion recovery sequence. We determined an ECV age- and sex-adjusted cutoff value (33%) in 26 controls.

Results: Mean ECV was significantly higher in HFpEF patients versus healthy controls ($32.9 \pm 4.8\%$ vs $28.2 \pm 2.4\%$, $P < 0.001$). Multivariate logistic regression showed that body mass index (BMI) (odds ratio (OR) $=0.92$ [0.86–0.98], $P = 0.011$), diabetes (OR $= 2.62$ [1.11–6.18], $P = 0.028$), and transmitral peak E wave velocity (OR $= 1.02$ [1.00–1.03], $P = 0.022$) were significantly associated with abnormal ECV value. During a median follow-up of 11 ± 6 months, the primary outcome (all-cause mortality or first heart failure hospitalization) occurred in 38 patients. In multivariate Cox regression analysis, diabetes (hazard ratio (HR) $=1.98$ [1.04; 3.76], $P = 0.038$) and hemoglobin level (HR $= 0.81$ [0.67; 0.98], $P = 0.028$) were significant predictors of composite outcome. The ECV ability to improve this model added significant prognostic information. We then developed a risk score including diabetes, hemoglobin and ECV $> 33\%$ demonstrating significant prediction of risk and validated this score in a validation cohort of 53 patients. Kaplan–Meier curves showed a significant difference according to tertiles of the probability score ($P < 0.001$).

Conclusion: Among HFpEF patients, high ECV, likely reflecting abnormal diffuse myocardial fibrosis, was associated with a higher rate of all-cause death and first HF hospitalization in short term follow up.

Keywords: Diffuse myocardial fibrosis, Cardiac magnetic resonance, Prognosis

* Correspondence: clotilderoy23@gmail.com
[1]Division of Cardiology, Department of Cardiovascular Diseases, Cliniques Universitaires St. Luc UCL, Av Hippocrate 10/2806, B-1200 Woluwé St. Lambert, Belgium
[2]Pôle de Recherche Cardiovasculaire (CARD), Institut de Recherche Expérimentale et Clinique (IREC), Université Catholique de Louvain, Brussels, Belgium

Background

Heart failure (HF) with preserved ejection fraction (HFpEF) has been established as a major cause of cardiovascular morbidity and mortality, especially among the elderly [1, 2]. Prevalence is increasing, affecting half of the patients with clinical signs of heart failure [3]. However, compared to HF with reduced ejection fraction (HFrEF), survival in HFpEF has not improved over time, and to date, no treatment effectively improves outcomes, probably because of the phenotypic heterogeneity of this syndrome [4].

Several mechanisms have been implicated in HFpEF, including advanced age and cardiovascular, metabolic, and pro-inflammatory comorbidities such as hypertension, diabetes, obesity, chronic obstructive pulmonary disease), coronary disease and renal failure [1, 4–6]. The exact pathophysiology of HFpEF remains unclear as a result of the absence of a proper animal model and the presence of numerous confounding effects. Recently, several studies using autopsies or myocardial biopsies have highlighted the key role of myocardial extracellular matrix abnormalities (fibrosis [7–9]) and myocardial structural changes such as altered cardiomyocyte function (hypertrophy [7]), systemic and coronary microvascular inflammation, and endothelial dysfunction (oxidative stress) as all being involved in myocardial stiffness and diastolic dysfunction [10, 11].

Quantification of extracellular volume fraction (ECV) by cardiovascular magnetic resonance (CMR) has recently emerged as a novel non-invasive diagnostic tool to assess myocardial fibrosis [12–14]. Recently, some studies have demonstrated the importance of diffuse or focal fibrosis estimated by biopsies or/and by CMR in patients with HFpEF [15, 16].

The aim of our study was to evaluate the presence, associations, and prognostic significance of ECV, likely reflecting diffuse myocardial fibrosis, in HFpEF patients.

Methods

Study population

Between December 2014 and October 2016, consecutive patients with suspected HFpEF were prospectively evaluated for inclusion in the study. The local ethics committee approved the study, and all patients gave written informed consent before study enrollment (Clinical trial NCT03197350).

The following criteria had to be fulfilled for study inclusion: New York Heart Association functional (NYHA) class ≥II, typical signs of HF, NT-proBNP > 350 pg/ml and/or a hospitalization for HF in the previous 12 months, left ventricular (LV) ejection fraction (EF) ≥50%, and relevant structural heart disease (LV hypertrophy/left atrial (LA) enlargement) and/or diastolic

dysfunction by echocardiography [17]. Ischemic cardiomyopathy was defined as history of myocardial infarction or revascularization by either coronary artery bypass graft surgery (CABG) or coronary artery angioplasty. Diabetes was defined as an abnormal fasting glycaemia (> 126 mg/dl) or the use of antidiabetic drugs.

The exclusion criteria were any contraindications to CMR (pacemaker, estimated glomerular filtration rate (eGFR) < 30 ml/min/m², claustrophobia), severe valvular disease, infiltrative (ie amyloidosis, sarcoidosis or hypertrophic cardiomyopathy, acute coronary syndrome in the last 30 days, chronic obstructive pulmonary disease GOLD 3 or 4, congenital heart disease, pericardial disease, atrial fibrillation with a ventricular response > 140 bpm, and severe anemia (hemoglobin < 7 g/dl). Patients with severe cognitive disorder were also excluded. One patient screened for the study was excluded due to presence of unknown cardiac amyloidosis.

Patients were compared to 26 age- and sex-matched controls without history of cardiovascular disease. Controls were recruited by advertisement in the community. All subjects underwent a full clinical exam, electrocardiogram (ECG), transthoracic echocardiography and exercise stress test, which all had to be normal prior to inclusion.

Controls and patients underwent blood sampling, complete transthoracic echocardiography and a CMR.

Echocardiography

All subjects underwent a two-dimensional (2D) transthoracic echocardiography at inclusion (iE33 system Philips Healthcare, Best, The Netherlands) with parasternal long- and short-axis views and apical views to assess LV and right ventricular (RV) systolic and diastolic functions and measurements of LA and right atrial (RA) volumes, as well as a valvular evaluation. Mitral valve inflow pattern (E and A velocity) and septal and lateral mitral valve annular velocities (e') were recorded.

RV function was assessed by systolic annular tissue velocity of the lateral tricuspid annulus, tricuspid annular plane systolic excursion (TAPSE), and tracing the RV endocardium in the apical four-chamber view in systole and diastole to obtain fractional area change (RV FAC%) [18]. All measurements were averaged over three beats in atrial fibrillation.

Cardiovascular magnetic resonance

CMR was performed using a 3 Tesla system (Ingenia, Philips Hearlthcare). Briefly, after localization of the heart, to assess LV and RV myocardial function and mass, 10–12 consecutive short-axis (SAX) images and 2-, 3-, and 4-chamber long-axis images of the LV were acquired using a cine balanced steady-state free precession sequence (bSSFP). Then, mid-ventricular short-axis modified Look-Locker inversion recovery (MOLLI) images were acquired for T1 determination using an 11-image, 18-heartbeat 3-(3)-3-(3)-5 bSSFP sequence. A total dose of 0.2 mmol/kg gadobutrol (Gadavist, Bayer Healthcare Leverkusen, Germany) was injected, and 10–15 min after contrast injection, short- and long-axis 2D inversion recovery late gadolinium enhancement (LGE) images were acquired to evaluate focal myocardial fibrosis. Finally, 15-min post-contrast, MOLLI T1 mapping was repeated in a protocol identical to that used for pre-contrast T1 mapping. The presence of LGE was visually assessed.

Pre- and post-contrast MOLLI images were processed using the open-source software MRmap v1.4 [19] under IDL. Images were corrected for respiratory motion when needed. T1 maps were exported to Osirix 5.7 (Pixmeo, Geneva, Switzerland) and pre- and post-myocardial T1 times were measured in six regions-of-interest (ROI) in the myocardium (anterior, anterolateral, inferolateral, inferior, inferoseptal, anteroseptal). We calculated the average T1 time of the six different ROIs. Areas of ischemic focal fibrosis identified by late gadolinium enhancement were excluded from the analysis. The partition coefficient lambda (λ) and ECV were then computed according to the formula [20].

End-diastolic and end-systolic LV and RV volumes as well as LV mass and presence of LGE were analyzed using the freely available software Segment 2.0 (Medviso, Lund, Sweden), as previously described. LGE was considered present if myocardial enhancement was observed on both short-axis and long-axis views. The total LGE volume was calculated by summing the LGE volume of all slices, and the ratio (%) of LGE was then calculated using the same software.

Follow-up

Patients were prospectively followed by ambulatory visits and telephone calls at 6-month intervals. Clinical and survival status was obtained by follow up visits and by phone contact with the patients, their relatives, and their physician if necessarily. The primary outcome was a composite of all-cause mortality or a first hospitalization for HF. Vital status was ascertained by medical record review. First HF hospitalization was defined as patients treated in the emergency room or admitted to a hospital and requiring intravenous diuretics. Patients had at least one symptom and 2 signs of HF (peripheral edema, pulmonary crackles, high NT-proBNP level, radiological signs of pulmonary congestion or hemodynamic evidence).

Statistical analysis

Statistical analyses were performed using SPSS version 22 (International Business Machines, Inc., Armonk, New York, USA) and STATA version 11 (Stata Corporation, College Station, Texas, USA) software. All tests were two-sided, and a $P < 0.05$ was considered statistically significant. Continuous variables were expressed as mean ± 1 SD if normally distributed or as medians (25th and 75th percentiles) if not normally distributed. Categorical variables were expressed as counts and percentages. Comparison between groups was performed using ANOVA, chi-square test, or unpaired t-tests when appropriate. We determined an ECV age and sex-adjusted cutoff value corresponding to the upper 95% confidence interval of 26 age- and sex matched volunteers (ECV ≥ 33%).

Logistic regression was performed to determine predictors of abnormal diffuse fibrosis (ECV above or below 95% confidence intervals in controls). For this purpose, after univariate comparison of the two groups, parameters with a $P < 0.10$ were proposed for inclusion in the multiple logistic regression analysis with a backward selection procedure.

Event-free survival was estimated using Kaplan–Meier methods and Cox regression analysis. All baseline and imaging variables were initially proposed for inclusion in a univariate Cox proportional hazard model. To avoid colinearity in the Cox regression model, the correlation coefficients between covariates were examined. In cases of colinearity ($r > 0.50$), only the strongest of the two covariates was proposed for inclusion into the multivariate model. After univariate Cox regression analysis, all significant variables ($P < 0.10$) were entered into a stepwise forward multivariate Cox regression model. Two different models were evaluated using ECV as either a continuous or a categorical variable (ECV ≥ 33%).

A prognostic score was established in patients followed up for at least 6 months. The accuracy of ECV, risk score or LGE to predict composite outcome were evaluated by area under the receiver operator curve (ROC) curves. This score was validated in 53 consecutive HFpEF patients recruited between October 2016 and July 2017.

Results

Baseline characteristics

Between December 2014 and October 2016, a total of 118 consecutive HFpEF patients (78 ± 8 years, 63% women) and 26 age- and sex-matched controls (76 ± 5 years, 62% women) were included in the study. The demographic, clinical, and laboratory characteristics of HFpEF patients and controls are summarized in Table 1. We observed a high prevalence of established cardiovascular risk factors in our HFpEF population; including arterial hypertension (93%), diabetes (39%), hypercholesterolemia (67%), and higher body mass index (BMI). HFpEF patients had worse renal

Table 1 Baseline characteristics of HFpEF patients and age- and sex-matched controls

	HFpEF ($n = 118$)	Healthy Controls ($n = 26$)	P
Age (years)	78 ± 8	76 ± 5	0.28
Body mass index (kg/m^2)	29 ± 7	25 ± 4	0.011
Female (n, %)	74 (63)	16 (62)	0.91
Heart rate (bpm)	73 ± 14	67 ± 9	0.040
Systolic blood pressure (mmHg)	136 ± 21	144 ± 22	0.069
Diastolic blood pressure (mmHg)	75 ± 13	82 ± 12	0.014
NYHA functional class III-IV (n, %)	53 (45)	0 (0)	< 0.001
Medical history			
Atrial fibrillation (n, %)	73 (62)	0 (0)	< 0.001
Ischemic cardiomyopathy (n, %)	39 (33)	0 (0)	< 0.001
Previous valvular surgery (n, %)	12 (10)	0 (0)	0.12
Previous heart failure episode	84 (71)	0 (0)	< 0.001
Cardiovascular risk factors			
Smoking (n, %)	47 (40)	6 (23)	0.10
Hypertension (n, %)	109 (93)	16 (62)	< 0.001
Diabetes (n, %)	46 (39)	1 (4)	< 0.001
Family history of cardiovascular disease (n, %)	24 (21)	3 (12)	0.40
Hypercholesterolemia (n, %)	78 (67)	23 (88)	0.027
Medication			
Diuretics other than MRA (n, %)	94 (80)	2 (8)	< 0.001
MRA (n, %)	23 (19)	0 (0)	0.01
Beta-blockers (n, %)	76 (64)	3 (12)	< 0.001
ACE-I or ARB (n, %)	76 (64)	9 (35)	0.005
Statins (n, %)	54 (46)	5 (19)	0.01
Laboratory characteristics			
eGFR (ml/min/1.73 m^2)	59 ± 23	70 ± 18	0.018
Hemoglobin (g/dl)	11.8 ± 1.9	14.0 ± 1.3	< 0.001
NT-proBNP (pg/ml)	1747 [374; 34,306] £	111 [29; 393] £	0.001

£ Median [min; max]

ACE-I angiotensin converting enzyme inhibitor, *ARB* angiotensin receptor blocker, *eGFR* estimated glomerular filtration rate; MRA:

function and lower hemoglobin and hematocrit levels than healthy controls, and 62% of patients had a history of atrial fibrillation.

Table 2 summarizes echocardiographic and CMR measurements. As expected, compared to age- and sex-matched healthy controls, HFpEF patients had higher E/e' ratio, higher indexed LA and RA volumes, higher RV/RA gradient, and worse RV function as evaluated by TAPSE and FAC. Prevalence of pulmonary hypertension (RV–RA gradient > 35 mmHg) in our population was 39% ($n = 46$). By CMR, HFpEF patients had a slightly lower LVEF and higher indexed LV mass than age- and sex-matched healthy controls. Twenty-six HFpEF patients had LGE (8 = focal spots, 18 = ischemic pattern). When present, the average percentage of LGE was 5.5 ± 2.9%.

ECV was significantly higher in HFpEF patients than in the healthy control group (Fig. 1). Forty-nine (42%) HFpEF patients had significant diffuse fibrosis based on the ECV cutoff (defined as ≥33%). Sixteen (14%) HFpEF patients had impaired RV systolic function defined as RVEF≤45% by CMR. HFpEF patients with RV dysfunction had higher ECV (36 ± 6% vs. 32 ± 4%, $P < 0.001$), higher indexed LA volume (81 ± 26 ml/m^2 vs. 64 ± 28 ml/m^2, $P = 0.03$), lower LVEF (59 ± 7% vs. 64 ± 8%, $P = 0.010$), lower TAPSE (14 ± 5 mm vs. 19 ± 5 mm, $P < 0.001$), lower FAC (32 ± 6% vs. 43 ± 8%, $P < 0.001$), and higher septal E/e' ratio (24 ± 9 vs. 17 ± 7, $P = 0.001$).

Diabetic HFpEF patients were younger (75 ± 9 vs. 80 ± 7 years, $P = 0.002$), had a higher body mass index (BMI) (31.2 ± 6.9 vs. 27.3 ± 6.1, $P = 0.002$), a lower atrial fibrillation

Table 2 Echocardiographic and CMR parameters of HFpEF patients and age- and sex-matched controls

	HFpEF (n = 118)	Healthy Controls (n = 26)	P
Echocardiography			
LV ejection fraction (%)	64 ± 7	64 ± 5	0.93
Transmitral peak E velocity max (m/s)	91 ± 29	55 ± 9	< 0.001
Transmitral E deceleration time (ms)	160 ± 62	197 ± 35	0.004
E/e' septal ratio	18.1 ± 7.3	9.4 ± 1.7	< 0.001
RV/RA gradient (mmHg)	32 ± 11	19 ± 5	< 0.001
RA volume index (ml/m^2)	35 ± 20	18 ± 5	< 0.001
RV fractional area change (%)	41 ± 9	47 ± 8	0.008
RV FAC ≤ 35% (n, %)	32 (27)	0 (0)	< 0.001
TAPSE (mm)	19 ± 5	24 ± 4	< 0.001
TAPSE≤16 mm (n, %)	47 (40)	1 (4)	< 0.001
Cardiac MR			
LVM index (g/m^2)	68 ± 15	58 ± 12	0.003
LV EDV index (ml/m^2)	73 ± 18	63 ± 11	0.006
LVEF (%)	63 ± 8	67 ± 5	0.024
RV EDV index (ml/m^2)	82 ± 28	67 ± 11	0.005
RVEF (%)	57 ± 9	60 ± 6	0.052
RVEF≤45% (n, %)	16 (14)	2 (8)	0.41
LV mass/volume ratio	0.96 ± 0.20	0.94 ± 0.19	0.71
LA volume index (ml)	66 ± 29	32 ± 10	< 0.001
Myocardium native T1 time (ms)	1109 ± 82	1144 ± 47	0.038
Myocardium post contrast T1 time (ms)	353 ± 56	381 ± 64	0,028
ECV (%)	32.9 ± 4.8	28.2 ± 2.4	< 0.001
Lambda coefficient	0.52 ± 0.08	0.49 ± 0.05	0.051
ECV ≥ 33% (n, %)	49 (42)	0 (0)	< 0.001
Late gadolinium enhancement (n, %)	26 (22)	0 (0)	0.022

Values are mean ± SD. *LA* left atrium, *LV* left ventricle, *RV* right ventricle, *RA* right atrium, *BMI* body mass index
TAPSE tricuspid annular plane systolic excursion, *LVM* left ventricular mass, *EF* ejection fraction, *EDV* end-diastolic volume, *ECV* extracellular volume

history rate (48% vs. 71%, $P = 0.012$), and more known ischemic cardiomyopathy (43% vs. 26%, $P = 0.055$) than non-diabetic HFpEF patients. Echocardiographic and CMR parameters were quite similar except for a trend to higher indexed LV mass in diabetics (71.0 ± 12.6 vs. 65.6 ± 16.1 g/m^2, $P = 0.056$). Diabetic HFpEF patients presented more frequently ECV ≥33% than non-diabetic patients (52% vs. 35%, $P = 0.061$).

Predictors of high ECV

Table 3 compares HFpEF patients with high and low ECV values. ECV and the lambda coefficient were different between the two groups, demonstrating that the difference in ECV was not solely the result of a significant difference in hematocrit level..

HFpEF patients with ECV ≥ 33% had lower BMI, lower hematocrit, higher prevalence of diabetes, higher transmitral peak E wave velocity and higher E/e' ratio. A higher proportion of HFpEF patients with ECV ≥ 33%

had an impaired RV systolic function (CMR RVEF ≤45% (20% vs. 9%, $P = 0.073$). There were no differences in NT-proBNP and LGE in HFpEF patients between the two groups.

In multivariate logistic regression, BMI (OR = 0.92 [0.86–0.98], $P = 0.011$), presence of diabetes (OR = 2.62 [1.11–6.18], $P = 0.028$), and higher transmitral peak E wave velocity (OR = 1.02 [1.00–1.03], $P = 0.022$) were significantly associated with high ECV value.

Outcomes

During a mean follow-up of 11 ± 6 months, we observed 43 events (11 deaths and 32 hospitalizations for HF) (Fig. 2a). The primary outcome (all-cause mortality or first hospitalization for HF) occurred in 38 patients (32%). Only one patient was lost to follow up. The percentage of combined event at 18 months in our population was 50%.

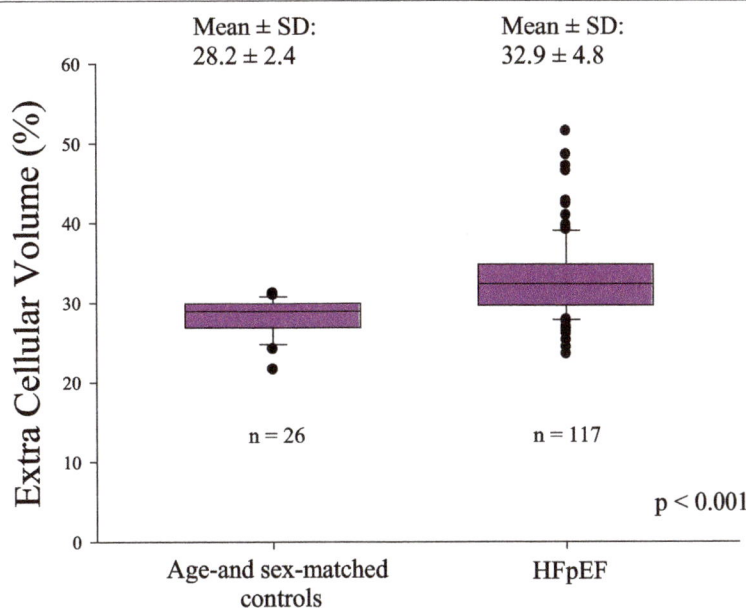

Fig. 1 Extracellular volume fraction (ECV) values between age- and sex-matched healthy controls and heart failure with preserved ejection fraction (HFpEF) patients

In univariate Cox regression analysis, lower eGFR, lower hemoglobin, presence of diabetes, higher transmitral E wave velocity, and ECV ≥ 33% were significant predictors of the composite outcome (Table 4). In multivariate Cox regression analysis, only the presence of diabetes (HR = 1.98 [1.04; 3.76], $P = 0.038$) and hemoglobin level (HR = 0.81 [0.67; 0.98], $P = 0.028$) were significantly associated with the composite outcome (Table 5). The ability of either ECV as a continuous variable or ECV as a categorical variable (ECV > 33%) to improve this model was then tested and added significant prognostic information (χ^2 4.33, $P = 0.037$ and χ^2 4.46, $P = 0.035$, respectively), as opposed to transmitral peak E wave velocity and eGFR (χ^2 3.00, $p = 0.083$ and χ^2 2.86, $p = 0.091$ respectively). The ability of the model to discriminate outcome was good with an area under the curve (AUC) of 0.76. Kaplan–Meier event-free survival curves showed that HFpEF patients with ECV ≥ 33% had poorer one-year prognosis than those with ECV < 33% (56 ± 8% vs 82 ± 5%, $P = 0.001$, Fig. 2b).

A prognostic score was established based on the significant predictors of composite outcome in patients with at least 6 months of follow up ($n = 97$). Diabetes, hemoglobin, and ECV > 33% were thus used to build the risk score. ROC curves showed a better discrimination with the prognostic score and ECV (c-statistic of 0,76 and 0,67 respectively) compared to LGE (c statistic 0,51) (Additional file 1). In the validation cohort of 53 patients, 2 deaths and 9 HF hospitalizations were observed during a mean follow up of 11 ± 5 months.

Our risk score based on the initial cohort and applied in the validation cohort had an AUC of 0.71 to predict primary outcome.

Discussion

We sought to evaluate the presence, associations, and prognostic significance of quantification of ECV using 3 T CMR in a prospective and well-characterized HFpEF cohort. The salient findings of our study are as follows. Mean ECV by T1-mapping was significantly higher in HFpEF patients than in age-matched healthy controls; ECV in HFpEF patients was related to the presence of anemia and diabetes and associated with altered diastolic function by echocardiography and lower CMR RV systolic function; and finally, increased ECV and the presence of anemia and diabetes were independent risk markers of short-term poor prognosis with increased rehospitalization or all-cause mortality in HFpEF.

HFpEF

HFpEF is a heterogeneous disease observed mainly in the aging population. We and others demonstrated that aging is associated with structural changes in the heart, such as alterations of diastolic function, increased stiffening, LV and atrial remodeling characterized by decreased LV and RV volumes and mass, increased atrial volumes, and an increase in ECV [21]. It is crucial to separate age-related changes from disease-related processes associated with HFpEF. Therefore, we compared our population to carefully

Table 3 Baseline characteristics of HFpEF patients with ECV < or ≥ 33%

	HFpEF with ECV < 33% (n = 68)	HFpEF with ECV ≥ 33% (n = 49)	P
Baseline characteristics			
Age (years)	78 ± 8	79 ± 9	0.49
Body mass index (kg/m²)	30 ± 7	28 ± 7	0.082
Female (n, %)	41 (60)	33 (67)	0.44
Systolic blood pressure (mmHg)	137 ± 21	135 ± 21	0.54
Diastolic blood pressure (mmHg)	76 ± 12	74 ± 14	0.45
NYHA functional class III-IV (n, %)	28 (41)	24 (49)	0.57
Laboratory characteristics			
eGFR (ml/min/1.73 m²)	58 ± 20	60 ± 28	0.56
Hemoglobin (g/dl)	12.1 ± 1.8	11.3 ± 2.0	0.020
NT-proBNP (pg/ml)	1584[432; 34,306] £	1889 [374; 27,736] £	0.40
Medical history			
Atrial fibrillation (n, %)	42 (62)	30 (61)	0.90
Ischemic cardiomyopathy (n, %)	23 (34)	16 (33)	0.94
Previous valvular surgery (n, %)	8 (12)	4 (8)	0.76
Cardiovascular risk factors			
Smoking (n, %)	29 (43)	18 (37)	0.52
Hypertension (n, %)	64 (94)	44 (92)	0.37
Diabetes (n, %)	22 (33)	24 (49)	0.069
Family history of cardiovascular disease (n, %)	14 (21)	10 (20)	0.98
Hypercholesterolemia (n, %)	47 (70)	30 (61)	0.29
Echocardiography			
Left ventricular ejection fraction (%)	64 ± 7	63 ± 8	0.66
Transmitral peak E velocity max (m/s)	86 ± 29	98 ± 26	0.025
Transmitral E deceleration time (ms)	155 ± 62	167 ± 63	0.35
E/e' septal ratio	16 ± 6	20 ± 8	0.004
RV/RA gradient (mmHg)	31 ± 11	34 ± 11	0.13
RA volume index (ml/m²)	34 ± 19	36 ± 22	0.75
RV fractional area change (%)	42 ± 8	42 ± 11	0.84
TAPSE (mm)	19 ± 5	18 ± 5	0.11
Cardiac MR			
LVM index (g/m²)	67 ± 14	66 ± 16	0.81
LV EDV index (ml/m²)	71 ± 16	72 ± 20	0.58
LVEF (%)	63 ± 8	63 ± 8	0.997
RV EDV index (ml/m²)	77 ± 22	86 ± 32	0.097
RVEF (%)	56 ± 7	56 ± 10	0.98
RVEF≤45% (n, %)	6 (9)	10 (20)	0.073
LV mass/volume ratio	0.97 ± 0.21	0.94 ± 0.19	0.43
LA volume index (ml/m²)	65 ± 29	68 ± 28	0.68
Myocardium native T1 time (ms)	1109 ± 83	1107 ± 82	0.88
Myocardium post contrast T1 time (ms)	362 ± 58	340 ± 52	0.036
ECV (%)	30.0 ± 2.2	37.0 ± 4.3	< 0.001
Lambda coefficient	0.48 ± 0.05	0.57 ± 0.08	< 0.001
Late gadolinium enhancement	13 (19)	13 (28)	0.29

Values are mean ± SD. £: median (min, max); *LA* left atrium, *LV* left ventricle, *RV* right ventricle, *RA* right atrium, *BMI* body mass index, *TAPSE* tricuspid annular plane systolic excursion, *LVM* left ventricular mass, *EF* ejection fraction, *EDV* end-diastolic volume, *ECV* extracellular volume

age- and sex-matched healthy subjects, allowing for a better understanding of these two processes. As compared to previous work [22, 23], our HFpEF population was older and had more comorbidities, probably reflecting a less selected population but a more advanced stage because patients were highly symptomatic with high NT-proBNP levels (45% NYHA III/IV). Overall, and in accordance with prior reports, we observed relatively poor outcomes with a high rehospitalization rate and high mortality despite optimal medical treatment.

Role of extracellular matrix abnormalities in HFpEF

Extracellular matrix abnormalities causing LV stiffening and secondary LV diastolic dysfunction are probably among the main potential pathophysiologic mechanisms involved in HFpEF. Previous studies using endomyocardial biopsies or autopsies have already shown that the extent of fibrosis is higher in HFpEF patients than in controls [7].Studies have demonstrated that ECV closely correlates with histologically determined diffuse interstitial fibrosis, providing a non-invasive estimation for its quantification; however, only a few studies have

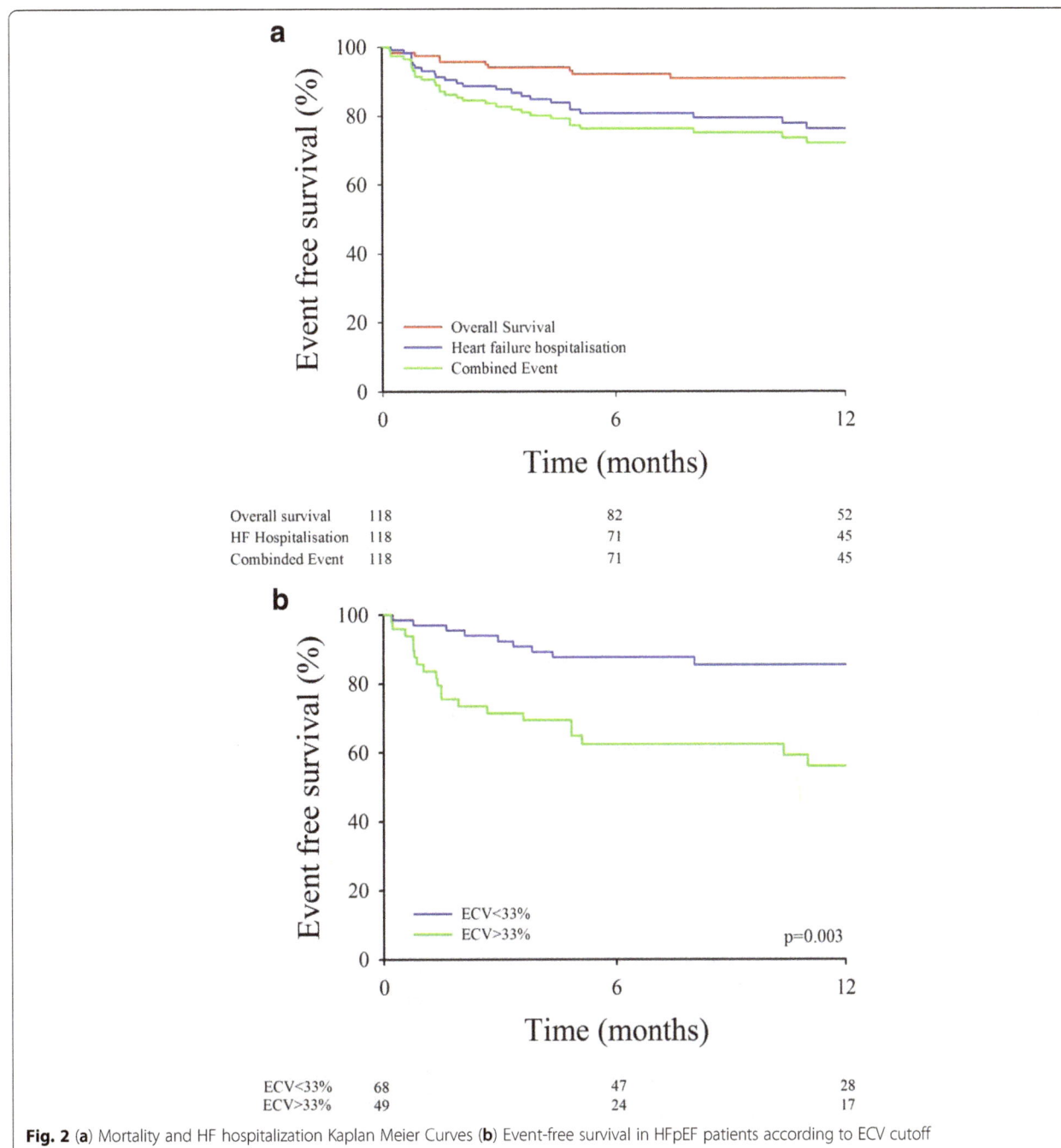

Fig. 2 (a) Mortality and HF hospitalization Kaplan Meier Curves (b) Event-free survival in HFpEF patients according to ECV cutoff

Table 4 Univariate Cox analysis for composite event (death and first HF)

	Composite outcome (death or first HF)	
	HR [95%IC]	P
Age (years)	1.00 [0.96; 1.04]	0.96
Body surface area (m^2)	0.29 [0.08; 1.08]	0.065
Female (n, %)	1.63 [0.79; 3.36]	0.19
Heart rate (bpm)	1.02 [1.00; 1.04]	0.086
Systolic blood pressure (mmHg)	0.99 [0.97; 1.01]	0.18
Diastolic blood pressure (mmHg)	0.97 [0.95; 1.00]	0.064
NYHA functional class III-IV	1.18 [0.62; 2.26]	0.62
Laboratory characteristics		
eGFR (ml/min/1.73 m^2)	0.98 [0.96; 0.99]	0.040
Hemoglobin (g/dl)	0.80 [0.66; 0.96]	0.020
NT-proBNP (pg/ml)	1.12 [0.82; 1.55]	0.48
Medical history		
Atrial fibrillation (n, %)	1.15 [0.58; 2.25]	0.69
Ischemic cardiomyopathy (n, %)	1.03 [0.52; 2.04]	0.94
Previous valvular surgery (n, %)	1.16 [0.35; 3.83]	0.81
Previous heart failure episode	1.17 [0.50; 2.73]	0.72
Cardiovascular risk factors		
Smoking (n, %)	0.99 [0.51; 1.92]	0.98
Hypertension (n, %)	0.81 [0.25; 2.68]	0.73
Diabetes (n, %)	2.15 [1.13; 4.08]	0.020
Family history of cardiovascular disease (n, %)	0.97 [0.45; 2.12]	0.94
Hypercholesterolemia (n, %)	1.04 [0.51; 2.11]	0.91
Echocardiography		
LV ejection fraction (%)	1.03 [0.98; 1.08]	0.20
Transmitral peak E velocity max (m/s)	1.01 [1.00; 1.02]	0.025
E/e' septal ratio	1.02 [0.98; 1.06]	0.42
RV/RA gradient (mmHg)	1.01 [0.98; 1.04]	0.60
RA volume index (ml/m^2)	1.00 [0.99; 1.02]	0.53
RV fractional area change (%)	2.01 [0.06; 73.25]	0.70
TAPSE (mm)	0.94 [0.89; 1.00]	0.064
Cardiac MR		
LVM index (g/m^2)	0.99 [0.98; 1.01]	0.62
LV EDV index (ml/m^2)	0.99 [0.98; 1.01]	0.58
LVEF (%)	1.03 [0.99; 1.07]	0.19
RV EDV index (ml/m^2)	1.00 [0.99; 1.01]	0.59
RVEF (%)	0.99 [0.96; 1.04]	0.81
LV mass/volume ratio	1.24 [0.06; 25.3]	0.89
LA volume index (ml/m^2)	1.00 [0.98; 1.02]	0.87
Myocardium native T1 (ms)	1.01 [0.99; 1.01]	0.23
ECV (%)	1.07 [1.01; 1.12]	0.015
ECV ≥ 33%	2.62 [1.35; 5.09]	0.005
LGE (%)	1.08 [0.96; 1.21]	0.22

Table 5 Multivariate Cox analysis for event-free survival in HFpEF

	HR ([95% CI]	P	X² to remove	X² to enter	P
Diabetes mellitus	1.98 [1.04; 3.76]	0.038	4.327		
Hemoglobin	0.81 [0.67; 0.98]	0.028	4.961		
Mean E wave				3.00	0.083
eGFR				2.86	0.091
Model 1: ECV (continuous variable)	1.07 [1.00; 1.13]			4.33	0.037
Model 2: ECV 33%	2.00 [1.00; 4.03]			4.46	0.035

CI confidence interval

evaluated ECV in HFpEF patients [15, 22, 23]. Our findings confirm that high ECV likely reflecting diffuse extracellular matrix abnormalities, a potential surrogate for myocardial fibrosis, may play a key role in the pathophysiology of HFpEF. Indeed, ECV was significantly increased relative to the age-matched population, yet only 42% of our HFpEF patients had high ECV, suggesting that other mechanisms are involved in HFpEF pathophysiology. Assessment of ECV allows for a direct evaluation of the extracellular space, reflecting interstitial disease. However, it lacks the ability to provide information about the relative contribution of edema, fibrosis, inflammation, or deposition of other extracellular proteins such as amyloid [13] and therefore may not allow for a full understanding of the pathophysiological mechanisms underlying HFpEF. In our study, low BMI, diabetes, and high transmitral peak E wave velocity were significant determinants of high ECV. High transmitral peak E wave velocity is a good surrogate for high filling pressures, and it could be easily anticipated as an important determinant of fibrosis.

Surprisingly, we observed that a higher BMI was associated with lower ECV values, suggesting that diffuse fibrosis is not the sole mechanism involved in HFpEF pathogenesis in the obese population. Indeed, adiposity-induced inflammation has considerable adverse effects, including endothelial dysfunction, capillary rarefaction, and mitochondrial dysfunction in both the cardiac and systemic beds [24].

Diabetic cardiomyopathy could be considered as a form of HFpEF, explaining the increased incidence of HF in the diabetic population [25]. This cardiomyopathy is characterized by insulin resistance and a loss of metabolic flexibility, and subsequently by cardiomyocyte hypertrophy and increased fibrosis. Increased reactive oxygen species production is one of the major pathophysiological mechanisms triggered by hyperglycemia and high free fatty acid level.

Finally, native T1 time was surprisingly significantly lower in HFpEF patients than in healthy controls. We can only speculate on the explanation. Possible explanation could be that HFpEF patients have slightly higher intramyocadial iron concentration or more intramyocardial fat, particularly related to presence of diabetes.

Prognosis in HFpEF

As demonstrated in our study, the prognosis of HFpEF patients is still quite poor. Many studies have compared HFpEF and HFrEF prognosis and demonstrated the same or even a worse mortality and morbidity rate [26, 27] for HFpEF than for HFrEF. Our study identified high ECV, hemoglobin and diabetes as independent prognostic predictors for the short-term composite outcome. This result is in accordance with observations by Redfield et al. [28], who showed that profibrotic pathways may contribute to adverse outcomes in diabetic HFpEF patients. However, in our work, presence of LGE was not a significant predictor of the composite outcome (HR = 1.08 [0.96; 1.21], p = 0.22) in univariate analysis, in contrast to another recent study [16]. A potential explanation was that patients in this pre cited study had significantly higher percentage of LGE quantification (13 ± 8%), as opposed to our population where only 26 patients had small amounts of LGE (5.5 ± 2.9%).

The prognostic role of anemia has already been demonstrated in large HFpEF studies (SENIOR [29], MAGGIC [30], ARIC [26], respectively).

Clinical implications

Because HFpEF syndrome is a heterogeneous disease, better characterization of HFpEF phenotypes based on clinical presentation and biological and/or imaging data is crucial for better designing therapies [31]. In particular, the identification of anemia is relevant because its association with composite outcome could suggest a potential beneficial effect of iron-replacement therapy in HFpEF patients, and this hypothesis could be evaluated in larger randomized trials. Our study contributes to a better understanding of the heterogeneous and complicated nature of HFpEF [32]. Larger studies are needed to confirm our findings and prospectively validate our risk markers in other populations.

Study limitations

Our study is a single-center study of relatively small size, and its power is limited by a modest number of events, which bears a risk of overfitting in multivariable models. Yet our study was prospective, and the echocardiographic and CMR imaging, as well as biomarker sampling, were standardized. Because we excluded patients with contraindications to CMR, in particular renal failure, our conclusions cannot be generalized to all patients with HFpEF. Although we validated ECV assessment by T1 mapping in other populations against histopathology [15] with reasonably good correlation, in this fragile elderly population, we did not sample cardiac biopsies and thus could not ascertain the pathophysiological correlates of increased ECV in our patients. Another limitation is the lack of others SAX slices for the MOLLI acquisition to have a better idea of ECV value in the rest of the myocardium.

Focal fibrosis is probably also very important in HFpEF patients but only 26 patients had LGE.

Moreover, we interpreted CMR data from patients in atrial fibrillation but the impact of atrial fibrillation on MOLLI sequences has not been fully studied yet.

In addition, our study was performed mainly in a white population, and findings might differ in other groups, particularly in African American or other populations. Finally, the presence of different comorbidities is an important confounding factor in HFpEF. Thus, findings might be affected by selection criteria and presence of comorbidities in such HFpEF populations.

Conclusions

Among HFpEF patients, high ECV likely reflecting increased myocardial fibrosis was associated with BMI, diabetes, and transmitral peak E wave velocity. Among HFpEF patients, abnormal diffuse myocardial fibrosis estimated by ECV was associated with a higher rate of all-cause death and first HF hospitalization in the short term follow up.

Abbreviations

2D: Two dimensional; AUC: Area under the curve; BMI: Body mass index; bSSFP: Balanced steady state free precession; CMR: Cardiovascular magnetic resonance; ECG: Electrocardiogram; ECV: Extracellular volume fraction; EDV: End-diastolic volume; EF: Ejection fraction; eGFR: Estimated glomerular filtration rate; ESV: End-systolic volume; FAC: Fractional area change; HF: Heart failure; HFpEF: Heart failure with preserved ejection fraction; HFrEF: Heart failure with reduced ejection fraction; LA: Left atrium/left atrial; LV: Left ventricle/left ventricular; LVM: Left ventricular mass; MOLLI: Modified Look-Locker inversion recovery; NYHA: New York Heart Association; RA: Right atrium/right atrial; ROC: Receiver operator curve; ROI: Region-of-interest; RV: Right ventricle/right ventricular; SAX: Short axis; TAPSE: Tricuspid annular plane systolic excursion

Funding

This work was funded by a grant of the Fondation Nationale de la Recherche Scientifique of the Belgian Government (FRMS CDR 23597851). ACP is sponsored by a Post-doctorate Clinical Master Specialist of the Fondation Nationale de la Recherche Scientifique of the Belgian Government (FRSM: SPD 10844948). Dr. Roy is supported by Fondation Damman and Fondation Saint Luc for her fellowship. This work was funded by an unrestricted grant from Astra Zeneca.

Authors' contributions

CR conceived the study, recruited patients, acquired and analysed CMR data and drafted the manuscript. AS and CDM acquired CMR data and performed statistical analysis. MA, BG and ACP participated in study coordination and acquired and analysed MR studies. JLVO, AP, DVC, CB and ACP participated in design and coordination of the study. ACP conceived the study, participated in its design and coordination and helped to draft the manuscript. All authors read and approved the final manuscript.

Competing interests

The Cliniques St. Luc UCL has a master clinical research agreement with Philips Medical Instruments, and the MOLLI patch was supplied by Philips Healthcare under the terms of this agreement. The authors declare that they have no competing interests.

References

1. Kanwar M, Walter C, Clarke M, Patarroyo-Aponte M. Targeting heart failure with preserved ejection fraction: current status and future prospects. Vasc Health Risk Manag. 2016;12:129–41.
2. Gerber Y, Weston SA, Redfield MM, Chamberlain AM, Manemann SM, Jiang R, Killian JM, Roger VL. A contemporary appraisal of the heart failure epidemic in Olmsted County, Minnesota, 2000 to 2010. JAMA Intern Med. 2015;175:996–1004.
3. Steinberg BA, Zhao X, Heidenreich PA, Peterson ED, Bhatt DL, Cannon CP, Hernandez AF, Fonarow GC. Trends in patients hospitalized with heart failure and preserved left ventricular ejection fraction: prevalence, therapies, and outcomes. Circulation. 2012;126:65–75.
4. Paulus WJ, Tschope C. A novel paradigm for heart failure with preserved ejection fraction: comorbidities drive myocardial dysfunction and remodeling through coronary microvascular endothelial inflammation. J Am Coll Cardiol. 2013;62:263–71.
5. Mohammed SF, Borlaug BA, Roger VL, Mirzoyev SA, Rodeheffer RJ, Chirinos JA, Redfield MM. Comorbidity and ventricular and vascular structure and function in heart failure with preserved ejection fraction: a community-based study. Circ Heart Fail. 2012;5:710–9.
6. Fang JC. Heart failure with preserved ejection fraction: a kidney disorder? Circulation. 2016;134:435–7.
7. Mohammed SF, Hussain S, Mirzoyev SA, Edwards WD, Maleszewski JJ, Redfield MM. Coronary microvascular rarefaction and myocardial fibrosis in heart failure with preserved ejection fraction. Circulation. 2015;131:550–9.
8. Campbell KS, Sorrell VL. Cell- and molecular-level mechanisms contributing to diastolic dysfunction in HFpEF. J Appl Physiol (1985). 2015;119:1228–32.
9. Borlaug BA, Lam CS, Roger VL, Rodeheffer RJ, Redfield MM. Contractility and ventricular systolic stiffening in hypertensive heart disease insights into the pathogenesis of heart failure with preserved ejection fraction. J Am Coll Cardiol. 2009;54:410–8.
10. van Heerebeek L, Paulus WJ. Understanding heart failure with preserved ejection fraction: where are we today? Neth Heart J. 2016;24:227–36.
11. Mohammed SF, Majure DT, Redfield MM. Zooming in on the microvasculature in heart failure with preserved ejection fraction. Circ Heart Fail. 2016;9(7):e003272. https://doi.org/10.1161/CIRCHEARTFAILURE.116. 003272.
12. Flett AS, Hayward MP, Ashworth MT, Hansen MS, Taylor AM, Elliott PM, McGregor C, Moon JC. Equilibrium contrast cardiovascular magnetic resonance for the measurement of diffuse myocardial fibrosis: preliminary validation in humans. Circulation. 2010;122:138–44.
13. Moon JC, Messroghli DR, Kellman P, Piechnik SK, Robson MD, Ugander M, Gatehouse PD, Arai AE, Friedrich MG, Neubauer S, Schulz-Menger J, Schelbert EB. Myocardial T1 mapping and extracellular volume quantification: a Society for Cardiovascular Magnetic Resonance (SCMR) and

CMR working Group of the European Society of cardiology consensus statement. J Cardiovasc Magn Reson. 2013;15:92.

14. de Meester de Ravenstein C, Bouzin C, Lazam S, Boulif J, Amzulescu M, Melchior J, Pasquet A, Vancraeynest D, Pouleur AC, Vanoverschelde JL, Gerber BL. Histological validation of measurement of diffuse interstitial myocardial fibrosis by myocardial extravascular volume fraction from modified look-locker imaging (MOLLI) T1 mapping at 3 T. J Cardiovasc Magn Reson. 2015;17:48.

15. Duca F, Kammerlander AA, Zotter-Tufaro C, Aschauer S, Schwaiger ML, Marzluf BA, Bonderman D, Mascherbauer J. Interstitial fibrosis, functional status, and outcomes in heart failure with preserved ejection fraction: insights from a prospective cardiac magnetic resonance imaging study. Circ Cardiovasc Imaging. 2016;9

16. Kato S, Saito N, Kirigaya H, Gyotoku D, Iinuma N, Kusakawa Y, Iguchi K, Nakachi T, Fukui K, Futaki M, Iwasawa T, Taguri M, Kimura K, Umemura S. Prognostic significance of quantitative assessment of focal myocardial fibrosis in patients with heart failure with preserved ejection fraction. Int J Cardiol. 2015;191:314–9.

17. Ponikowski P, Voors AA, Anker SD. 2016 ESC guidelines for the diagnosis and treatment of acute and chronic heart failureThe task force for the diagnosis and treatment of acute and chronic heart failure of the European Society of Cardiology (ESC) developed with the special contribution of the heart failure association (HFA) of the ESC. Eur Heart J. 2016;37:2129–200.

18. Rudski LG, Lai WW, Afilalo J, Hua L, Handschumacher MD, Chandrasekaran K, Solomon SD, Louie EK, Schiller NB. Guidelines for the echocardiographic assessment of the right heart in adults: a report from the American Society of Echocardiography endorsed by the European Association of Echocardiography, a registered branch of the European Society of Cardiology, and the Canadian Society of Echocardiography. J Am Soc Echocardiogr. 2010, 23:685–713. quiz 786–8

19. Messroghli DR, Rudolph A, Abdel-Aty H, Wassmuth R, Kuhne T, Dietz R, Schulz-Menger J. An open-source software tool for the generation of relaxation time maps in magnetic resonance imaging. BMC Med Imaging. 2010;10:16.

20. Kellman P, Wilson JR, Xue H, Ugander M, Arai AE. Extracellular volume fraction mapping in the myocardium, part 1: evaluation of an automated method. J Cardiovasc Magn Reson. 2012;14:63.

21. Loffredo FS, Nikolova AP, Pancoast JR, Lee RT. Heart failure with preserved ejection fraction: molecular pathways of the aging myocardium. Circ Res. 2014;115:97–107.

22. Rommel KP, von Roeder M, Latuscynski K, Oberueck C, Blazek S, Fengler K, Besler C, Sandri M, Lucke C, Gutberlet M, Linke A, Schuler G, Lurz P. Extracellular volume fraction for characterization of patients with heart failure and preserved ejection fraction. J Am Coll Cardiol. 2016;67:1815–25.

23. Su MY, Lin LY, Tseng YH, Chang CC, Wu CK, Lin JL, Tseng WY. CMR-verified diffuse myocardial fibrosis is associated with diastolic dysfunction in HFpEF. JACC Cardiovasc Imaging. 2014;7:991–7.

24. Kitzman DW, Shah SJ. The HFpEF obesity phenotype: the elephant in the room. J Am Coll Cardiol. 2016;68:200–3.

25. From AM, Scott CG, Chen HH. The development of heart failure in patients with diabetes mellitus and pre-clinical diastolic dysfunction a population-based study. J Am Coll Cardiol. 2010;55:300–5.

26. Caughey MC, Avery CL, Ni H, Solomon SD, Matsushita K, Wruck LM, Rosamond WD, Loehr LR. Outcomes of patients with anemia and acute decompensated heart failure with preserved versus reduced ejection fraction (from the ARIC study community surveillance). Am J Cardiol. 2014;114:1850–4.

27. Gupta DK, Shah AM, Castagno D, Takeuchi M, Loehr LR, Fox ER, Butler KR, Mosley TH, Kitzman DW, Solomon SD. Heart failure with preserved ejection fraction in African Americans: the ARIC (atherosclerosis risk in communities) study. JACC Heart Fail. 2013;1:156–63.

28. Lindman BR, Davila-Roman VG, Mann DL, McNulty S, Semigran MJ, Lewis GD, de las Fuentes L, Joseph SM, Vader J, Hernandez AF, Redfield MM. Cardiovascular phenotype in HFpEF patients with or without diabetes: a RELAX trial ancillary study. J Am Coll Cardiol. 2014;64:541–9.

29. von Haehling S, van Veldhuisen DJ, Roughton M, Babalis D, de Boer RA, Coats AJ, Manzano L, Flather M, Anker SD. Anaemia among patients with heart failure and preserved or reduced ejection fraction: results from the SENIORS study. Eur J Heart Fail. 2011;13:656–63.

30. Berry C, Poppe KK, Gamble GD, Earle NJ, Ezekowitz JA, Squire IB, McMurray JJ, McAlister FA, Komajda M, Swedberg K, Maggioni AP, Ahmed A, Whalley GA, Doughty RN, Tarantini L. Prognostic significance of anaemia in patients with heart failure with preserved and reduced ejection fraction: results from the MAGGIC individual patient data meta-analysis. QJM. 2016;109:377–82.

31. Vazir A, Solomon SD. Management strategies for heart failure with preserved ejection fraction. Heart Fail Clin. 2014;10:591–8.

32. Shah SJ, Katz DH, Selvaraj S, Burke MA, Yancy CW, Gheorghiade M, Bonow RO, Huang CC, Deo RC. Phenomapping for novel classification of heart failure with preserved ejection fraction. Circulation. 2015;131:269–79.

23

Quantitative myocardial first-pass cardiovascular magnetic resonance perfusion imaging using hyperpolarized [1-^{13}C] pyruvate

Maximilian Fuetterer[1], Julia Busch[1], Julia Traechtler[1], Patrick Wespi[1], Sophie M. Peereboom[1], Mareike Sauer[2], Miriam Lipiski[2], Thea Fleischmann[2], Nikola Cesarovic[2], Christian T. Stoeck[1] and Sebastian Kozerke[1*]

Abstract

Background: The feasibility of absolute myocardial blood flow quantification and suitability of hyperpolarized [1-^{13}C] pyruvate as contrast agent for first-pass cardiovascular magnetic resonance (CMR) perfusion measurements are investigated with simulations and demonstrated in vivo in a swine model.

Methods: A versatile simulation framework for hyperpolarized CMR subject to physical, physiological and technical constraints was developed and applied to investigate experimental conditions for accurate perfusion CMR with hyperpolarized [1-^{13}C] pyruvate. Absolute and semi-quantitative perfusion indices were analyzed with respect to experimental parameter variations and different signal-to-noise ratio (SNR) levels. Absolute myocardial blood flow quantification was implemented with an iterative deconvolution approach based on Fermi functions. To demonstrate in vivo feasibility, velocity-selective excitation with an echo-planar imaging readout was used to acquire dynamic myocardial stress perfusion images in four healthy swine. Arterial input functions were extracted from an additional image slice with conventional excitation that was acquired within the same heartbeat.

Results: Simulations suggest that obtainable SNR and B_0 inhomogeneity in vivo are sufficient for the determination of absolute and semi-quantitative perfusion with ≤25% error. It is shown that for expected metabolic conversion rates, metabolic conversion of pyruvate can be neglected over the short duration of acquisition in first-pass perfusion CMR. In vivo measurements suggest that absolute myocardial blood flow quantification using hyperpolarized [1-^{13}C] pyruvate is feasible with an intra-myocardial variability comparable to semi-quantitative perfusion indices.

Conclusion: The feasibility of quantitative hyperpolarized first-pass perfusion CMR using [1-^{13}C] pyruvate has been investigated in simulations and demonstrated in swine. Using an approved and metabolically active compound is envisioned to increase the value of hyperpolarized perfusion CMR in patients.

Keywords: Perfusion imaging, Myocardial blood flow, Perfusion quantification, Hyperpolarization, 13C pyruvate

* Correspondence: kozerke@biomed.ee.ethz.ch
[1]Institute for Biomedical Engineering, University and ETH Zurich, Gloriastrasse, 35 8092 Zurich, Switzerland
Full list of author information is available at the end of the article

Background

Qualitative and semi-quantitative myocardial perfusion cardiovascular magnetic resonance (CMR) imaging using gadolinium based contrast agents is a clinically established modality for diagnosing coronary artery disease and ischemia [1, 2]. To reduce operator dependence during analysis and to enable the assessment of triple-vessel disease, microvascular obstruction and other conditions that present themselves by global or diffuse perfusion deficits, absolute myocardial blood flow (MBF) quantification is promoted [3, 4]. Absolute MBF quantification requires an accurate estimation of the impulse response function (IRF), which links the concentration of an arterial input function (AIF) and the response concentration in the myocardium, and scales linearly with the MBF. In conventional first-pass perfusion CMR bolus administration of chelated gadolinium-based contrast agents is used to accelerate spin-lattice relaxation subject to contrast agent concentration. The resulting dynamic contrast enhancement (DCE) provides contrast between ischemic and normally perfused myocardial tissue [5, 6] with commonly used saturation recovery sequences [7]. However, determination of contrast agent concentrations from measured signal intensities is complicated by the non-linearity of spin-lattice relaxation and saturation effects during acquisition. To address these issues, dual-bolus [5, 8] or variable saturation delay [9] approaches have been proposed at the cost of additional bolus administrations and/or non-trivial correction steps.

Dissolution dynamic nuclear polarization enables the production of highly polarized endogenous ^{13}C labelled molecules in solution with $> 10,000$-fold enhanced signal relative to thermal equilibrium [10]. We have previously demonstrated the feasibility of hyperpolarized first-pass perfusion CMR using ^{13}C urea in porcine models [11]. Due to the lack of thermal background signal, hyperpolarized contrast agents benefit from high contrast to noise ratio (CNR) compared with gadolinium-based measurements, as well as linear dependency of signal intensity with respect to concentration, which makes them promising alternatives for absolute MBF quantification. To avoid unwanted effects from metabolic conversion, hyperpolarized perfusion imaging has so far been limited to ^{13}C urea and other metabolically inert substrates such as HP001 [12], tert-butanol [13] or α-trideuteromethyl $[^{15}N]$ glutamine [14].

Pyruvate is metabolically active and a vital intermediate in the process of glycolysis, where it is converted into lactate, carbon dioxide (CO_2)/ bicarbonate and alanine. As a hyperpolarized substrate, $[1\text{-}^{13}C]$ pyruvate has been widely used to probe the glycolytic pathway in various organs of the body, including the heart [15–17]. To better understand the pathological alterations in metabolism and to improve diagnostic value, quantification of the metabolic conversion rates in form of kinetic modelling has been applied in tumours [18, 19] and the isolated and in-vivo rat heart [20, 21]. This approach however requires accurate knowledge of the bolus input in the target organ for quantification and discrimination of metabolic and perfusion related signal variations. To this end tailored blood suppressing sequences and co-polarized administration of $[^{13}C]$ urea have been proposed [22, 23].

With recent progress in the translation of hyperpolarized $[1\text{-}^{13}C]$ pyruvate into clinical application [24] and first successful administrations in the human heart [25], the need for accurate perfusion assessment without additional measurements has been highlighted. Extensive alterations and global as well as diffuse deficits are only detectable by quantitative assessment of metabolic processes with kinetic modelling and knowledge of the underlying perfusion. As regulatory approval of hyperpolarized substrates for human administration is limited to $[1\text{-}^{13}C]$ pyruvate for the foreseeable future, previously proposed perfusion substrates are currently not suited for clinical trials.

In this work we therefore explore the feasibility and accuracy of absolute and semi-quantitative perfusion CMR using $[1\text{-}^{13}C]$ pyruvate. By administration of a sharp contrast agent bolus and using velocity-selective excitation [11], we show that myocardial perfusion can rapidly be assessed before metabolic conversion significantly alters myocardial pyruvate signal intensities. Extensive simulations including MBF, metabolic conversion and physical imaging constraints inform on the limitations and requirements for accurate determination of absolute and semi-quantitative perfusion indices. In vivo feasibility and absolute MBF quantification is demonstrated in a swine model.

Methods
Simulation framework

A high resolution computational model of a short axis view of the heart was generated from the MRXCAT phantom [26] at a field-of-view (FOV) of 120×120 mm^2. To account for limited sampling resolution and intra-slice effects, the initial phantom consists of three slices of 3 mm thickness with an in-plane resolution of 1×1 mm^2. A total of eight anatomical compartments were defined based on the mid left ventricular (LV) slice of the American Heart Association (AHA) segmentation [27]: right ventricular (RV) blood pool, LV blood pool and six myocardial segments. K-space sampling subject to several physical and physiological effects were then modeled as illustrated in Fig. 1. The full signal model for the presented simulation framework for sampling one 2D slice consisting of 3 isochromat sub-slices is given by:

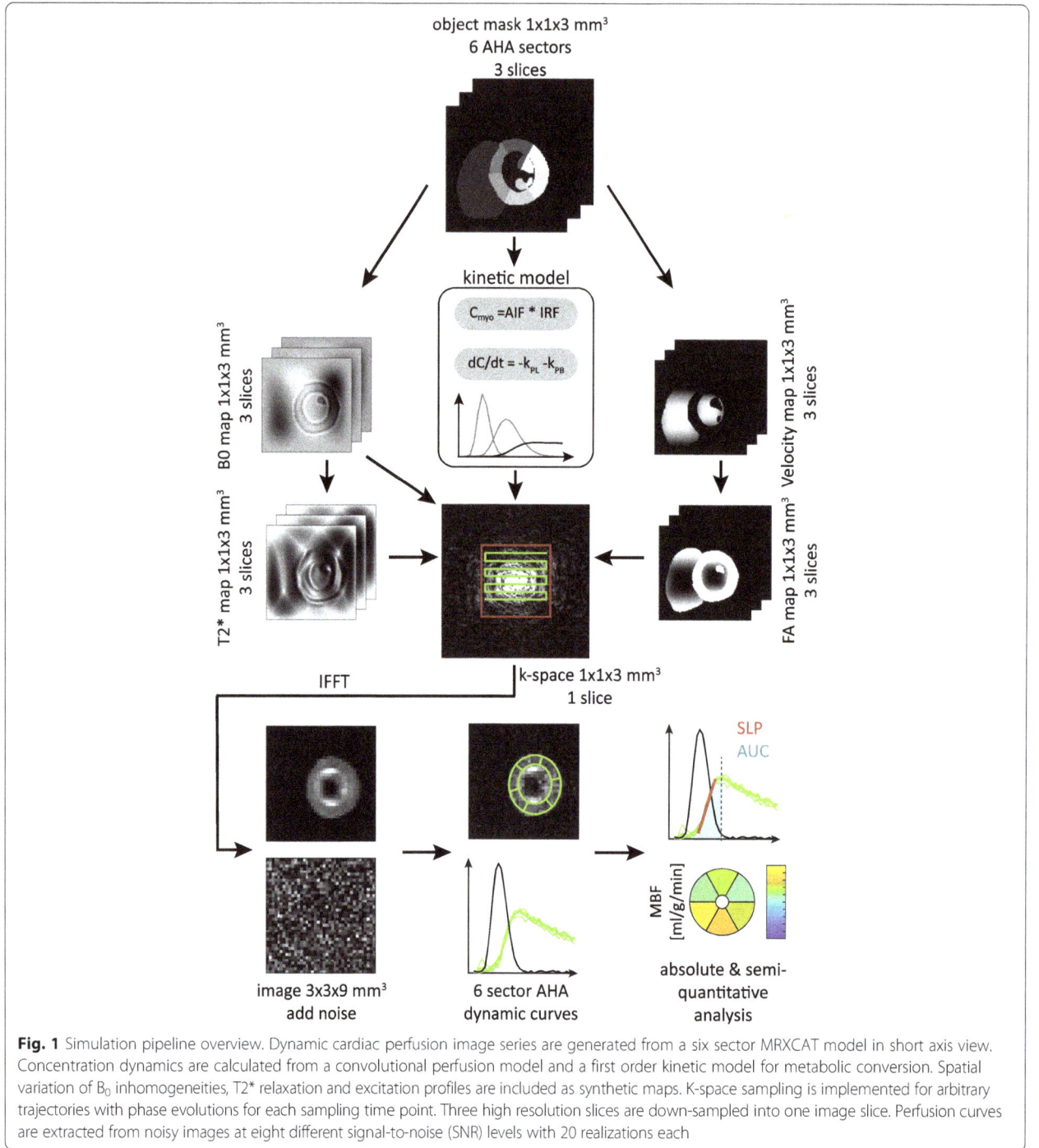

Fig. 1 Simulation pipeline overview. Dynamic cardiac perfusion image series are generated from a six sector MRXCAT model in short axis view. Concentration dynamics are calculated from a convolutional perfusion model and a first order kinetic model for metabolic conversion. Spatial variation of B_0 inhomogeneities, T2* relaxation and excitation profiles are included as synthetic maps. K-space sampling is implemented for arbitrary trajectories with phase evolutions for each sampling time point. Three high resolution slices are down-sampled into one image slice. Perfusion curves are extracted from noisy images at eight different signal-to-noise (SNR) levels with 20 realizations each

$$S\left(\vec{k}, t_d\right) = \sum_{\vec{r}} \sum_{t_s} e^{j\vec{k}(t_s)\vec{r}} \cdot \sin\left(\alpha\left(\vec{r}\right)\right)$$

$$\cdot \sum_{m=1}^{M} \left[C_m\left(\vec{r}, t_d\right) \cdot e^{j2\pi f_m t_s} \cdot e^{-t_d/T_{1,m}} \cdot e^{-t_s/T_{2,m}^*(\vec{r})} \right] \cdot e^{j2\pi\bar{\gamma}dB_o(\vec{r})t_s}$$

$$\text{(1)}$$

where $\vec{r} = (x, y, z)^T$ and $\vec{k} = (k_x, k_y, k_z)^T$ denote the spatial coordinates in image space and k-space respectively, t_d the time point in the dynamic series, α the spatially varying flip angle, C_m, f_m, $T_{1,m}$ the concentration, frequency offset and longitudinal relaxation time of metabolite m, and B_0, $T_{2,m}^*$ the off-resonance and apparent transverse relaxation times. The time dependent k-space trajectory $k(t_s)$ with sampling time points t_s enables k-space sampling along arbitrary trajectories and at arbitrary resolutions considering dephasing effects during the readout.

Dynamic pyruvate concentrations were simulated in a two-step process: Firstly, MBF was modeled by convolution of a generic AIF from the MRXCAT model in the LV with a Fermi function shaped IRF:

$$C_{myo}(t) = IRF(t) * AIF_{LV}(t)$$
$$IRF(t) = MBF \cdot \frac{1+\beta}{1+\beta e^{\alpha t}} \tag{2}$$

with shape parameters α, $\beta = 0.25$, temporal sampling interval 0.5 s (heart rate 120 bpm) and varying MBF. In a second step, a forward kinetic model was employed to account for metabolic conversion of pyruvate (Pyr) into lactate (Lac) and bicarbonate (Bic):

$$\frac{d}{dt}\begin{bmatrix} C_{Pyr}(t) \\ C_{Lac}(t) \\ C_{Bic}(t) \end{bmatrix} = \begin{bmatrix} -k_{PL}-k_{PB} & k_{LP} & 0 \\ k_{PL} & -k_{LP} & 0 \\ k_{PB} & 0 & 0 \end{bmatrix}$$
$$\cdot \begin{bmatrix} C_{Pyr}(t) \\ C_{Lac}(t) \\ C_{Bic}(t) \end{bmatrix} + \begin{bmatrix} \frac{d}{dt}C_{myo}(t) \\ 0 \\ 0 \end{bmatrix} \tag{3}$$

Where k_{PL}, k_{PB} denote the kinetic forward conversion rates from pyruvate into lactate and bicarbonate, respectively. Reverse conversion from lactate to pyruvate was assumed negligible ($k_{LP} = 0$).

Off-resonances were simulated as a high resolution B_0 map generated from a superposition of a three-dimensional second order polynomial and a filtered replica of the anatomical model. A convolution of the anatomical object with a Laplacian of Gaussian filter (width 8 mm, $\sigma = 2$ mm) was used to create an object that mimics strong susceptibility gradients at tissue interfaces as described in [28]. The combined B_0 map was then scaled to the desired maximum in-plane and through-slice off-resonance.

$$B_0(x,y,z) = LoG(x,y) * Myo_z(x,y)$$
$$+ f_{poly}(x,y,z) + B_{dz}(z) \tag{4}$$

where LoG denotes the filter kernel, Myo_z the myocardial object mask, f_{poly} the 3D 2nd order polynomial and B_{dz} the B_0 through-slice gradient.

Spatially varying T2* relaxation was calculated from the first order derivative of the B_0 map along phase and measurement direction using a 2D Gaussian kernel ($\sigma = 3$):

$$\frac{1}{T_{2,m}^*(x,y)} = \frac{1}{T_{2,m}} + G_{\Delta x} * B_0(x,y) + G_{\Delta y}$$
$$* B_0(x,y) \tag{5}$$

With $T_{2,m}$ the native T_2 of metabolite m, and $G_{\Delta x}$, $G_{\Delta y}$ the 2D Gaussian kernels along x and y, respectively.

Velocity-selective excitation [11] was simulated assuming a parabolic velocity distribution in the RV and LV according to:

$$v(x,y) = v_{max}\sqrt{\left(\frac{1}{2w}(x-x_c)^2\right)^2 + \left(\frac{1}{2w}(y-y_c)^2\right)^2} \tag{6}$$

where w denotes the width of the distribution and (x_c, y_c) the center of mass of the respective blood compartment. Based on the velocity distribution, the effective spatially dependent flip angle of the selective excitation is given by:

$$\alpha_{eff}(x,y) = \alpha \cdot \left| \sin\left(\frac{v_{enc}-v(x,y)}{v_{enc}}\frac{\pi}{2}\right) \right| \tag{7}$$

where α denotes the nominal flip angle and v_{enc} the encoding velocity of the excitation.

An echo planar imaging (EPI) trajectory for k-space sampling was generated from gradient waveforms with hardware limits in accordance to in vivo experiments on a clinical 3 T system (slew rate 195 T/m/s, amplitude 30 mT/m). Using Partial Fourier acquisition (factor 0.65) the effective number of profiles was reduced from 39 to 25, resulting in a readout duration of 35 ms for the target in-plane resolution of 3×3 mm^2 and a 120×120 mm^2 FOV.

Computationally the proposed model as described by Equation (1) is challenging, due to the inclusion of the phase evolution stemming from B_0 inhomogeneities. Consequently, the resulting phase maps need to be calculated for each k-space sampling time point t_s, which significantly increases the memory requirements. The simulation of a dynamic k-space series with 40 dynamics took approximately 5 min on a workstation equipped with a hexa-core Xeon X5670 processor and 256 GB of memory.

In order to assess the sensitivity and to inform on practical limitations of hyperpolarized perfusion measurements, pivotal simulation parameters were varied over their respectively expected value ranges in vivo. Table 1 shows the parameters in the defined reference case (BASE) as well as their respective sweep ranges.

Static parameters were set to: $\alpha = 60°$, $v_{enc} = 0.35$ m/s, $w = 0.2$ m. T_1/T_2 values for pyruvate, lactate and bicarbonate were set to 30/0.1 s, 20/0.1 s and 20/0.15 s, respectively. T1 values were chosen based on separate experiments outlined below. In absence of available T2 values for cardiac tissue, conservative estimations were used based on hepatic tissue in rats [29]. For each simulation according to Equation (1) and Table 1, a second simulation was performed with a constant flip angle of

Table 1 Parameters investigated by simulations. BASE values refer to the respective parameter value used for the reference simulation. Range refers to the respectively investigated value range for each parameter

Parameter	BASE value	Range [min, max]	Step size
MBF [mL/min/g]	2.5	[0.5, 5.0]	0.5
B_0 in-plane [ppm]	0.25	[0.0, 2.0]	0.5
B_{dz} through-plane [ppm]	0.0	[0.0, 1.0]	0.5
k_{PL} [s^{-1}]	0.0	[0.0, 0.2]	0.05
v_{max} [m/s]	0.35	[0.175, 0.7]	0.175

$5°$ to assess the parameter impact on AIF measurements in vivo.

Simulation post-processing

A total of 8 signal-to-noise ratio (SNR) levels were simulated: 5, 7.5, 10, 15, 20, 30, 40, 50. For each SNR level 20 realizations of noise were computed with respect to mean peak myocardial signal. Signal curves for the six AHA sectors and the AIF were then extracted, corrected for T_1 relaxation and baseline corrected. AIF signals were scaled to compensate for the flip angle difference. For all myocardial sectors, the area-under-the-curve (AUC) and upslope parameters were calculated. The AUC was calculated by signal integration from AIF peak to myocardial peak, whereas upslope was determined by fitting a linear slope over 5 time points centered between AIF peak and myocardial peak signal.

MBF quantification was performed by iterative fitting of the IRF in Equation (2) for varying time shifts as proposed by Wissmann et al. [30]. Prior to quantification, a three-parameter gamma variate function was fitted to the AIF signal according to Equation (8) to compensate for the insufficient sampling rate and to reflect the treatment of in vivo data described in the data post-processing section. Absolute MBF was then calculated from fitted AIF signals and up-sampled myocardial signals as described below for in vivo data post-processing.

Hyperpolarization and in vivo CMR

In vivo measurements were performed on a clinical 3 T wide-bore scanner (Ingenia, Philips Healthcare, Best, The Netherlands) equipped with a gradient system delivering 30 mT/m maximum amplitude at 195 T/m/s slew rate. A custom coil array with 6 ^{13}C and 2 ^{1}H receive channels was used for signal reception (Rapid Biomedical, Rimpar, Germany). Animals were placed in right recumbency inside the scanner and an electrocardiogram (ECG) unit was used for cardiac synchronization.

Samples of 0.75 mL neat pyruvic acid were doped with 15 mM AH111501 trityl radical and polarized for 3.5 h in a commercial 5 T SpinLab Polarizer (General Electric Healthcare, Waukesha, Wisconsin, USA) before dissolution

in a buffer of 25 mL 0.1% EDTA water solution. Upon sample collection, the prepared solution was neutralized and diluted with 10.85 g of 0.72 M NaOH solution and 4.5 mL buffer solution at 0 °C to achieve a final injection medium with a pH value of 7 at body temperature. 25 mL of the final 300 mM ^{13}C pyruvate solution were bolus injected over 2 s through femoral venous catheters 20 s after dissolution. Polarization levels and T_1 relaxation times of the neat solution inside the 3 T magnetic field were established in separate experiments as $54 \pm 3\%$ and 71 ± 3 s, respectively. In vivo T_1 relaxation times were determined to 32 ± 3 s, based on 3 measurements of hyperpolarized pyruvate solution diluted in porcine blood at a ratio of 1:10.

Animal handling

Four healthy female swine (Edelschwein, weight 30–35 kg) were used for the experiments. After induction of general anesthesia, all swine were intubated and sheaths (5 F) were introduced into both femoral arteries and veins. 100 IU/kg unfractionated heparin was given intravenously and repeated every hour. General anesthesia was maintained with isoflurane (2–3%) by positive pressure ventilation with 100% oxygen. Heart rate, rhythm and variability, inspiratory and expiratory gases (CO_2, O_2, isoflurane), pulse oximetry, temperature, direct arterial blood pressure, urine output, and arterial and venous blood gases were monitored throughout the procedure. Cardiac stress was pharmacologically induced by intravenous administration of dobutamine (Dobutrex, TEVA Pharma AG, Basel, Switzerland) at increasing infusion rates until a heart rate of 120 bpm was reached (from a baseline heart rate between 70 and 85 bpm). Upon reaching the target heart rate, the dobutamine infusion rate was maintained during all imaging experiments. Three animals received a second injection of hyperpolarized pyruvate to assess reproducibility. After the procedure, all animals were euthanized in deep anesthesia by lethal injection of pentobarbital.

CMR imaging

Dynamic series of ^{13}C perfusion images in late systole were acquired with electrocardiogram (ECG) triggering starting five heartbeats after the start of injection to minimize bolus saturation in the RV blood pool. Ventilation was suspended for the first 45 s of imaging to avoid misregistration between individual time frames. Velocity selective excitation [11] was followed by an EPI readout with parameters: FOV = 120×120 mm^2, slice thickness 15 mm, in-plane resolution 3.0×3.0 mm^2, TE = 13.5 ms, TR = 1 heartbeat, FA: 60°, partial Fourier factor 0.65, readout duration 32 ms. An additional image stack in an apically adjacent slice with conventional excitation (FA: 5°) was interleaved in diastole of the same heart beat to provide AIF signal curves for absolute MBF quantification.

All in vivo images were reconstructed from raw data using MRecon (GyroTools LLC, Zurich, Switzerland) and zero-filled to a common resolution of 1×1 mm^2. ^{1}H images were then rotated, aligned and cropped to the FOV of the ^{13}C images. Nyquist-ghosts of the EPI readout were removed by first order phase correction maximizing signal intensity in a predefined region of interest (e.g. LV blood pool). ^{13}C coil combination was implemented as root of weighted sum of squares [31].

Data post-processing

LV myocardium and LV blood pool were manually segmented on overlays of ^{13}C perfusion and ^{1}H reference images. The myocardium was subsequently divided into six segments corresponding to the basal / mid-ventricular slices in the 16 segment AHA model [27].

Magnitude coil sensitivities were estimated by fitting a plane over the entire FOV, using only regions with myocardial signal. A time point 3 s after myocardial bolus passage was selected to prevent overfitting of the sensitivities to local perfusion deficits. The resulting sensitivity plane was then visually inspected for plausibility and used to correct signal intensities in all previous image frames. [1-^{13}C] pyruvate signal intensities were calculated as mean values over each segment in the dynamic image series, as well as the LV blood pool from the AIF scan (scaled to compensate for different flip angles). Myocardial signals were corrected for T_1 relaxation ($T_1 = 32$ s) and cropped 1 s after myocardial peak signal for quantification. Baseline offsets were corrected for by subtraction of mean noise levels prior to bolus arrival.

Three-parameter gamma-variate functions

$$s(t) = at^b e^{-\frac{t}{c}} \qquad (8)$$

were fitted to the measured time curves $s(t)$ for further analysis. Area under the curve (AUC) and up-slope were extracted from the fitted curves as semi-quantitative perfusion measures [3]. SNR / CNR was calculated as mean signal intensities divided by the standard deviation over a noise frame after ^{13}C signal decay [32].

Absolute MBF quantification of in vivo data was performed by iterative fitting of a Fermi function as the impulse response for varying time shifts between 0 and 5 s. The first point in the time domain representation of the solution with the smallest fitting error was taken as the absolute MBF value and scaled to units of mL/min/g.

^{1}H gadolinium DCE imaging

DCE perfusion CMR image series using ^{1}H gadolinium were acquired in three of the four subjects for preliminary validation of the proposed method. Measurements were performed within 5 min after the last [1-^{13}C] pyruvate injection. Between the ^{13}C and ^{1}H measurements, dobutamine stress CMR was maintained constant. To facilitate MBF quantification, a dual-bolus approach with 0.025 mmol/kg and 0.075 mmol/kg gadolinium (Gadovist 1.0, Bayer Healthcare, Berlin, Germany) was chosen [33]. Dynamic image series were acquired every heart beat using a saturation-recovery spoiled gradient echo sequence with parameters: FOV = 220×220 mm2, slice thickness 10 mm, in-plane resolution 3.0×3.0 mm2, TR = 1.9 ms, TE = 0.7 ms, FA = 15°, WET saturation [34] delay = 80–100 ms. A total of 100 dynamics were acquired during suspended ventilation. Post-processing, extraction of semi-quantitative perfusion indices and absolute MBF quantification was performed analogous to the ^{13}C data.

Results

Simulations

Figure 2 qualitatively illustrates the effects of limited sampling resolution as well as variations of key parameters. Increased metabolic conversion results in reduced myocardial [1-^{13}C] pyruvate signal with chemically

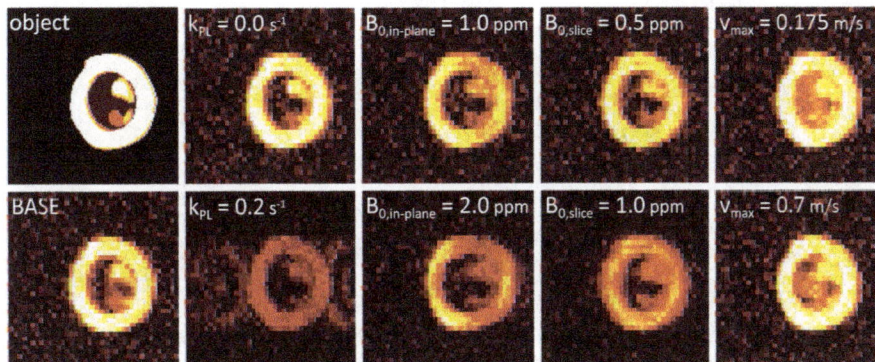

Fig. 2 Simulated perfusion images at myocardial signal peak for signal-to-noise ratio (SNR) = 15. Effects of limited sampling resolution and variation of simulation parameters are illustrated. BASE case simulation values were: myocardial blood flow (MBF) = 2.5 mL/g/min, B$_0$ in-plane = 0.25 ppm, B$_0$ through-plane = 0.0 ppm, k$_{PL}$ = 0.0 s^{-1}, v$_{max}$ = 0.35 m/s, flip-angle = 60°, in-plane resolution = 3×3 mm^2, field-of-view 120×120 mm^2

shifted contamination from [^{13}C] bicarbonate and [1-^{13}C] lactate. In-plane B$_0$ inhomogeneities give rise to EPI related geometrical distortions as well as signal loss due to intra-voxel dephasing. Through-plane B$_0$ gradients retain geometrical accuracy but contribute to dephasing and signal loss. Deviations between encoding and actual blood velocities result in reduced blood pool suppression and partial volume effects.

SNR dependency of absolute and semi-quantitative perfusion measures are illustrated in Fig. 3 for the BASE case. SNR levels ≥15 appear sufficient for absolute MBF quantification within a 25% uncertainty window. A systematic under-estimation towards lower SNR levels is apparent. Upslope appears largely insensitive to SNR variations with accurate results at SNR ≥ 7.5. AUC values exhibit systematic underestimation of ≥10% with outliers even at high SNR levels.

Metabolic conversion is analyzed in Fig. 4. Increasing kinetic rates k$_{PL}$ result in a reduced myocardial response signal. For k$_{PL}$ ≤ 0.05 s^{-1} the up-slope remains within 25% of the reference value and the relative error of absolute MBF quantification is ≤20%. AUC appears to be linearly dependent on k$_{PL}$ and more strongly affected by increased metabolic conversion than the upslope parameter.

Figure 5 shows the results obtained for simulated absolute MBF values between 0.5 and 5.0 mL /min/g. Low simulated MBF values between 0.5 and 1.0 mL/g/min lead to an SNR independent overestimation of 80 and

26% respectively. At higher simulated MBF values ≥3.5 mL/g/min underestimation for SNR levels < 30 is apparent. Semi-quantitative perfusion indices upslope and AUC present excellent linear dependency on simulated MBF with little SNR dependent variation. The respective linear regression models were calculated as MBF = 0.44 * upslope + 0.30 for upslope-to-MBF conversion (R = 0.999 at SNR = 50) and $MBF = 0.053 \cdot AUC - 0.224$ for AUC-to-MBF conversion (R = 0.999 at SNR = 50).

Impact of B$_0$ inhomogeneities and blood pool velocities is illustrated in Fig. 6. B$_0$ inhomogeneities show similar impact for in-plane and through-plane directions: Up to 0.5 ppm, mean absolute and semi-quantitative perfusion measures are within 25% of the respective reference values for SNR ≥ 15. For stronger field gradients, absolute MBF quantification appears to be more robust than semi-quantitative measures. Misadjusted velocity encoding has little effect on the analysis of perfusion indices in the simulated case.

In vivo

An example of a dynamic perfusion image series is shown in Fig. 7. Myocardial peak signal is observed 5–6 s after start of the scan (7–8 s after start of injection). The three main cardiac arteries (left anterior descending (LAD), left circumflex (LCx), right coronary artery (RCA)) are visible after 4 s. Summation over two time frames at myocardial peak signal is shown for qualitative assessment of perfusion. The LV and RV myocardium is clearly visible. Arterial

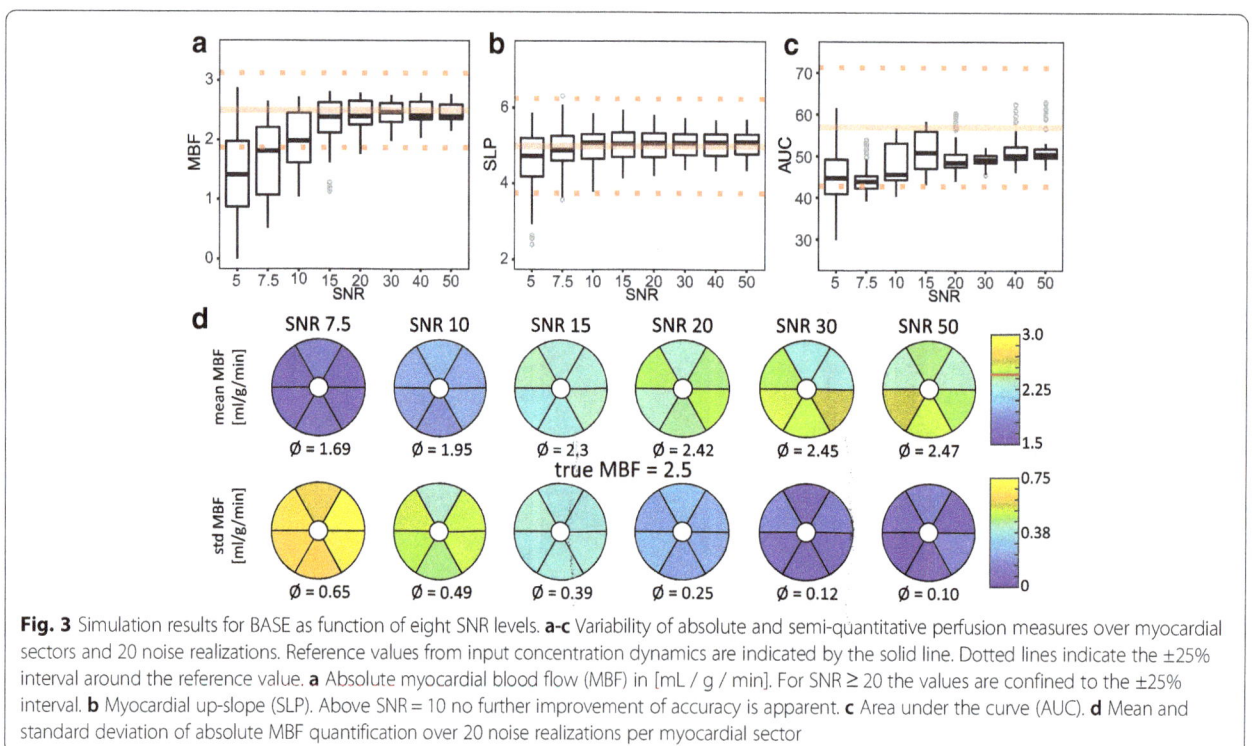

Fig. 3 Simulation results for BASE as function of eight SNR levels. **a-c** Variability of absolute and semi-quantitative perfusion measures over myocardial sectors and 20 noise realizations. Reference values from input concentration dynamics are indicated by the solid line. Dotted lines indicate the ±25% interval around the reference value. **a** Absolute myocardial blood flow (MBF) in [mL / g / min]. For SNR ≥ 20 the values are confined to the ±25% interval. **b** Myocardial up-slope (SLP). Above SNR = 10 no further improvement of accuracy is apparent. **c** Area under the curve (AUC). **d** Mean and standard deviation of absolute MBF quantification over 20 noise realizations per myocardial sector

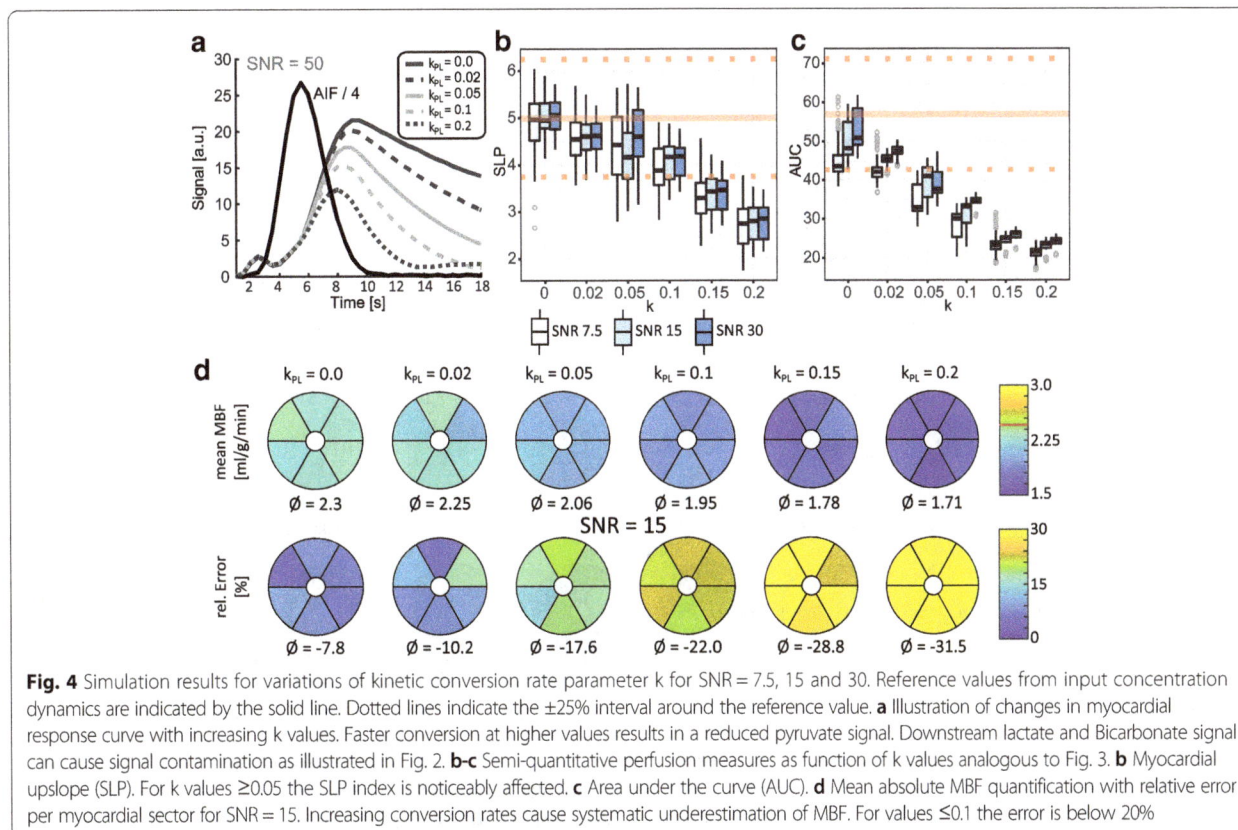

Fig. 4 Simulation results for variations of kinetic conversion rate parameter k for SNR = 7.5, 15 and 30. Reference values from input concentration dynamics are indicated by the solid line. Dotted lines indicate the ±25% interval around the reference value. **a** Illustration of changes in myocardial response curve with increasing k values. Faster conversion at higher values results in a reduced pyruvate signal. Downstream lactate and Bicarbonate signal can cause signal contamination as illustrated in Fig. 2. **b-c** Semi-quantitative perfusion measures as function of k values analogous to Fig. 3. **b** Myocardial upslope (SLP). For k values ≥0.05 the SLP index is noticeably affected. **c** Area under the curve (AUC). **d** Mean absolute MBF quantification with relative error per myocardial sector for SNR = 15. Increasing conversion rates cause systematic underestimation of MBF. For values ≤0.1 the error is below 20%

signal leads to local hyper-intensities around the respective vessels.

Figure 8 shows the absolute and semi-quantitative perfusion analysis for seven stress measurements in 4 swine. Under in vivo conditions, the myocardial SNR across the myocardium ranges from 11.0 ± 1.4 to 19.3 ± 2.1. Absolute MBF quantification yielded values between 2.85 ± 0.45 and 3.74 ± 0.75 mL/g/min, with mean variations ≤10% in repeat measurements. Normalized upslope values ranged from 0.07 ± 0.02 to 0.09 ± 0.1 (mean intra-subject variation ≤15%), and normalized AUC values from 0.04 ± 0.01 to 0.06 ± 0.01 (mean intra-subject variation ≤40%). Intra-myocardial coefficients of variance for MBF, upslope, AUC and CNR were determined as $29 \pm 19\%$, $22 \pm 15\%$, $21 \pm 13\%$ and $11 \pm 4\%$, respectively.

Figure 9 shows preliminary validation data obtained from ^{1}H gadolinium DCE imaging in three of the four subjects. Absolute MBF quantification yielded values between 2.90 ± 0.08 and 3.75 ± 0.44 mL/g/min, with myocardial SNR values ranging from 10.7 ± 0.4 to 20.6 ± 0.5. Bland-Altman analysis revealed good agreement between quantitative perfusion measures derived from ^{13}C and ^{1}H DCE image series.

Discussion

In this study, we employed extensive simulations to assess experimental requirements and limitations for absolute and semi-quantitative myocardial CMR perfusion imaging using hyperpolarized [1-^{13}C] pyruvate. We have demonstrated that for rapid bolus injections, the metabolic conversion into [1-^{13}C] lactate and [^{13}C] bicarbonate can largely be neglected as the information related to perfusion is contained in a very short window of a few seconds. In vivo stress measurements in swine suggest feasibility for the obtainable SNR and expected parameter range with respect to metabolic kinetics and B_0 inhomogeneities.

Metabolic conversion of hyperpolarized [1-^{13}C] pyruvate into the downstream metabolites [1-^{13}C] lactate, [^{13}C] bicarbonate and [1-^{13}C] alanine is a potential hindrance to accurate perfusion assessment. The presented simulations, however, indicate that the myocardial response signal is only weakly affected for rate constants $k_{PL} < 0.1$ s^{-1}. Based on measurements in rat hearts [20, 21], skeletal muscle [35] and tumor cell cultures [36] the expected in vivo values for k_{PL} are in the range of 0.01 s^{-1} to 0.1 s^{-1}. Absolute MBF quantification and the upslope perfusion index generally appear more robust towards metabolic conversion than the AUC index. In order to improve the robustness over a wider range of kinetic rate constants or to allow slower bolus injection, combining the chemically shifted signals of individual metabolites is envisioned.

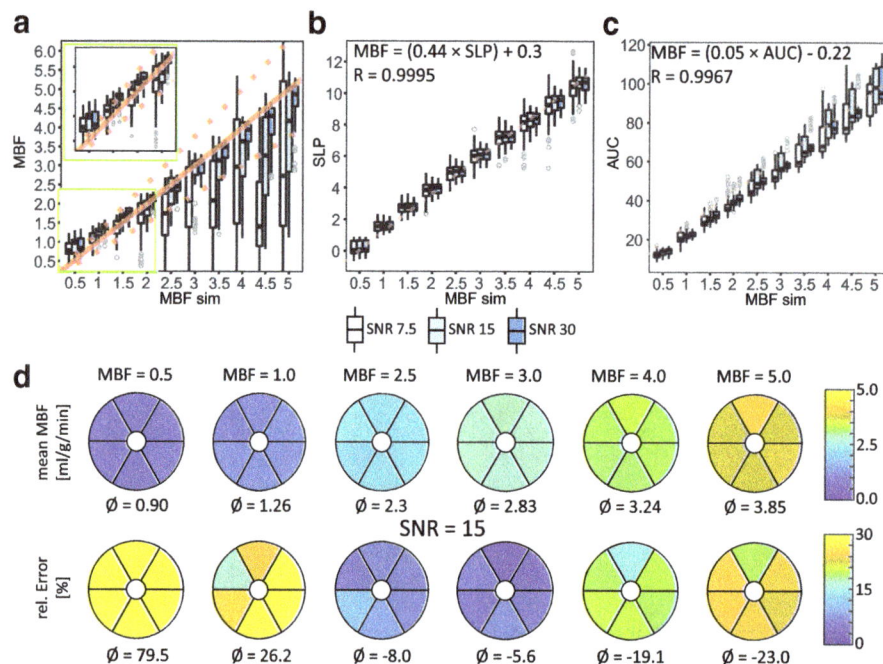

Fig. 5 Simulation results for variations of myocardial blood flow (MBF) in units of mL/g/min for SNR = 7.5, 15 and 30. **a** Calculated MBF after reconstruction vs. simulated MBF value. Reference values used to calculate input concentration dynamics are indicated by the solid line. Dotted lines indicate the ±25% interval around the reference value. Simulated MBF values ≤1.0 result in overestimation for all SNR levels, whereas higher simulated MBF values are only underestimated for lower SNR levels. **b-c** Semi-quantitative perfusion measures as function of absolute MBF values analogous to Fig. 3. The dotted line represents the linear regression model calculated at SNR = 50 (top left corner). **b** Myocardial upslope (SLP). **c** Area under the curve (AUC). **d** Mean absolute MBF quantification with relative error per myocardial sector for SNR = 15. Strong overestimation at low MBF values, and moderate underestimation at high MBF values is apparent

As described previously, the velocity-selective excitation employed in this study is tailored for measurements under stress condition with increased heart rates, contractility and therefore enhanced blood velocities inside the LV blood pool [11]. This potentially limits applicability in patient cohorts that cannot tolerate dobutamine infusion. Diagnostically, however, quantitative measurements under stress are considered of prime diagnostic value as early stage perfusion deficits only present at maximum workload/vasodilation [37]. A similar workload dependency can also be expected for the onset of metabolic alterations.

B$_0$ inhomogeneities are a common problem in hyperpolarized imaging, since relatively long readout trajectories such as EPI are used. The lower gyromagnetic ratio of the ^{13}C nucleus results in comparatively long readouts with low bandwidth in phase encoding direction. Phase offsets from B$_0$ inhomogeneities, as well as motion, can cause significant signal loss due to dephasing and geometric distortions. Different approaches for geometric distortion correction for hyperpolarized EPI acquisitions have been proposed. Inverting the readout direction in additional echoes [38] or by alternating the blip direction [39] enables the calculation of distortion maps for correction.

These methods however require tailored pulse sequences and full k-space sampling, as well as accurate image-based registration of distorted images for deriving a B$_0$ map estimate. Without distortion correction, the presented simulations indicate underestimations up to 30% on semi-quantitative perfusion indices for typically achievable B$_0$ variations of < 1.0 ppm over the imaging volume. Absolute MBF quantification appears more robust towards B$_0$ inhomogeneities at higher SNR levels with respect to mean values. However, larger B$_0$ inhomogeneities give rise to pronounced signal variations over the myocardium which potentially limits the diagnostic value. The observed robustness towards B$_0$ inhomogeneities in simulations is therefore contingent on similar signal dephasing effects inside the AIF and myocardial compartments. Under in vivo conditions fast flowing blood near the aortic valve (aortic jet) and strong off-resonances in the proximity of venous vessels can cause signal pile-up or dephasing in the septal and lateral inferior sectors respectively, which results in larger intra-myocardial variability. Additionally, phase accrual due to blood flow can significantly dampen the apparent amplitude of the AIF signal and result in underestimations of absolute MBF. Fat shift direction,

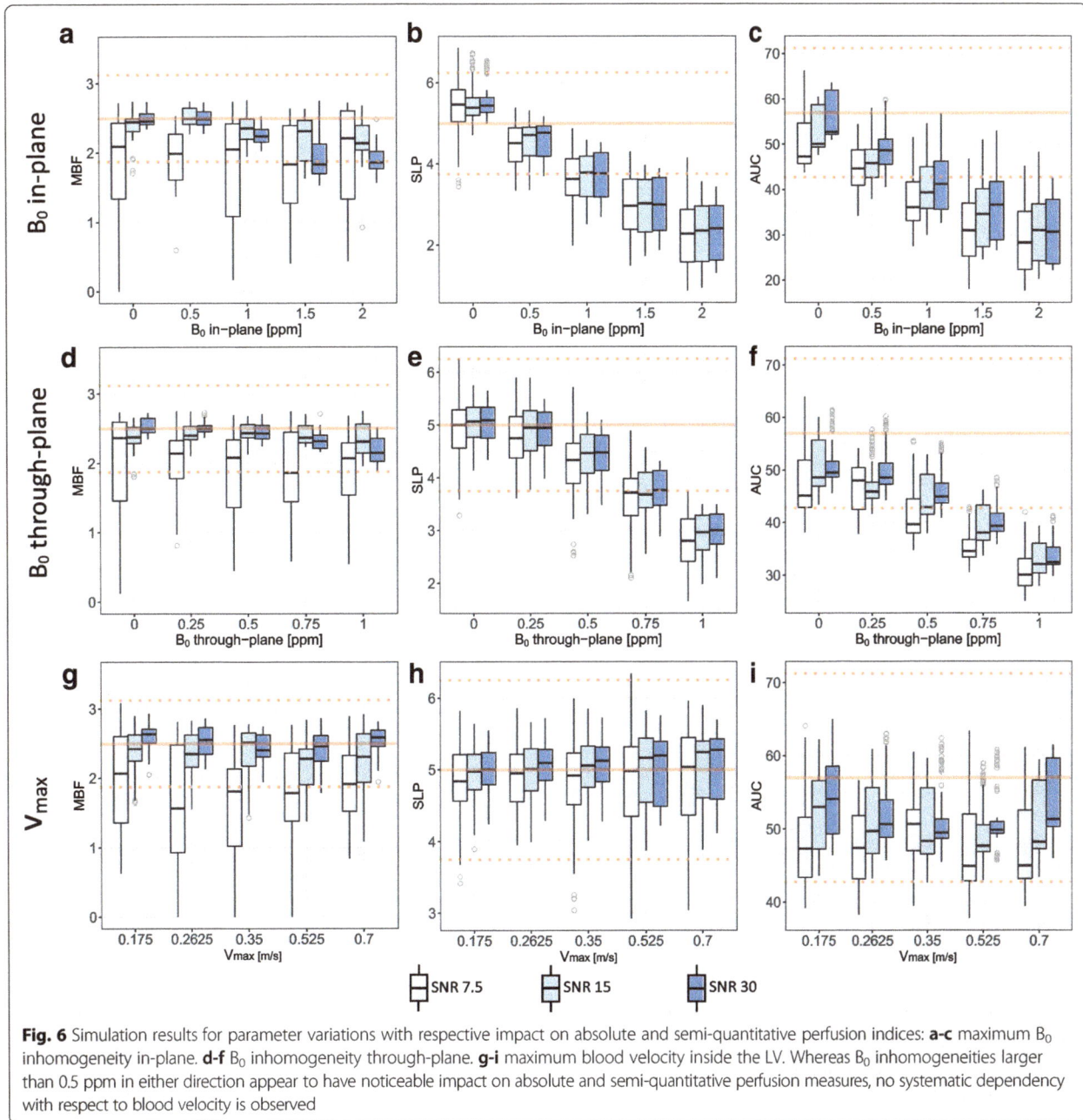

Fig. 6 Simulation results for parameter variations with respective impact on absolute and semi-quantitative perfusion indices: **a-c** maximum B_0 inhomogeneity in-plane. **d-f** B_0 inhomogeneity through-plane. **g-i** maximum blood velocity inside the LV. Whereas B_0 inhomogeneities larger than 0.5 ppm in either direction appear to have noticeable impact on absolute and semi-quantitative perfusion measures, no systematic dependency with respect to blood velocity is observed

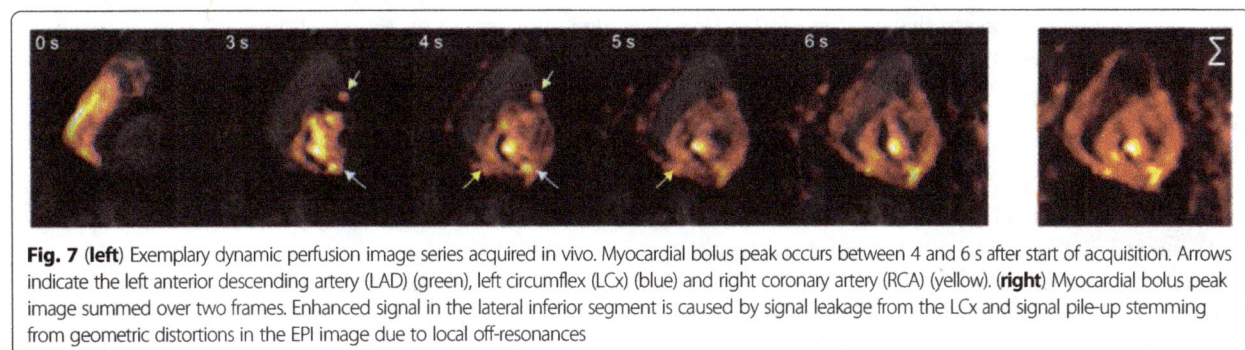

Fig. 7 (**left**) Exemplary dynamic perfusion image series acquired in vivo. Myocardial bolus peak occurs between 4 and 6 s after start of acquisition. Arrows indicate the left anterior descending artery (LAD) (green), left circumflex (LCx) (blue) and right coronary artery (RCA) (yellow). (**right**) Myocardial bolus peak image summed over two frames. Enhanced signal in the lateral inferior segment is caused by signal leakage from the LCx and signal pile-up stemming from geometric distortions in the EPI image due to local off-resonances

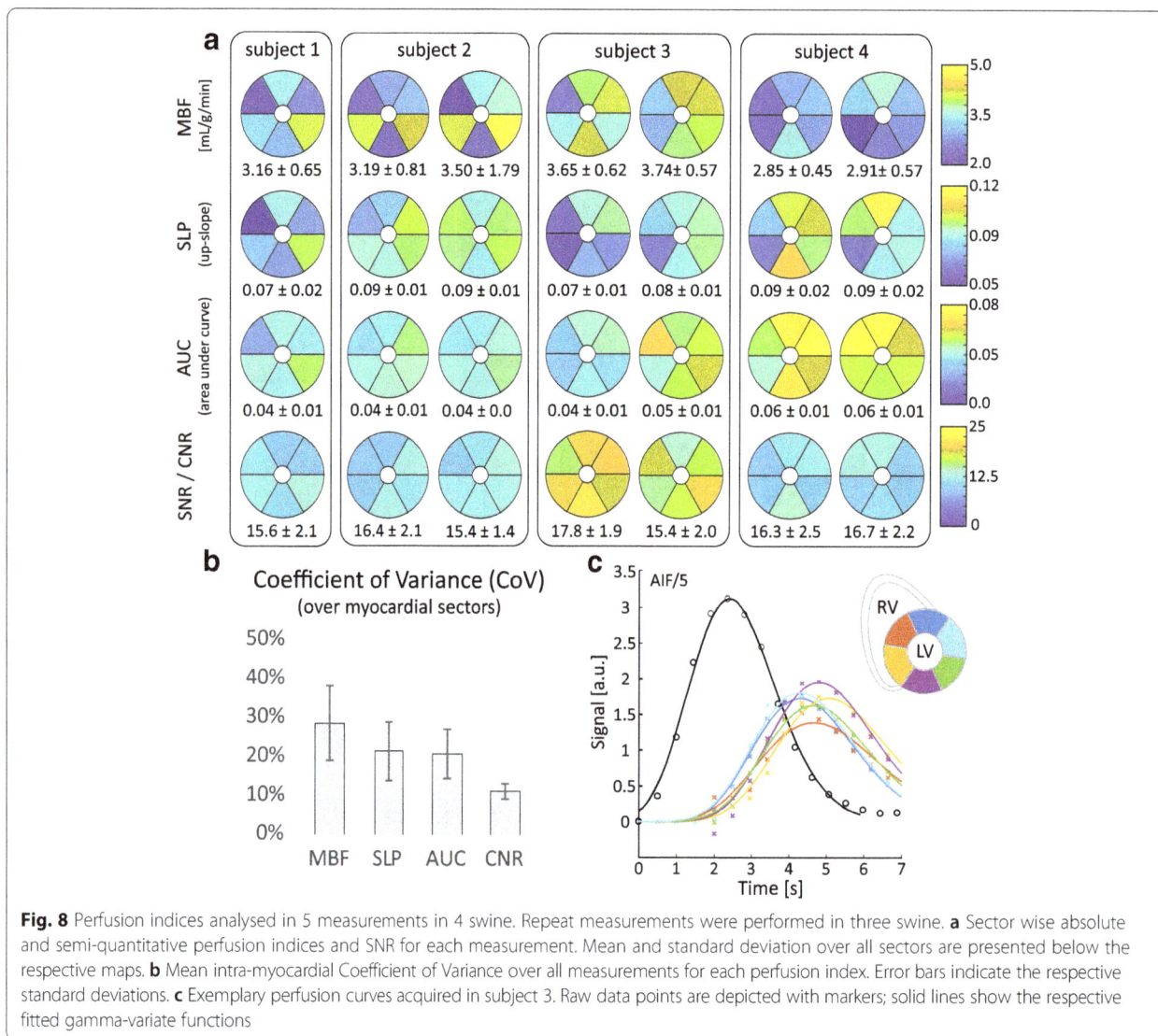

Fig. 8 Perfusion indices analysed in 5 measurements in 4 swine. Repeat measurements were performed in three swine. **a** Sector wise absolute and semi-quantitative perfusion indices and SNR for each measurement. Mean and standard deviation over all sectors are presented below the respective maps. **b** Mean intra-myocardial Coefficient of Variance over all measurements for each perfusion index. Error bars indicate the respective standard deviations. **c** Exemplary perfusion curves acquired in subject 3. Raw data points are depicted with markers; solid lines show the respective fitted gamma-variate functions

phase encoding direction and the trigger delay need therefore be considered carefully during planning in vivo to avoid unnecessary artifacts.

Comparison of absolute and semi-quantitative perfusion measures in simulations revealed excellent linear relationship between MBF and upslope and AUC, respectively. This confirms previous findings based on conventional contrast agents that upslope [40, 41] and AUC [42] are suitable surrogate indices to assess MBF and perfusion reserve. Based on simulation results, the upslope index appears superior to AUC for hyperpolarized [1-^{13}C] pyruvate, due to lower parameter dependency overall and less bias introduced by baseline correction steps. Of all the derived perfusion indices, MBF showed the strongest SNR dependent variability, especially for higher MBF values > 4 mL/g/min. These findings suggest that in vivo measurements obtained in this range are only accurate for relatively high SNR

values. The practically reliable measurement range for MBF quantification is therefore subject to the achievable SNR with a given experimental setup.

Using a plane fit for the correction of spatial variance in receive coil sensitivity inherently assumes homogeneous signal intensities over the region of interest. By choosing a time frame after initial myocardial bolus passage, the effect of impaired perfusion is reduced, as hypo-perfused areas are characterized by delayed contrast agent uptake. Estimated sensitivity maps were visually inspected to ensure that the resulting sensitivity gradient was plausible with respect to coil placement. For clinical applications with possibly vast perfusion deficits, a different sensitivity correction strategy might be required.

Although the presented simulation framework reflects image acquisition more accurately than previous work [43], acquisitions in vivo are aggravated by additional

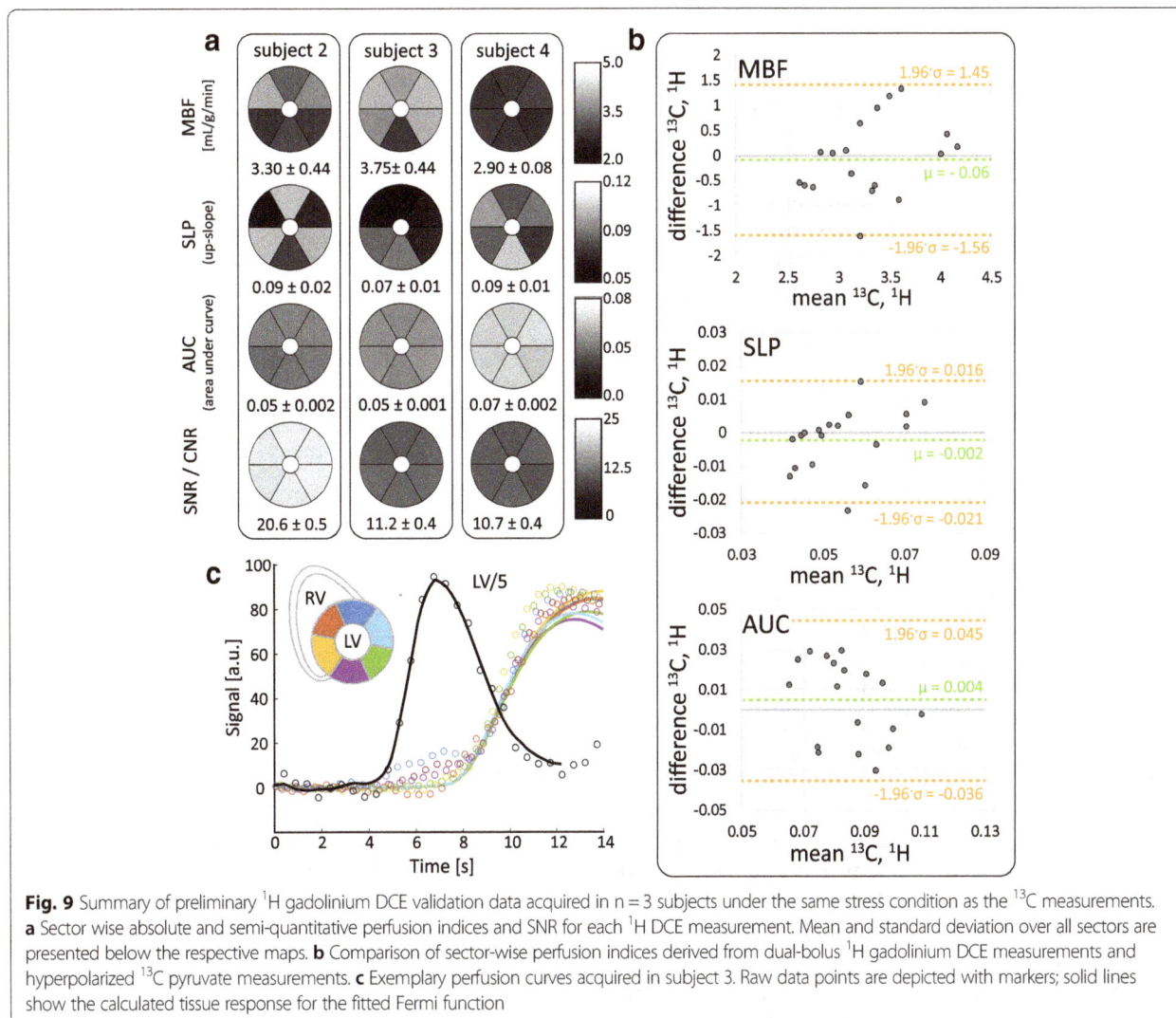

Fig. 9 Summary of preliminary ^{1}H gadolinium DCE validation data acquired in n = 3 subjects under the same stress condition as the ^{13}C measurements. **a** Sector wise absolute and semi-quantitative perfusion indices and SNR for each ^{1}H DCE measurement. Mean and standard deviation over all sectors are presented below the respective maps. **b** Comparison of sector-wise perfusion indices derived from dual-bolus ^{1}H gadolinium DCE measurements and hyperpolarized ^{13}C pyruvate measurements. **c** Exemplary perfusion curves acquired in subject 3. Raw data points are depicted with markers; solid lines show the calculated tissue response for the fitted Fermi function

effects: Firstly, cardiac motion and hemodynamics can introduce additional dephasing and distortions as well as misregistration between image frames. Hemodynamics are particularly important for hyperpolarized contrast agents, as each excitation of the imaging slice saturates part of the contrast agent bolus magnetization in the blood compartment. In the presented simulation, this effect was neglected as the dynamics of bolus localization and concentration are not available and would require extensive 3D computational fluid dynamics. Improper adjustment of the velocity selective excitation may therefore have stronger impact on perfusion measurements in vivo than indicated by simulations. Other common obstacles in hyperpolarized imaging in general, such as coil combination strategies at low SNR levels without measured sensitivity maps and flip-angle miscalibration were also omitted in this study.

Feasibility of cardiac perfusion CMR with interleaved AIF sampling using hyperpolarized [1-^{13}C] pyruvate was

demonstrated in vivo in swine. As predicted by simulations, the achievable SNR, B_0 homogeneity and expected kinetic conversion rates appear feasible for absolute and semi-quantitative perfusion assessment. Overall data quality was comparable to a previous study using hyperpolarized [^{13}C] urea [11]. Localized phase variations caused by the aortic jet resulted in geometric distortion and signal pile-up artifacts in the septal region which compromised accurate analysis in this sector. Optimizing the readout strategy is believed to be crucial in improving overall quality of hyperpolarized perfusion CMR. The phase sensitivity of EPI readouts could be reduced by increasing the bandwidth along the phase encoding direction if higher gradient system performance becomes available. Similarly, spiral readouts that are inherently insensitive to flow artifacts require gradient specifications beyond most current clinical systems in order to achieve sufficient resolution. Flow-compensated EPI [44] could minimize motion induced artifacts, yet results in prohibitively long readout durations and echo times.

Full validation regarding the accuracy of quantitative perfusion CMR using hyperpolarized pyruvate with a gold-standard method remains to be performed. However, preliminary ^{1}H gadolinium DCE data obtained from the same subjects under maintained stress condition have been processed and are presented in Fig. 9. Good agreement between the two modalities with respect to mean values is found, variability is however relatively high in both cases due to current experimental limitations. Our current combined ^{13}C TxRx/^{1}H Rx coil setup is limited in particular regarding ^{1}H sensitivity which in turn compromised the quality of ^{1}H perfusion data. In order to acquire state-of-the-art ^{1}H images during the same stress protocol, future validation studies need to improve the experimental setup with respect to ^{1}H receive coil architecture.

Although adenosine is often used as a vasodilator in clinical stress CMR, administration protocols in swine are still being established. The required adenosine doses are significantly higher compared to humnan protocols and cause systemic vasodilation and hypotension in the porcine model [45]. These systemic side-effects warrant additional pharmacological intervention, e.g. with α_1-adrenergic receptor agonists [46, 47]. In this proof-of-principle study, dobutamine was hence used for the ease of inducing a strong vasodilatory response [48, 49]. Accordingly, the ^{1}H perfusion protocols had to be adjusted to cope with high heart rates during dobutamine stress CMR, which also required compromises regarding the optimal saturation delay in the ^{1}H perfusion sequence. Upon translation of our work to humans, adenosine will be the preferred stressor and hence clinically tested ^{1}H perfusion protocols are applicable.

The quantification methods used for ^{13}C pyruvate data in this study have been directly adopted from existing methods for ^{1}H gadolinium enhanced perfusion stress CMR. Although initial comparison between both modalities looks promising, further work is required in the development of tailored perfusion models for ^{13}C pyruvate. Such improved models should not only account for differences in molecular size and therefore permeability, but also entail active transport over cell membranes and possible metabolic conversion.

Conclusion

In this study, a comprehensive simulation framework to assess requirements for accurate absolute and semi-quantitative cardiac perfusion CMR using hyperpolarized [1-^{13}C] pyruvate has been presented along with demonstration of in vivo feasibility. With the current translation of dissolution dynamic nuclear polarization

into humans, the assessment of myocardial perfusion CMR with hyperpolarized [1-^{13}C] pyruvate holds potential for the diagnosis of coronary artery and microvascular disease.

Abbreviations

AHA: American Heart Association (segmentation); AIF: Arterial input function; AUC : Area under the curve; CMR: Cardiovascular magnetic resonance; CNR: Contrast-to-noise ratio; CoV: Coefficient of variance; DCE: Dynamic contrast enhancement; ECG: Electrocardiogram; EPI: Echo planar imaging; FA: Flip angle; FOV: Field-of-view; IRF: Impulse response function; LAD: Left anterior descending coronary artery; LCx: Left circumflex coronary artery; LV: Left ventricle/left ventricular; MBF: Myocardial blood flow; RCA: Right coronary artery; RF: Radio-Frequency; RV: Right ventricle/right Ventricular; SNR: Signal-to-noise ratio; TE: Echo time; TR: Repetition time

Funding

This research was funded in parts by the Clinical Research Priority Program for Molecular Imaging of the University of Zurich (MINZ) and the Swiss National Science Foundation, grant SNF 320030_153014.

Authors' contributions

MF, JB: study design, CMR sequence programming. MF: image reconstruction and post-processing, manuscript drafting, participation in animal preparation. MF, JT, PW: implementation of simulation framework. MF, JB, JT, SMP, CTS: in-vivo measurements, participation in animal preparation. MF, JB, JT, SMP: preparation of hyperpolarized ^{13}C urea solution. MF,JB,JT,PW,SMP,ML,MS,TF,NC,CTS,SK: manuscript revision. ML, MS, TF, NC: preparation and monitoring of animals, ethics approval. CTS: study coordination, study design. SK: study coordination, study design. All authors read and approved the final manuscript.

Competing interests

The authors declare that they have no competing interests.

Author details

^{1}Institute for Biomedical Engineering, University and ETH Zurich, Gloriastrasse, 35 8092 Zurich, Switzerland. ^{2}Division of Surgical Research, University Hospital Zurich, Sternwartstrasse, 14 8091 Zurich, Switzerland.

References

1. Gerber BL, Raman SV, Nayak K, Epstein FH, Ferreira P, Axel L, et al. Myocardial first-pass perfusion cardiovascular magnetic resonance: history, theory, and current state of the art. J Cardiovasc Magn Reson. 2008;10:18.
2. Greenwood JP, Maredia N, Younger JF, Brown JM, Nixon J, Everett CC, et al. Cardiovascular magnetic resonance and single-photon emission computed tomography for diagnosis of coronary heart disease (CE-MARC): a

prospective trial. Lancet. 2012;379:453–60. https://doi.org/10.1016/S0140-6736(11)61335-4.

3. Jerosch-Herold M. Quantification of myocardial perfusion by cardiovascular magnetic resonance. J Cardiovasc Magn Reson. 2010;12:57. https://doi.org/10.1186/1532-429X-12-57.

4. Engblom H, Xue H, Akil S, Carlsson M, Hindorf C, Oddstig J, et al. Fully quantitative cardiovascular magnetic resonance myocardial perfusion ready for clinical use: a comparison between cardiovascular magnetic resonance imaging and positron emission tomography. J Cardiovasc Magn Reson. 2017;19:1–9.

5. Köstler H, Ritter C, Lipp M, Beer M, Hahn D, Sandstede J. Prebolus quantitative MR heart perfusion imaging. Magn Reson Med. 2004;52:296–9. https://doi.org/10.1002/mrm.20160.

6. Epstein FH, London JF, Peters DC, Goncalves LM, Agyeman K, Taylor J, et al. Multislice first-pass cardiac perfusion MRI: validation in a model of myocardial infarction. Magn Reson Med. 2002;47:482–91 http://www.ncbi.nlm.nih.gov/pubmed/11870835.

7. Kellman P, Arai AE. Imaging sequences for first pass perfusion - a review. J Cardiovasc Magn Reson. 2007;9:525–37. https://doi.org/10.1080/10976640601187604.

8. Christian TF, Rettmann DW, Aletras AH, Liao SL, Taylor JL, Balaban RS, et al. Absolute myocardial perfusion in canines measured by using dual-bolus first-pass MR imaging. Radiology. 2004;232:677–84. https://doi.org/10.1148/radiol.2323030573.

9. Gatehouse PD, Elkington AG, N a A, Yang G-Z, Pennell DJ, Firmin DN. Accurate assessment of the arterial input function during high-dose myocardial perfusion cardiovascular magnetic resonance. J Magn Reson Imaging. 2004;20:39–45. https://doi.org/10.1002/jmri.20054.

10. Ardenkjaer-Larsen JH, Fridlund B, Gram A, Hansson G, Hansson L, Lerche MH, et al. Increase in signal-to-noise ratio of > 10,000 times in liquid-state NMR. Proc Natl Acad Sci U S A. 2003;100:10158–63 http://www.pnas.org/content/100/18/10158.short. Accessed 16 Oct 2014.

11. Fuetterer M, Busch J, Peereboom SM, von Deuster C, Wissmann L, Lipiski M, et al. Hyperpolarized 13C urea myocardial first-pass perfusion imaging using velocity-selective excitation. J Cardiovasc Magn Reson. 2017;19:46. https://doi.org/10.1186/s12968-017-0364-4.

12. von Morze C, Larson PEZ, Hu S, Yoshihara HAI, Bok RA, Goga A, et al. Investigating tumor perfusion and metabolism using multiple hyperpolarized 13C compounds: HP001, pyruvate and urea. Magn Reson Imaging. 2012;30:305–11. https://doi.org/10.1016/j.mri.2011.09.026.

13. Grant AK, Vinogradov E, Wang X, Lenkinski RE, Alsop DC. Perfusion imaging with a freely diffusible hyperpolarized contrast agent. Magn Reson Med. 2011;66:746–55. https://doi.org/10.1002/mrm.22860.

14. Durst M, Chiavazza E, Haase A, Aime S, Schwaiger M, Schulte RF. α-Trideuteromethyl[15N]glutamine: a long-lived hyperpolarized perfusion marker. Magn Reson Med. 2016;76:1900–4. https://doi.org/10.1002/mrm.26104.

15. Dodd MS, Ball V, Bray R, Ashrafian H, Watkins H, Clarke K, et al. In vivo mouse cardiac hyperpolarized magnetic resonance spectroscopy. J Cardiovasc Magn Reson. 2013;15:19. https://doi.org/10.1186/1532-429X-15-19.

16. Golman K, Petersson JS, Magnusson P, Johansson E, Akeson P, Chai C-M, et al. Cardiac metabolism measured noninvasively by hyperpolarized 13C MRI. Magn Reson Med. 2008;59:1005–13. https://doi.org/10.1002/mrm.21460.

17. Ball DR, Cruickshank R, C a C, Stuckey DJ, Lee P, Clarke K, et al. Metabolic imaging of acute and chronic infarction in the perfused rat heart using hyperpolarised [1-13C]pyruvate. NMR Biomed. 2013;26:1441–50. https://doi.org/10.1002/nbm.2972.

18. Bankson JA, Walker CM, Ramirez MS, Stefan W, Fuentes D, Merritt ME, et al. Kinetic modeling and constrained reconstruction of hyperpolarized [1-13C]-pyruvate offers improved metabolic imaging of tumors. Cancer Res. 2015;75:4708 17. https://doi.org/10.1158/0008-5472.CAN-15-0171.

19. Harris T, Eliyahu G, Frydman L, Degani H. Kinetics of hyperpolarized 13C1-pyruvate transport and metabolism in living human breast cancer cells. Proc Natl Acad Sci U S A. 2009;106:18131–6. https://doi.org/10.1073/pnas.0909049106.

20. Mariotti E, Orton MR, Eerbeek O, Ashruf JF, Zuurbier CJ, Southworth R, et al. Modeling non-linear kinetics of hyperpolarized [1- 13 C] pyruvate in the crystalloid-perfused rat heart. NMR Biomed. 2016;29:377–86. https://doi.org/10.1002/nbm.3464.

21. Gómez Damián PA, Sperl JI, Janich MA, Khegai O, Wiesinger F, Glaser SJ, et al. Multisite kinetic modeling of 13C metabolic MR using [1- 13C] pyruvate. Radiol Res Pract. 2014;2014:1–10. https://doi.org/10.1155/2014/871619.

22. Lau AZ, Miller JJ, Robson MD, Tyler DJ. Cardiac perfusion imaging using hyperpolarized 13C urea using flow sensitizing gradients. Magn Reson Med. 2016;75:1474–83. https://doi.org/10.1002/mrm.25713.

23. Lau AZ, Miller JJ, Robson MD, Tyler DJ. Simultaneous assessment of cardiac metabolism and perfusion using copolarized [1- 13C]pyruvate and 13C-urea. Magn Reson Med. 2017;77:151–8. https://doi.org/10.1002/mrm.26106.

24. Rider OJ, Tyler DJ. Clinical implications of cardiac hyperpolarized magnetic resonance imaging. J Cardiovasc Magn Reson. 2013;15:93. https://doi.org/10.1186/1532-429X-15-93.

25. Cunningham CH, Lau JYC, Chen AP, Geraghty BJ, Perks WJ, Roifman I, et al. Hyperpolarized 13C metabolic MRI of the human heart: initial experience. Circ Res. 2016;119:1177–82. https://doi.org/10.1161/CIRCRESAHA.116.309769.

26. Wissmann L, Santelli C, Segars WP, Kozerke S. MRXCAT: realistic numerical phantoms for cardiovascular magnetic resonance. J Cardiovasc Magn Reson. 2014;16:63. https://doi.org/10.1186/s12968-014-0063-3.

27. Cerqueira MD. Standardized myocardial segmentation and nomenclature for tomographic imaging of the heart: a statement for healthcare professionals from the cardiac imaging Committee of the Council on clinical cardiology of the American Heart Association. Circulation. 2002;105:539–42. https://doi.org/10.1161/hc0402.102975.

28. Khalidov I, Van De Ville D, Jacob M, Lazeyras F, Unser M. BSLIM: spectral localization by imaging with explicit B0 field inhomogeneity compensation. IEEE Trans Med Imaging. 2007;26:990–1000. https://doi.org/10.1109/TMI.2007.897385.

29. Yen Y-F, Le Roux P, Mayer D, King R, Spielman D, Tropp J, et al. T 2 relaxation times of 13 C metabolites in a rat hepatocellular carcinoma model measured in vivo using 13 C-MRS of hyperpolarized [1–13 C]pyruvate. NMR Biomed. 2010; May 2009:n/a-n/a. doi:https://doi.org/10.1002/nbm.1481.

30. Wissmann L, Niemann M, Gotschy A, Manka R, Kozerke S. Quantitative three-dimensional myocardial perfusion cardiovascular magnetic resonance with accurate two-dimensional arterial input function assessment. J Cardiovasc Magn Reson. 2015;17, 108. https://doi.org/10.1186/s12968-015-0212-3.

31. Roemer PB, Edelstein WA, Hayes CE, Souza SP, Mueller OM. The NMR phased array. Magn Reson Med. 1990;16:192–225. https://doi.org/10.1002/mrm.1910160203.

32. Firbank MJ, Coulthard A, Harrison RM, Williams ED. A comparison of two methods for measuring the signal to noise ratio on MR images. Phys Med Biol. 1999;44:N261–4. https://doi.org/10.1088/0031-9155/44/12/403.

33. Ishida M, Schuster A, Morton G, Chiribiri A, Hussain S, Paul M, et al. Development of a universal dual-bolus injection scheme for the quantitative assessment of myocardial perfusion cardiovascular magnetic resonance. J Cardiovasc Magn Reson. 2011;13:28. https://doi.org/10.1186/1532-429X-13-28.

34. Ogg RJ, Kingsley PB, Taylor JS. WET, a T1- and B1-insensitive water-suppression method for in vivo localized 1H NMR spectroscopy. J Magn Reson B. 1994;104:1–10.

35. Park JM, Josan S, Mayer D, Hurd RE, Chung Y, Bendahan D, et al. Hyperpolarized 13C NMR observation of lactate kinetics in skeletal muscle. J Exp Biol. 2015;218:3308–18. https://doi.org/10.1242/jeb.123141.

36. Hill DK, Orton MR, Mariotti E, Boult JKR, Panek R, Jafar M, et al. Model free approach to kinetic analysis of real-time hyperpolarized 13C magnetic resonance spectroscopy data. PLoS One. 2013;8:e71996. https://doi.org/10.1371/journal.pone.0071996.

37. Pfeffer MA, Braunwald E, Moyé LA, Basta L, Brown EJ, Cuddy TE, et al. Effect of captopril on mortality and morbidity in patients with left ventricular dysfunction after myocardial infarction. Results of the survival and ventricular enlargement trial. The SAVE investigators. N Engl J Med. 1992;327:669–77. https://doi.org/10.1056/NEJM199209033271001.

38. Geraghty BJ, Lau JYC, Chen AP, Cunningham CH. Dual-Echo EPI sequence for integrated distortion correction in 3D time-resolved hyperpolarized13C MRI. Magn Reson Med. 2018;79:643–53.

39. Miller JJ, Lau AZ, Tyler DJ. Susceptibility-induced distortion correction in hyperpolarized echo planar imaging. Magn Reson Med. 2018;79:2135–41.

40. Nagel E, Klein C, Paetsch I, Hettwer S, Schnackenburg B, Wegscheider K, et al. Magnetic resonance perfusion measurements for the noninvasive detection of coronary artery disease. Circulation. 2003;108:432–7. https://doi.org/10.1161/01.CIR.0000080915.35024.A9.

41. Jerosch-Herold M, Hu X, Murthy NS, Rickers C, Stillman AE. Magnetic resonance imaging of myocardial contrast enhancement with MS-325 and its relation to myocardial blood flow and the perfusion reserve. J Magn Reson Imaging. 2003;18:544–54.

42. Klocke FJ, Simonetti OP, Judd RM, Kim RJ, Harris KR, Hedjbeli S, et al. Limits of detection of regional differences in vasodilated flow in viable myocardium by first-pass magnetic resonance perfusion imaging. Circulation. 2001;104:2412–6.

43. Durst M, Koellisch U, Frank A, Rancan G, Gringeri CV, Karas V, et al. Comparison of acquisition schemes for hyperpolarised 13 C imaging. NMR Biomed. 2015;28:715–25. https://doi.org/10.1002/nbm.3301.

44. Duerk JL, Simonetti OP. Theoretical aspects of motion sensitivity and compensation in echo-planar imaging. J Magn Reson Imaging. 1991;1:643–50. https://doi.org/10.1002/jmri.1880010605.

45. Rossi A, Uitterdijk A, Dijkshoorn M, Klotz E, Dharampal A, Van Straten M, et al. Quantification of myocardial blood flow by adenosine-stress CT perfusion imaging in pigs during various degrees of stenosis correlates well with coronary artery blood flow and fractional flow reserve. Eur Heart J Cardiovasc Imaging. 2013;14:331–8.

46. Duncker DJ, Stubenitsky R, Verdouw PD. Autonomic control of vasomotion in the porcine coronary circulation during treadmill exercise: evidence for feed-forward beta-adrenergic control. Circ Res. 1998;82:1312–22.

47. Sorop O, Merkus D, De Beer VJ, Houweling B, Pistea A, McFalls EO, et al. Functional and structural adaptations of coronary microvessels distal to a chronic coronary artery stenosis. Circ Res. 2008;102:795–803.

48. Gebker R, Jahnke C, Manka R, Frick M, Hucko T, Kozerke S, et al. High spatial resolution myocardial perfusion imaging during high dose dobutamine/atropine stress magnetic resonance using k-t SENSE. Int J Cardiol. 2012;158: 411–6. https://doi.org/10.1016/j.ijcard.2011.01.060.

49. Gebker R, Jahnke C, Manka R, Hamdan A, Schnackenburg B, Fleck E, et al. Additional value of myocardial perfusion imaging during Dobutamine stress magnetic resonance for the assessment of coronary artery disease. Circ Cardiovasc Imaging. 2008;1:122–30. https://doi.org/10.1161/CIRCIMAGING. 108.779108.

24

Comparison of left ventricular strains and torsion derived from feature tracking and DENSE CMR

Gregory J. Wehner[1], Linyuan Jing[2,3], Christopher M. Haggerty[2,3], Jonathan D. Suever[2,3], Jing Chen[2], Sean M. Hamlet[4], Jared A. Feindt[2], W. Dimitri Mojsejenko[3], Mark A. Fogel[5] and Brandon K. Fornwalt[1,2,3,4,6]* (iD)

Abstract

Background: Cardiovascular magnetic resonance (CMR) feature tracking is increasingly used to quantify cardiac mechanics from cine CMR imaging, although validation against reference standard techniques has been limited. Furthermore, studies have suggested that commonly-derived metrics, such as peak global strain (reported in 63% of feature tracking studies), can be quantified using contours from just two frames – end-diastole (ED) and end-systole (ES) – without requiring tracking software. We hypothesized that mechanics derived from feature tracking would not agree with those derived from a reference standard (displacement-encoding with stimulated echoes (DENSE) imaging), and that peak strain from feature tracking would agree with that derived using simple processing of only ED and ES contours.

Methods: We retrospectively identified 88 participants with 186 pairs of DENSE and balanced steady state free precession (bSSFP) image slices acquired at the same locations across two institutions. Left ventricular (LV) strains, torsion, and dyssynchrony were quantified from both feature tracking (TomTec Imaging Systems, Circle Cardiovascular Imaging) and DENSE. Contour-based strains from bSSFP images were derived from ED and ES contours. Agreement was assessed with Bland-Altman analyses and coefficients of variation (CoV). All biases are reported in absolute percentage.

Results: Comparison results were similar for both vendor packages (TomTec and Circle), and thus only TomTec Imaging System data are reported in the abstract for simplicity. Compared to DENSE, mid-ventricular circumferential strain (Ecc) from feature tracking had acceptable agreement (bias: -0.4%, $p = 0.36$, CoV: 11%). However, feature tracking significantly overestimated the magnitude of Ecc at the base (bias: -4.0% absolute, $p < 0.001$, CoV: 18%) and apex (bias: -2.4% absolute, $p = 0.01$, CoV: 15%), underestimated torsion (bias: -1.4 deg/cm, $p < 0.001$, CoV: 41%), and overestimated dyssynchrony (bias: 26 ms, $p < 0.001$, CoV: 76%). Longitudinal strain (Ell) had borderline-acceptable agreement (bias: -0.2%, $p = 0.77$, CoV: 19%). Contour-based strains had excellent agreement with feature tracking (biases: -1.3–0.2%, CoVs: 3–7%).

(Continued on next page)

* Correspondence: bkf@gatech.edu
[1]Department of Biomedical Engineering, University of Kentucky, Lexington, KY, USA
[2]Department of Imaging Science and Innovation, Geisinger, 100 North Academy Avenue, Danville, PA 17822-4400, USA
Full list of author information is available at the end of the article

(Continued from previous page)

Conclusion: Compared to DENSE as a reference standard, feature tracking was inaccurate for quantification of apical and basal LV circumferential strains, longitudinal strain, torsion, and dyssynchrony. Feature tracking was only accurate for quantification of mid LV circumferential strain. Moreover, feature tracking is unnecessary for quantification of whole-slice strains (e.g. base, apex), since simplified processing of only ED and ES contours yields very similar results to those derived from feature tracking. Current feature tracking technology therefore has limited utility for quantification of cardiac mechanics.

Keywords: DENSE, Feature tracking, Strain, Torsion, Dyssynchrony,

Background

Cardiac mechanics, such as strain, torsion, and dyssynchrony, are important indicators of cardiac function and independent predictors of serious outcomes, even when accounting for traditional measures such as ejection fraction [1, 2]. Several advanced cardiovascular magnetic resonance (CMR) sequences have been developed to assess cardiac mechanics including tagging [3, 4], displacement encoding with stimulated echoes (DENSE) [5–7], strain encoding (SENC) [8], and tissue phase mapping (TPM) [9]. While these techniques can provide reference standard measurements of myocardial motion and deformation, their use is often clinically impractical. Furthermore, because they are specialized non-clinical techniques, there are few large datasets available that could be used to guide the clinical use of these techniques. As such, there has been growing interest in the use of feature tracking software to approximate the mechanics produced by reference standard techniques [10–12]. While feature tracking is simple to use and requires only standard anatomical cine sequences that are widely available, it is important to assess how well measures of cardiac mechanics such as left ventricular (LV) strain, torsion, and dyssynchrony derived from feature tracking agree with those derived from reference standard techniques.

While results from feature tracking have been compared to those from tissue tagging [10, 13–16] and TPM [17], many of these studies have been limited in scope. The largest study [10], with 191 patients with Duchenne's Muscular Dystrophy and 42 healthy controls, surveyed only mid-ventricular short-axis images, while other studies have had limited sample sizes (n = 18 [16], n = 20 [13]). Such studies have suggested that feature tracking may have poor reproducibility and poor agreement with reference standard techniques for some measures of cardiac mechanics [12, 13] due to the following potential limitations: 1) feature tracking derives displacement fields by propagating myocardial borders from frame to frame, which relies on quantification of local changes in signal intensity and therefore is likely to fail when quantifying motion parallel to or inside the myocardium where there are no features; 2) feature tracking only captures in-plane displacement, and through-plane motion of the myocardium violates the assumptions required to track pixel data.

DENSE, an advanced CMR technique, encodes a component of tissue displacement into the phase of the CMR image [5]. The reconstructed phase image measures displacements directly at the pixel-level with higher spatial resolution (2–3 mm) than myocardial tagging, which is limited by the number of tag lines that can be reliably tracked in the image. Therefore, motion within the myocardium can be accurately captured in all directions. Indeed, data from a deforming phantom demonstrated that DENSE has equal or better performance than tagged CMR, depending on the measured cardiac mechanic [18]. Several advancements in DENSE acquisition since its introduction, such as complementary spatial modulation of magnetization (CSPAMM) artifact suppression [6] and efficient spiral readouts [7], make it an ideal, highly reproducible and validated technique for reference standard measurements of myocardial motion and deformation used by numerous previous studies [18–24]. However, none of the feature tracking validation studies have been performed with DENSE. Indeed, a recent study [25] included data from both DENSE and feature tracking, but no direct comparisons were made.

Additionally, a literature review including 62 CMR feature tracking studies found that slice-wise strains (i.e. the average strain over an entire image, such as basal, mid-ventricular, or apical short-axis slices) are the most commonly reported measures derived from feature tracking (Table 1 and Additional file 1). In total, 39 studies (63%) reported either circumferential, longitudinal, or radial slice-wise strain, and 13 studies (21%) reported only those strains. However, slice-wise strains, which are reflective of the change in length of an entire contour between just two frames, end-diastole (ED) and end-systole (ES), should not require segmental motion tracking [26]. This suggests that the most commonly reported results from feature tracking could be easily assessed without performing tracking, by simply using the ED and ES contours which are already generated during most clinical CMR scans.

We hypothesized that LV strains, torsion, and dyssynchrony estimated from feature tracking would not agree well with those measured by DENSE as a reference standard. We also hypothesized that slice-wise strains

Table 1 Reported mechanics from 62 CMR feature tracking studies

Mechanics	Number of Studies
Circumferential Strain – slice-wise	36
Longitudinal Strain – slice-wise	28
Radial Strain – slice-wise	21
Circumferential Strain – segmental	18
Longitudinal Strain – segmental	12
Radial Strain – segmental	12
Systolic Strain Rate	5
Diastolic Strain Rate	6
Torsion	8
Torsion Rate	5
Synchrony	6
Atrial Strain	8
Right Ventricular Strain - any	13
Right Ventricular Strain - segmental	7
Other[a]	3

[a]Feature tracking in non-CMR modality

from measuring the change in length of entire contours between the ED and ES frames ("contour-based" strains) would agree well with strains reported by feature tracking.

Methods

Study population

We reviewed our database of CMR participant datasets that were acquired from 2013 to 2016 at two institutions (University of Kentucky and the Children's Hospital of Philadelphia) for all instances where both spiral cine DENSE and balanced steady state free precession (bSSFP) were acquired at the same slice location either in basal, mid-ventricular, or apical short-axis image planes or in the four-chamber image plane. The studies were approved by the local IRBs and all participants gave informed consent. During the review, no exclusions for diagnosis or the presence of cardiovascular risk factors were applied.

Image acquisition

All datasets from the University of Kentucky were acquired on a 3 T system (Trio, Siemens Healthineers, Erlangen, Germany) while datasets from the Children's Hospital of Philadelphia were acquired on a 1.5 T system (Avanto, Siemens Healthineers). Spiral cine DENSE images with displacements encoded in at least the two in-plane dimensions were acquired with an established spiral sequence [7, 18, 21] using the following parameters: 6 spiral interleaves with 2 spiral interleaves acquired per temporal frame, 250×250 to 360×360 mm^2 field of view, 128×128

image matrix, 1.95×1.95 to 2.81×2.81 mm^2 pixel size, 8 mm slice thickness, 1.08 ms echo time, 15 to 17 ms repetition time, 17 to 34 ms temporal resolution. Simple or balanced encoding [19] with an encoding frequency between 0.04 and 0.10 cycles/mm [20] was used to measure in-plane displacements, while through-plane dephasing [27] and CSPAMM [6] were used for echo suppression. Cine bSSFP images were acquired at the same locations as the DENSE images using the following parameters: 1.15×1.15 to 1.77×1.77 mm^2 pixel size, 7 to 10 mm slice thickness, 1.15 to 1.51 ms echo time, 2.70 to 3.43 ms repetition time, 8 to 15 k-space segments (true number of frames, 14–30 reconstructed frames), 20.2 to 49.7 ms temporal resolution.

DENSE strain analysis

Cardiac strains were derived from the DENSE images as previously described using *DENSEanalysis*, an open-source application [28] written in MATLAB (The Mathworks Inc., Natick, Massachusetts, USA) [22]. Examples of image analysis for DENSE as well as feature tracking are shown in Fig. 1. The post-processing steps for each cine DENSE slice included manual segmentation of the LV myocardium and semi-automated phase unwrapping to obtain the 2D displacements within each cardiac frame [22]. Following the unwrapping, spatial smoothing and temporal fitting of displacements (10th order polynomial) were performed as previously described to obtain smooth trajectories for all tissue points beginning at end-diastole and continuing through systole and into mid-diastole [22]. Circumferential (Ecc) and longitudinal (Ell) strains were calculated from short-axis and four-chamber images, respectively, using the Lagrangian Green finite strain tensor. Both circumferential and longitudinal strain were defined as negative for tissue shortening. For participants ($n = 38$) that had all three short-axis images (basal, mid-ventricular, and apical), cardiac torsion was calculated as the gradient of twist down the long axis of the left ventricle by finding the slope of the linear regression line between twist and longitudinal position. Twist was defined as positive for counter-clockwise rotation relative to the centroid of the LV when viewing a short-axis image from the apex towards the base. Torsion was positive when the apex was twisting more positively than the base. Dyssynchrony was quantified in these same participants ($n = 38$). To quantify dyssynchrony, cross-correlation delays for each segmental circumferential strain curve from the basal, mid-ventricular, and apical short-axis slices were calculated relative to a patient-specific reference curve [29]. Dyssynchrony was defined as the standard deviation of the segmental delays.

Feature tracking strain analysis

Strain and twist were derived from bSSFP imaging with Diogenes feature tracking software (2D CPA MR, version 1.1.2.36, TomTec Imaging Systems, Munich,

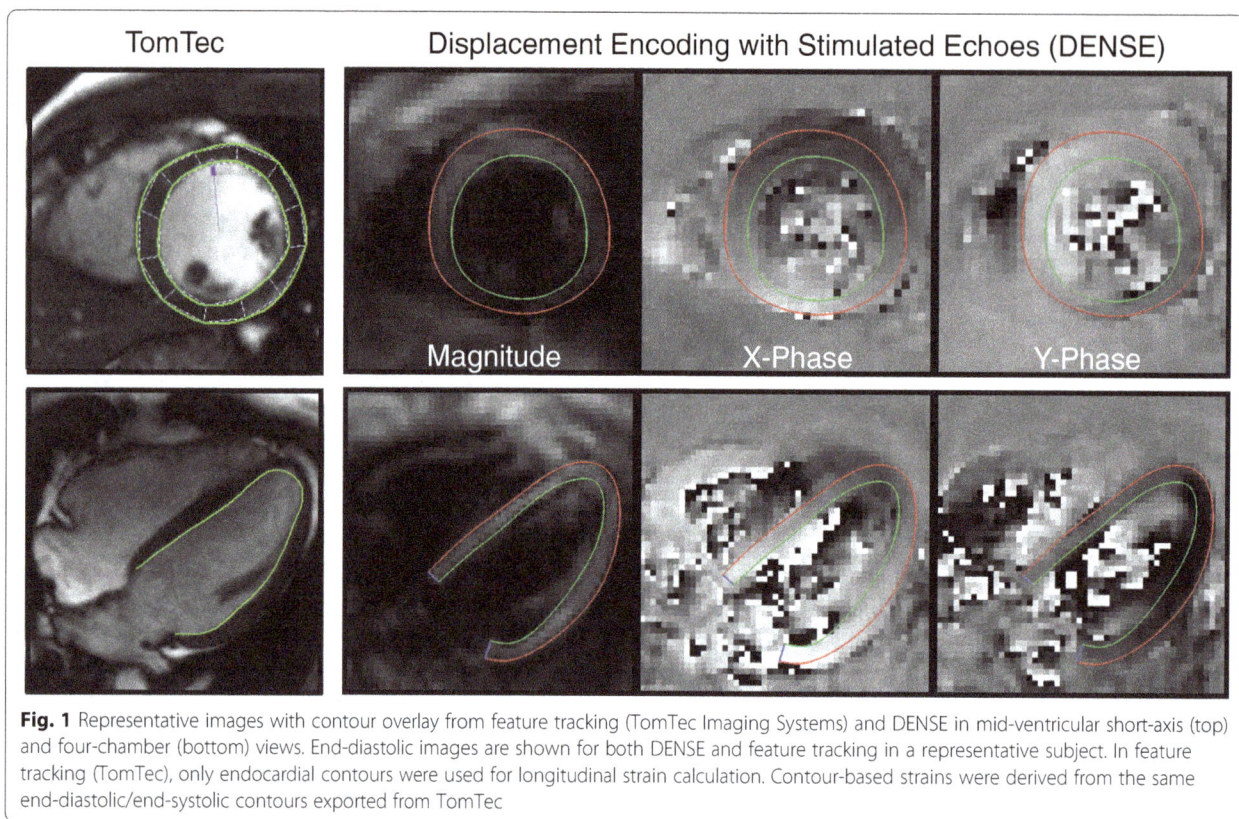

Fig. 1 Representative images with contour overlay from feature tracking (TomTec Imaging Systems) and DENSE in mid-ventricular short-axis (top) and four-chamber (bottom) views. End-diastolic images are shown for both DENSE and feature tracking in a representative subject. In feature tracking (TomTec), only endocardial contours were used for longitudinal strain calculation. Contour-based strains were derived from the same end-diastolic/end-systolic contours exported from TomTec

Germany). For short-axis images, both endocardial and epicardial contours were manually drawn at ED and the software automatically propagated the contours through the remaining frames. For the four-chamber image, only an endocardial contour was drawn before propagation, since there is minimal transmural difference in longitudinal strain (Ell) between the endocardium and epicardium as compared to the typical transmural differences seen in circumferential strain (Ecc). In the case of poor tracking, ED contours were redrawn and the propagation repeated until the tracking was visually acceptable. Ecc, Ell, and twist were derived from output files generated by the software. In short-axis slices and for appropriate comparisons to DENSE, which measures strain and twist throughout the myocardial wall, the endocardial and epicardial strains and twist from feature tracking were averaged together to obtain a single transmural value. Additional file 2 contains comparisons between just the endocardial strain from feature tracking and DENSE. Torsion and dyssynchrony were computed using the same calculations as above for DENSE imaging. Studies using feature tracking have stated that strains were derived using the 1D Lagrangian calculation [14, 30, 31], and this was reaffirmed through email correspondence with the vendor.

To assess Ecc and Ell via the change in length of entire contours, the contour position data reported in the

output files for only the ED and ES frames from feature tracking using the bSSFP images were used. The frame with the smallest contour circumference was defined as the ES frame. By using these contours, rather than having an observer draw them separately, any intra- and inter-observer variability was removed for the comparison between contour-based strains and feature tracking. However, there should be no fundamental difference in manually-drawn contours and the TomTec propagated contours. This enabled a pure assessment of whether regional tracking information, which would be known to the TomTec strain calculation, is different from just using the lengths of the ED and ES contours. Contour-based strains were derived from the 1D Lagrangian strain calculation.

Finally, it is important to consider the mathematics of the strain calculations if they are different between two techniques. A full derivation of the difference between strains computed from the 2D Lagrangian Green strain tensor of DENSE and the 1D Lagrangian strain from feature tracking and contours is provided in Additional file 3. The relationship can also be found throughout the literature on deformation mechanics (e.g. see chapter 3, page 119, eq. 3.24.12 [32]). From this relationship, we propose that a correction can be applied to the 1D Lagrangian strain results to allow a proper comparison with the DENSE strain results from the 2D Lagrangian Green strain tensor. Specifically, given a 1D

Lagrangian strain, ε, we propose to adjust that value by adding $(1/2)\,\varepsilon^2$ to account for differences in the strain calculations per the following equation:

$$2D\ Lagrangian\ Green\ Strain = \varepsilon + \left(\frac{1}{2}\right)(\varepsilon)^2.$$

In order to validate our findings in feature tracking, we also analyzed all data using a separate commercial feature tracking software (cvi[42], Circle Cardiovascular Imaging Inc., Calgary, Alberta, Canada). Detailed description of data analyses and results from this comparison are shown in Additional file 4. Since the results were not substantially different between the two vendor platforms, the term "feature tracking" refers to TomTec only in the primary results below for simplification.

Statistics

Agreement of strains and torsion between feature tracking and DENSE was assessed with Bland-Altman analyses and coefficients of variation (CoV). Based on similar analyses in previous studies [24, 33], CoVs less than 20% were interpreted as acceptable. Paired t-tests were utilized to determine whether biases were statistically significant from zero at a significance level of 0.05. Comparisons between feature tracking and DENSE were made both before and after adjusting the feature tracking results to account for the differences in strain calculations. Bland-Altman analyses and CoVs were also used to compare adjusted feature tracking strains to adjusted contour-based strains. Continuous data are presented as mean ± standard deviation.

Results

Study population

From the review of our database, 89 unique participants were identified that had spiral cine DENSE and bSSFP imaging at the same image locations. Of those, 1 participant had poor DENSE image quality due to aberrant prospective electrocardiogram (ECG) triggering and was therefore omitted from analyses. From these 88 participants, we obtained 186 independent image pairs, regionally distributed as follows: 39 basal short-axis, 69 mid-ventricular short-axis, 38 apical short-axis, and 40 four-chamber images. For torsion and dyssynchrony, 38 participants had all 3 of the necessary short-axis images (i.e. all participants that had an apical short-axis image also had the other short-axis images). Characteristics of the participants for each image location are reported in Table 2. Compared to other regions, there was a preponderance of healthy individuals in the four-chamber images due to only acquiring short-axis images in many patient studies.

Table 2 Participant characteristics

	Base (n = 39)	Mid (n = 69)	Apex/Torsion/ Dyssynchrony (n = 38)	Four-Chamber (n = 40)
Age, years	27 ± 12	26 ± 14	27 ± 12	22 ± 9
Male, n (%)	23 (59)	44 (64)	22 (58)	23 (58)
Diagnosis, n (%)				
Healthy	24 (62)	51 (74)	23 (61)	39 (98)
Tetralogy of Fallot	6 (15)	6 (9)	6 (16)	1 (3)
Duchennes	1 (3)	1 (1)	1 (3)	0 (0)
Hypertrophic CM	2 (5)	2 (3)	2 (5)	0 (0)
Ischemic CM	1 (3)	2 (3)	1 (3)	0 (0)
Other	5 (13)	7 (10)	5 (13)	0 (0)

CM: Cardiomyopathy

Comparison between feature tracking and DENSE

When using just the endocardial strain from feature tracking, Ecc was significantly overestimated compared to DENSE, which measured strain throughout the myocardial wall (Additional file 2). The remainder of the Ecc, torsion, and dyssynchrony results are based on the average of the endocardial and epicardial values from feature tracking in order to better approximate the DENSE results as described in the Methods.

Before adjusting for differences in the strain calculations, Ecc was significantly overestimated by feature tracking compared to DENSE by between 2.3 and 6.0% (absolute, Table 3). Similarly, feature tracking tended to over-estimate Ell by 1.4%, although the result was not statistically significant ($p = 0.08$).

After adjusting the feature tracking results to account for differences in the strain calculations, feature tracking strains all decreased in magnitude – closer to corresponding DENSE values – such that the mid-ventricular Ecc were no longer different (–17.5 vs –17.2%, $p = 0.36$). However, basal and apical Ecc remained significantly overestimated by feature tracking even after adjustment (by 4.1 and 2.5% absolute, respectively [$p < 0.001$ for both]). A physiologic gradient of increasing Ecc magnitude from the base to the mid-ventricle to the apex was observed in the DENSE results. This gradient was not present in the feature tracking results before or after adjustment. On Bland-Altman analyses, the 95% limits of agreement and CoVs were lower after the feature tracking results were adjusted (Table 4, Fig. 2). Ecc at the mid-ventricular level had the best agreement between adjusted feature tracking and DENSE (95% limits: ±6.3%, CoV: 10.9%). All other strains demonstrated CoVs above 20% before applying the adjustment. Those same CoVs dropped below 20% after the adjustment. The CoV for Ell was 19.3%.

Torsion was significantly underestimated by feature tracking compared to DENSE (2.1 vs 3.5 deg/cm, $p < 0.001$). Dyssynchrony was significantly overestimated by

Table 3 Summary of strains and torsion from feature tracking and DENSE

	Feature Tracking (Unadjusted)	Feature Tracking (Adjusted)	DENSE	p₁	p₂
Circumferential Strain (%)					
Base	−21.7 ± 4.2	−19.3 ± 3.3	−15.2 ± 3.7	< 0.001*	< 0.001*
Mid	−19.5 ± 4.3	−17.5 ± 3.5	−17.2 ± 3.4	< 0.001*	0.36
Apex	−25.4 ± 7.8	−21.9 ± 5.7	−19.4 ± 3.6	< 0.001*	0.01*
Longitudinal Strain (%)					
Four-Chamber	−15.4 ± 5.1	−14.1 ± 4.3	−13.8 ± 2.9	0.083	0.77
Torsion (deg/cm)	2.1 ± 1.2	–	3.5 ± 0.9	< 0.001*	–
Dyssynchrony (ms)	42 ± 22	–	16 ± 20	< 0.001*	–

Unadjusted and Adjusted indicate the feature tracking results before and after adjustment, respectively
p_1, Feature Tracking (Unadjusted) vs. DENSE; p_2, Feature Tracking (Adjusted) vs. DENSE
*Indicates statistical significance ($p < 0.05$)

feature tracking (42 vs 16 ms, $p < 0.001$). Both torsion and dyssynchrony had poor agreement with DENSE as demonstrated by wide 95% limits and large CoVs (Fig. 3).

Comparison between feature tracking and contour-based strain

Excellent agreement was observed between all Ecc and Ell from feature tracking and contour-based strains (Table 5, Fig. 4) with CoVs between 3.2 and 7.0%. Bland-Altman 95% limits (between ±2.2 and ± 3.8%) were substantially lower than those observed during the comparisons between feature tracking and DENSE.

While the agreement between feature tracking and contour-based strain was excellent, we investigated why it was not perfect. Specifically, we found discrepancies between the appearance of the propagated contours and the strains that feature tracking reported for them. For example, Fig. 5 shows propagated endocardial contours for frame 1 and frame 30 (the last frame) for a short-axis image from a representative subject. There are noticeable differences in the contour

lengths between those two frames, and the contour-based strain calculation would quantify a small strain for frame 30 relative to frame 1. However, the feature tracking software reported exactly zero strain for all segments in both frame 1 and frame 30, which is inconsistent with the noticeable differences between the contours.

Validation of feature tracking using circle

In summary, the results from Circle are similar to the findings from TomTec. Consistent with TomTec, Circle significantly overestimated basal and apical Ecc, Ell, and dyssynchrony compared to DENSE (all $p < 0.001$, Additional file 4 Table S3), and the amount of overestimation was in general larger than that of TomTec (Additional file 4 Table S4, Figure S4). Only mid-ventricular Ecc from Circle showed good agreement with DENSE (bias = 0.7%, CoV = 11%). Opposite to TomTec, torsion was overestimated in Circle compared to DENSE (bias = 1.5 deg/cm, CoV = 36%). The agreements of torsion and dyssynchrony between Circle and TomTec, as well as between Circle and DENSE, were

Table 4 Bland-Altman analyses and coefficients of variation comparing Feature Tracking to the reference (DENSE)

	Feature Tracking (Unadjusted) vs. DENSE			Feature Tracking (Adjusted) vs. DENSE		
	Bias	95% Limits	CoV	Bias	95% Limits	CoV
Circumferential Strain (Absolute %)						
Base	−6.5	±7.7	25.1	−4.0	±6.7	17.8
Mid	−2.3	±7.3	13.7	−0.4	±6.3	10.9
Apex	−6.0	±14.3	22.3	−2.4	±10.8	14.8
Longitudinal Strain (Absolute %)						
Four-Chamber	−1.5	±10.7	21.3	−0.2	±9.3	19.3
Torsion (deg/cm)	−1.4	±2.4	41.1	–	–	–
Dyssynchrony (ms)	26	±56	76.3	–	–	–

Unadjusted and Adjusted indicate the feature tracking results before and after adjustment, respectively
CoV indicates coefficient of variation (%)

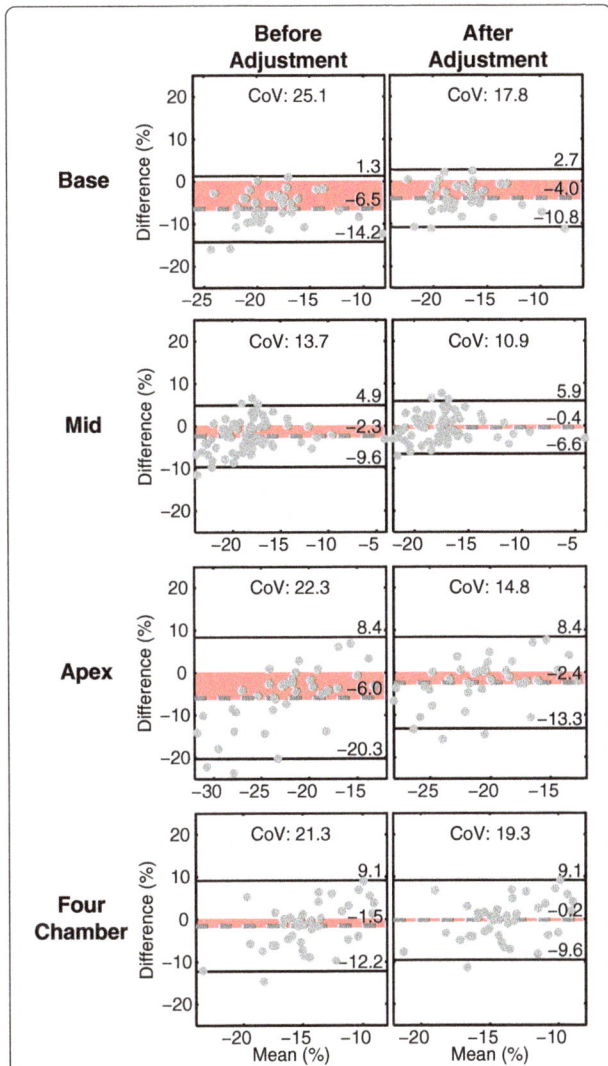

Fig. 2 Bland-Altman analyses for circumferential and longitudinal strains between feature tracking and DENSE. Analyses were performed both before (left column) and after (right column) adjusting the feature tracking results to account for differences in the strain calculation. All differences were calculated by subtracting the DENSE strain from the feature tracking strain. All biases and 95% limits of agreement improved after adjusting the feature tracking strains. The red shaded region highlights the bias. The best agreement was observed in mid-ventricular circumferential strain. CoV, coefficient of variation

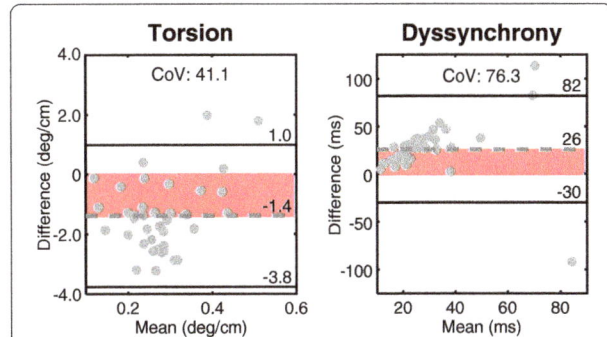

Fig. 3 Bland-Altman analyses for torsion and dyssynchrony between feature tracking and DENSE. All differences were calculated by subtracting the DENSE measurement from the feature tracking measurement. The red shaded region highlights the bias. Poor agreement between feature tracking and DENSE was observed for both measures as demonstrated by large biases, 95% limits, and CoVs. CoV, coefficient of variation

overestimated the magnitude of Ecc in basal and apical images, 3) feature tracking overestimated Ell in four-chamber images, 4) feature tracking significantly overestimated dyssynchrony and under- or over- estimated torsion depending on the vendor with unacceptable CoVs, and 5) slice-wise strains from the change in length of entire contours (contour-based strains) had excellent agreement with slice-wise strains reported by feature tracking.

Slice-wise strains from feature tracking and contour-based strains

Feature tracking has emerged as a simple and convenient tool for estimating cardiac mechanics from standard CMR imaging. However, we found that the most commonly-reported mechanics from feature tracking (slice-wise Ecc and Ell) can be reproduced by contour-based strains. Such agreement between feature tracking and contour-based strains has been previously reported along with the suggestion that manual border delineation could be a low-cost alternative to purchasing feature tracking software [26]. Because of the excellent agreement between feature tracking and contour-based strain, regional tracking capabilities

Table 5 Bland-Altman analyses and coefficients of variation for feature tracking compared to contour-based strains

	Feature Tracking vs. Contour Strain		
	Bias	95% Limits	CoV
Circumferential Strain (Absolute %)			
Base	−0.0	±2.8	3.6
Mid	−0.5	±2.2	3.2
Apex	0.2	±3.8	4.4
Longitudinal Strain (Absolute %)			
Four-Chamber	−1.3	±2.4	7.0

CoV indicates coefficient of variation (%)

very poor with unacceptable limits and CoVs (Fig. S5). Detailed results are included in Additional file 4.

Discussion

This study evaluated the utility of commercially available feature tracking software for quantifying measures of cardiac mechanics, including LV strains, torsion and dyssynchrony. Our primary findings included: 1) the only truly acceptable agreement between feature tracking and the reference standard (DENSE) was observed for mid-ventricular Ecc, 2) feature tracking significantly

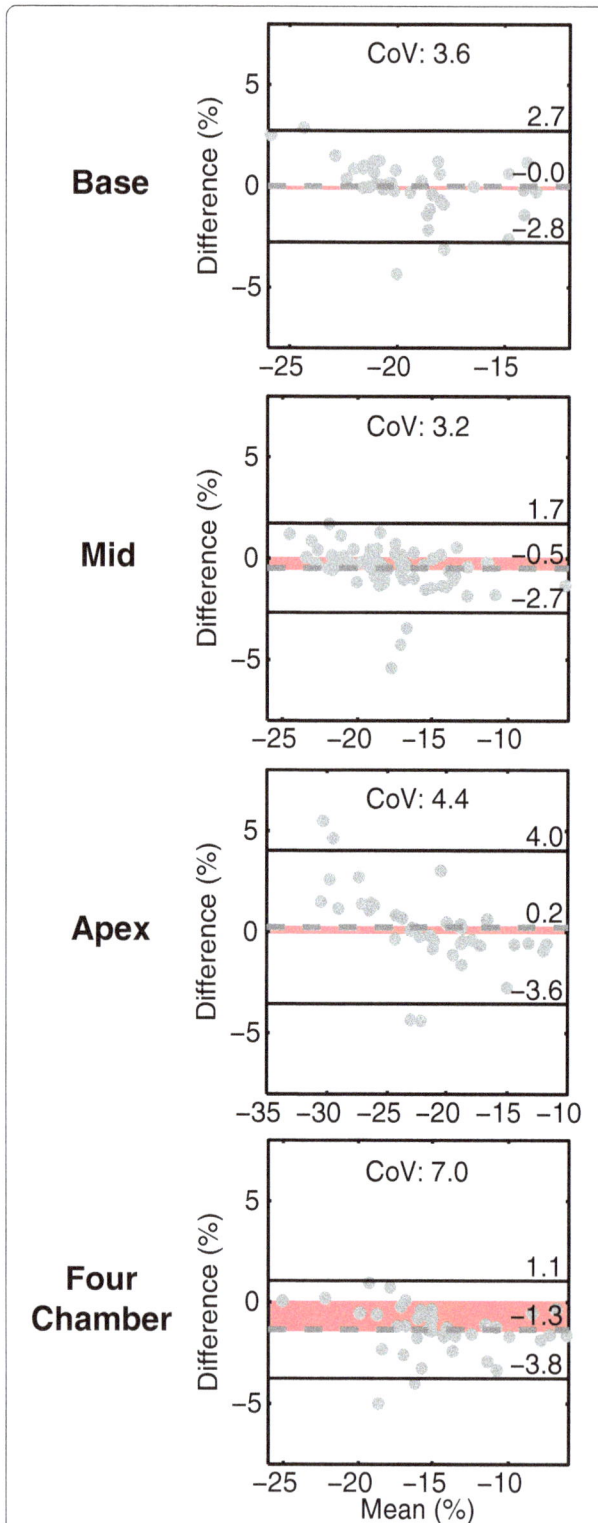

Fig. 4 Bland-Altman analyses for circumferential and longitudinal strains between feature tracking and contour-based strains. All differences were calculated by subtracting the feature tracking strain from the contour-based strain. The red shaded region highlights the bias. Excellent agreement (small biases and tight 95% limits) was observed for all circumferential and longitudinal strains. CoV, coefficient of variation

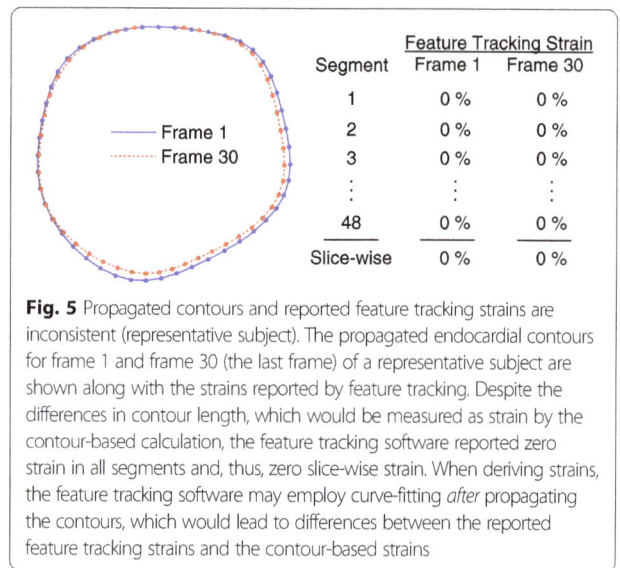

Fig. 5 Propagated contours and reported feature tracking strains are inconsistent (representative subject). The propagated endocardial contours for frame 1 and frame 30 (the last frame) of a representative subject are shown along with the strains reported by feature tracking. Despite the differences in contour length, which would be measured as strain by the contour-based calculation, the feature tracking software reported zero strain in all segments and, thus, zero slice-wise strain. When deriving strains, the feature tracking software may employ curve-fitting *after* propagating the contours, which would lead to differences between the reported feature tracking strains and the contour-based strains

and the cost of the feature tracking software are not required to assess these metrics. Many of the insights from previous feature tracking studies could have been easily produced without the software by the manual delineation of borders at two time points, ED and ES, which is already routine for most clinical examinations in which LV volumes are reported.

However, the use of feature tracking or manual delineation to assess slice-wise strains is not beyond reproach. Only mid-ventricular Ecc had good agreement between feature tracking and DENSE with 95% limits of agreement of ±6.3% and a CoV of 10.9%. Previous studies that assessed the agreement between feature tracking and myocardial tagging have shown 95% limits ranging from ±3.3% [10] to ±9.1% [16], with several other studies in between [13, 14, 31]. However, for Ecc in basal and apical images, we found significant biases and larger CoVs, which indicates that feature tracking and DENSE do not agree as well in those regions. In particular, apical Ecc had the largest 95% limits of agreement (±10.8%), which is consistent with a previous study that also observed that the apical region had the largest 95% limits (±12.8% at 1.5 T and ±9.2% at 3 T) [16]. The largest bias (−4.0%) was observed in basal Ecc. This bias was large enough to disrupt the physiologic gradient in Ecc from base to apex that was observed in the DENSE results and has been documented extensively [21, 34–36]. These inconsistencies between feature tracking and DENSE at the basal and apical levels are likely due to both through-plane motion, which is most prominent at the base and invalidates the fundamental assumption that a segment of tissue can be observed and tracked through the entire cardiac cycle in a single 2D image plane, and the difficulty in tracking the true endocardial contour, which may be more prominent at the apex due to papillary musculature and trabeculations. Inter-test variability in both techniques, while larger in feature tracking [12, 20], also contributes to imperfect agreement between them. Among the slice-wise strains quantified in this study, Ell had the highest CoV (19.3%) along with high 95% limits of agreement compared to DENSE (±9.3%). This is consistent with a previous comparison between feature tracking and myocardial tagging which found 95% limits of agreement to be ±9.5% [13].

To reiterate, for slice-wise strains in general, manual contour delineation at just ED and ES can replace results from feature tracking. However, neither agree strongly with a reference standard technique like DENSE with the exception of mid-ventricular Ecc.

Torsion, Dyssynchrony, and other mechanics

Less commonly-reported measures of mechanics from feature tracking include segmental strains, strain rates, torsion, and dyssynchrony. However, these are precisely the measurements for which accurate feature tracking would be most useful since none of these can be quantified by the manual delineation of contours at only ED and ES. Unfortunately, feature tracking has limited success in accurately and reproducibly quantifying these mechanics.

Previous studies of segmental strains and strain rates from feature tracking have demonstrated poor reproducibility and poor agreement with reference standards [12, 16]. Similar results were observed for torsion in the present study where torsion from feature tracking (TomTec) significantly underestimated DENSE by 1.4 deg/cm on average, while torsion from Circle overestimated DENSE by 1.5 deg./cm. This large bias is consistent with the literature as the torsion found by DENSE (3.5 ± 0.9 deg/cm) is similar to previous results from DENSE (3.1 to 3.9 deg./cm) [21] and myocardial tagging (3.4 to 3.7 deg/cm) [37] while the torsion result from TomTec (2.1 ± 1.2 deg/cm) is similar to previous feature tracking studies (2.3 ± 0.8 deg./cm) [33]. Furthermore, the CoV and 95% limits of agreement for comparing DENSE and feature tracking were high (41.1% and ± 2.4 deg/cm, respectively). Another previous study also found poor agreement and correlation between torsion derived from feature tracking and myocardial tagging as well as poor reproducibility from feature tracking [15]. The poor results from feature tracking using bSSFP images are likely due to the difficulty in tracking myocardial motion in the circumferential direction. While a strong gradient between the blood pool and the myocardium exists for accurately tracking the location of the endocardial contour in bSSFP imaging, the gradients in the orthogonal direction, which are necessary for tracking twist along that contour, are much weaker. Therefore, it is nearly impossible to track motion parallel to the myocardial wall unless additional features (such as papillary muscles) are present for tracking.

In the present study, dyssynchrony was significantly overestimated compared to DENSE (42 ± 22 vs 16 ± 20 ms) while demonstrating large 95% limits of agreement (±56 ms) and CoV (76.3%). A previous study has also demonstrated poor reproducibility for the quantification of dyssynchrony from segmental Ecc (CoV: 37.5%) [38]. The poor agreement between feature tracking and DENSE is largely due to the need for accurate segmental strains within the dyssynchrony calculation. Poor reproducibility of segmental strains, which has been demonstrated for feature tracking [12], likely resulted in both erroneously high measured dyssynchrony within volunteers (i.e. a bias) and greater variability in general.

Limitations

While this study evaluated the agreement between measurements derived from feature tracking and those same measures derived from a reference standard DENSE sequence, we could not evaluate the prognostic utility of the measures. While we observed imperfect agreement between the techniques, it is still possible that feature tracking (or manual contour delineation) produces useful results. However, careful consideration is required before generalizing results from reference standard techniques to feature tracking. There may be cases where only a reference standard technique is sufficient (e.g., identifying a gradient in Ecc from base to apex). Measures of radial strain were not included in this study due to well-known poor reproducibility [12, 13]. In addition, the current study did not evaluate all patient populations. Different populations will likely show different levels of agreement. In particular, populations with poor function and reduced through-plane motion would be expected to have better agreement between feature tracking and reference standard techniques. However, since changes in strains may precede changes in other functional measures, quantification of cardiac strains is likely most important in populations with healthy or nearly healthy function (e.g. pediatric obesity [23]). While it is common to assess the agreement between feature tracking and reference standard techniques with only healthy participants [13], we note that there was a preponderance of healthy subjects in the assessment of Ell compared to other strains in this study.

Conclusion

Compared to DENSE as a reference standard, feature tracking was inaccurate for quantification of apical and basal LV Ecc, Ell, torsion, and dyssynchrony. Feature tracking was only accurate for quantification of mid LV Ecc. Moreover, feature tracking is unnecessary for quantification of global peak strains, since simplified processing of only ED and ES contours yields very similar results to those derived from feature tracking. Current commercial feature tracking technology therefore has limited utility for quantification of cardiac mechanics.

Abbreviations
bSSFP: Balanced steady state free precession; CMR: Cardiovascular magnetic resonance; CoV: Coefficient of variation; CSPAMM: Complementary spatial modulation of magnetization; DENSE: Displacement encoding with stimulated echoes; Ecc: Circumferential strain; ED: End-diastole; Ell: Longitudinal strain; ES: End-systole; LV: Left ventricle/left ventricular; SENC: Strain encoding; TPM: Tissue phase mapping

Funding
This work was supported by a National Institutes of Health (NIH) Director's Early Independence Award (DP5 OD-012132), NIH T32 HL-072743, NIH P20 GM103527, and NIH grant number UL1TR000117 from the National Center for Research Resources and the National Center for Advancing Translational Sciences. The content is solely the responsibility of the authors and does not necessarily represent the official views of NIH.

Authors' contributions
GJW analyzed and collected data, assisted with study design and implementation, and drafted the manuscript. LJ and CMH analyzed and collected data, assisted with study design and implementation, and critical revision of the manuscript. JDS assisted with study design and implementation, and critical revision of the manuscript. JC, SMH, JAF and WDM analyzed and collected data, and assisted with critical revision of the manuscript. MAF collected data, assisted with study design and implementation, and critical revision of the manuscript. BKF conceived the study, assisted in study design and coordination, and assisted with drafting and critical revision of the manuscript. All authors read and approved the final manuscript.

Competing interests
The authors declare that they have no competing interests

Author details
[1]Department of Biomedical Engineering, University of Kentucky, Lexington, KY, USA. [2]Department of Imaging Science and Innovation, Geisinger, 100 North Academy Avenue, Danville, PA 17822-4400, USA. [3]Department of Pediatrics, University of Kentucky, Lexington, KY, USA. [4]Department of Electrical Engineering, University of Kentucky, Lexington, KY, USA. [5]Division of Cardiology, Department of Pediatrics, Children's Hospital of Philadelphia, Philadelphia, PA, USA. [6]Department of Radiology, Geisinger, Danville, PA, USA.

References
1. Stanton T, Leano R, Marwick TH. Prediction of all-cause mortality from global longitudinal speckle strain: comparison with ejection fraction and wall motion scoring. Circ Cardiovasc Imaging. 2009;2:356–64.
2. Choi E-Y, Rosen BD, Fernandes VRS, Yan RT, Yoneyama K, Donekal S, Opdahl A, Almeida ALC, Wu CO, Gomes AS, D a B, Lima J a C. Prognostic value of myocardial circumferential strain for incident heart failure and cardiovascular events in asymptomatic individuals: the multi-ethnic study of atherosclerosis. Eur Heart J. 2013;34:2354–61.
3. Axel L, Dougherty L. MR imaging of motion with spatial modulation of magnetization. Radiology. 1989;171:841–5.
4. Ibrahim el SH. Myocardial tagging by cardiovascular magnetic resonance: evolution of techniques--pulse sequences, analysis algorithms, and applications. J Cardiovasc Magn Reson. 2011;13:36.
5. Aletras AH, Ding S, Balaban RS, Wen H. DENSE: displacement encoding with stimulated echoes in cardiac functional MRI. J Magn Reson. 1999; 137:247–52.
6. Kim D, Gilson WD, Kramer CM, Epstein FH. Myocardial tissue tracking with two-dimensional cine displacement-encoded MR imaging: development and initial evaluation. Radiology. 2004;230:862–71.
7. Zhong X, Spottiswoode BS, Meyer CH, Kramer CM, Epstein FH. Imaging

three-dimensional myocardial mechanics using navigator-gated volumetric spiral cine DENSE MRI. Magn Reson Med. 2010;64:1089–97.
8. Osman NF, Sampath S, Atalar E, Prince JL. Imaging longitudinal cardiac strain on short-axis images using strain-encoded MRI. Magn Reson Med. 2001;46:324–34.
9. Simpson R, Keegan J, Firmin D. Efficient and reproducible high resolution spiral myocardial phase velocity mapping of the entire cardiac cycle. J Cardiovasc Magn Reson. 2013;15:34.
10. Hor KN, Gottliebson WM, Carson C, Wash E, Cnota J, Fleck R, Wansapura J, Klimeczek P, Al-Khalidi HR, Chung ES, Benson DW, Mazur W. Comparison of magnetic resonance feature tracking for strain calculation with harmonic phase imaging analysis. JACC Cardiovasc Imaging. 2010;3:144–51.
11. Claus P, Omar AMS, Pedrizzetti G, Sengupta PP, Nagel E. Tissue tracking Technology for Assessing Cardiac MechanicsPrinciples, normal values, and Clinical Applications. JACC Cardiovasc Imaging. 2015;8:1444–60.
12. Morton G, Schuster A, Jogiya R, Kutty S, Beerbaum P, Nagel E. Inter-study reproducibility of cardiovascular magnetic resonance myocardial feature tracking. J Cardiovasc Magn Reson. 2012;14:43.
13. Augustine D, Lewandowski AJ, Lazdam M, Rai A, Francis J, Myerson S, Noble A, Becher H, Neubauer S, Petersen SE, Leeson P. Global and regional left ventricular myocardial deformation measures by magnetic resonance feature tracking in healthy volunteers: comparison with tagging and relevance of gender. J Cardiovasc Magn Reson. 2013;15:8.
14. Harrild DM, Han Y, Geva T, Zhou J, Marcus E, Powell AJ. Comparison of cardiac MRI tissue tracking and myocardial tagging for assessment of regional ventricular strain. Int J Cardiovasc Imaging. 2012;28:2009–18.
15. Kuetting D, Sprinkart AM, Doerner J, Schild H, Thomas D. Comparison of magnetic resonance feature tracking with harmonic phase imaging analysis (CSPAMM) for assessment of global and regional diastolic function. Eur J Radiol. 2015;84:100–7.
16. Singh A, Steadman CD, Khan JN, Horsfield MA, Bekele S, Nazir SA, Kanagala P, Masca NGD, Clarysse P, McCann GP. Intertechnique agreement and interstudy reproducibility of strain and diastolic strain rate at 1.5 and 3 tesla: a comparison of feature-tracking and tagging in patients with aortic stenosis. J Magn Reson Imaging. 2015;41:1129–37.
17. Kuetting DLR, Sprinkart AM, Dabir D, Schild HH, Thomas DK. Assessment of cardiac dyssynchrony by cardiac MR: a comparison of velocity encoding and feature tracking analysis. J Magn Reson Imaging. 2015;43:940–46.
18. Young AA, Li B, Kirton RS, Cowan BR. Generalized spatiotemporal myocardial strain analysis for DENSE and SPAMM imaging. Magn Reson Med. 2012;67:1590–9.
19. Zhong X, Helm PA, Epstein FH. Balanced multipoint displacement encoding for DENSE MRI. Magn Reson Med. 2009;61:981–8.
20. Wehner GJ, Grabau JD, Suever JD, Haggerty CM, Jing L, Powell DK, Hamlet SM, Vandsburger MH, Zhong X, Fornwalt BK. 2D cine DENSE with low encoding frequencies accurately quantifies cardiac mechanics with improved image characteristics. J Cardiovasc Magn Reson. 2015;17:93.
21. Wehner GJ, Suever JD, Haggerty CM, Jing L, Powell DK, Hamlet SM, Grabau JD, Mojsejenko WD, Zhong X, Epstein FH, Fornwalt BK. Validation of in vivo 2D displacements from spiral cine DENSE at 3T. J Cardiovasc Magn Reson. 2015;17:5.
22. Spottiswoode BS, Zhong X, Hess a T, Kramer CM, Meintjes EM, Mayosi BM, Epstein FH. Tracking myocardial motion from cine DENSE images using spatiotemporal phase unwrapping and temporal fitting. IEEE Trans Med Imaging. 2007;26:15–30.
23. Jing L, Binkley CM, Suever JD, Umasankar N, Haggerty CM, Rich J, Nevius CD, Wehner GJ, Hamlet SM, Powell DK, Radulescu A, Kirchner HL, Epstein FH, Fornwalt BK. Cardiac remodeling and dysfunction in childhood obesity: a cardiovascular magnetic resonance study. J Cardiovasc Magn Reson. 2016;18:28.
24. Haggerty CM, Kramer SP, Binkley CM, Powell DK, Mattingly AC, Charnigo R, Epstein FH, Fornwalt BK. Reproducibility of cine displacement encoding with stimulated echoes (DENSE) cardiovascular magnetic resonance for measuring left ventricular strains, torsion, and synchrony in mice. J Cardiovasc Magn Reson. 2013;15:71.
25. Cao JJ, Ngai N, Duncanson L, Cheng J, Gliganic K, Chen Q. A comparison of both DENSE and feature tracking techniques with tagging for the cardiovascular magnetic resonance assessment of myocardial strain. J Cardiovasc Magn Reson. 2018;20:26.
26. Kempny A, Fernández-Jiménez R, Orwat S, Schuler P, Bunck AC, Maintz D, Baumgartner H, Diller G-P. Quantification of biventricular myocardial function using cardiac magnetic resonance feature tracking, endocardial

border delineation and echocardiographic speckle tracking in patients with repaired tetralogy of Fallot and healthy controls. J Cardiovasc Magn Reson. 2012;14:32.

27. Zhong X, Spottiswoode BS, E a C, Gilson WD, Epstein FH. Selective suppression of artifact-generating echoes in cine DENSE using through-plane dephasing. Magn Reson Med. 2006;56:1126–31.

28. Gilliam AD, Suever JD: DENSEanalysis. 2016.

29. Jing L, Haggerty CM, Suever JD, Alhadad S, Prakash A, Cecchin F, Skrinjar O, Geva T, Powell AJ, Fornwalt BK. Patients with repaired tetralogy of Fallot suffer from intra- and inter-ventricular cardiac dyssynchrony: a cardiac magnetic resonance study. Eur Heart J Cardiovasc Imaging. 2014;15:1333–43.

30. Wu L, Germans T, Güçlü A, Heymans MW, Allaart CP, van Rossum AC. Feature tracking compared with tissue tagging measurements of segmental strain by cardiovascular magnetic resonance. J Cardiovasc Magn Reson. 2014;16:10.

31. Moody WE, Taylor RJ, Edwards NC, Chue CD, Umar F, Taylor TJ, Ferro CJ, Young AA, Townend JN, Leyva F, Steeds RP. Comparison of magnetic resonance feature tracking for systolic and diastolic strain and strain rate calculation with spatial modulation of magnetization imaging analysis. J Magn Reson Imaging. 2015;41:1000–12.

32. Lai WM, Rubin D, Krempl E. Chapter 3 – kinematics of a continuum. In: Introduction to continuum mechanics. Volume 3; 2010. p. 69–153.

33. Kowallick JT, Morton G, Lamata P, Jogiya R, Kutty S, Lotz J, Hasenfuß G, Nagel E, Chiribiri A, Schuster A. Inter-study reproducibility of left ventricular torsion and torsion rate quantification using MR myocardial feature tracking. J Magn Reson Imaging. 2015;43:128–37.

34. Moore CC, Lugo-Olivieri CH, McVeigh ER, E a Z. Three-dimensional systolic strain patterns in the normal human left ventricle: characterization with tagged MR imaging. Radiology. 2000;214:453–66.

35. Feng L, Donnino R, Babb J, Axel L, Kim D. Numerical and in vivo validation of fast cine displacement-encoded with stimulated echoes (DENSE) MRI for quantification of regional cardiac function. Magn Reson Med. 2009;62:682–90.

36. Leitman M, Lysiansky M, Lysyansky P, Friedman Z, Tyomkin V, Fuchs T, Adam D, Krakover R, Vered Z. Circumferential and longitudinal strain in 3 myocardial layers in normal subjects and in patients with regional left ventricular dysfunction. J Am Soc Echocardiogr. 2010;23:64–70.

37. Donekal S, Ambale-Venkatesh B, Berkowitz S, Wu CO, Choi EY, Fernandes V, Yan R, A a H, D a B, J a L. Inter-study reproducibility of cardiovascular magnetic resonance tagging. J Cardiovasc Magn Reson. 2013;15:37.

38. Kowallick JT, Morton G, Lamata P, Jogiya R, Kutty S, Hasenfuss G, Lotz J, Chiribiri A, Nagel E, Schuster A. Quantitative assessment of left ventricular mechanical dyssynchrony using cine cardiovascular magnetic resonance imaging: inter-study reproducibility. J Cardiovasc Magn Reson. 2016; 18(Suppl 1):P40.

Permissions

All chapters in this book were first published in JCMR, by BioMed Central; hereby published with permission under the Creative Commons Attribution License or equivalent. Every chapter published in this book has been scrutinized by our experts. Their significance has been extensively debated. The topics covered herein carry significant findings which will fuel the growth of the discipline. They may even be implemented as practical applications or may be referred to as a beginning point for another development.

The contributors of this book come from diverse backgrounds, making this book a truly international effort. This book will bring forth new frontiers with its revolutionizing research information and detailed analysis of the nascent developments around the world.

We would like to thank all the contributing authors for lending their expertise to make the book truly unique. They have played a crucial role in the development of this book. Without their invaluable contributions this book wouldn't have been possible. They have made vital efforts to compile up to date information on the varied aspects of this subject to make this book a valuable addition to the collection of many professionals and students.

This book was conceptualized with the vision of imparting up-to-date information and advanced data in this field. To ensure the same, a matchless editorial board was set up. Every individual on the board went through rigorous rounds of assessment to prove their worth. After which they invested a large part of their time researching and compiling the most relevant data for our readers.

The editorial board has been involved in producing this book since its inception. They have spent rigorous hours researching and exploring the diverse topics which have resulted in the successful publishing of this book. They have passed on their knowledge of decades through this book. To expedite this challenging task, the publisher supported the team at every step. A small team of assistant editors was also appointed to further simplify the editing procedure and attain best results for the readers.

Apart from the editorial board, the designing team has also invested a significant amount of their time in understanding the subject and creating the most relevant covers. They scrutinized every image to scout for the most suitable representation of the subject and create an appropriate cover for the book.

The publishing team has been an ardent support to the editorial, designing and production team. Their endless efforts to recruit the best for this project, has resulted in the accomplishment of this book. They are a veteran in the field of academics and their pool of knowledge is as vast as their experience in printing. Their expertise and guidance has proved useful at every step. Their uncompromising quality standards have made this book an exceptional effort. Their encouragement from time to time has been an inspiration for everyone.

The publisher and the editorial board hope that this book will prove to be a valuable piece of knowledge for researchers, students, practitioners and scholars across the globe.

List of Contributors

Victoria M. Stoll, Margaret Loudon, Malenka M. Bissell, Saul G. Myerson, Stefan Neubauer and Aaron T. Hess
University of Oxford Centre for Clinical Magnetic Resonance Research (OCMR), Division of Cardiovascular Medicine, Radcliffe Department of Medicine, Oxford, UK

Jonatan Eriksson, Petter Dyverfeldt, Tino Ebbers and Carl- Johan Carlhäll
Division of Cardiovascular Medicine, Linköping University, Linköping, Sweden

Sowmya Balasubramanian, David M. Harrild, Basavaraj Kerur, Edward Marcus, Tal Geva and Andrew J. Powell
Department of Cardiology, Boston Children's Hospital, Boston, USA

Sowmya Balasubramanian, David M. Harrild, Edward Marcus, Tal Geva and Andrew J. Powell
Department of Pediatrics, Harvard Medical School, Boston, USA

Pedro del Nido
Department of Cardiac Surgery, Boston Children's Hospital, Boston, USA
Department of Surgery, Boston Children's Hospital, Boston, USA

Mun Hong Cheang, Nathaniel J. Barber, Abbas Khushnood, Jakob A. Hauser, Gregorz T. Kowalik, Jennifer A. Steeden, Michael A. Quail and Vivek Muthurangu
Centre for Cardiovascular Imaging, UCL Institute of Cardiovascular Science, 30 Guilford Street, London WC1N 1EH, UK

Mun Hong Cheang, Nathaniel J. Barber, Abbas Khushnood, Jakob A. Hauser, Michael A. Quail, Kjell Tullus, Daljit Hothi and Vivek Muthurangu
Great Ormond Street Hospital, London, UK

Karl P. Kunze, Markus Schwaiger, Christoph Rischpler and Stephan G. Nekolla
Nuklearmedizinische Klinik und Poliklinik, Klinikum rechts der Isar, Technische Universität München, Ismaninger Straße 22, 81675 Munich, Germany

Ralf J. Dirschinger, Hans Kossmann, Franziska Hanus, Tareq Ibrahim and Karl-Ludwig Laugwitz
Klinik und Poliklinik für Medizin I, Klinikum rechts der Isar, Technische Universität München, Ismaninger Straße 22, 81675 Munich, Germany

Tareq Ibrahim, Karl-Ludwig Laugwitz, Markus Schwaiger, Christoph Rischpler and Stephan G. Nekolla
DZHK (Deutsches Zentrum für Herz-Kreislauf-Forschung e.V.)partner site Munich Heart Alliance, Munich, Germany

Adrienne E. Campbell-Washburn, Toby Rogers, Annette M. Stine, Jaffar M. Khan, Rajiv Ramasawmy, William H. Schenke, Delaney R. McGuirt, Jonathan R. Mazal, Laurie P. Grant, Elena K. Grant, Daniel A. Herzka and Robert J. Lederman
Adrienne E. Campbell-Washburn and Toby Rogers contributed equally to this work. Cardiovascular Branch, Division of Intramural Research, National Heart, Lung, and Blood Institute, National Institutes of Health, Building 10, Room 2C713, Bethesda, MD 20892-1538, USA

Philippa R. P. Krahn, Sheldon M. Singh, Venkat Ramanan, Labonny Biswas, Nicolas Yak, Kevan J. T. Anderson, Jennifer Barry, Mihaela Pop and Graham A. Wright

Philippa R. P. Krahn, Mihaela Pop and Graham A. Wright
Department of Medical Biophysics, University of Toronto, Toronto, ON, Canada

Philippa R. P. Krahn, Venkat Ramanan, Labonny Biswas, Nicolas Yak, Kevan J. T. Anderson, Jennifer Barry, Mihaela Pop and Graham A. Wright
Sunnybrook Research Institute, Toronto, ON, Canada

Sheldon M. Singh, Mihaela Pop and Graham A. Wright
Schulich Heart Research Program, Sunnybrook Research Institute, Toronto, ON, Canada

Sheldon M. Singh
Division of Cardiology, Schulich Heart Centre, Sunnybrook Health
Sciences Centre, Toronto, ON, Canada
Faculty of Medicine, University of Toronto, Toronto, ON, Canada

Seung-Hoon Pi, Jin-Oh Choi, Eun Kyoung Kim, Sung-A Chang, Sang-Chol Lee and Eun-Seok Jeon
Department of Internal Medicine, Heart Vascular Stroke Institute, Samsung Medical Center, Sungkyunkwan University School of Medicine, 81 Irwon-ro, Gangnam-gu, Seoul 06351, Republic of Korea

Sung Mok Kim and Hyeon Choe
Department of Radiology, Cardiovascular Imaging Center, Samsung Medical Center, Sungkyunkwan University School of Medicine, Seoul, Republic of Korea

Thomas Wehrum, Thomas Lodemann, Paul Hagenlocher and and Andreas Harloff
Department of Neurology and Neuroscience, Medical Center - University of Freiburg, Faculty of Medicine, University of Freiburg, Breisacher Straße 64, 79106 Freiburg, Germany

Judith Stuplich, Ba Thanh Truc Ngo and Sebastian Grundmann
Department of Cardiology, University Heart Center Freiburg, Faculty of Medicine, University of Freiburg, Freiburg, Germany

Anja Hennemuth
Charité – Universitätsmedizin Berlin, Institute for Imaging Science and Computational Modelling in Cardiovascular Medicine, Berlin, Germany

Jürgen Hennig
Department of Diagnostic Radiology – Medical Physics, Medical Center, University of Freiburg, Faculty of Medicine, University of Freiburg, Freiburg, Germany

Amol S Pednekar
Department of Radiology, Texas Children's Hospital, 6701 Fannin Street, Suite D470.09, Houston, TX 77030-2399, USA

Hui Wang
Philips Healthcare, Gainesville, FL, USA

Benjamin Y. Cheong and Raja Muthupillai
Department of Radiology, Baylor St. Luke's Medical Center, Houston, TX, USA

José Fernando Rodríguez-Palomares, Lydia Dux-Santoy, Andrea Guala, Raquel Kale, Giuliana Maldonado, Laura Galian, Filipa Valente, Laura Gutiérrez and Teresa González-Alujas
Hospital Universitari Vall d'Hebron, Department of Cardiology. Vall d'Hebron Institut de Recerca (VHIR), Universitat Autònoma de Barcelona, Paseo Vall d'Hebron 119-129, 08035 Barcelona, Spain

Marina Huguet
Cardiac Imaging Department, CETIR-ERESA, Clínica del Pilar-Sant Jordi, Barcelona, Spain

Kevin M. Johnson and Oliver Wieben
Departments of Medical Physics and Radiology, University of Wisconsin – Madison, Madison, WI, USA

Allison D. Ta, Li-Yueh Hsu, Hannah M. Conn, Susanne Winkler, Anders M. Greve, Sujata M. Shanbhag, Marcus Y. Chen, W. Patricia Bandettini and Andrew E. Arai
National Heart, Lung and Blood Institute, National Institutes of Health, Department of Health and Human Services, Bldg 10, Rm B1D416, MSC 1061, 10 Center Drive, Bethesda, MD 20892-1061, USA

Allison D. Ta
Duke University School of Medicine, Durham, North Carolina, USA

Susanne Winkler
Medical University of Vienna, Vienna, Austria

Kihei Yoneyama, Bharath A. Venkatesh, Nathan Mewton, Ola Gjesdal, Satoru Kishi and João A. C. Lima
Department of Cardiology, Johns Hopkins University, Baltimore, MD, USA

Colin O. Wu
Offices of Biostatistics Research, National Heart, Lung, and Blood Institute, Bethesda, MD, USA

Robyn L. McClelland
Department of Biostatistics, University of Washington, Seattle, WA, USA

David A. Bluemke
National Institute of Biomedical Imaging and Bioengineering, National Institutes of Health Clinical Center, Bethesda, MD, USA

João A. C. Lima
Radiology and Epidemiology, Johns Hopkins University, Blalock 524D1, Johns Hopkins Hospital, 600 North Wolfe Street, Baltimore, MD 21287, USA

Na Zhang, Hairong Zheng and Xin Liu
Paul C. Lauterbur Research Center for Biomedical Imaging, Shenzhen
Institutes of Advanced Technology, Chinese Academy of Sciences, 1068
Xueyuan Ave., Shenzhen University Town, Shenzhen 518055, China

Na Zhang, Fan Zhang, Zixin Deng, Qi Yang, Debiao Li and Zhaoyang Fan
Biomedical Imaging Research Institute, Department of Biomedical Sciences, Cedars-Sinai Medical Center, 8700 Beverly Blvd., PACT 400, Los Angeles, CA 90048, USA

Na Zhang, Hairong Zheng and Xin Liu
Shenzhen College of Advanced Technology, University of Chinese Academy of Sciences, Shenzhen, China

Zixin Deng and Debiao Li
Department of Bioengineering, University of California, Los Angeles, CA, USA

Marcio A. Diniz
Biostatistics and Bioinformatics Research Center, Cedars-Sinai Medical Center, Los Angeles, CA, USA

Shlee S. Song and Konrad H. Schlick
Department of Neurology, Cedars-Sinai Medical Center, Los Angeles, CA, USA

Nestor Gonzalez
Department of Neurosurgery, Cedars-Sinai Medical Center, Los Angeles, CA, USA

Debiao Li and Zhaoyang Fan
Department of Medicine, University of California, Los Angeles, CA, USA

Shiteng Suo, Hui Tang, Suqin Li, Haimin Mao, Xiangyu Liu, Shengyun He, Qing Lu and Jianrong Xu
Department of Radiology, Renji Hospital, School of Medicine, Shanghai Jiao Tong University, No. 160, Pujian Rd, Shanghai 200127, China

Lan Zhang and Qihong Ni
Department of Vascular Surgery, Renji Hospital, School of Medicine, Shanghai Jiao Tong University, Shanghai, China

Jianxun Qu
GE Healthcare China, Shanghai, China

Hanwei Chen, Xueping He, Jianke Liang, Yufeng Ye, Wei Deng, Zhuonan He and Dexiang Liu
Department of Radiology, Guangzhou Panyu Central Hospital, Guangzhou 511400, Guangdong, China

Hanwei Chen and Xueping He
Medical Imaging Institute of Panyu, Guangzhou 511400, Guangdong, China

Guoxi Xie
The Sixth Affiliated Hospital, Guangzhou Medical University, Xinzao, Panyu District, Qingyuan 511518, Guangdong, China
Department of Biomedical Engineering of Basic Medical School, Guangzhou Medical University, Guangzhou 511436, Guangdong, China

Debiao Li and Zhaoyang Fan
Biomedical Imaging Research Institute, Cedars-Sinai Medical Center, Los Angeles, CA 90048, USA

Xin Liu
Lauterbur Research Center for Biomedical Imaging, Shenzhen Institutes of Advanced Technology, Chinese Academy of Sciences, Shenzhen 518055, Guangdong, China

Sean Robison, Gauri Rani Karur, Rachel M. Wald, Paaladinesh Thavendiranathan, Andrew M. Crean and Kate Hanneman
Department of Medical Imaging, Toronto General Hospital, University Health Network, University of Toronto, 585 University Ave, 1PMB-298, Toronto, ON M5G 2N2, Canada

Rachel M. Wald, Paaladinesh Thavendiranathan and Andrew M. Crean
Division of Cardiology, Department of Medicine, Peter Munk Cardiac Center, Toronto General Hospital, University of Toronto, Toronto, Canada

Masafumi Nii, Hiroaki Tanaka, Eiji Kondo and Tomoaki Ikeda
Department of Obstetrics and Gynecology, Mie University Hospital, 2-174 Edobashi, Tsu, Mie 514-8507, Japan

Kaoru Dohi
Department of Cardiology and Nephrology, Mie University Hospital, 2-174 Edobashi, Tsu, Mie 514-8507, Japan

Adriana D. M. Villa, Laura Corsinovi, Ioannis Ntalas, Xenios Milidonis, Cian Scannell, Gabriella Di Giovine, Nicholas Child, Muhummad Sohaib Nazir, Julia Karady, Viola De Francesco, Tevfik F. Ismail, Reza Razavi and Amedeo Chiribiri
School of Biomedical Engineering and Imaging Sciences, King's College London, King's Health Partners, 4th Floor Lambeth Wing, St Thomas' Hospital, London SE1 7EH, UK

Laura Corsinovi
Cardiology Department of the Basingstoke and North Hampshire Hospital, Basingstoke, UK

Ioannis Ntalas
Cardiology Department, St.Thomas' Hospital, Guy's and St Thomas' NHS Foundation Trust, London, UK

Catarina Ferreira
Faculdade de Ciências da Saúde CICS, UBI, Covilhã, Portugal

Esmeralda Eshja
Radiology Department, ICS Maugeri IRCCS, Porto, Italy

Andreas Schuster
Department of Cardiology, Royal North Shore Hospital, The Kolling Institute, Northern Clinical School, University of Sydney, Sydney, Australia
Department of Cardiology and Pneumology, University Medical Center Göttingen, Georg-August University, Göttingen, Germany
German Center for Cardiovascular Research (DZHK), Partner Site Göttingen, Göttingen, Germany

Fourat Ridouani, Vania Tacher, Haytham Derbel, François Legou, Islem Sifaoui, Alain Rahmouni and Jean-François Deux
Radiology Department, Henri Mondor Hospital, University Paris Est Créteil, Assistance Publique-Hôpitaux de Paris, 51 av Mal de Lattre de Tassigny, 94000 Créteil, France

Thibaud Damy and Diane Bodez
Cardiology Department, Henri Mondor Hospital, University Paris Est Crétei, Assistance Publique-Hôpitaux de Paris, Créteil, France

Thibaud Damy, Diane Bodez and Jean-François Deux
National Referal Centre for Cardiac Amyloidoses, Henri Mondor Hospital, Créteil, France

Etienne Audureau
Public Health Department, Henri Mondor Hospital, CEpiA EA7376, University Paris Est Créteil, Assistance Publique-Hôpitaux de Paris, Créteil, France
Valentina O. Puntmann, Silvia Valbuena, Rocio Hinojar4, Steffen E. Petersen, John P. Greenwood, Christopher M. Kramer, Raymond Y. Kwong, Gerry P. McCann, Colin Berry Eike Nage and on behalf of SCMR Clinical Trial Writing Group

Valentina O. Puntmann and, Eike Nagel
1Institute of Experimental and Translational Cardiovascular Imaging, Goethe University Hospital Frankfurt, Frankfurt, Germany

Valentina O. Puntmann
Department of Cardiology, Goethe University Hospital Frankfurt, Frankfurt, Germany

Silvia Valbuena
Department of Cardiology, University Hospital La Paz, Madrid, Germany

Rocio Hinojar
Department of Cardiology, University Hospital Ramón y Cajal, Madrid, Spain

Steffen E. Petersen
William Harvey Research Institute, Queen Mary University of London, Barts and the London
NIHR Biomedical Research Centre at Barts, London, UK

Christopher M. Kramer
Department of Medicine (Cardiology) and Radiology, Cardiovascular
Imaging Center, University of Virginia Health System, Charlottesville, Virginia, USA

Raymond Y. Kwong
Cardiovascular Division, Department of Medicine, Brigham and Womens' Hospital, Boston, Massachusetts, USA

Gerry P. McCann
Department of Cardiovascular Sciences, University of Leicester, Leicester, UK. the NIHR Leicester Cardiovascular Biomedical Centre, University Hospitals of Leicester NHS Trust, Glenfield Hospital, Leicester, UK

Colin Berry
British Heart Foundation Glasgow Cardiovascular Research Centre, University of Glasgow, Glasgow, UK
West of Scotland Heart and Lung Centre, Golden Jubilee National Hospital, Clydebank, UK

Rajiv Ramasawmy, Toby Rogers, Miguel A. Alcantar, Delaney R. McGuirt, Jaffar M. Khan, Peter Kellman, Hui Xue, Anthony Z. Faranesh, Adrienne E. Campbell-Washburn, Robert J. Lederman and Daniel A. Herzka
Division of Intramural Research, National Heart Lung and Blood Institute, National Institutes of Health, Building 10, Room 2C713, 10 Center Drive, Bethesda, MD 20892, USA

Clotilde Roy, Alisson Slimani, Christophe de Meester, Mihaela Amzulescu, Agnes Pasquet, David Vancraeynest, Christophe Beauloye, Jean-Louis Vanoverschelde, Bernhard L. Gerber and Anne-Catherine Pouleur
Division of Cardiology, Department of Cardiovascular Diseases, Cliniques Universitaires St. Luc UCL, Av Hippocrate 10/2806, B-1200 Woluwé St.Lambert, Belgium
Pôle de Recherche Cardiovasculaire (CARD), Institut de Recherche Expérimentale et Clinique (IREC), Université Catholique de Louvain, Brussels, Belgium

Maximilian Fuetterer, Julia Busch, Julia Traechtler, Patrick Wespi, Sophie M. Peereboom, Christian T. Stoeck and Sebastian Kozerke
Institute for Biomedical Engineering, University and ETH Zurich, Gloriastrasse, 35 8092 Zurich, Switzerland

Mareike Sauer, Miriam Lipiski, Thea Fleischmann and Nikola Cesarovic
Division of Surgical Research, University Hospital Zurich, Sternwartstrasse, 14 8091 Zurich, Switzerland

Gregory J. Wehner and Brandon K. Fornwalt
Department of Biomedical Engineering, University of Kentucky, Lexington, KY, USA

Linyuan Jing, Christopher M. Haggerty, Jonathan D. Suever, Jing Chen, Jared A. Feindt and Brandon K. Fornwalt
Department of Imaging Science and Innovation, Geisinger, 100 North Academy Avenue, Danville, PA 17822-4400, USA

Linyuan Jing, Christopher M. Haggerty, Jonathan D. Suever, W. Dimitri Mojsejenko and Brandon K. Fornwalt
Department of Pediatrics, University of Kentucky, Lexington, KY, USA

Brandon K. Fornwalt
Department of Electrical Engineering, University of Kentucky, Lexington, KY, USA
Department of Radiology, Geisinger, Danville, PA, USA

Mark A. Fogel
Division of Cardiology, Department of Pediatrics, Children's Hospital of Philadelphia, Philadelphia, PA, USA

Index